Autoimmune Reactions

Contemporary Immunology

Autoimmune Reactions

Edited by

Sudhir Paul

Health Science Center
University of Texas Medical School
Houston, TX

Humana Press ✳ Totowa, New Jersey

© 1999 Humana Press Inc.
999 Riverview Drive, Suite 208
Totowa, New Jersey 07512

This publication is printed on acid-free paper. ∞
ANSI Z39.48-1984 (American National Standards Institute) Permanence of Paper for Printed Library Materials.

Cover illustration: Fig. 1(**A**) from Chapter 17, "Kidney Damage in Autoimmune Disease," by Gerald C. Groeggel.
Cover design by Patricia F. Cleary.

For additional copies, pricing for bulk purchases, and/or information about other Humana titles, contact Humana at the above address or at any of the following numbers: Tel.: 973-256-1699; Fax: 973-256-8341; E-mail: humana@humanapr.com or visit our Web site: http://humanapress.com

Printed in the United States of America. 10 9 8 7 6 5 4 3 2 1
Library of Congress Cataloging in Publication Data

Autoimmune Reactions / edited by Sudhir Paul.
     p. cm. — (Contemporary immunology)
    Includes bibliographical references and index.
    ISBN 0-89603-550-6 (alk. paper)
    1. Autoimmunity. 2. Autoimmune diseases. I. Paul, Sudhir. II. Series.
    [DNLM: 1. Autoimmune Diseases — immunology. 2. Autoimmunity. WD
305A9385 1998]
QR188.3.A96 1998
616.97'8—dc21
DNLM/DLC
for Library of Congress   98-28423

Preface

The development of immunological mechanisms that destroy harmful microbes with minimal or no damage to "self" constituents has been an important factor in the survival and evolution of higher organisms. Contrary to initial expectations, it is now evident that self-tolerance is not a state of immunological inertia. Many immune responses to self-antigens, in fact, participate in maintaining immunological homeostasis.

No life system, however, is perfect. Autoimmune diseases can be viewed as derangements in the ability of the body to distinguish self from nonself. Genetic factors are often involved in such derangements, and environmental stimuli can also induce autoimmune diseases. Substantial advances have been achieved in understanding autoimmune diseases, and the underlying nature of the immunological defects are slowly becoming comprehensible. Certain authors have even attempted mathematical modeling of autoimmune disease (e.g., *1,2),* raising expectations that it may eventually be possible to understand the disease process as a discrete set of quantifiable variables.

Where possible, the contributing authors in *Autoimmune Reactions* have translated the phenomenological data to a mechanistic account of the disease process. If the reader of our book concludes, however, that the verifiable causes and theories of autoimmune disease remain unclear, the conclusion is a much shared one. This statement does not indict the reductionist scientific methods upon which we rely. Rather, it reflects our incomplete understanding of the means by which multiple and seemingly disparate molecular and cellular events combine to generate disease.

As the editor of *Autoimmune Reactions*, I was privileged to share the thoughts of leading immunologists, for which I am grateful. Tom Lanigan of Humana Press provided encouraging comments while reviewing the format and contents of this book. I thank Marcy Bigner and Esmeralda Garcia for efficient secretarial assistance, and the editorial staff of Humana for their contributions.

Sudhir Paul

REFERENCES

1. Morris, J. A. (1987) Autoimmunity: a decision theory model. *J. Clin. Pathol.* **40,** 210–215.
2. Waniewski, J. and Prikrylova, D. (1988) Autoimmunity and its therapy: math-

Contents

Contributors

R. A. AJJAN • *Department of Medicine, University of Sheffield Clinical Science Center, North General Hospital, Sheffield, UK*

YARON BAR-DAYAN • *Research Unit of Autoimmune Diseases, Department of Medicine B, Chaim Sheba Medical Center, Tel-Aviv University Medical School, Tel-Hashomer, Israel*

CONSTANTIN A. BONA • *Department of Microbiology, Mount Sinai School of Medicine, New York, NY*

ANNE DAVIDSON • *Department of Medicine, Albert Einstein College of Medicine, Bronx, NY*

GUILLAUME DIGHIERO • *Unité d'Immunohématologie et d'Immunopathologie, Institut Pasteur, Paris, France*

EDWARD DWYER • *Department of Medicine, Columbia University College of Physicians and Surgeons, New York, NY*

KRISTINE GARZA • *Department of Pathology, University of Virginia, Charlottesville, VA*

GERALD GROGGEL • *Department of Internal Medicine–Nephrology, University of Nebraska Medical Center, Omaha, NE*

MICHAEL HOLLINGSWORTH • *Departments of Biochemistry and Molecular Biology, College of Medicine and Pathology/ Microbiology, University of Nebraska Medical Center, Omaha, NE*

SRINIVAS KAVERI • *INSERM U28, Hôpital Broussais, Paris, France*

MARGUERITE M. B. KAY • *Department of Microbiology and Immunology and Department of Veterans Affairs, University of Arizona College of Medicine, Tucson, AZ*

MICHEL D. KAZATCHKINE • *INSERM U28, Hôpital Broussais, Paris, France*

LYNELL W. KLASSEN • *Department of Internal Medicine, University of Nebraska Medical Center, Omaha, NE*

HEINZ K. KOHLEr • *Lucille P. Markey Cancer Center, University of Kentucky Medical Center, Lexington, KY*

HANS LINK • *Division of Neurology, Huddinge Hospital, Huddinge, Sweden*

YA-HUAN LOU • *Department of Pathology, University of Virginia, Charlottesville, VA*

MICHAEL P. MADAIO • *Department of Medicine, University of Pennsylvania, Philadelphia, PA*

JOHN J. MARCHALONIS • *Microbiology and Immunology, University of Arizona College of Medicine, Tucson, AZ*

TONY MARION • *Department of Microbiology and Immunology, University of Tennessee, Memphis, TN*

KINJI MATSUURA • *Department of Biochemistry, Kinki University School of Medicine, Osaka-Sayama, Osaka, Japan*

SYBILLE MULLER • *Lucille P. Markey Cancer Center, University of Kentucky Medical Center, Lexington, KY*

CHIHIRO MURAI • *Department of Microbiology, Mount Sinai School of Medicine, New York, NY*

K. A. NAGENDRA PRASAD • *INSERM U28, Hôpital Broussais, Paris, France*

ISAO NISHIMORI • *Departments of Biochemistry and Molecular Biology, College of Medicine and Pathology/Microbiology, University of Nebraska Medical Center, Omaha, NE*

SUDHIR PAUL • *Department of Pathology and Laboratory Medicine, Health Sciences Center, University of Texas Medical School, Houston, TX*

DAVID N. POSNETT • *Division of Immunology, Department of Medicine, Cornell University Medical College, New York, NY*

OTTO PRITSCH • *Unité d'Immunohématologie et d'Immunopathologie, Institut Pasteur, Paris, France*

MORRIS REICHLIN • *Immunology Section, Department of Medicine, Oklahoma Medical Research Foundation, Oklahoma City, OK*

NOEL R. ROSE • *Department of Immunology and Infectious Diseases, School of Hygiene and Public Health, Johns Hopkins University, Baltimore, MD*

ISRAEL RUBENSTEIN • *Section of Respiratory and Critical Care Medicine, Department of Medicine, University of Illinois at Chicago, Chicago, IL*

TAKESHI SASAKI • *Department of Microbiology, Mount Sinai School of Medicine, New York, NY*

SAMUEL SCHLUTER • *Department of Microbiology and Immunology, University of Arizona College of Medicine, Tucson, AZ*

YANIV SHERER • *Research Unit of Autoimmune Diseases, Department of Medicine B, Chaim Sheba Medical Center, Tel-Aviv University Medical School, Tel-Hashomer, Israel*

YEHUDA SHOENFELD • *Research Unit of Autoimmune Diseases, Department of Medicine B, Chaim Sheba Medical Center, Tel-Aviv University Medical School, Tel-Hashomer, Israel*

HYOGO SINOHARA • *Department of Biochemistry, Kinki University School of Medicine, Osaka-Sayama, Osaka, Japan*

CONNIE SIVINSKI • *Departments of Biochemistry and Molecular Biology, College of Medicine and Pathology/Microbiology, University of Nebraska Medical Center, Omaha, NE*

HARALDINE STAFFORD • *Immunology Section, Department of Medicine, Oklahoma Medical Research Foundation, Oklahoma City, OK*

RICHARD TEMPERO • *Departments of Biochemistry and Molecular Biology, College of Medicine and Pathology/Microbiology, University of Nebraska Medical Center, Omaha, NE*

GOEFFREY M. THIELE • *Department of Internal Medicine, UMA, University of Nebraska Medical Center, Omaha, NE*

DEAN J. TUMA • *Department of Internal Medicine, University of Nebraska Medical Center, Omaha, NE*

KENNETH S. K. TUNG • *Department of Pathology, University of Virginia, Charlottesville, VA*

MICHELLE VANLITH • *Departments of Biochemistry and Molecular Biology, College of Medicine and Pathology/Microbiology, University of Nebraska Medical Center, Omaha, NE*

Anthony P. Weetman • *Department of Medicine, University of Sheffield Clinical Science Center, North General Hospital, Sheffield, UK*

RICHARD H. WEISBART • *Department of Medicine, Division of Rheumatology, Sepulveda Veterans Administration Medical Center, Sepulveda, CA*

BAO-GUO XIAO • *Division of Neurology, Huddinge Hospital, Huddinge, Sweden*

KUMIKO YANASE • *Penn Center for Molecular Studies of Kidney Diseases, University of Pennsylvania, Philadelphia, PA*

DAVID YOCUM • *Microbiology and Immunology, University of Arizona College of Medicine, Tucson, AZ*

DEBRA JESKE ZACK • *Department of Medicine, Division of Rheumatology, Sepulveda Veterans Administration Medical Center, Sepulveda, CA*

Diversity of Immunological Defects in Autoimmune Diseases

Sudhir Paul

The primary function of the immune system in higher organisms is generally thought to be defense against microbial infection. The sites of the defensive immunological reactions are the extracellular and intracellular compartments into which microbial organisms gain entry. Immunological effector agents elaborated against foreign microbial constituents must also inevitably contact various self-constituents, thus rendering the latter vulnerable to destruction. The self–nonself discrimination problem for the immune system is compounded by the fact that the sequence of essential proteins is often highly conserved across the species.

How, then, does the immune system in healthy humans manage to kill microorganisms without destroying self-constituents? The answer resides in three unique capabilities of the immune system. First, it elaborates humoral and cellular effector mechanisms that specifically recognize foreign structural components while minimizing crossreactivity with self-constituents. Second, harmful immunological reactions to self-constituents are inhibited by various suppressor mechanisms. Third, development of the defensive effector mechanisms occurs on demand, i.e., when the immune system is exposed to the foreign antigen, thus limiting the possibility of damage to self-constituents arising from chance crossreactivities.

The last two decades of research have conclusively shown that the immune system can mount responses to self-constituents without causing autoimmune disease. It can even be argued that some of these antiself responses are better classified as being "pro"-self, in that they fulfill essential homeostatic functions. Binding of foreign antigenic peptides by T-cells, for example, invariably occurs in the context of recognition of self major histocompatibility antigens. Autoantibodies capable of serving a physiological function, such as removal of senescent red blood cells, have been demonstrated. "Natural" antibodies found in healthy individuals are capable of binding many self-antigens and have been suggested to fulfill a metabolic role in removal of excess autoantigens. Autoantibodies directed to idiotopes found in other antibodies are postulated to regulate the synthesis of the latter as mediators of the idiotypic network.

Contemporary Immunology: Autoimmune Reactions
Edited by: S. Paul © Humana Press Inc., Totowa, NJ

The contents of this book are a reflection of the empirical nature of the our current understanding of autoimmune disease. These diseases are a heterogeneous class of disorders with varying symptoms, organ involvements, and biochemical and cellular markers. The heterogeneity of the disease forms is not surprising given the complexity of the molecular and cellular phenomena underlying immunological homeostasis (Fig. 1). There is so much that can go wrong, that eventually something or the other does go wrong. A unifying explanation for the initiation of the various autoimmune diseases, such as a global loss of the abilities to delete or anergize lymphocytes to self-constituents, does not appear plausible. Likewise, the tissue damage seen in autoimmune diseases does not occur by a single effector pathway. This is to be anticipated, since there is a plethora of destructive humoral and cellular effectors that can potentially turn against the self, and alterations in the production, activity levels, and life cycle of each of these effectors could potentially be involved in harmful autoimmune reactions. These considerations have necessitated empirical and individualized approaches in the study and treatment of the autoimmune diseases. The main order of business has been to systematically catalog the clinical symptoms; establish the diagnostic markers of the disease; evaluate the statistical and mechanistic contribution of individual immunological effectors such as antibodies, T-cells, and inflammatory cells as the mediators of tissue damage; and analyze individual afferent immunological events, such as antigen presentation, cytokine release, and T-cell receptor activity levels, as being responsible for the establishment of the harmful antiself immune responses.

Intensive studies of the type described in the preceding paragraph support the idea that most autoimmune diseases are polyfactorial disorders, involving qualitative and quantitative changes in various effector and afferent pathways of the immune response. Systemic lupus erythematosus (SLE), for instance, is associated with immune complex deposition in the kidney; activation of various inflammatory pathways in multiple tissues; an apparent tendency toward increased polyclonal B-cell activation resulting in autoantibody formation to nucleic acids, polypeptides, and low molecular weight antigens; derangements in the idiotype–antiidiotype network; and possible defects in clonal deletion of self-reactive T-cells as a result of decreased apoptotic activity. Even comparatively organ-specific diseases, such as autoimmune thyroiditis, display several different immunological derangements, i.e., infiltration of the thyroid by inflammatory cells, increased production of autoantibodies to various thyroid-associated antigens, and intrathyroidal development of cytotoxic T-cell response. On the other hand, such diseases as autoimmune hemolytic anemia and myasthenia gravis appear mainly to involve antibodies to cell-surface antigens as the mediators of damage.

Notwithstanding the complexity and multiplicity of deranged immunological functions known to occur in autoimmune diseases, comparatively general theories of autoimmune disease have been proposed. Since microbial antigens are often structurally similar to self-constituents, fortuitous crossreactivity of

Immune Effector Mechanisms
(each susceptible to dysfunction)

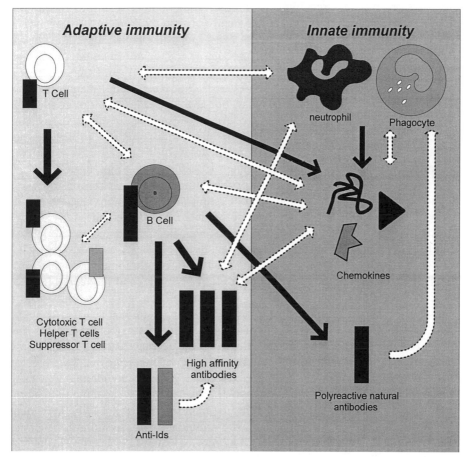

Fig. 1. Multiple immunological effector mechanisms susceptible to dysfunction in autoimmune disease. Solid arrows lead to mediators derived from immature and differentiated T- and B-cells and from cells like neutrophils and macrophages. Broken arrows show interacting species: cells like neutrophils, phagocytes and dendritic cells present antigens to T-cells and secrete chemokines (e.g., interleukins and prostanoid mediators) that can facilitate the differentiation and proliferation of B- and T-cells; antibodies produced by B-cells can bind to Fc receptors on various cells, including phagocytes, facilitating the effector functions of the latter; B-cells can also modulate T-cell activity via antigen presentation and by producing antibodies that modulate antigen presentation; antibodies to chemokines and antibodies to antibodies (anti-idiotypic antibodies) offer further regulatory possibilities.

immunological responses intended to destroy microbes has been suggested as the cause of autoimmune disease. A vivid example is the acute induction of heart lesions by cross-reactive antibodies formed against a streptococcal antigen. A retroviral origin for lupus has been suggested based on the presence of antiviral antibodies in lupus patients. The induction of autoimmune disease caused by this type of crossreactivity need not be an acute phenomenon. Cumulative exposure to various microbes over a long period of time may be necessary to break tolerance and induce disease. The aging theory of autoimmune disease, which was once quite popular, but has now fallen into disfavor, holds that destructive immune responses are mounted as a result of cumulative errors either in the structure of self-antigens or in immunoregulatory processes. For instance, accumulation of structural errors caused by processes such as somatic mutation or free radical-induced damage of self proteins may permit antiself reactivities to exceed the threshold for the compensatory capabilities of tissue repair mechanisms. In this view, the occurrence of autoimmune disease can be viewed as an adjunct of a series of minor catastrophes, the cumulative effect of which is the loss of balance between the maintenance of immunological defense and the suppression of destructive self reactivity.

These propositions do not imply that prevention of autoimmune disease must await such global solutions as the prevention of aging or of the recognition of foreign antigens as being structurally similar to self-antigens. To the contrary, further collection of the mechanistic facts concerning autoimmune disease can be predicted to permit the development of immunoregulatory interventions that allow restoration of self-tolerance, even if they are not directly related to the cause of the disease. Because there are so many mechanisms that are involved in maintenance of tolerance, it is perfectly conceivable to the optimist that each represents an opportunity to restore self-tolerance without fundamentally compromising the readiness to defend against the intruder. This will readily be evident to the practicing pharmacologist, i.e., the redundancy of physiological mechanisms geared to achieve the same aim permits exploitation of one mechanism to redress the problems created by a different pathway. For instance, β-adrenergic agonists are the mainstay of asthma therapy, even though the pathological events underlying reversible airway constriction in asthma do not appear to involve the smooth muscle effects of catecholamines. Therapy is possible because of the presence of excess β-adrenergic receptors in airways.

2

Insights into Mechanisms of Autoimmune Disease Based on Clinical Findings

Noel R. Rose

1. INTRODUCTION

The first example of a human autoimmune disease, paroxysmal cold hemoglobinuria (PCH) described by Donath and Landsteiner in 1903 *(1)*, still serves as a prototype for our understanding of the mechanisms of pathogenesis in autoimmune disease. In PCH, the patient produces an antibody that binds his own red blood cells. At the time of its discovery, the specificity of this antibody was unknown. In more recent times, it was found that the PCH antibody is usually directed to a widely distributed alloantigen of the P bloodgroup system. It is remarkable that the target antigen is actually an alloantigen to which autoantibodies are produced under the special circumstances of this disease. In the field of immunohematology, alloantigens are often the targets of autoimmune responses.

In the instance of PCH, the antibody has another significant attribute; that is, it binds its red blood cell antigen only at lowered temperatures, i.e., temperatures below 37°C. At low temperatures, the autoantibodies have no apparent adverse effect. When the blood is restored to the neighborhood of 37°C, however, the autoantibody activates the complement cascade. The consequent enzymatic reaction lyses the antibody-coated red blood cells. The symptomatology of PCH is due to the release of hemoglobin.

The phenomonology of PCH was duplicated by Ehrlich *(2)* using a simple in vivo experiment. He tied a ligature around the finger of a patient and immersed the finger in cold water. Under these conditions, the PCH antibody fixed to the patient's own red blood cells. Removing the finger from its cold environment and allowing it to warm, Ehrlich showed that hemoglobin was present in the plasma of the finger, indicating the in vivo lysis of the red cells through the agency of complement.

Putting together the information derived from the original Donath/Landsteiner *(1)* discovery and Ehrlich's *(2)* subsequent investigations, we can derive several fundamental generalities about the mechanisms of damage in autoimmune disease. First, the presence of autoantibodies is not necessarily indicative of disease.

Contemporary Immunology: Autoimmune Reactions
Edited by: S. Paul © Humana Press Inc., Totowa, NJ

Naturally occurring autoantibodies, especially to intracellular macromolecules, are present in all normal humans *(3)*. They are generally, but not always, low-affinity IgMs and do not cause any harm. Natural antibodies may even be useful as early mediators of protection. Some investigators have considered the possibility that natural autoantibodies play a physiological role in removing damaged or effete body constituents. The second important lesson to be learned from PCH is that the harmful effects of autoimmunity require progression or escalation of the initial autoimmune response, frequently involving mobilization of nonspecific effector mechanisms. These mechanisms are the same as those responsible for protective immunity against invading pathogens. In the case of PCH, for example, there is activation of the complement cascade, a response valuable in protective immunity against certain gram-negative bacteria.

The body normally goes to some lengths to avoid activating these potentially harmful effector mechanisms. Ehrlich epitomized this principle in his famous dictum *horror autotoxicus*. It should be emphasized that Ehrlich was not denying the existence of autoimmunity. Quite the contrary! He recognized, from the earlier experiments of Metalnikoff *(4)*, that autoimmunity is possible. Rather, Ehrlich suggested that the body will mobilize a number of "contrivances" to avoid the harmful consequences of autoimmunity. Thus, we can affirm, based on our present understanding of the immune response, that autoimmunity is common, but autoimmune disease is unusual. It is attributable to the breakdown of a number of homeostatic safeguards designed to prevent the harmful consequences of autoimmunity.

In this chapter, we will review the circumstances that favor the development of harmful or pathogenic autoimmunity as well as the underlying mechanisms known to cause, or contribute to, autoimmune disease.

2. AUTOIMMUNITY AND AUTOIMMUNE DISEASE

The initiation of autoimmune diseases of humans depends upon two types of risk factors, genetic and environmental. Genetic factors provide a disposition, whereas the environmental agent is the immediate trigger of disease.

Multiple genes are involved in producing the heightened susceptibility to autoimmune diseases. Following our original discovery of the association of the murine major histocompatibility complex (MHC) H-2 with experimental thyroiditis *(5)*, many studies in animals demonstrated an association of particular MHC haplotypes with autoimmune disease. In most human autoimmune diseases, there is a significant skewing of the MHC repertoire toward particular HLA haplotypes; for example, Graves' disease is associated with the HLA B8/DR3 haplotype; insulin-dependent diabetes associates most closely with HLA B8/DR3/DR4 with DR2 serving as a protective allele *(6)*. Although these associations are statistically valid, the biological basis of the connection of an autoimmune disease with a particular Class II MHC haplotype is uncertain. It may be that the Class II MHC gene product is involved in presentation by an antigen-presenting cell of a particular "pathogenic" epitope of the self-antigen.

Alternatively, MHC expression in the thymus may affect the T-cell repertoire of the host.

Although statistically significant, the HLA association with human autoimmune diseases is relatively modest and not generally close enough to be of clinical value. An exception is the disease ankylosing spondylitis, which shows a close association with HLA-B27 *(7)*. The autoimmune origin of this disease, however, has not been established and the connection may be on some different basis than the other diseases. HLA haplotypes, therefore, should be considered harbingers, but not genetic requirements for the initiation of autoimmune responses. Equally significant is the observation that HLA associations for a particular disease differ among different racial and ethnic groups; for example, among the Japanese, Graves' disease is associated with HLA-B35 rather than HLA-B8 *(8)*. An even more dramatic instance is the juvenile form of chronic lymphocytic (Hashimoto's) thyroiditis. In this disease, there is a close association of the HLA haplotype of the proband with disease within a particular family, but the haplotype incriminated differs from family to family *(9)*.

In our investigations of experimentally induced thyroiditis, we further showed that the MHC association with autoimmune disease is heterogeneous with respect to the subloci involved *(10)*. Susceptibility to experimental thyroiditis in mice, for example, depends upon at least two Class II MHC loci, I-A and I-E. While $H-2^k$ alleles at I-A increase susceptibility to thyroid autoimmunity, I-E appears to modulate the autoimmune process. Equally interesting is the role of Class I MHC, which modifies the severity of thyroid inflammation in the experimental disease *(11)*. Thus, the MHC is involved in this autoimmune process on three levels. First, the two principal Class II MHC determinants control the initiation of the autoimmune response, regulating the recognition of the "pathogenic" epitopes of thyroglobulin. Given the vigorous recognition of the requisite "pathogenic" epitopes, Class I MHC determines the severity of thyroid cell damage, possibly through the effect on cytotoxic T-lymphocytes (CTL).

In addition to genes of the MHC, a number of non-MHC genes regulate the development of a pathogenic autoimmune response. In the spontaneous form of autoimmune thyroiditis in the OS chicken, for example, at least two additional, non-MHC genetic traits have been identified *(12)*. They involve differences in the development of the thymus and probably the ratio of different thymic cell subpopulations. Another non-MHC gene controls the organification of iodine by the thyroid follicle cells.

Undoubtedly, additional genetic traits affect the susceptibility of humans as well as of experimental animals to the development of autoimmune disease. We have proposed in the past that the genetic predisposition is best viewed as the chance aggregation of a number of unrelated normal genetic traits in an individual or in an inbred strain of animals. The genes act in diverse ways, often having little or no obvious relationship to the development of the particular autoimmune disorder. It is rather the interaction of such normally occurring genetic traits rather than distinct "disease susceptibility genes" that produce the genetic predisposition of some individuals to develop autoimmune disease.

In all of the human autoimmune diseases studied, genetic traits account for about half of the risk of developing an autoimmune disease. This evidence is based primarily on a comparison of genetically identical monozygotic twins with nonidentical, dizygotic twins *(13,14)*. We must conclude, therefore, that the other half of the risk of developing autoimmune disease resides in factors not encoded by germline genes. Since lymphocytes are notoriously hypermutable, it is possible that somatic mutation or epigenetic changes contribute to increased genetic susceptibility. A preponderance of evidence, however, suggests that extrinsic environmental factors play a major role in the development of human autoimmune diseases.

Unfortunately, we have relatively little information about the environmental factors involved in most autoimmune diseases and even less understanding of their mechanisms of action *(15)*. Several drugs, including hydralizines and procainamide, are known to induce a lupus-like disorder in genetically susceptible individuals. Penicillamine has been associated with myasthenia gravis as well as with a number of other autoimmune diseases. Exposure of miners to silica is described as a precipitating factor in the autoimmune disease, scleroderma, and mercury salts have been associated with autoimmune glomerulonephritis. One of the best documented environmental factors related to autoimmune disease is dietary iodine, which is known to induce autoimmune thyroid disease. This association is seen not only in human populations, but in the spontaneous forms of thyroiditis described in the OS chicken, BB/Wor rat, and NOD H-2^{h4} mouse *(16)*. In the latter case, increasing the amount of iodine hastens the development of thyroiditis and increases the severity of lymphocytic infiltration of the thyroid. Preliminary evidence suggests that iodinated haptens in the thyroglobulin molecule, probably the active thyroid hormone tetraiodothyronine, increase the immunoreactivity of thyroglobulin.

The foregoing discussion assumes that self-reactive lymphocytes are not deleted during prenatal or neonatal development as the original clonal selection theory of Burnet predicted *(17)*. Intrathymic clonal deletion has been convincingly demonstrated with a few potent antigens, particularly MHC and MHC-like antigens, such as H-Y, and with superantigens *(18)*. In the case of most other tissue antigens, however, clonal deletion is ineffective or incomplete, probably because these antigens are not present in the thymus in requisite quantities. Self-reactive T-cells, therefore, can readily be demonstrated to a large number of self-antigens, such as thyroglobulin *(19)*. Because of their relatively low affinity, these T-cells are generally not activated unless a powerful adjuvant, such as Freund's complete adjuvant (FCA) or lipopolysaccharide (LPS), is co-administered with the autologous protein *(20)*.

Usually, CD4+ self-reactive T-helper cells must be activated in order to induce an autoimmune disease, whether the disease is owing directly to T-cell-mediated immunity or to antibody-mediated immunity. On the other hand, the presence of antibody has been an invariable sign of autoimmune disease in humans. There are, as yet, no examples reported of an autoimmune disease produced by cell-mediated immunity in the absence of antibody, even though the antibody may play no pathogenic role. For this reason, the presence of autoantibody in the serum is the most readily available tool for the diagnosis of autoimmune disease in human subjects.

Most human autoimmune diseases are complex, involving a number of antigens of the target tissue. Part of the complexity is owed to epitope spread; that is, the enlargement of the immune response to include increasing numbers of epitopes of the initiating antigen. Another common feature of human autoimmune disease is the presence of antibodies to a number of unrelated, organ-specific antigens, a phenomenon we previously described as immunologic escalation *(21)*. It may be that an initial inflammatory response owing to autoimmunity recruits additional organ-specific antigens into the autoimmune response. For example, in chronic thyroiditis, one commonly finds antibodies not only to thyroglobulin, the antigen responsible for initiation of the disease process, but to thyroid peroxidase, another antigenically unrelated constituent of the thyroid gland.

There is strong evidence that T-cell-mediated immunity is of major importance in the pathogenesis of many autoimmune diseases, based primarily on adoptive transfer studies in experimental animals. The statement holds for insulin-dependent diabetes or for multiple sclerosis *(22,23)*. These findings, however, do not exclude a role for antibody. The human disease, myocarditis, can be replicated by immunization of genetically susceptible strains of mice with purified cardiac myosin *(24)*. The experimental disease has been adoptively transferred by CD4[+] T-cells. However, human patients with myocarditis, produce an autoimmune response to another cardiac antigen, the adenine nucleotide transporter *(25)*. Antibody to this cardiac antigen may produce a functional defect in the cardiac myocyte and play an important role in the cardiac failure associated with this disease. Thus, multiple mechanisms participate in the pathogenesis of autoimmune disease.

3. B-CELL EFFECTOR MECHANISMS

The critical role of autoantibody initiating PCH can be viewed as a prototype of the pathological processes of autoimmune disease. In the more common forms of hemolytic anemia, autoantibody to erythrocytes is also a key factor in initiating disease. In the warm-type hemolytic anemia, utoantibody fixes to the red blood cell at body temperatures *(26)*. Often this antibody is directed to one of the alloantigens of the Rh bloodgroup system *(27)*. This antibody may not initiate complement-mediated lysis; rather, it shortens the survival of the red cell by enhancing uptake of the antibody-coated erythrocyte by phagocytic cells of the spleen and liver. In cold antibody hemolytic anemia, the union of antibody with erythrocyte is demonstrable at laboratory temperatures, but difficult to demonstrate in the patient. Sometimes, one actually finds the third component of complement, C3a, on the erythrocyte in the absence of immunoglobulin, presumably because the antibody that initiated the complement fixation eluded spontaneously from the erythrocyte *(28)*. This form of hemolytic anemia is also not owing to intervascular hemolysis, but rather to increased uptake of the opsonized erythrocytes by phagocytic cells. The other major cells of the blood, leukocytes and platelets, may also be depleted by autoimmune mechanisms *(29,30)*. Autoimmune leukopenias and autoimmune thrombocytopenias, however, are more difficult to diagnose than autoimmune hemolytic anemias for a variety of technical reasons, involving the spontaneous attachment of immunoglobulins to the cell surfaces.

Recently, the presence of antibodies to clotting factors is receiving increased attention. The lupus anticoagulant was originally described many years ago *(31)* and was associated with the bleeding diathesis of that disease. The presence of antibody to phospholipids or to beta-2-glycoprotein-I is a valuable clinical indicator of thrombotic problems *(32)*. They may be manifest as repeated spontaneous abortions, stroke, or other thrombocytic phenomena. The mechanisms by which the antiphospholipid antibody produces these syndromes is still unclear, but may well involve some catalytic function of the autoantibody in the clotting cascade.

Another possible pathological consequence of autoantibody production is the development in vivo of immune complexes. Antigen/antibody aggregates tend to localize in capillary beds in several locations, such as lung, brain and skin. The most damaging problems generally arise from immune complexes deposited in the glomeruli of the kidneys. In lupus nephritis, complexes of native DNA/anti-DNA are important mediators of renal injury *(33)*. However, in most cases in which immune complexes can be demonstrated directly in the kidney, it is not possible to identify the corresponding antigen. For that reason, some investigators have suggested that these immune complexes may represent idiotype/anti-idiotype combinations or other antibodies to immunoglobulins. Regardless of the inciting antigen, immune complex-mediated glomerular damage can be distinguished from glomerulonephritis produced by autoantibody to antigens of the glomerular or tubular basement membranes *(34)*. The latter antibodies directly attack a kidney antigen and show a different pattern of distribution by direct immunofluorescence or electron microscopy. The damage inflicted by immune complexes or by direct antibody attack is mediated through complement activation and the generation of inflammatory mediators.

A topic receiving a great deal of discussion recently is the ability of antibody to produce damage to intracellular or even intranuclear antigens *(35)*. Although the notion that antibody can penetrate living cells runs contrary to much historical dogma, evidence that some classes of antibody can bind to cell-surface F_c receptors, and be taken in by endocytosis, is now quite persuasive. Whether such antibody can remain functional within the cell is still debated, but the implications of intracellular activity of antinuclear antibodies in lupus is enormous.

Another mechanism by which autoantibody may produce autoimmune tissue damage is through the cooperative action with lymphoid cells. This mechanism, referred to as antibody-dependent, cell-mediated cytotoxicity, involves the attachment of antibody to a lymphocyte or macrophage through F_c receptors *(36)*. The antibody then provides the directional specificity, whereas the cell is the actual mediator of damage. Such reactions have been demonstrated in the test tube, but it is not known how important this mechanism is in the body.

Antireceptor antibodies occur in a number of autoimmune diseases. In myasthenia gravis, antibodies to acetylcholene receptor reduce the number of receptors available on the myocyte and possibly interfere with neuromuscular transmission of impulses *(36)*. The resultant muscular weakness is the major manifestation of the disease. In Graves' disease, antibodies to the thyrotropin receptor are present *(37)*. Some of these antibodies actually stimulate the receptor, producing the sustained hyperthyroidism that is the major manifestation of Graves' disease. Other antibodies bind the receptor without producing stimulation, but may actually block its binding to thyrotropin. Antibodies to the tissue antigen R_o are responsible for congenital heart block *(38)*. When these antibodies are produced by a mother with lupus, they may be able to traverse the placenta and act upon the heart of the newborn. Yet the antibodies do not appear to injure the heart of the mother.

4. T-CELL EFFECTOR MECHANISMS

Although antibody is clearly of primary importance in dealing with antigens accessible to the circulation or intracellular fluids, T-cells have the major responsibility of dealing with antigens located within cells. In order to serve this function, it is essential that T-cells not be triggered by an encounter with circulating antigens. Were they to recognize free antigens, T-cells might be activated in the bloodstream before they were able to reach their cellular targets. Not only would such an event lead to useless or "sterile" activation of the T-cell, it may well cause the release of soluble mediators, cytokines, that may produce adverse reactions upon the host.

In order to avoid such "sterile" activation, T-cells are engineered to recognize antigenic determinants only in context of the syngeneic MHC. CD8 T-cells are restricted by the Class I MHC determinants found on all nucleated tissue cells *(39)*. When they encounter their corresponding antigen in conjunction with a congruent Class I MHC, the CD8 T-cells are effective as cytotoxic T-lymphocytes (CTLs). CTLs are the major effectors of cell-mediated immunity in both protective immune reactions and immunopathological reactions. They recognize the corresponding antigenic determinant at the cell surface in the presence of Class I MHC. Since human red blood cells do not express Class I MHC, they are unaffected by CTLs. Certain tissues normally express only low levels of Class I MHC, including the thyroid gland. The amount of Class I MHC, however, is up-regulated during inflammation, probably as the result of the local production of cytokines such as interferon γ *(40)*. Thus the inflammatory process itself may make tissues more vulnerable to CTL attack.

Another important limitation of CTL function is the ability of the circulating T-cell to localize in the relevant tissue. This function is controlled primarily by adhesion molecules expressed on the vascular endothelium, such as V-CAM, and the presence of corresponding ligands on the lymphocyte, such as LFA-3 *(41)*. The up-regulation of these molecules enhances the migration of CTLs to sites of inflammation.

CTLs kill target cells, using at least two effector pathways. One pathway requires direct contact of the CTL with its target and the other involves the secretion of effector molecules. By direct contact, the CTL produces lesions in the target cell membrane through the activation of perforins *(42)*. The pores produced appear to be quite similar to those seen in complement-mediated cell lysis. Another direct cytotoxic mechanism involves the interaction of *Fas* ligand *(FasL)* with *Fas (43)*. In this reaction, surface *FasL* on the CTL crosslinks *Fas* on target cells. The crosslinking induces apoptotic changes in target cell nuclei, resulting in programmed cell death.

The second indirect T-cell effector mechanism involves the production of cytotoxic cytokines. Tumor necrosis factor-α is the best characterized of these substances *(44)*. This cytokine is capable of inducing target cell death by activating preformed granules within the cell and triggering the apoptotic events. Thus, both CTL pathways may lead to similar endpoints of target cell elimination by apoptosis.

Among human autoimmune diseases, there is general consensus that CTLs are the major effectors of damage in the organ-localized autoimmune disorders. They include such diseases as insulin-dependent diabetes, chronic thyroiditis and multiple sclerosis. The evidence for the primary role of CTLs in these diseases is based upon studies of the analogous animal models, where the disease can be transferred with T-cells and not with antibody. It is not ethical or possible to do such experiments in humans because of MHC restriction. Therefore, evidence for the primary role of CTLs in human autoimmune disease is necessarily indirect. Moreover, the finding in animals that an autoimmune disease can be transferred with lymphocytes and not with serum does not exclude a role of antibody in augmenting the disease.

5. MACROPHAGE EFFECTOR MECHANISMS

Macrophages are proficient phagocytic cells and provide a large measure of protective immunity against infections, particularly chronic infections. In a similar fashion, they contribute to the chronic pathological consequences of autoimmune reactions. The extensive network of monocytic phagocytes in organized lymphoid tissues is sometimes referred to collectively as the reticuloendothelial system. These cells are particularly important in removing from the bloodstream damaged cells or altered protein molecules. Consequently, the reticuloendothelial system plays the major role in removing red blood cells that have been opsonized by autoantibody as in cases of hemolytic anemia. Reticuloendothelial cells also attempt to remove immune complexes from the circulation and thereby reduce the potential injury produced by these complexes in capillary beds throughout the body. The phagocytic functions of the macrophage population are greatly enhanced when the particles, be they cellular or subcellular, are coated with antibody. Macrophages present F_c receptors that bind antibody and facilitate phagocytic uptake *(45)*. There is, then, close cooperation between antibody-mediated immunity and macrophage effector mechanisms.

Following phagocytic uptake, macrophages become activated. During this process, the production of proteolytic and other hydrolytic enzymes within the macrophages is increased, allowing the phagocyte to digest many of the injected particles. The accumulation of lytic enzymes with phagocytic vesicles results in phagolysosomes, structures in which degradation of the phagocytized particles occurs *(46)*.

The activated macrophage is an important effector mechanism in cell-mediated immunopathologic reactions. Macrophages are a source of cytokines, such as IL-12, that enhance the production of the T_H1 subset of CD4 T-cells *(47)*. IL-12 is particularly important, because it enhances T-cell-mediated immunity as well as the production of complement-fixing isotypes of antibody. Another important product of activated macrophages is interferon γ (IFN-γ) *(48)*. There is some evidence that this cytokine is directly responsible for damage of certain epithelial cells, such as thyroid follicular cells *(49,50)*. Moreover, IFN-γ enhances the activity of nitric acid synthase. Nitric acid is a mediator of protective immunity and cardiovascular tone *(51)*. It can also have tissue-damaging effects alone or by the interaction with reactive oxygen intermediates *(52)*. These substances are potential agents of cellular necrosis. Although the role of nitric acid and reactive oxygen intermediates is not yet firmly established in the pathological changes of autoimmune diseases, there is reason to suppose that they will turn out to be major effector agents *(53)*.

6. OTHER EFFECTOR MECHANISMS

The several mechanisms described in the previous section do not fully justify to the large repertory of potential immunopathological effectors available in the body. Although it is traditional to draw a distinction between innate and adaptive immune responses, the cells and mediators of these reactions overlap. Many of the mechanisms of innate immunity are involved in the damaging effects of autoimmune responses; for example, natural killer (NK) cells are important in the early stages of resistance to viral infection *(54)*. NK cells are common in many autoimmune responses, such as autoimmune myocarditis *(55)*. They are attracted by the production of interferon γ by the infiltrating inflammatory cells. In turn, NK cells produce additional IFN-γ, with the potential immunopathological consequences ascribed to this cytokine *(56)*. In addition to NK cells, polymorphonuclear neutrophils are attracted by cell injury and necrosis. They may also join in producing immunopathological responses. Similar statements can be made for the complement cascade, which may be activated through alternative as well as classic pathways. Thus, all of the agents of innate immunity may be engaged in autoimmune disease.

7. SUMMARY AND CONCLUSIONS

Multiple mechanisms produce the immunopathological changes of autoimmune diseases. They involve the same mechanisms responsible for protective immunity. The target of these responses, however, is the host itself rather than an invading pathogen. The particular mechanisms involved are determined first by the location of the autologous antigen. For example, the immunopathological mechanisms injuring antigens present in the bloodstream often differ from those attacking antigens in cells. Antibody is generally of primary importance in accessible antigen. On the other hand, antigens within cells are generally dealt with by T-cells. It is likely, however, that both categories of effector mechanisms, humoral and cellular, play a role in most human autoimmune diseases. The important determinant is the method of induction. It may influence the balance of T_H1 and T_H2 T-cell populations which, in turn, determines the relative involvement of cell-mediated and humoral immune responses and the final outcome of the autoimmune process *(57,58)*.

REFERENCES

1. Donath, J., and Landsteiner, K. (1904) Ueber paroxysmale Hämoglobinurie. *Münch.med.Wochenschr.* **51**, 1590–1593.
2. Ehrlich, P. (1881) Ueber paroxysmale Hämoglobinurie. *Deutsch. med. Wochenschr.* **7**, 224–225.
3. Dighiero, G., Lymberi, P., Holmberg, D., Lundquist, I., Coutinho, A., and Avrameas, S. (1985) High frequency of natural autoantibodies in normal newborn mice. *J. Immunol.* **134**, 765–771.
4. Metalnikoff, S. (1900) Etudes sur la spermotoxine. *Ann. Inst. Pasteur* **14**, 577–590.
5. Vladutiu, A. O. and Rose, N. R. (1971) Autoimmune murine thyroiditis. Relation to histocompatibility (H-2) type. *Science* **174**, 1137–1139.
6. Tiwari, T. L. and Terasaki, P. I. (Eds.) (1985) *HLA and Disease Association.* Springer-Verlag, New York.
7. Nepom, G. T. and Concannon, P. (1992) Molecular genetics of autoimmunity, in *The Autoimmune Diseases II* (Rose, N. R. and Mackay, I. R., eds.), Academic Press, San Diego, CA. pp. 127–152.
8. Farid, N. R. (1981) Graves' disease, in *Endocrine and Metabolic Disorders* (Farid, N. R., ed.), Academic, New York, pp. 85–143.
9. Rose, N. R. and Burek, C. L. (1991) The interaction of basic science and population-based research: autoimmune thyroiditis as a case history. *Am. J. Epidemiol.* **14**, 1073–1078.

10. Rose, N. R., Kong, Y. M., and Sundick, R. S. (1980) The genetic lesions of auto-immunity. *Clin. Exp. Immunol.* **39,** 545–550.
11. Kong, Y. M., David, C. S., Giraldo, A. A., ElRehewy, M., and Rose, N. R. (1979) Regulation of autoimmune response to mouse thyroglobulin: influence of H-2D-end genes. *J. Immunol.* **123,** 15–18.
12. Rose, N. R. (1994) Avian models of autoimmune disease: lessons from the birds. *Poultry Science* **73,** 984–990.
13. Sinha, A. A., Lopez, M. T., and McDevitt, H. O. (1990) Autoimmune diseases: the failure of self tolerance. *Science* **248,** 1380–1388.
14. Worthington, J. and Silman, A.J. (1995) Genetic control of autoimmunity, lessons from twin studies. *Clin. Exp. Immunol.* **101,** 390–392.
15. Rose, N. R. and Caturegli, P. P. (1997) Environmental and drug-induced autoimmune diseases of humans, in *Comprehensive Toxicology* (Sipes, I. G., McQueen, C. A., and Gandolfi, A. J., eds.) / *Vol. 5 - Toxicology of the Immune System* (Lawrence. D. A., ed.), Elsevier Science, Oxford, UK, pp. 381–390.
16. Rasooly, L., Burek, C. L., and Rose, N. R. (1996) Iodine-induced autoimmune thyroiditis in NOD-H-2^{h4} mice. *Clin. Immunol. Immunopathol.* **81,** 287–292.
17. Burnet, F. M. (1959) *The Clonal Selection Theory of Acquired Immunity.* Cambridge University Press, Cambridge, UK.
18. Mondino, A., Khoruts, A., and Jenkins, M. K. (1996) The anatomy of T-cell activation and tolerance. *Proc. Natl. Acad. Sci. USA* **93,** 2245–2252.
19. Esquivel, P. S., Kong, Y. M., and Rose, N. R. (1978) Evidence for thyroglobulin-reactive T cells in good responder mice. *Cell. Immunol.* **37,** 14–19.
20. Rose, N. R., Kong, Y. M., Okayasu, I., Giraldo, A. A., Beisel, K., and Sundick, R. S. (1981) T-cell regulation in autoimmune *thyroiditis. Immunol. Rev.* **55,** 299–314.
21. Rose, N. R., Skelton, F. R., Kite, J. H., Jr., and Witebsky, E. (1966) Experimental thyroiditis in the rhesus monkey. III. Course of the disease. *Clin. Exp. Immunol.* **1,** 171–188.
22. Katz, J. D., Benoist, C., and Mathis, D. (1995) T helper cell subsets in insulin-dependent diabetes. *Science* **268,** 1185–1188.
23. Zanvil, S. S. and Steinman, L. (1990) The T lymphocyte in experimental allergic encephalomyelitis. *Annu. Rev. Immunol.* **8,** 579–621.
24. Rose, N. R. and Hill, S. L. (1996) The pathogenesis of postinfectious myocarditis. *Clin. Immunol. Immunopathol.* **80,** S92–S99.
25. Schultheiss, H.-P. and Bolte, H.-D. (1985) Immunological analysis of autoantibodies against the adenine nucleotide translocator in dilated cardiomyopathy. *Mol. Cell. Cardiol.* **17,** 603–617.
26. Englefriet, C. P., Overbeek, M. A., and von dem Borne, A. E. (1992) Autoimmune hemolytic anemia. *Seminars Hematol.* **29,** 3–12.
27. Leddy, J. P., Falang, J. L., Kissel, G. E., Passadar, S. T. and Rosenfeld, S. I. (1993) Erythrocyte membrane proteins reactive with human (warm-reacting) anti-red cell autoantibodies. *J. Clin. Invest.* **91,** 1672–1680.
28. Garratty, G. (1994) Autoimmune hemolytic anemia, in *Immunobiology of Transfusion Medicine* (Garratty, G., ed.), Marcel Dekker, New York, pp. 493–521.
29. Waters, A. H. (1992) Autoimmune thrombocytopenia: clinical aspects. *Seminars Hematol.* **29,** 18–25.
30. Bux, J. and Mueller-Eckhardt, C. (1992) Autoimmune neutropenia. *Seminars Hematol.* **29,** 45–53.

31. Conley, E. L. and Hartmann, R. C. (1952) A hemolytic disorder caused by circulating anticoagulants in patients with disseminated lupus erythematosus. *J. Lab. Clin. Med.* **31,** 621–622.

32. Jones, J. V., James, H., Mansour, M., and Eastwood, B. J. (1995) β_2 glycoprotein-I is a cofactor for antibodies reacting with 5 anionic phospholipids. *J. Rheumatol.* **22,** 2009.

33. Tan, E. M. (1989) Antinuclear antibodies: diagnostic markers for autoimmune diseases and probes for cell biology. *Adv. Immunol.* **44,** 93–151.

34. Herody, M., Bobric, G., Gourin, G., Grundfeld, J. P., and Noel, L. H. (1993) Anti-GBM disease: predictive value of clinical, histological and serological data. *Clin. Nephrol.* **40,** 249–255.

35. Alarcon-Segovia, D., Leorente, L., and Ruiz-Arguellar, A. (1996) Broken dogma: autoantibodies to intracellular constituents penetrate live cells, reach their target, alter function and cause death. *Immunol. Today* **17,** 163–164.

36. Rodien, P., Madec, A. M., Morel, Y., Stefanutti, A., Bornet, H., and Orgiazzi, J. (1992) Assessment of antibody dependent cell cytotoxicity in autoimmune thyroid disease using porcine thyroid cells. *Autoimmunity* **13,** 177-185.

37. Newsom-Davis, J., Pinching, A. J., Vincent, A., and Wilson, S. G. (1978) Function of circulating antibody to acetylcholine receptor in myasthenia gravis: investigation by plasma exchange. *Neurology* **28,** 266–272.

38. McGregor, A. M. (1990) Autoantibodies to the TSH receptor in patients with autoimmune thyroid disease. *Clin. Endocrinol. (Oxf.)* **33,** 683–685.

39. Reichlin, M., Brucato, A., Frank, M. B., Maddison, P. J., McCubbin, V. R., Wolfson-Reichlin, M., et al. (1994) Concentration of autoantibodies to native 60-kD Ro/SS-A and 52-kD Ro/SS-A in eluates from the heart of a child who died with congenital complete heart block. *Arthritis Rheum.* **37,** 1698–1703.

40. Norment, A. M., Salter, R. D., Parham, P., Engelhard, V. H., and Littman, D. R. (1988) Cell-cell adhesion mediated by CD8 and MHC class I molecules. *Nature* **336,** 79–81.

41. Molne, J., Nilsson, M., Jansson, S., Hansson, G., and Ericson, L. E. (1991) Non-polarized cell surface expression of HLA-A,B,C and HLA-DR antigens in Graves' thyroid follicle cells. *Autoimmunity* **10,** 189–199.

42. Kuchroo, V. K., Martin, C. A., Greer, J. M., Ju, S. T., Sobel, R. A., and Dorf, M. E. (1993) Cytokines and adhesion molecules contribute to the ability of myelin proteolipid protein-specific T cell clones to mediate experimental allergic encephalommyelitis. *J. Immunol.* **151,** 4371–4382.

43. Young, J. D.-E., Cohn, Z. A., and Podack, E. R. (1986) The ninth component of complement and the pore-forming protein (perforin) from cytotoxic T cells: structural, immunological and functional similarities. *Science* **233,** 184–190.

44. Henkart, P. A. (1996) Lymphocyte-mediated cytotoxicity: two pathways and multiple effector molecules. *Immunity* **1,** 343–346.

45. Sharief, M. K. and Hentges, R. (1991) Association between tumor necrosis factor-α and disease progression in patients with multiple sclerosis. *N. Engl. J. Med.* **325,** 467–472.

46. Ravetch, J. V. and Kinet, J.-P. (1991) Fc receptor. *Annu. Rev. Immunol.* **9,** 457.

47. Nathan, C. F. (1983) Macrophage microbiocidal mechanism. *Trans. Roy. Soc. Trop. Med. Hyg.* **77,** 620–630.

48. Wolf, S. F., Sieburth, D., and Sypek, J. (1994) Interleukin 12: a key modulator of immune function. *Stem Cells* **12,** 154–168.
49. Gately, M. K., Wolitzky, A. G., Quinn, P. M., and Chizzonite, R. (1992) Regulation of human cytolytic lymphocyte responses by interleukin-12. *Cell. Immunol.* **143,** 127–142.
50. Magram, J., Connaughton, S. E., Warrier, R. R., Carvajal, D. M., Wu, C.-Y., Ferrante, J., et al. (1996) IL-12-deficient mice are defective in IFN-γ production and type 1 cytokine responses. *Immunity* **4,** 471–481.
51. Frohman, M., Francfort, J. W., and Cowing, C. (1991) T-dependent destruction of thyroid isografts exposed to IFN-γ. *J. Immunol.* **146,** 2227–2234.
52. Babior, B. M., Kipnes, R. S., and Curnette, J. T. (1973) Biological defense mechanisms. The production by leukocytes of superoxide, a potential bacteriocide. *J. Clin. Invest.* **52,** 741.
53. Rabinovitch A., Suarez-Pinzon, W. L., Strynadka, K., Lakey, J. R. T., and Rajotte, R. V. (1996) Human pancreatic islet β-cell destruction by cytokines involves oxygen free radicals and aldehyde production. *J. Clin. Endocrinol. Metab.* **81,** 3197–3202.
54. Vladutiu, A. O. (1995) Role of nitric oxide in autoimmunity. *Clin. Immunol. Immunopathol.* **76,** 1–11.
55. Lancaster, J. R., Jr. (1992) Nitric oxide in cells. *Am. Scientist* **80,** 248–259.
56. Gauntt, C. J. (1988) The possible role of viral variants in pathogenesis, in *Coxsackievirus: a General Update on Infectious Agents and Pathogenesis* (Bendinelli, M. and Friedman, H., eds.), Plenum, New York, pp. 159–179.
57. Godeny, E. K. and Gauntt, C. J. (1987) Murine natural killer cells limit coxsackie virus B3 replication. *J. Immunol.* **139,** 913.
58. Romagnani, S. T-Cell Subsets (T_H1, T_H2) and cytokines in autoimmunity, in *The Autoimmune Diseases,* 3rd ed. (Rose, N. R. and Mackay, I. R., eds.), Academic Press, San Diego, CA, in press.

3

Autoimmunity and B-Cell Malignancies

Otto Pritsch and Guillaume Dighiero

1. INTRODUCTION

The historical concept of humoral immunity is based on three major properties of antibodies: nonself specificity, monospecificity, and immune memory. In 1900, Metchnikoff suggested the idea of autoimmunization by demonstrating the presence of autoantibodies in normal conditions (1,2). This finding directly opposed the concept of *horror autotoxicus* raised by Ehrlich (3,4) where nearly at the same time, Landsteiner described the rules governing blood compatibility (5). He showed that a subject will never be able to produce autoantibodies against the major blood group antigens, which provided strong support to Ehrlich's idea. Although Metchnikoff (1) clearly demonstrated that animals were able to produce autoantibodies against spermatozoids, their significance was soon jailed into the convenient explanation of a pathological process. The influence of Ehrlich's ideas was so strong that these experiments were forgotten, and when Donath and Landsteiner (6) described for the first time an auto-antibody, the biphasic hemaglutinin responsible for paroxysmal cold hemoglobinuria, they failed to call it an autoantibody.

In 1949 Burnet proposed the clonal deletion theory (7). This theory was strongly influenced by the experiments done by Owen with dizygotic calves sharing a single placenta (8). The red blood cells from these two calves were mixed but, despite the fact that they expressed different blood groups, each was unable to produce alloantibodies against the blood group from the other. The interpretation of these experiments led Burnet and Fenner to elaborate the clonal deletion theory. This was a magnificent theory explaining tolerance and autoimmunity in a simple way. Autoimmunity, according to this theory, would only arise as a consequence of somatic mutation, which is an unusual phenomenon (7).

During recent years, evidence has emerged, however, indicating that the autoreactive repertoire is an important component of the normal B-cell repertoire and this repertoire is frequently involved in malignant transformation. In this chapter, we will develop these two points.

Contemporary Immunology: Autoimmune Reactions
Edited by: S. Paul © Humana Press Inc., Totowa, NJ

2. THE AUTOREACTIVE REPERTOIRE IS AN IMPORTANT COMPONENT OF THE NORMAL B-CELL REPERTOIRE

In 1956 for the first time, Witebsky and Rose were able to induce an experimental autoimmune disease mediated by autoantibodies: autoimmune thyroiditis *(9)*. They succeeded in inducing this disease by injecting thyroglobulin in the presence of Freund's adjuvant. Since they were able to produce autoantibodies, it is logical to conclude that the precursor B-cells capable of producing these antibodies were not deleted. More recently, considerable data have accumulated raising doubts concerning the clonal deletion theory as a unique and sufficient explanation for tolerance

1. Autoimmune diseases can be induced by injecting organ extracts *(9)*.
2. Numerous autoantibodies have been demonstrated under normal condiions *(10-12)*.
3. Autoantibody synthesis by normal B-lymphocytes has been induced upon mitogenic stimulation *(13,14)*.

In the early 1980s, several groups demonstrated naturally occurring polyreactive autoantibodies in the serum of all normal subjects *(15–17)*. Further, myeloma proteins frequently corresponded to expansion of the polyreactive autoantibodies *(18,19)*. We also demonstrated that a high frequency of precursor B-cells secrete natural autoantibodies (NAA), i.e., antibodies displaying low affinity binding of self antigens *(20,21)*. These data were confirmed, and extended through several functional and structural studies [reviewed in *(22,23)*].

We have evolved in our thinking, thus, from Ehrlich's *horror autotoxicus* notion, to Burnet's forbidden clones hypothesis, to now reach the view that autoimmunity is a normal physiological phenomenon. But how can we reconcile the experiments from Metchnikoff with those from Ehrlich and Landsteiner? Recent transgenic mice studies allow the integration of the expermental evidence. Nemazee's group has created transgenic mice expressing an Ig transgene with antibody activity against class-I antigens of the major histocompatibility complex (MHC) *(24)*. This is a very critical experiment, since the transgene recognizes a determinant of a polymorphic and true self antigen. In keeping with Burnet's prediction, the transgene was found to be deleted. However, in mice expressing autoantibody transgenes against nonpolymorphic self determinants (e.g., DNA and lysozyme), the transgenes are not deleted; they are simply down-regulated or anergized *(25,26)*. These experiments throw light on the apparent discrepancy between Ehrlich, Landsteiner, and Metchnikoff. Indeed, the rule that a subject expressing the A or B blood group antigen will never produce autoantibodies against these determinants is widely accepted. We know of no cases of autoimmune hemolytic anemias displaying autoantibodies with this specificity. On the other hand, the production of autoantibodies against public antigens, like the I blood group antigen, is a common phenomenon (public antigens are defined here as nonpolymorphic conserved antigens shared by all members of a species). Autoantibodies found in hemolytic anemia are all directed against the public antigens. So, the B-cell repertoire directed against polymorphic determinants will probably be submitted to a very stringent negative selection, i.e., a deletion process, whereas the repertoire directed against public determinants is probably not deleted, and may be an important component of the *normal* immune repertoire. Autoantibodies to the public determinants have come to be grouped under the term NAA. The NAA are characterized, thus, by their reactivity to widespread self antigens, but their affinity for the self antigens is usually low.

These results suggested that in normal serum, a substantial proportion of circulating Igs are indeed NAA, and that the cellular precursors of this autoreactive repertoire account for a substantial proportion of the available B-cells. As these autoantibodies express recurrent idiotopes, express V genes frequently in germinal configuration and predominate early in life, they are the expression of the germinal repertoire *(27–30)*. They are autoantibodies since they bind autoantigens. However, they are not self-specific, since they have never been reported to react with critical self antigens like the A and B red blood cells groups. On the contrary, these autoantibodies bind public epitopes shared by all individuals belonging to a given species, and even bind antigens that are well-conserved during evolution. Pathogenic autoantibodies observed in autoimmune diseases can also bind public epitopes. For instance, anti-red blood cell autoantibodies recognize public antigens, anti-DNA from systemic lupus erythematous (SLE) patients recognize human, rat and murine DNA, and anti-AChR autoantibodies recognize human and even fish receptors *(22)*. Pathogenic autoantibodies, unlike the NAA, usually display high affinity binding to their antigens.

One of the major characteristics of the NAA is their broad specificity, which allows them to bind both self and nonself antigens such as microbial molecules. Interestingly, the NAA repertoire is shared across phylogenetically distant species, e.g., in several species of fish and batracians *(31)*, permitting conception of NAAs in immune defenses against infections *(32)*. We know that these species are unable to mutate their antibody V genes somatically or to produce highly specific, high-affinity antibodies. Hence, their antibody repertoire is much less diverse *(32)*. When the repertoire cannot be expanded by mutational diversification, the only possible strategy is to produce the polyreactive, low-affinity antibodies. The reason why the NAA activity is conserved during evolution is probably to serve as the first-line barrier of defense. Even when an immunological memory exists to a foreign antigen, it takes five to six days to obtain high-affinity antibodies over the course of the secondary immune response. The polyreactive NAA repertoire might be the system that copes with microbial aggression during this time of weakness, i.e., the initial five to six days. It has been theorized that the polyreactive NAAs constitute partly specialized templates upon which Ag driven selection and somatic mutation operate to ultimately derive the highly specific immune antibodies *(20,22)*. This hypothesis, however, requires experimental verification.

3. NAA CLONES ARE FREQUENTLY COMMITTED TO MALIGNANT TRANSFORMATION

Evidence has accumulated indicating that the autoreactive B repertoire frequently undergoes malignant transformation, derived from the study of monoclonal immunoglobulins (MIg) in multiple myeloma, chronic lymphocytic leukemia (CLL) and follicular non-Hodgkin lymphomas (FNHL).

3.1. Antibody Activity of MIg

MIg are the structurally normal synthetic products of malignant B-cells, whose counterparts can usually be found as subpopulations present in the heterogenous normal Ig compartment. The antibody-like activity of MIg has been observed against a large number of antigens, e.g., bacterial antigens, plasma proteins, tissue antigens and nonbiological haptens *(33)*. An impressive and unexpectedly large frequency of MIg activity has been reported against certain autoantigens:

1. Blood group antigen I (cold agglutinins, [CA])
2. The Fc fragment of IgG (rheumatoid factor [RF])
3. Cytoskeleton proteins and DNA (polyreactive autoantibodies)
4. Antimyelin associated glycoproteins (MAG).

3.1.1. MIg with CA Activity

The anti-Ii cold agglutinins are an interesting exception to the diverse usage of multiple VH segments for synthesis of pathogenic human autoantibodies. Pioneering work by Williams et al. *(34)* demonstrated that these cold agglutinins shared certain recurrent idiotopes. This suggested the presence of common V region structures shared by these pathogenic autoantibodies responsible for hemolytic anemia. Recent structural studies have substantiated this conclusion by demonstrating that anti-Ii autoantibodies are invariably encoded by the VH4-21 gene segment, which is frequently associated to a VκIII gene *(35–37)*. The structural basis of the recurrent idiotope detected in the cold agglutinins by rat anti-idiotypic antibody 9G4, which inhibits the binding of the agglutinins to red blood cells, was recently elucidated by Potter et al. *(38)*. This group found that the AVY motif at positions 23–25 of the VH FR1 region constituted the reactive site of the idiotope. The structural relationship between the idiotope and the antigen binding site has yet to be clarified. The cold agglutinins are similar in gross antigenic specificity but differ in their fine antigenic specificity. According to Silberstein et al. *(36)*, the gross anti-Ii specificity is regulated by the overall VH4-21 structure, whereas the fine specificity is determined by the CDR3 regions, which differ among the different cold agglutinins. CA paraproteins are almost invariably IgMκ paraproteins, and they usually react with a set of antigenic determinants expressed by the Ii system, or with compound antigens including Ii (AI, HI, and so on). Their binding activity is increased by cold temperatures, but the range of temperatures over which they are active is variable *(39)*.

3.1.2. MIg with RF Activity

Since the first report by Kritzman et al. *(40)* of a monoclonal IgMκ parapro-tein with anti-IgG activity (RF activity), an increasing number of similar examples have been reported, and the frequency of this antigenic specificity has been estimated at more than 10% of total IgM paraproteins *(41)*. Most mono-clonal components with RF activity were found to form a cryoprecipitate. Almost all cases corresponded to IgMκ MIg, but rare cases of human monoclonal IgG and IgA with RF activity and cryoprecipitables have been described. Agnello et al. *(42)* first reported the presence of cross-reactive idiotopes (CRI) in the MIg. Sixty percent of the MIg displaying RF activity were found to share a major CRI, designated Wa; 20% belonged to a less common CRI, designated Po, and a few expressed a rare CRI, named Bla.

Considerable work emanating from the group of Dennis Carson has contrib-uted important information concerning this type of MIg, by precisely defining their genetic origin in serological and structural terms *(43)*. These studies were mainly focused on MIg sharing the Wa CRI. It was found that

1. Almost all Wa$^+$ RF share the 17109 CRI related to the light chains and the G6 idiotype related to the heavy chains
2. The RF invariably express the comparatively rare subgroup VκIIIb light chain
3. The Vκ light chain is derived from a single germinal gene (*Hum*κv325), since most Wa$^+$ paraproteins display an identical or nearly identical light chain sequence, evident from study of 13 complete light chain sequences
4. There is strong sequence homology among μ chains expressing the Wa idiotype
5. Most Wa$^+$ MIg with RF activity use the VH1 family (80%) and the minor-ity use VH2 and VH3 families. Although information derived from Po$^+$ RF MIg is less extensive, they appear to invariably use the Vκ germline gene *Hum*κv328 and a conserved VH3 sequence *(43,44)*. More recently, it has been demonstrated that the idiotype Bla was encoded by a gene of the VH4 family *(45)*.

3.1.3. MIg with Polyreactive Activity

Prompted by our results on normal human serum in the early 1980s, we screened 612 MIg for the presence of antibody activity directed against cyto-skeleton proteins and DNA. Our results indicated that approx six percent of all MIg and 10% of the IgM paraproteins bound to these antigens, and that most displayed a polyreactive pattern of binding comparable to normal human serum Ig *(18,19)*. It appears, therefore, that MIg frequently correspond to the expan-sion of a B-cell clone normally producing a NAA *(18,19)*. Dellagi et al. *(46)* reported the presence of IgM paraproteins capable of binding to intermediate fila-ments, and Shoenfeld et al. *(47)* found more than 10% MIg to shared the 16-6 CRI initially identified in a monoclonal Ig with anti-DNA activity. Only 25% of the MIg, however, were demonstrated to possess anti-DNA activity. Another anti-idiotypic reagent (F4) was present in 12% of the MIg and was strongly associated with an IgG isotype and an anti-DNA activity *(48)*. The sequences the immunoglobulin genes expressed in multiple myeloma reveal considerable information about the stage in the B-cell differentiation pathway at which the oncogenic event might have taken place. The presence of nonrandomly distributed somatic mutations and the absence of intraclonal variation in the V genes has led to the conclusion that the precursor myeloma cell could not possibly be a pre-B-cell or stem cell, but must be a mature B-cell that has been in contact with antigen and has passed through the phase of somatic hypermutation, like a memory B-cell or a plasmablast *(49)*.

3.1.4. MIg with Anti-MAG Activity

A peripheral neuropathy is observed in about 5% of Waldenström's macroglobulinemia patients *(50,51)*. In the majority of these cases, the MIg display an antibody activity against a myelin associated glycoprotein (MAG). The epitope recognized by the MIg is a glycuronyl sulfate group. A pathogenic role of the MIg, however, is not established definitively. Brouet et al. *(51)* reported a recurrent idiotype in 9 MIg with anti-MAG activity. Six of the seven MIgs subjected to further analysis belonged to the VH3 family, and one belonged to the VH2 family. Interestingly, the rare VκIV family was found in 3 MIgs, the VκI family in 2 MIgs and the VκII family in 1 MIg. The remaining MIg contained a λ light chain.

3.2. Antibody Activity of the CD5+ CLL B-Lymphocytes

One of the main difficulties in working with CLL B-lymphocytes is that these cells are highly resistant to transformation by Epstein-Barr virus (EBV). Only a few EBV cell lines have been obtained from CLL B-lymphocytes *(52)*. Given this difficulty, recent work was performed by applying the alternative of mitogenic stimulation of the CLL B-lymphocytes. The work succeeded in demonstrating autoantibody production by these cells *(53,54)*. With the aim of obtaining stable cell lines capable of producing Ig at high levels and permitting studies at the molecular level, we fused leukemic lymphocytes from 27 different CLL patients with the nonsecreting X-63 mouse myeloma. We found that 11 of 19 patients for which study of antibody activity was possible expressed autoantibody activities *(55)*. These results indicated that CD5+ B-CLL lymphocytes to be frequently committed to the production of natural autoantibodies. Further, the surprisingly high frequency of autoantibody activities in CLL-B lymphocytes favors the idea that these cells express a restricted set of V genes. Kipps et al. *(56,57)* found a high proportion of B-CLL cells to express κ chains reacting with an anti-idiotypic antibody to the rheumatoid factor idiotope Wa. Further analysis of Vκ genes expressed by the leukemic cells with the shared idiotope Wa showed that the light chains contained the unmutated *Hum*κv325 germline gene. Humphries et al. *(58)* reported that 30% of CLL patients expressed the *VH251* gene, which is one of the two germline sources of the *VH5* gene family. Logtenberg et al. *(59)* found the heavy chains expressed in CLL B-lymphocytes to belong to the VH4 family in 50% of Igs, VH5 family in 20% and VH6 family in 15%. Further evidence for restricted VH gene use consists of the observation of the germinal V1–69 gene in 20% of CLL cases *(57)*.

We studied VH family expression in 40 CD5$^+$ B-CLL, and found VH1 to be present in 17% of the Igs, VH2 in 8%, VH3 in 36%, VH4 in 17%, VH5 in 8%, and VH6 in 14% (60). The VH4, VH5 and VH6 are small families containing only a few members. These families are clearly over-represented in B-CLL. These results confirm that CD5$^+$ B-CLL lymphocytes are frequently committed to the production of natural autoantibodies. With Harry Schroeder *(61)*, we recently reviewed 75 V region sequences published to be expressed in CLL *(61–69)*. We found that the use of 27 different VH genes has been reported. However, four genes are over-represented. One is the V1–69 gene, which is the same gene found in Wa$^+$ cryoglobulins. This gene accounts for about half of the reported genes in the VH1 family, which derives from about 30 different germline genes. The VH4 family expresses from 11 different genes. In CLL, the 4–34 and the 4–39 genes are overrepresented, being expressed in 13 of the 17 VH4 family members we reviewed. Of the 20 reported B-CLL antibodies of the VH5 family, 15 are derived from the V5–51 germline gene. If the use of these germline genes was stochastic, their frequencies should be approx four percent. Their actual frequency is approx 50%, however, indicating that there is a 10-fold over-representation *(61)*. The JH family usage and the CDR3 length characteristics suggest that CLL B-cells express H chain variable domains typical of postnatal rather than the fetal lymphocytes. Our review of B-CLL also showed that some genes like V1–69 and V4–39 were in most cases expressed in a germline configuration, whereas others like V4–39 and V5–51 contained somatic mutations in most cases. It is an open question whether CLLs expressing genes in the germinal configuration represent immature B-cells and CLLs expressing genes containing somatic mutations represent a more mature population selected through an antigen-driven process. Recent work from Chiorazzi's laboratory on seven IgG-expressing CLLs indicates that the switch in use of the heavy chain is biased in favor of γ1, and that at least in some of these cases, there is evidence favoring an antigen-driven process *(62)*.

3.3. Antibody Activity of the CD5$^-$ B Lymphocyte from Follicular Non-Hodgkin Lymphomas (FNHL)

Our results on CLL patients support the hypothesis that CD5$^+$ B mostly secrete autoantibodies. In a related study on 40 murine hybridomas displaying natural autoantibody activity, however, we observed that both Ly1$^+$ and Ly1$^-$ B lymphocyte subsets were involved in the production of natural autoantibodies, as evaluated by the detection of mRNA transcripts of the Ly gene *(70)*. To gain better insight into this problem, we studied 31 hybridomas obtained in the laboratories of R.A. Miller and R. Levy from the CD5$^-$ B-cell non-Hodgkin lymphoma (NHL). Eight of the 31 hybridomas displayed rheumatoid factor activity and two of these displayed a polyreactive activity *(71)*. The results support the idea that CD5⁻ B-cells are also involved in the production of natural autoantibodies. Unlike CLL and Acute Lymphoblastic Leukemia, in which a bias in expression of VH4, VH5, and VH6 families has been demonstrated *(72)*, the CD5⁻ B-cells proliferating in NHL appear to employ VH gene families in a more stochastic way, by privileging the use of multigenic VH3 families. Further, an active somatic mutational process in B-cell follicular NHL is evident, which is rarely observed in B-CLL.

4. CONCLUSION

There is consistent evidence indicating that autoreactive B-cells constitute a substantial part of the B-cell repertoire. This autoreactive repertoire secretes natural autoantibodies, which are germline encoded, display a widespread reactivity against very well-conserved public epitopes. Their germinal origin is suggested by their early appearance during ontogeny, their expression of crossreactive idiotopes, and structural studies of their V region sequences. The natural autoantibodies may play an important physiological role as a first barrier of defense. It is presently unknown whether the polyreactive B-cell repertoire constitutes a preimmune template, which through an antigen-driven process may be involved in the production of high affinity antibodies.

It is evident from studies in monoclonal gammopathies, chronic lymphocytic leukemia and follicular lymphomas, that the autoreactive B-cell repertoire frequently undergoes malignant transformation, although there is controversy concerning the reasons for this phenomenon. It has been postulated that the continuous challenge of the autoreactive repertoire by self-antigens could create propitious conditions for the occurrence of malignant transformation. Alternatively, it can be hypothesized that overexpression of certain V genes responsible for autoreactivity reflects the normal ontogenetic events, since V gene expression is a developmentally regulated phenomenon and not all V genes are expressed during fetal life *(73–74)*. Some of the genes found to be recurrently expressed by malignant B-cells are also overexpressed in the fetal repertoires, and even in the normal adult B-cell repertoire. We do not know with certainty, therefore, the factors that impart selective advantages for malignization (i.e., the challenge by self-antigens or biased V gene expression).

REFERENCES

1. Metchnikoff, S. (1900) Etudes sur la spermotoxine. *Ann. Inst. Pasteur* **9,** 577–589.
2. Besredka, M. (1901) Les anti-hémolysines naturelles. *Ann. Inst. Pasteur* **15,** 785–807.
3. Ehrlich, P. and Morgenroth, J. (1957) *On haemolysins: Third Communication in The Collected Papers of Paul Ehrlich* vol 2. Pergamon, London, pp. 205–212.
4. Ehrlich, P. and Morgenroth, J. (1957) *On haemolysins: Fifth communication in The Collected Papers of Paul Ehrlich* vol 2. Pergamon, London, pp. 246–255.
5. Landsteiner, K. (1900) *The specificity of serological reactions.* Harvard Univ. Press, Cambridge, MA, pp. 357–371.
6. Donath, J. and Landsteiner, K. (1904) Uber paroxysmale hamoglobinurie. *Munch. Med. Wochenschr.* **51,** 1590–1595.

7. Burnet, F. M. and Fenner, F. (1949) *The production of antibodies.* Macmillan, London.
8. Owen, R. D. (1945) Immunogenetic consequences of vascular anastomoses between bovine cattle twins. *Science* **102**, 400–404.
9. Rose, N. R. and Witebsky, E. (1956) Studies on organ specificity: V changes in the thyroid glands of rabbits following acute immunization with rabbit thyroid extracts. *J. Immunol.* **76**, 417–428.
10. Martin, S. E. and Martin, W. J. (1975) Interspecies brain antigen detected by naturally occurring mouse anti-brain auto-antibody. *Proc. Natl. Acad. Sci. USA* **72**, 1036–1041.
11. Martin, W. J. and Martin, S. E. (1975) Thymus reactive IgM auto-antibodies in normal mouse sera. *Nature* **254**, 716–718.
12. Sela, B. A., Wang, J. L., and Edelman, G. M. (1975) Antibodies reactive with cell surface carbohydrates. *Proc. Natl. Acad. Sci. USA* **72**, 1127–1132.
13. MacKay, I. R. (1983) Natural autoantibodies to the fore - forbidden clones to the rear? *Immunol. Today* **4**, 340–342.
14. Izui, S., Lambert, P. H., and Founie, G. L. (1977) Features of systemic lupus erythematosus in mice infected with bacterial lipopolysaccharides. *J. Exp. Med.* **145**, 1115–1128.
15. Guilbert, B., Dighiero, G., and Avrameas, S. (1982) Naturally occurring antibodies against nine common antigens in human sera: I. Detection, isolation and characterization. *J. Immunol.* **128**, 2779–2787.
16. Lutz, H. U. and Wipf, G. (1982) Naturally occurring auto-antibodies to skeletal proteins from human red blood cells. *J. Immunol.* **128**, 1695–1701.
17. Haspel, M. V., Onodera, T., Prabhakar, B. S., McClintock, K. E., Ray, U. R., Yagihashi, S., et al. (1983) Multiple organ-reactive monoclonal autoantibodies. *Nature* **304**, 74–76.
18. Dighiero, G., Guilbert, B., and Avrameas, S. (1982) Naturally occurring antibodies against nine common antigens in human sera: II. High incidence of monoclonal Ig exhibiting antibody activity against actin and tubulin and sharing antibody specificities with natural antibodies. *J. Immunol.* **128**, 2788–2792.
19. Dighiero, G., Guilbert, B., Fermand, J. P., Lymberi, P., Danon, F., and Avrameas, S. (1983) Thirty-six human monoclonal immunoglobulins (MIg) with antibody activity against cytoskeleton proteins, thyroglobulin and native DNA, immunological studies and clinical correlations. *Blood* **62**, 264–270.
20. Dighiero, G., Lymberi, P., Mazié, J. C., Rouyre, S., Butler-Browne, G. S., Whalen, R. G., et al. (1983) Murine hybridomas secreting natural monoclonal antibodies reacting with self antigens. *J. Immunol.* **131**, 2267–2272.
21. Dighiero, G., Lymberi, P., Holmberg, D., Lundquist, I., Coutinho, A., and Avrameas, S. (1985) High frequency of natural autoantibodies in normal newborn mice. *J. Immunol.* **134**, 765–771.
22. Dighiero, G. (1995) Natural autoantibodies in humans: their relevance in auto-immunity and lymphoproliferative disorders. Forum. *Trends Exp. Clin. Med.* **5**, 58–71.
23. Casali, P. and Notkins, A. L. (1988) Probing the human B-cell repertoire with EBV. Polyreactive antibodies and CD5+ B lymphocytes. *Ann. Rev. Immunol.* **7**, 513–535.
24. Nemazee, D. and Burki, K. (1989) Clonal deletion of B lymphocytes in a transgenic mouse bearing anti-MHC class antibody genes. *Nature* **337**, 562–566.
25. Goodnow, C. C., Brink, R., and Adams, E. (1991) Breakdown of self-tolerance in anergic B lymphocytes. *Nature* **352**, 532–536.

26. Erikson, J., Radic, M. Z., Camper, S. A., Hardy, R. R., Carmack, C., and Weigert, M. (1991) Expression of anti-DNA immunoglobulin transgenes in non-autoimmune mice. *Nature* **349,** 331–335.
27. Holmberg, D., Forsgren, S., Ivars, F., and Coutinho, A. (1984) Reactions among IgM antibodies derived from normal, neonatal mice. *Eur. J. Immunol.* **14,** 435–440.
28. Lymberi, P., Dighiero, G., Ternynck, T., and Avrameas, S. (1985) A high incidence of cross-reactive idiotypes among murine natural autoantibodies. *Eur. J. Immunol.* **5,** 702–707.
29. Kearney, J. F. and Vakil, M. (1986) Idiotype directed interactions during ontogeny play a major role in the establishment of the adult B cell repertoire. *Immunol. Rev.* **94,** 39–62.
30. Baccala, R., Quang, T. V., Gilbert, M., Ternynck, T., and Avrameas, S. (1989) Two murine natural polyreactive autoantibodies are encoded by nonmutated germline genes. *Proc. Natl. Acad. Sci. USA* **86,** 4624–4628.
31. Gonzalez, R., Charlemagne, J., Mahana, W., and Avrameas, S. (1988) Specificity of natural serum antibodies present in phylogenetically distinct fish species. *Immunology* **63,** 31–36.
32. Du Pasquier, L. (1993) Evolution of the immune system, in *Fundamental Immunology,* 3rd ed. (Paul, W., ed.), Raven, New York, pp. 199–235.
33. Seligmann, M. and Brouet, J. C. (1973) Antibody activity of human myeloma globulins. *Semin. Hematol.* **10,** 163–177.
34. Williams, R. C., Kunkel, H. G., and Capra, J. D. (1968) Antigenic specificities related to the cold agglutinin activity of gamma M globulins. *Science* **161,** 379–384.
35. Pascual, V., Victor, K., Lelsz, D., Spellerberg, M. B., Hamblin, T. J., Thompson, K. M., et al. (1991) Nucleotide sequence analysis of the V region of two IgM cold agglutinins. Evidence that the VH4-21 gene segment is responsible for the major cross-reactive idiotype. *J. Immunol.* **146,** 4385–4392.
36. Silberstein, L. E., Jefferies, L. C., Goldman, J., Friedman, D., Moore, J. S., Nowell, P. C., et al. (1991) Variable region gene analysis of pathologic human autoantibodies to the related I and I red blood cell antigens. *Blood* **78,** 2372–2379.
37. Stevenson, F. K., Wrightham, M., Glennie, M. J., Jones, D. B., Cattan, A. R., Feizi, T., et al. (1986) Antibodies to shared idiotypes as agents for analysis and therapy for human B cell tumors. *Blood* **68,** 430–437.
38. Potter, K. N., Li, Y., Pascual, V., Williams, R. C., Byres, L. C., Spellerberg, M., et al. (1993) Molecular characterization of a cross-reactive idiotope on human immunoglobulins utilizing the VH4-21 gene segment. *J. Exp. Med.* **178,** 1419–1428.
39. Pruzanski, W. and Shumak, K. H. (1977) Biologic activity of cold reacting autoantibodies. *N. Engl. J. Med.* **297,** 538–542.
40. Kritzman, J., Kunkel, H. G., McCarthy, J., and Mellors, R. C. (1961) Studies of a Waldenström-type macroglobulin with rheumatoid factor properties. *J. Lab. Clin. Med.* **57,** 905–912.
41. Crowley, J. J., Goldfien, R. D., Schrohenlober, R. E., Spiegelberg, H. L., Silverman, G. J, Mageed, R. A., et al. (1988) Incidence of three cross-reactive idiotypes on human rheumatoid factor paraproteins. *J. Immunol.* **40,** 3411–3418.
42. Agnello, V., Joslin, F. G., and Kunkel, H. G. (1972) Cross idiotypic specificity among monoclonal IgM anti-gammaglobulins. *Scand. J. Immunol.* **1,** 283–292.
43. Chen, P. P., Robbins, D. L., Jirik, F. R., Kipps, T. J., and Carson, D. A. (1987) Isolation and characterization of a light chain variable region gene for human rheumatoid factors. *J. Exp. Med.* **66,** 1900–1912.

44. Silverman, G. J., GoBi, F., Fernandez, J., Chen, P. P., Frangione, B., and Carson, D. A. (1988) Distinct patterns of heavy chain variable region subgroup use by human monoclonal autoantibodies of different specificity. *J. Exp. Med.* **168**, 2361–2366.

45. Silverman, G. J., Schrohenholer, R. E., Achavitti, M. A., Koopman, W. J., and Carson, D. A. (1990) Structural characterization of the second major cross-reactive idiotype group of human rheumatoid factors: association with the VH4 gene family. *Arthritis Rheum.* **33**, 1347–1360.

46. Dellagi, K., Brouet, J. C., and Danon, F. (1979) Cross idiotypic antigens among monoclonal immunoglobulin M from patients with Waldenström's macroglobulinemia and polyneuropathy. *J. Clin. Invest.* **64**, 1530–1539.

47. Shoenfeld, Y., Amital Teplizki, H., Mendlovic, S., Blank, M., Mozes, E., and Isenberg, D. A. (1989) The role of the human anti-DNA idiotype 16/6 in autoimmunity. *Clin. Immunol. Immunopathol.* **51**, 313–325.

48. Davidson, A., Smith, A., Katz, J., Preud'homme, J. L., Salomon, A., and Diamond, B. (1989) A cross-reactive idiotype on anti-DNA antibodies define a H chain determinant present almost exclusively on IgG antibodies. *J. Immunol.* **143**, 174–180.

49. Bakkus, M. H., Van Riet, I., Van Camp, B., and Thielemans, K. (1994) Evidence that the clonogenic cell in multiple myeloma originates from a pre-switched but somatically mutated B cell. *Brit. J. Haematol.* **87**, 68–74.

50. Saito, T., Sherman, W., and Latov, N. (1983) Specificity and idiotype of M-proteins that react with MAG in patients with neuropathy. *J. Immunol.* **130**, 2496–2502.

51. Brouet, J. C., Dellagi, K., Gendron, M. C., Chevalier, A., Schmitt, C., and Mihaesco, E. (1989) Expression of a public idiotype by human monoclonal IgM directed to myelin-associated glycoprotein and characterization of the variability subgroup of their heavy and light chains. *J. Exp. Med.* **170**, 1551–1558.

52. Dighiero, G., Travade, P., Chevret, S., Fenaux, P., Chastang, C., and Binet, J. L. (1991) B-cell Chronic Lymphocytic Leukemia: present status and future directions. *Blood* **78**, 1901–1914.

53. Bröker, B. M., Klajman, A., Youinou, P., Jouquan, J., Worman, C. P., Murphy, J., et al. (1988) Chronic lymphocytic leukemic (CLL) cells secrete multispecific autoantibodies. *J. Autoimmun.* **1**, 469–481.

54. Sthoeger, Z. M., Wakai, M., Tse, D. B., Vinciguerra, V. P., Allen, S. L., Budman, D. R., et al. (1989) Production of autoantibodies by CD5-expressing B lymphocytes from patients with chronic lymphocytic leukemia. *J. Exp. Med.* **169**, 255–268.

55. Borche, L., Lim, A., Binet, J. L., and Dighiero, G. (1990) Evidence that chronic lymphocytic leukemia B lymphocytes are frequently committed to productions of natural autoantibodies. *Blood* **76**, 562–569.

56. Kipps, T. J., Tomhave, E., Chen, P. P., and Carson, D. A. (1988) Autoantibody associated K light chain variable region gene expressed in chronic lymphocytic leukemia with little or no somatic mutation, implications for etiology and immunotherapy. *J. Exp. Med.* **167**, 840–852.

57. Kipps, T. J., Tomhave, E., Pratt, L. F., Duffy, S., Chen, P. P., and Carson, D. A. (1989) Developmentally restricted immunoglobulin heavy chain variable region gene expressed at high frequency in chronic lymphocytic leukemia. *Proc. Natl. Acad. Sci. USA* **86**, 5913–5917.

58. Humphries, C. G., Shen, A., Kuziel, W. A., Capra, J. D., Blattner, F. R., and Tucker, P. W. (1988) A new human immunoglobulin VH family preferentially rearranged in immature B-cell tumors. *Nature* **331**, 446–449.

59. Logtenberg, T., Schutte, M. E. M., Inghirami, G., Berman, J. E., Gmelig-Meyling, F. H. J., Insel, R. A., et al. (1989) Immunoglobulin VH gene expression in human B-cells lines and tumors: biased VH expression in chronic lymphocytic leukemia. *Int. Immunol.* **1,** 362–370.

60. Mayer, R., Logtenberg, T., Strauchin, J., Dimitriu-Bona, A., Mayer, L., Mechanic, S., et al. (1991) CD5 and immunoglobulin V gene expression in B-cell lymphomas and Chronic Lymphocytic Leukemia. *Blood* **75,** 1518–1524.

61. Schroeder, H. W. and Dighiero, G. (1994) Clues to the pathogenesis of CLL through analysis of B-cell CLL antibody repertoires. *Immunol. Today* **15,** 288–294.

62. Hashimoto, S., Wakai, M., Silver, J., and Chiorazzi, N. (1992) Biased usage of variable and constant region Ig genes by IgG$^+$ CD5$^+$ human leukemic B cells. *Ann. NY Acad. Sci.* **651,** 477–479.

63. Ebeling, S. B., Schutte, M. E. M., Akkermans Koolhaas, E., Bloem, A. C., Gmelig-Meyling, F. H. J., and Lotenberg, T. (1992) Expression of members of the immunoglobulin VH3 gene families is not restricted at the level of individual genes in human chronic lymphocytic leukemia. *Int. Immunol.* **4,** 313–320.

64. Shen, A. C., Humprhies, P. W., Tucker. P. W., and Blattner, F. R. (1987) Human heavy-chain gene family nonrandomly rearranged in familial chronic lymphocytic leukemia. *Proc. Natl. Acad. Sci. USA* **84,** 8563–8567.

65. Cai, J., Humphries, C., Lutz, C., and Tucker, P. W. (1992) Analysis of VH 251 gene mutation in chronic lymphocytic leukemia and normal B-cell subsets. *Ann. NY Acad. Sci.* **651,** 384–392.

66. Meeker, T. C., Grimaldi, J. C., O'Rourke, R., Loeb, J., Juliusson, G., and Einhorn, S. (1988) Lack of detectable somatic hypermutation in the V region of Ig H chain gene of a human chronic B lymphocytic leukemia. *J. Immunol.* **141,** 3994–3998.

67. Rassenti, L. Z. and Kipps, T. J. (1993) Lack of extensive mutations in the VH5 genes used in common B cell chronic lymphocytic leukemia. *J. Exp. Med.* **177,** 1039–1046.

68. Deane, M. and Norton, J. D. (1990) Immunoglobulin heavy chain variable region family usage is independent of tumor cell phenotype in human B lineage leukemias. *Eur. J. Immunol.* **20,** 2209–2217.

69. Pritsch, O., Magnac, C., Dumas, G., Egile, C., and Dighiero, G. (1993) V gene usage by seven hybrids derived from CD5+ B-cell Chronic Lymphocytic Leukemia and displaying autoantibody activity. *Blood* **82,** 3103–3112.

70. Kaushik, A., Mayer, R., Fidanza, V., Zaghouani, H., Lim, A., Bona, C., et al. (1990) Ly1 and V-gene expression among hybridomas secreting natural autoantibody. *J. Autoimmun.* **3,** 687–700.

71. Dighiero, G., Hart, S., Lim, A., Borche, L., Levy, R., and Miller, R. A. (1991) Autoantibody activity of immunoglobulins isolated from B-cell follicular lymphomas. *Blood* **78,** 581–586.

72. Cleary, M. L., Meeker, T. C., Levy, S., Lee, E., Trela, M., Sklar, J., et al. (1986) Clustering of extensive somatic mutations in the variable region of an immunoglobulin heavy chain gene from a human B cell lymphoma. *Cell* **44,** 97–105.

73. Schroeder, H. W., Hillson, J. L., and Perlmutter, R. M. (1987) Early restriction of the human antibody repertoire. *Science* **238,** 791–793.

74. Schroeder, H. W. and Wang, J. Y. (1990) Preferential utilization of conserved immunoglobulin heavy chain variable gene segments during human fetal life. *Proc. Natl. Acad. Sci. USA* **87,** 6146–6150.

4

Pathogenesis of Autoimmune Thyroid Disease

Ramzi A. Ajjan and Anthony P. Weetman

1. INTRODUCTION

Autoimmune thyroid disease (ATD), the archetypal example of organ-specific autoimmune disease, comprises several disorders which as a group constitute the commonest clinically relevant autoimmune disease, affecting up to one percent of the population (1). Both hypothyroidism and hyperthyroidism are consequences of thyroid autoimmunity.

1.1. Clinical Disorders

Autoimmune hypothyroidism is a common disease affecting one percent of women but no more than 0.1% of men (1). It is generally divided into a goitrous form (Hashimoto's thyroiditis-HT), affecting middle aged women predominantly, and a nongoitrous form (primary myxedema-PM) affecting the elderly more commonly. Pathologically, HT is characterized by a dense accumulation of lymphocytes, plasma cells and macrophages with the formation of germinal centers. The thyroid follicles are small, containing some macrophages, plasma cells and occasional multinucleated giant cells. The epithelial cells are enlarged with a distinctive eosinophilic cytoplasm owing to increased number of mitochondria (Hürthle or Askanazy cells). A variable amount of fibrosis can be identified. The PM variant shows extensive replacement by fibrous tissue and atrophy of the gland, with much less inflammatory infiltrate.

Hyperthyroidism affects nearly two percent of women, and 0.2% of men (1). Approximately 80% of hyperthyroid patients have Graves' disease (GD), characterised by the presence of thyroid stimulating antibodies (TSAb), which activate the thyroid stimulating hormone receptor (TSH-R), resulting in hyperthyroidism. Lymphoid infiltration in the interfollicular stroma, sometimes with germinal center formation, is often seen in GD. The follicles show marked epithelial cell hyperplasia, whereas fibrosis is unusual (2).

An autoimmune-mediated transient thyroid dysfunction may occur after childbirth, termed postpartum thyroiditis. The population prevalence is five percent in the 12 months following delivery, although this figure includes many patients diagnosed during surveys of biochemical changes postpartum; clinically

Contemporary Immunology: Autoimmune Reactions
Edited by: S. Paul © Humana Press Inc., Totowa, NJ

apparent disease is much less common. The pathology resembles that of HT or PM. Postpartum thyroiditis starts usually with a thyrotoxic phase at two to three months postpartum, followed by a hypothyroid phase at five to six months. The thyrotoxic or hypothyroid phase can occur alone. After a euthyroid interval, up to a quarter of patients become hypothyroid three to four years after the onset of postpartum thyroiditis *(3)*.

Thyroid-associated ophthalmopathy (TAO) and pretibial myxedema (PTM) are almost always associated with some evidence of thyroid autoimmunity *(4)*. At present it seems most likely that this association is a consequence of auto-antigenic cross reactivity in the target tissues, although the target autoantigen is unclear *(5)*.

1.2. Thyroid Autoantigens

There are three major autoantigens in ATD: the TSH-R, thyroid peroxidase (TPO) and thyroglobulin (TG). In addition, recent evidence indicates that the sodium/iodide symporter is a potential autoantigen.

TSH-R, which forms the binding site for TSH, is a member of the G-protein-coupled receptor family. It is composed of three extracellular loops containing the amino terminus, seven transmembrane segments and three intracellular loops ending with a carboxyl terminus. Stimulation of the receptor by TSH causes generation of cAMP, stimulating both growth and function of thyroid follicular cells (TFC). High concentrations of TSH can also stimulate the phosphatidyl inositol (PI) cascade, but this pathway seems to have only a minor role in signal transduction in the thyroid *(6)*. Human TSH-R is encoded by 10 exons situated on chromosome 14. The extracellular domain of 398 amino acids is encoded by nine exons, whereas exon 10 encodes for both the transmembrane and the intracellular domains of 266 and 83 amino acids respectively *(7,8)*. TSH-R mRNA variants have been identified, but seem to have little physiological significance, apart from mutations responsible for the development of some toxic adenomas *(9)*. TSAb acting on the TSH-R are the hallmark of GD, whereas the role of TSH-R blocking antibodies in the pathogenesis of autoimmune hypothyroidism is less pronounced.

TPO, previously known as the microsomal antigen, is the primary enzyme involved in iodination of tyrosine residues, and in their coupling to form thyroid hormones *(10)*. In human, TPO is a membrane-associated protein of 933 amino acids with five potential glycosylation sites, and is encoded by a single gene on chromosome 2, spanning 17 exons. TPO gene mutations, leading to both qualitative and quantitative abnormalities in enzyme activity, are rare causes of thyroid dysfunction *(11)*.

TG serves as the precursor and storage form of thyroid hormones, and is the major intrathyroidal store of organified iodide. It consists of two monomers of 2750 amino acids extensively disulfide-linked to form a globular homodimer. TG is primarily secreted into the thyroid follicles, although small amounts gain access to the circulation. Several hormonogenic sites (tyrosine acceptors) are present on each subunit and seem to have a role in TG antigenicity *(12)*. Although some studies have suggested abnormal TG structure in patients with ATD, others failed to confirm these findings *(13,14)*. Antibodies to TPO and TG, detected in all types of ATD, are thought to contribute to the inflammatory process through several mechanisms detailed in Subheadings 3.1. and 4.1.

A second colloid antigen (besides TG) was first described in 1961 *(15)*, and antibodies against this molecule have continued to be identified in patients with ATD *(16)*, but their role in disease pathogenesis remains unknown. Additionally, ATRA-1 *(17)*, heat shock protein *(18)*, and 64 kDa antigens *(19)* have all been suggested to play a role in ATD. Most recently, attention has focused on the sodium/iodide symporter (NIS) as a potential autoantigen with the demonstration of the inhibition of thyroidal ^{125}I uptake by (albeit rare) serum autoantibodies *(16)*. Moreover, autoantibodies binding to the symporter have been detected in 85% of GD and 15% of HT patients by immunoblotting *(20)*. The latter study employed recombinant rat NIS to screen patient sera, and these results remain to be confirmed using the human counterpart.

2. PREDISPOSING FACTORS

An interaction of genetics and environment, in addition to endogenous factors such as age and sex, predisposes to ATD.

2.1. Immunogenetics

As with most autoimmune diseases, HLA alleles have been studied extensively in ATD (Table 1; 21–40), and an association of HLA-DR3 with GD and autoimmune hypothyroidism has been recognised in most Caucasian studies. Recently, studies on Caucasian populations have described HLA-DQA1*0501 as an important risk factor in GD, over and above that of HLA-DR3 *(23,27)*. In addition to DR3, autoimmune hypothyroidism and postpartum thyroiditis may be associated with HLA-DR4 and -DR5, while negative associations (HLA-DQ), offering protection from the disease, have also been reported *(29)*. However, variability has been identified between different ethnic groups, and in all cases, these associations have been rather weak with inconsistent linkage results, suggesting that HLA genes play only a minor role in the susceptibility to ATD *(41,42)*.

Non-HLA loci have also been studied, including polymorphisms of immunoglobulin and T-cell receptor (TCR) genes, but have given conflicting and inconsistent results *(40)*. A TSH-R codon 52 polymorphism has been shown to confer an increased risk for GD, especially when associated with HLA-DR3, suggesting a synergism between these two alleles *(28)*. However, the latter association was documented in only six GD patients, and therefore, a larger study is warranted. An autosomal dominant trait for thyroid autoantibody production has been proposed, but was subsequently refuted using more refined assays *(43)*.

A NcoI restriction fragment length polymorphism in the tumor necrosis factor-β (TNFβ) gene resulting from nucleotide substitution in the TNFB1*

Table 1
Summary of HLA Association Studies Based
on Molecular Methods in Autoimmune Thyroid Disease

Study	Population	DR	DQB1	DDQA1	DR
1. Graves' disease					
Susceptibility					
Mangklabruks et al. *(21)*	Caucasians				DR3
Chen et al. *(22)*	Caucasians				DRB3*0101
Yanagawa et al. *(23)*	Caucasians		0301(M)	501	DR3(F)
Ratanachaiyavong et al. *(24)*	Caucasians	B1*0402			
Onuma et al. *(25)*[a]	Japanese	B1*0501			
Badenhoop et al. *(26)*	Caucasians			0501 Arg. 52 positive	
Barlow et al. *(27)*	Caucasians			0501	
Cuddihy et al. *(28)*	Caucasians			None with 501	DR3 None with DRB3*0101
Protection					
Yanagawa et al. *(23)*	Caucasians			0201	DR7
Badenhoop et al. *(26)*	Caucasians		0602		
Tamai et al. *(29)*	Japanese		0501		
Cavan et al. *(30)*	Chinese		0301	0401	DR12
2. Hashimoto's thyroiditis					
Susceptibility					
Badenhoop et al. *(31)*	Caucasians	None	0301(DQw7)		
Tandon et al. *(32)*	Caucasians	None	0201(DQw2)		DR3
Shi et al. *(33)*	Caucasians		0201	0301	
Wu et al. *(34)*	Caucasians	None	0301	0301/2	
Santamaria et al. *(35)*	Caucasians		0201		
Badenhoop et al. *(26)*	Caucasians		0301	0301, 0501 Arg. 52 positive	
Protection					
Tamai et al. *(29)*	Japanese		0602	0102	
Santamaria et al. *(35)*	Caucasians		0302		
3. Primary myxedema					
Susceptibility					
Bogner et al. *(36)*	Caucasians			0301	
Badenhoop et al. *(26)*	Caucasians			0301 Arg. 52 positive	
Cho et al. (37)	Koreans		0302		
4. Postpartum thyroiditis					
Susceptibility					
Parkes et al. *(38)*	Caucasians				DR3, DR5
Protection					
Parkes et al. *(38)*	Caucasians		DQ6		DR2
5. Autoimmune hypothyroidism associated with Down's syndrome					
Susceptibility					
Nicholson et al. *(39)*	Caucasians			0301	

[a] Early onset.

allele was associated with GD in Caucasian patients and was still evident after excluding DR3 positive patients, despite linkage disequilibrium between the TNFB*1 allele and DR3 haplotype *(44)*. However, this association was not confirmed in Chinese GD patients *(45)*. The interleukin-1 receptor antagonist (IL-1ra) is related to IL-1α and IL-1β, and competes with these molecules for occupancy of the common cell surface receptor but does not deliver a stimulus for signal transduction, thus acting as a competitive inhibitor of IL-1 action *(46)*. The IL1RN*2 allele is associated with a number of autoimmune and inflammatory diseases, as either a risk factor or as a marker of disease severity *(47)*. In a case control study of ATD, IL-1RN*2 was found to be associated with GD but not HT *(48)*. Given the role of IL-1RN*2 as a severity factor, the allele distribution was also analysed with respect to TAO but no additional association was found. The cytokine and cytokine receptor gene polymorphisms represent an interesting group of potential susceptibility and modifying factors in autoimmune and inflammatory disease, study of which may offer new therapeutic approaches in the future.

Finally, CTLA-4 is a T-cell surface molecule that binds the B7 family of receptors, thereby regulating T-cell activation. An association between a polymorphism of the CTLA-4 gene (allele106) and both GD and HT in Caucasian patients has been shown *(49,50)*.

These results indicate the complexity of the immunogenetics in ATD, with several condidate loci being identified but, so far, without compelling evidence of linkage based on family studies. The development of automated DNA screening now allows the analysis of a huge number of polymorphisms scattered throughout the human genome, thus enabling determination of susceptibility loci *(51)*. Application of this methodology should improve our understanding of the genetic basis of ATD.

2.2. Environmental Factors

2.2.1. Infection

Age plays an important role in susceptibility by increasing the exposure to environmental agents, in addition to the changes in the immunoregulation associated with ageing *(52)*. The implication of infectious agents in the etiology of autoimmune diseases has always been an attractive concept, and there are accumulating data suggesting that viruses and bacteria may play a role in GD and, to a lesser extent, in HT *(53)*. Several mechanisms have been suggested by which infectious agents can trigger ATD. The possible incorporation of viruses into the human genome renders the virus a source of persistent endogenous antigen. Molecular mimicry between infectious organisms and host cells can also play a role, while the production of superantigens by invading microorganisms and the induction of heat shock protein (HSP) synthesis may exert important immunomodulatory effects. Finally, viral infections can induce interferon-γ (IFNγ) production, which in turn induces HLA class II expression in non-immune cells (e.g., TFC), discussed in Subheading 3.3.

Yersinia enterocolitica was one of the first agent to be implicated in the etiology of GD. Patients with *Y. enterocolitica* infections have antibodies to thyroid epithelium *(54)*, and a large proportion of GD patients have antibodies to *Yersinia* antigens, proposed to be owing to TSH-R crossreactivity *(55)*. Furthermore, lymphocytic thyroiditis can be induced in rats by immunization with *Y. enterocolitica* outer membrane protein *(56)*. However, most patients with *Yersinia* infection do not develop GD and the role of this organism in the pathogenesis of ATD is still controversial.

Multiple viruses have also been implicated in the initiation of thyroid immunity, including measles, influenza, adenovirus, Epstein-Barr, coxsackie and, most importantly, retroviruses. Retroviral sequences have been detected in both the thyroid and peripheral blood mononuclear cells of patients with GD *(57,58)*. Furthermore, thyroid biopsies from GD patients showed reactivity to human foamy virus antibodies in another study *(59)*. As an area of 66% homology (across a 166bp region) has been identified between HIV-1 and TSH-R, it is tempting to speculate that GD can be induced in susceptible individuals as a result of molecular mimicry. However, such virus-like particles have been also detected in normal thyroids and other tissues, and therefore their importance in the development of ATD is currently unknown. Recently, a role for environmental allergens has been suggested after the induction of GD by an attack of allergic rhinitis *(60)*.

2.2.2. Iodide

Epidemiological data point to iodide as an important factor in enhancing thyroid autoimmunity *(61)*. Iodine supplementation has been shown both to increase the incidence of ATD and to exacerbate preexisting thyroiditis *(62,63)*. The involvement of iodine in ATD has been further emphasised by showing that a high iodine diet exacerbates thyroiditis in animal models of ATD, whereas a low iodine diet results in amelioration of the disease *(64,65)*. The mechanism of these effects is unclear, but high concentrations of iodide are directly toxic to TFC *(66)*, which could lead to release of autoantigens. In addition, iodide could form highly toxic species with oxygen metabolites that could precipitate autoimmunity in a genetically predisposed individual.

2.2.3. Toxins

Exposure to radiation predisposes to thyroid autoimmunity *(67)*, and lithium exacerbates autoimmune thyroiditis *(68)*, both probably acting on T-cell regulation. Treatment with amiodarone can result in thyroid dysfunction, particularly in the presence of pre-existing thyroid abnormalities. Thyroid dysfunction is mainly a result of metabolic abnormalities, arising from a disturbance of iodide organification, or secondary to the high iodine load. However, direct toxic effects of the drug on TFC have been repeatedly shown, but without clear evidence of autoimmune involvement *(69–71)*. Therapeutic doses of cytokines, particularly IL-2 and IFNα, may initiate ATD in susceptible individuals, by mechnisms that presumably involve altered immunoregulation *(72,73)*.

2.2.4. Stress

Stress in the form of adverse life events has also been suggested as an important factor in the development of ATD *(74)*. The implication of stress in ATD must be interpreted carefully, because unfavorable life events could be a consequence rather than a cause of the disease, but Sonino et al. *(75)* have shown that such events precede the onset of GD and disease-independent life events are more frequent (albeit only slightly) than disease-dependent life events in patients *(76)*. Stress causes stimulation of the hypothalamic-pituitary-adrenal axis and the sympathetic autonomic nervous system, and this type of neuroendocrine disturbance has been suggested to alter the immune responses that predispose to autoimmunity.

2.3. Endogenous Factors

Sex hormones are highly likely to be involved in the etiology of ATD, as this primarily affects women and pregnancy ameliorates the disease, with subsequent exacerbation of thyroiditis (or even *de novo* appearance of disease) in the postpartum period *(3)*. Moreover, estrogens can be shown to exacerbate experimental autoimmune thyroiditis whereas testosterone ameliorates it *(77)*. In addition to sex hormones, prolactin may play a role, as autoimmune thyroiditis is more common in women with hyperprolactinemia *(78)*.

3. PATHOGENIC MECHANISMS IN AUTOIMMUNE HYPOTHYROIDISM

3.1. Humoral Immunity

Most patients with autoimmune hypothyroidism have serum antibodies (Ab) to TG and TPO, and occasionally to TSH-R. Although TGAb are found mainly in patients with ATD, they are also commonly detected in normal individuals, especially in the elderly or following viral infections *(1,52)*. However, the titers and affinities of TGAb are higher in the ATD group compared to the TGAb positive group without ATD, and they are mainly of the IgG class rather than IgM *(77)*. Subclass restriction of TGAb is suggested by the predominance of IgG_1 and IgG_4, although all four subclasses are typically present, with IgG_2 showing the highest functional activity *(79)*. TGAb are restricted to two major and one minor epitope on each subunit, but this restriction is only relative; many more epitopes are recognised by the TGAb as titers rise. There is no light chain restriction and a wide range of variable (V) region gene families is used by both heavy and light chains *(80)*. However, a recent study has shown highly restricted heavy chain usage, with only a moderate restriction of light chain usage *(81)*.

The detection of TGAb in apparently normal individuals, together with the inability of TGAb to fix complement (probably due to wide separation of epitopes on the TG molecule, thus preventing IgG cross-linking) casts some doubt on their importance in ATD. However, TGAb can mediate antibody-dependent cell-mediated cytotoxicity (ADCC) in vitro *(82)*, and additionally a catalytical role for TGAb has been recently described *(83)*. It appears that TGAb-positivity alone is not sufficient to cause thyroid dysfunction, but a role for TGAb in the perpetuation of the disease cannot be ruled out.

TPOAb are also detected in a small percentage of clinically normal individuals. As with TGAb, IgG_1, and IgG_4 subclasses predominate in TPOAb *(79)*, and although a clear restriction in light chains is not evident, a predominance of κ light chain usage has been observed in the majority of patients. TPOAb are able to mediate ADCC, and unlike TGAb, they can also fix complement *(84,85)*. ADCC is mediated by the interaction of NK cells with the *Fc* portion of the TPOAb that are in turn attached to TFC. Despite initial suggestions of more ADCC activity in PM compared to HT *(82)*, a recent study was unable to find differences in ADCC activity between sera from patients with HT, PM, and GD *(86)*. Terminal complement complexes (TCC), the fluid phase products released after formation of membrane attack complexes (MAC), surround the thyroid follicles in ATD, and their levels are elevated in patient sera, suggesting a major role for complement-mediated cell damage in ATD. The ability of TPOAb to cause enzymatic inhibition in vitro indicates a potential direct mechanism for these antibodies in disease pathogenesis, but this remains controversial *(87)*. TPOAb from GD and HT patients exhibit similarity in sequences and reactivities to native TPO, indicating a similar Ab response in both types of ATD. Bispecific Abs interacting with both TG and TPO have been termed TGPOAb. These Abs are present in sera with high TGAb and TPOAb titers, and they are more frequently detected in patients with HT than in patients with other ATD *(88)*. Their role in the pathogenesis remains to be resolved.

Several types of Ab to TSH-R have been identified. TSAb are dominant in patients with GD, whereas thyroid blocking antibodies (TBAb) are mainly found in patients with HT or PM. A minority of patients with autoimmune hypothyroidism and patients with GD have reactivity to TSAb and TBAb, respectively. Assays for TSH binding inhibiting immunoglobulins (TBII) detect the broad range of TSH-R antibodies and TBII present in all of the above diseases, but the levels of the TBII do not correlate with TSAb or TBAb activities; the latter two activities can only be determined by bioassay. The existence of TBAb was first demonstrated by the development of transient neonatal hypo-thyroidism secondary to transplacental transfer of these antibodies *(89)*. Subsequent studies have shown the association of TBAb with PM in Japanese and Korean patients, and, at a lower frequency, with both PM and HT in Caucasians *(40)*. The discrepancy in the results between the Oriental and the Caucasian groups could be related to immunogenetic differences, or to different sensitivities of the assays used. It is worth noting that GD can develop in patients with hypothyroidism (and vice versa), and this appears to be related to the balance between TBAb and TSAb. The existence of autoantibodies that increase or inhibit TFC growth independently of the TSH-R remains debatable *(90–92)*.

Several difficulties have been encountered in the study of TSH-R antibodies. TSAb, sometimes associated with an increase in thyroid hormone levels, have been produced by immunising different mammalian species with TSH peptides, but a satisfactory animal model of GD remains to be established *(93,94)*. Rather than using primary cell cultures or cell lines as a source of autoantigen, prokaryotic and eukaryotic expression systems for TSH-R have been developed, but none of them is ideal for the assay of antibodies. TSH-R expressed in *E. coli* does not bind TSH *(95)*. The TSH-R extracellular domain expressed in baculovirus remains intracellular and must be purified from cell homogenates, and again, does not bind TSH, although it binds to serum antibodies from patients with GD *(96)*. In addition, TSH-R expressed in the various systems has often shown inconsistent or insufficient binding of autoantibodies, which has recently been attributed to the important relationship between autoantibody recognition and TSH-R maturation associated with glycosylation *(97)*. Developing methods to produce the native, functional TSH-R in quantity is critical to elucidating the exact properties of autoantibodies against the receptor in ATD.

3.2. Cellular Immunity

T-cells play a critical role in the development of ATD. These cells migrate from the periphery to the thyroid gland where they interact with TFC and extracellular matrix. Many studies have found a reduction in the proportion of circulating CD8+ T cells in ATD, leading to the concept that a T-suppressor cell defect as a key factor in the development of ATD *(98)*, although this has not gone unchallenged *(99)*. Defects in the putative T-suppressor cell response to TPO and TG (but not to irrelevant antigens) have been demonstrated in both autoimmune hypothyroidism and GD, but the results have not been consistently confirmed by others *(100)*.

Restricted usage of TCR by intrathyroidal T-cells has been the focus of several recent studies. If T-cell autoreactivity is clonally limited, this would permit the application of novel therapeutic approaches, such as the targeted inactivation of selected subpopulations of T-cells. Davies et al. *(101)* have reported a marked restriction in variable (V) α gene usage (encoding the α chain of TCR) by intrathyroidal T-cells in ATD. Others have failed to confirm these findings, even by analysing the IL-2 receptor positive T-cells *(102,103)*. Using cell fractionation studies, Vα restriction in the intrathyroidal CD8+ T-cells from three HT patients has been observed, suggesting a role for clonally restricted T-cell-mediated cytotoxicity in HT *(104)*.

T-cells may destroy TFC in HT and PM by direct cytotoxicity, or indirectly via cytokine secretion. The presence of perforin in HT-derived CD8+ T-cells indicates that these cells are activated *in situ (105)*. Furthermore, CD8+ cytotoxic T-cell clones, capable of killing autologous TFC in an HLA class I-restricted fashion, have been raised from different HT patients. However, T-cell stimulation in culture by IL-2 favors the expansion of the nonspecific NK cells, rendering the study of thyroid-specific CD8+ cells difficult and often inconclusive *(106–108)*.

Several groups have demonstrated the ability of infiltrating T-cells in HT to produce cytokines both in vitro and in vivo. These molecules modulate TFC growth and function, and alter the immunological properties of TFC, including the induction of HLA class II and adhesion molecule expression *(109)*. In vitro studies have shown that HT-derived T-cells have a high potential for TNFα and IFNγ production *(110–112)*. On the other hand, IL-4 levels produced by T-cell clones derived from ATD tissue are low *(113)*, suggesting a Th1 pattern of cytokine production in HT, which may be capable of mediating delayed-type hypersensitivity and cytotoxicity. Studies in experimental autoimmune thyroiditis (EAT) have further shown a Th1-like pattern of cytokine production by both CD4+ and CD8+ TFC- reactive T-cell clones *(114,115)*. Others have found that HT-derived CD4+ T-clones produce a mixed Th1/Th2 cytokine pattern, suggesting that the T-cells from ATD cannot be classified simply into two distinct subsets *(116)*.

The reverse transcription-polymerase chain reaction (RT-PCR) technique has demonstrated the in vivo expression of IL-1, IL-2, IL-4, IL-6, IL-8, IL-10, IFNγ, and TNFα in HT tissue samples, in keeping with a mixed Th1/Th2 response *(117,118)*. However, a quantitative RT-PCR study has shown the predominance of a Th1 response *(119)*. By the application of cell fractionation techniques to HT-derived lymphocytes, mRNA for all the above cytokines has been detected in infiltrating CD4+ and CD8+ T-cells, except for IL-1, which seems to be produced by cells other than lymphocytes, most probably macrophages *(118)*. When interpreting the results of such studies, it is worth bearing in mind that even a short period in culture may radically alter the cellular properties, and hence, cytokine production, whereas in cell fractionation analysis, complete resolution of the different populations is difficult and contamination of an apparently purified population with only a few cells highly expressing a particular cytokine can lead to artefacts.

Peripheral and intrathyroidal T-cell responses to thyroid antigens has been studied in vitro, and epitope mapping have been carried out using a series of overlapping peptides. As TG generates only a weak proliferative response in HT-derived T-cells, attention has focused on TPO and TSH-R. The latter molecule is considered in detail in the section on GD below. In general, T-cell proliferation to TPO epitopes was found to be heterogeneous both within and between patients *(120–123)*. Furthermore, no clear differences between the HT and GD groups could be demonstrated in T-cell responses, which is probably owing to "determinant spreading," whereby diversification of the immune response to antigenic epitopes occurs as disease progresses *(124)*. These observations make it unlikely that therapeutic intervention with modified TPO peptides is an option in ATD.

3.3. The Role of TFC

In normal thyroid tissue, TFC express low concentrations of HLA class I and no HLA class II molecules. In contrast, ATD-derived TFC show increased expression of HLA class I and II, which is regulated by cytokines, most importantly IFNγ. Expression of class I and II molecules, possibly after a viral infection, has been suggested as one mechanism for the induction of ATD *(12,125)*. In particular, hyperinducibility of class II on TFC from GD patients *(126)* suggests a role for these cells in antigen presentation. Recent evidence indicates that class II expression may in some circumstances be protective through the induction of peripheral tolerance, as TFC fail to express costimulatory signals (B7-1 and B7-2) necessary for naive T-cell activation (through CD28 and CTLA-4), and thus class II expression by TFC may result in anergy *(127)*. However, there is a possible role for TFC in perpetuation of the disease, after autoimmunity is firmly established and B7-dependence is no longer important for continued T-cell responses.

Adhesion between T-cells and their targets is a fundamental component of any immune response. Therefore, TFC expression of adhesion molecules, including intercellular adhesion molecule-1 (ICAM-1), Hermes-1, lymphocyte function-associated molecule-3 (LFA-3) and neural cell adhesion molecule (NCAM) *(128–131)*, may play a central role in ATD through leukocyte activation and localization to the inflammatory sites. Cytokine-mediated modulation of such adhesion molecule expression in the thyroid could be crucial to the perpetuation, if not initiation, of the inflammatory process.

TFC express different cytokines (IL-1, IL-6, IL-8, IL-12, IL-13, IL-15, TGFβ1, and TNF), and this expression is in turn upregulated by IL-1, TNF, IFNγ, and sublethal complement attack *(132–136)*. Therefore, cytokines released by the lymphocytic infiltrate may stimulate TFC to produce more cytokines, which in turn might increase the size and activity of the infiltrate, creating a vicious cycle that augments the inflammatory reaction (Fig. 1).

In addition to the above proinflammatory effects, TFC have protective mechanisms against immune damage. The expression of complement activation regulators by TFC render the cells resistant to complement-mediated cell lysis. These protective proteins comprise MAC-inhibitory protein/homologous restriction factor (MIP/HRF), CD46, CD55 and most importantly CD59. The expression of these proteins is regulated by cytokines *(137,138)*. On the other hand, sublethal complement attack impairs TFC function, and induces the release of proinflammatory molecules, including reactive oxygen metabolites, prostaglandins, IL-1 and IL-6 *(139)*. HLA class II induction on TFC by IFNγ is an another possible protective mechanism as discussed above. Other protective effects of cytokines include TFC resistance to cell-mediated cytotoxicity after IFNγ and TNF treatment in vitro *(140–141)*, and the inhibition of T-cell proliferation after TGFβ1 treatment in culture *(142)*. Figure 2 shows the potential effector mechanisms operating in TFC in ATD, and Fig. 3, the possible protective mechanisms.

4. PATHOGENIC MECHANISMS IN GD

4.1. Humoral Immunity

It is now accepted that TSH and TSH-RAb interact mainly with the extracellular domain of the receptor *(143)*, but the existence of antibody-reactive epitopes on the extracellular surface of the transmembrane domain cannot be ruled out. Substitution studies have shown that epitopes for TSAb and TBII in

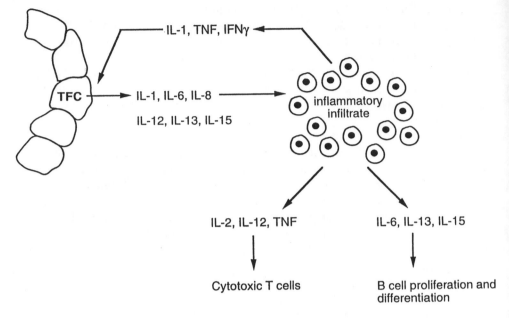

Fig. 1. The cytokine cascade in autoimmune thyroid disease. TFC, thyroid follicular cells; IFN, interferon; TNF, tumor necrosis factor.

GD are primarily located in the N-terminal region of the extracellular domain, whereas TBAb and high affinity TSH binding sites are found in the C-terminal portion of TSH-R *(12)*. Mutagenesis studies suggest that residues 30–61 are important for both TSAb and GD TBII activities, whereas residues 90–110 are only critical for TSAb binding. Furthermore, peptide studies implicate residues 90–110 as important epitopes for TSAb binding. In keeping with these results, immunization of animals with peptides from the N-terminal site can induce TSAb (but not TBAb) formation *(144,145)*, and immunization with peptides in the C-terminus can induce the synthesis of TBAb (but not TSAb) *(146,147)*. TSH-R Abs are often light chain restricted and predominantly of the IgG1 subclass *(148,149)*, suggesting an oligoclonal B-cell origin for these antibodies. On the other hand, TSAb activity (detected based on cAMP and phosphatidyl inositol production) is variable from one patient to another, with antibodies activating both signal transduction pathways found in patients with the most severe disease, implying a heterogeneity in the composition of TSAb *(150)*.

Residues 303–382 comprise the immunodominant portion of TSH-R, which is flanked by residues important for TSH and TBAb activity. More than 80% of the antibodies generated by immunization of rabbits with the extracellular domain of TSH-R react with peptides 352–366 and 357–372 *(151)*. Moreover, peptide 352–366 reacts with IgG preparations from around 80% of GD patients *(151,152)*. The immunodominant peptide does not seem to have an intrinsic

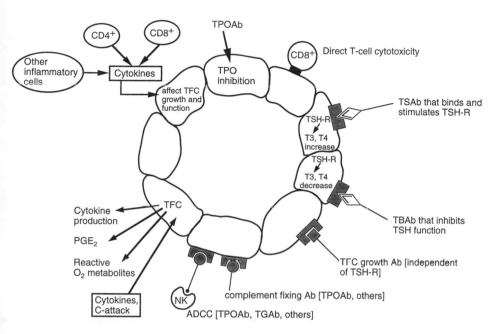

Fig. 2. Possible effector mechanisms in autoimmune thyroid disease. ADCC, antibody dependent cell mediated cytotoxicity; C, complement; NK, natural killer cells; PG, prostaglandin; TBAb, thyroid blocking antibodies; TFC, thyroid follicular cells; TPO, thyroid peroxidase; TG, thyroglobulin; TSAb, thyroid stimulating antibodies.

biological function but is important for the formation of both TSAb and TBAb. The ability of residues 352–377 to adsorb TSAb activity, together with the inhibition of this activity by peptides located between residues 30 and 90, indicates that TSAb can interact with the N-terminal region of the receptor, presumably because the N terminus is in close proximity to the immunodominant peptide *(152-155)*.

Although such studies have advanced our understanding of TSH-R interactions, we should be cautious in their interpretation. The majority of TSH-R B cell epitopes appear to be conformational, rendering the results of the peptide studies questionable *(156)*. In addition, chimeric substitution studies in a particular region of TSH-R may induce overall conformational changes in the remaining receptor molecule, making it possible to obtain false negative results in antibody binding assays.

4.2. Cellular Immunity

A TSH-R-specific defect in T-suppressor cells has been proposed in GD, but not HT *(98)*, yet clear evidence is so far lacking and the exact mechanism of suppression is poorly defined. As in HT, TCR restriction has been investi-

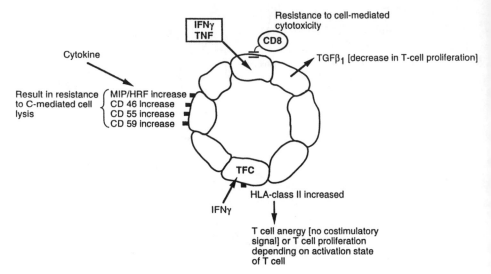

Fig. 3. Possible protective mechanisms in autoimmune thyroid disease. C, complement; IFN, interferon; MIP/HRF, MAC-inhibitory protein/homologous restriction factor; TFC, thyroid follicular cells; TGF, transforming growth factor; TNF, tumor necrosis factor.

gated in GD with contradictory results *(101–103)*. A recent study has shown similarities in the intrathyroidal, pretibial and retroocular Vα and Vβ TCR repertoire in two patients, which were restricted to 7–8 families, indicating recognition of similar antigenic determinants in the different sites of GD complications, but there was a heterogeneity in TCR usage between the two patients *(157)*. Thyroid-infiltrating CD8$^+$ cells in GD do not seem to have a role in cell-mediated cytotoxicity as they fail to express perforin, whereas GD-derived αβ$^+$, CD4$^-$ CD8$^-$ T-cells do contain perforin. In addition, TFC-reactive cytotoxic γδ$^+$ T-cells have been grown from the GD infiltrate, which are not HLA restricted and preferentially express IL-4, indicating a Th2-like phenotype *(158)*. The importance of these cells to pathogenesis is unclear.

Earlier studies suggested that GD-derived CD4$^+$ T-clones produce a mixed Th1/Th2 cytokine pattern *(116)*. Using EBV-transformed B-cell lines transfected with TPO or TSH-R as the antigen presenting cells, it has been recently demonstrated that GD-derived TPO-specific T-cell clones have Th1 characteristics, whereas the Th2 cells predominate in TSH-R-specific T-cell clones *(159–160)*. However, IL-4 mRNA is often not detected in GD thyroid tissue samples in vivo, and no distinct Th1 or Th2 response can be identified *(117,161)*. This discrepancy could reflect the influence of antithyroid drug treatment on the cytokine profiles, or it may be due to the culture conditions used for T-cell growth, which might favor the expansion of Th2 cells. A third possibility is the mediation of the Th2 response in vivo by another cytokine such as IL-13. Indeed we have shown IL-13 expression by the majority of GD thyroid tissue samples *(136)*. On balance, the predominance of a Th2 response in GD is likely, as the local formation of TSAb is important in the pathogenesis of the disease.

Using recombinant techniques, T-cell responses in GD to full length TSH-R extracellular domain have also been reported, but the positive reactivity was also evident in patients with focal thyroiditis (albeit at lower levels) *(162)*. To define T-cell epitopes on TSH-R, the peripheral, and intrathyroidal T-cell responses to a series of overlapping peptides covering the entire extracellular domain of TSH-R have been investigated in proliferation assays. A heterogeneous response is generally detected, and occasional responses are even found in T-cells obtained from normal individuals *(163,164)*. Recent studies suggest that peptide 158–176 may he an immunodominant epitope in GD both in vitro and in vivo *(165,166)*. Furthermore, a loss of T-cell reactivity to this peptide has been demonstrated after the treatment of GD by thyroidectomy or radioiodine administration *(167)*. Extensions of this work may eventually lead to the use of TSH-R peptides in GD treatment.

4.3. Complications of GD

A detailed discussion of the pathogenic mechanisms in TAO and PTM is beyond the scope of this chapter and these have been reviewed extensively elsewhere *(168–170)*. In both conditions, there is infiltration of the affected site (extraocular muscle or skin) by activated T-cells. A variety of cytokines can be detected by immunohistochemistry and RT-PCR, including IL-1, TNF, and IFNγ. In vitro these cytokines can activate fibroblasts to secrete glycosaminoglycans (GAGs). The accumulation of GAGs is a cardinal feature of TAO and PTM, and this is thought to cause water trapping and edema. The resulting swelling accounts for most of the clinical features of these complications (Fig 4).

Late in disease, continued fibroblast activation may lead to fibrosis. At this stage, some muscle fiber damage may be detectable in TAO. In the early stage of disease, the muscle cells are intact. The key target, therefore, is most likely the fibroblast of the extraocular muscles and the skin. An enhanced susceptibility to cytokine-mediated induction of GAG production may be a feature of the fibroblasts from these particular sites, explaining the morphological localisation of the autoimmune process. Hypoxia enhances GAG production in vitro, which may be the reason for the adverse effect of smoking on TAO.

A key outstanding question is the relationship between the thyroid and the extrathyroid immune responses. A shared autoantigen at these sites is still the most likely explanation, but its nature remains elusive. One possible candidate is the TSH-R, but the evidence for expression of full-length receptor protein by fibroblasts is at present equivocal. The detection of the receptor mRNA by RT-PCR could simply represent illegitimate transcription *(171)*. A wide variety of eye muscle autoantibodies have been described in TAO, but these are heterogeneous, and none has so far been accepted as having a critical role in disease. The strongest autoantigen candidate is a 64 kDa protein identified by Wall

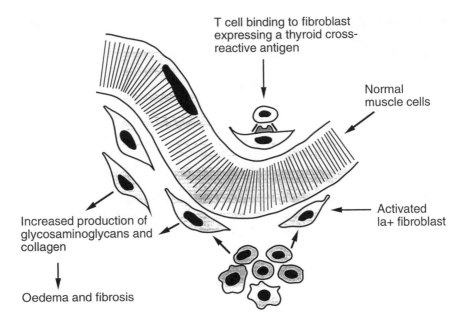

Fig. 4. Possible pathogenic mechanisms in thyroid associated ophthalmopathy. (Reproduced from ref. *168* with permission)

et al. *(172)*, which is the target of autoantibodies in over half of TAO patients. Molecular characterisation of this protein is awaited with interest.

5. PATHOGENIC MECHANISMS IN POSTPARTUM THYROIDITIS (PPT)

A significant increase in B-cells within the thyroid has been demonstrated in PPT *(173)*, together with an increase in serum TPOAb levels in almost all cases. Occasionally, TGAb accompany TPOAb. Very rarely, the TGAb represent the only marker of the disease. Studies on TPOAb IgG subclass restriction have given conflicting results. One study has shown an increase in IgG_1 and IgG_4 levels, whereas another found elevated IgG_2 and IgG_3 levels, and a third demonstrated an increase in IgG_1 and IgG_2 accompanied by decreased IgG_3 *(174–176)*. These contradictory results may well be due to the different methodologies applied in the various studies. The role of the TPOAb in the pathogenesis of the disease is unclear, but one possible mechanism is the mediation by complement fixation. Although TCC levels are not elevated in patient sera *(177)*, several lines of evidence indicate a role for complement in disease pathogenesis. Particularly significant is the fact that complement activation is related to the extent of thyroiditis and correlated with the severity of thyroid dysfunction *(178,179)*.

PPT is associated with an elevated $CD4^+:CD8^+$ ratio, both during pregnancy and in the postpartum period. Furthermore, in the antenatal period an increase in the $CD45RA^+$ lymphocyte subset has been found in women who subsequently developed PPT *(180)*, indicating the involvement of cellular immune reactions in disease pathogenesis. Elevated levels of CD45RA$^+$ T-cells have been found in individuals in the predisease state *(181)*. This T-cell subset may serve, therefore, as a predictive marker of the disease.

6. SUMMARY

ATD has been studied intensively for 40 yr and a considerable body of literature has accumulated which has defined the major pathogenic mechanisms. Autoimmune hypothyroidism results from thyroid cell destruction, most probably initiated by cytotoxic T-cells and exacerbated by a number of mechanisms including ADCC and complement-mediated injury. TFC themselves seem to participate in the autoimmune process at a number of points by expression of cell surface molecules such as class II and by secretion of cytokines and other phlogistic mediators. It remains unclear how important this coributuion by TFC actually is to the destructive process, but differences between individuals, either genetic or environmental, in TFC behavior could be critical in determining the initiation or subsequent tempo of the autoimmune process. Similar mechanisms, although temporary, seem likely to underlie PPT and some patients progress to permanent hypothyroidism. Determining how this progression occurs in certain patients but is prevented in others could provide critical insights into the control of thyroid autoimmunity.

While autoimmune hypothyroidism is relatively simple to treat, GD often poses a more significant clinical problem for which an immunotherapeutic solution would be welcome. Defining further the autoantibody response against the TSH-R may reveal novel approaches to treatment, particularly if there is an oligoclonal B-cell response. At the time of diagnosis, however, the T-cell response is heterogeneous in terms of TCR usage and epitope recognition, and T-cell-based treatment at present seems unlikely to be feasible. In TAO, however, there is considerable evidence that the process is mediated by T-cell-derived cytokines, and therapy using cytokine or receptor antagonists offer a real prospect of improvement for this distressing complication of GD.

REFERENCES

1. Tunbridge, W. M. G, Evered, D. C., Hall, R., Appleton, D., Brewis, M., and Smith, P. A. (1977) The spectrum of thyroid disease in the community; the Whickham survey. *Clin. Endocrinol.* 7, 481–492.
2. LiVolsi, V.A. (1994) The pathology of autoimmune thyroid disease: a review. *Thyroid* 4, 333–339.
3. Hall, R. (1995) Pregnancy and autoimmune endocrine disease. *Bailliere's Clin. Endocrinol. Metab.* 9, 137–155.
4. Salvi, M., Zhang, Z-G, Haegert, D., Woo, M., Liberman, A., Cadarso, L., et al. (1990) Patients with endocrine ophthalmopathy not associated with overt thyroid disease have multiple thyroid immunological abnormalities. *J. Clin. Endocrinol. Metab.* 70, 89–93.

5. Perros, P. and Kendall-Taylor, P. (1995) Thyroid associated ophthalmopathy: pathogenesis and clinical management. *Bailliere's Clin. Endocrinol. Metab.* **9,** 115–135.
6. Paschke, R., Van Sande, J., Parma, J., and Vassart, G. (1996) The TSH receptor and thyroid diseases. *Bailliere's Clin. Endocrinol. Metab.* **10,** 9–27.
7. Libert, F., Passage, E., Lefort, A., Vassart, G., and Mattei, M. G. (1990) Localization of human thyrotropin receptor gene to chromosome region 14q31 by in situ hybridization. *Cytogen Cell Genet.* **54,** 82–83.
8. Gross, B., Misrahi, M., Sar, S., and Milgrom, E. (1991) Composite structure of the human thyrotropin receptor gene. *Biochem. Biophys. Res. Commun.* **177,** 679–687.
9. Parma, J., Duprez, L., Van Sande, J., Cochaux, P., Gervy, C., Mockel, J., et al. (1993) Somatic mutations in the thyrotropin receptor gene cause hyperfunctioning thyroid adenomas. *Nature* **365,** 649–651.
10. McLachlan, S. M. and Rapoport, B. (1992) The molecular biology of thyroid peroxidase: cloning, expression and role as autoantigen in autoimmune thyroid disease. *Endocr. Rev.* **13,** 192–206.
11. Bikker, H., Vulsma, T., Baas, F., and De Vijlder, J. J. M. (1995) Identification of five novel inactivating mutations in the human thyroid peroxidase gene by denaturing gradient gel electrophoresis. *Hum. Mutation.* **6,** 9–16.
12. Kohn, L. D., Giuliani, C., Montani, V., et al. (1995) Antireceptor immunity, in *Thyroid Autoimmunity* (Rayner, D. C. and Champion, B. R., eds.), Springer-Verlag, Heidelberg, Germany, pp. 115–170.
13. Chan, C. T. J., Byfield, P. G. H., Himsworth, R. L., and Shepherd, P. (1987) Human autoantibodies to thyroglobulin are directed towards a restricted number of human specific epitopes. *Clin. Exp. Immunol.* **70,** 516 –523.
14. Medeiros-Neto, G., Targovnik, H. M., and Vassart, G. (1993) Defective thyroglobulin synthesis and secretion causing goiter and hypothyroidism. *Endocr. Rev.* **14,** 165–183.
15. Balfour, P. M., Doniach, D., Roitt, I. M., and Couchman, K. G. (1961) Fluorescent antibody studies in human thyroiditis: autoantibody to an antigen of the thyroid colloid distinct from thyroglobulin. *Brit. J. Exp. Pathol.* **42,** 307-316.
16. Raspé, E., Costagliola, S., Ruf, J., Mariotti, S., Dumont, J. E., and Ludgate, M. (1995) Identification of the thyroid Na^+/I^- cotransporter as a potential autoantigen in thyroid autoimmune disease. *Eur. J. Endocrinol.* **132,** 399–405.
17. Hirayu, H., Seto, P., Magnusson, R. P., Filetti, S., and Rapoport, B. (1987) Molecular cloning and partial characterization of a new autoimmune thyroid disease-related antigen. *J. Clin. Endocrinol. Metab.* **64,** 578–584.
18. Heufelder, A. E., Goellner, J. R., Wenzel, B. E., and Bahn, R. S. (1992) Immunohistochemical detection and localization of a 72-kilodalton heat-shock protein in autoimmune thyroid-disease. *J. Clin. Endocrinol. Metab.* **74,** 724–731.
19. Dong, Q., Ludgate, M., and Vassart, G. (1991) Cloning and sequencing of a 64kDa autoantigen recognised by patients with autoimmune thyroid disease. *J. Clin. Endocrinol. Metab.* **72,** 1375–1381.
20. Endo, T., Kogai, T., Nakazato, M., Saito, T., Kaneshige, M., and Onaya, T. (1996) Autoantibody against Na^+/I^- symporter in the sera of patients with autoimmune thyroid disease. *Biochem. Biophys. Res. Commun.* **224,** 92–95.
21. Mangklabruks, A., Cox, N., and Degroot, L. J. (1991) Genetic-factors in autoimmune thyroid-disease analyzed by restriction fragment length polymorphisms of candidate genes. *J. Clin. Endocrinol. Metab.* **73,** 236–244.

22. Chen, M. C., Maerz, W., Manfras, B. J., Kuehnl, P., Usadel, K. H., and Boehm, B. O. (1993) Rapid and simple subtyping of the HLA-DRB3 gene in Graves' disease by using temperature-gradient gel-electrophoresis. *Hum. Immunol.* **36,** 199–203.

23. Yanagawa, T., Mangklabruks, A., and Degroot, L. J. (1994) Strong association between HLA-DQA1*0501 and Graves' disease in a male Caucasian population. *J. Clin. Endocrinol. Metab.* **79,** 227–229.

24. Ratanachaiyavong, S., Lloyd, L., Darke, C., and McGregor, A. M. (1993) MHC-extended haplotypes in families of patients with Graves' disease. *Hum. Immunol.* **36,** 99–111.

25. Onuma, H., Ota, M., Sugenoya, A., and Inoko, H. (1994) Association of HLA-DPB1* 0501 with early-onset Graves-disease in Japanese. *Hum. Immunol.* **39,** 195–201.

26. Badenhoop, K., Walfish, P. G., Rau, H., Fischer, S., Nicolay, A., Bogner, U., et al. (1995) Susceptibility and resistance alleles of human-leukocyte antigen (HLA) DQA1 and HLA DQB1 are shared in endocrine autoimmune-disease. *J. Clin. Endocrinol. Metab.* **80,** 2112–2117.

27. Barlow, A. B. T., Wheatcroft, N., Watson, P., and Weetman, A. P. (1996) Association of HLA-DQA1*0501 with Graves' disease in English Caucasian men and women. *Clin. Endocrinol.* **44,** 73–77.

28. Cuddihy, R. M., Schaid, D. S., and Bahn, R. S. (1996) Multivariate-analysis of IILA loci in conjunction with a thyrotropin receptor codon-52 polymorphism in conferring risk of Graves' disease. *Thyroid* **6,** 261–265.

29. Tamai, H., Kimura, A., Dong, R. P., Matsubayashi, S., Kuma, K., Nagataki, S., et al. (1994) Resistance to autoimmune thyroid disease is associated with HLA-DQ. *J. Clin. Endocrinol. Metab.* **78,** 94–97.

30. Cavan, D. A., Penny, M. A., Jacobs, K. H., Kelly, M. A., Jenkins, D., Mijovic, C., et al. (1994) The HLA association with Graves' disease is sex-specific in Hong-Kong Chinese subjects. *Clin. Endocrinol.* **40,** 63–66.

31. Badenhoop, K., Schwarz, G., Walfish, P. G., Drummond, V., Usadel, K. H., and Bottazzo, G. F. (1990) Susceptibility to thyroid autoimmune-disease: molecular analysis of HLA-D region genes identifies new markers for goitrous Hashimoto's thyroiditis. *J. Clin. Endocrinol. Metab.* **71,** 1131–1137.

32. Tandon, N., Zhang, L., and Weetman A. P. (1991) HLA association with Hashimoto's thyroiditis. *Clin. Endocrinol.* **34,** 383–386.

33. Shi, Y. F., Zou, M. J., Robb, D., and Farid, N. R. (1992) Typing for MHC class II antigens in thyroid-tissue blocks: association of Hashimoto's thyroiditis with HLA-DQA0301. *J. Clin. Endocrinol. Metab.* **75,** 943–946.

34. Wu, Z. L., Stephens, H. A., Sachs, J. A., Biro, P. A., Cutbush, S., Magzoub, M. M., et al. (1994) Molecular analysis of HLA-DQ and HLA-DP genes in Caucasoid patients with Hashimotos' thyroiditis. *Tissue Antigens* **43,** 116–119.

35. Santamaria, P., Barbosa, J. J., Lindstrom, A. L., Lemke, T. A., Goetz, F. C., and Rich, S. S. (1994) HLA-DQB1-associated susceptibility that distinguishes Hashimoto's thyroiditis from Graves' disease in type-I diabetic-patients. *J. Clin. Endocrinol. Metab.* **78,** 878–883.

36. Bogner, U., Badenhoop, K., Peters, H., Schmieg, D., Mayr, W. R. Usadel, K. H., et al. (1992) HLA-DR/DQ gene variation in nongoitrous autoimmune-thyroiditis at the serological and molecular-level. *Autoimmunity* **14,** 155–158.

37. Cho, B. Y., Chung, J. H., Shong, Y. K., Chang, Y. B., Han, H., Lee, J. B., et al. (1993) A strong association between thyrotropin receptor-blocking antibody-positive atrophic autoimmune-thyroiditis and HLA-DR8 and HLA-DQB1*0302 in Koreans. *J. Clin. Endocrinol. Metab.* **77,** 611–615.

38. Parkes, A. B., Darke, C., Othman, S., Thomas, M., Young, N., Richards, C. J., et al. (1996) Major histocompatibility complex class-II and complement polymorphisms in postpartum thyroiditis. *Eur. J. Endocrinol.* **134,** 449–453.

39. Nicholson, L. B., Wong, F. S., Ewins, D. L., Butler, J., Holland, A., Demaine, A. G., et al. (1994) Susceptibility to autoimmune-thyroiditis in Down's syndrome is associated with the major histocompatibility class II DQA-0301 allele. *Clin. Endocrinol.* **41,** 381–383.

40. Weetman, A. P. and McGregor, A. M. (1994) Autoimmune thyroid disease: further developments in our understanding. *Endocr. Rev.* **15,** 788–830.

41. Roman, S. H., Greenberg, D., Rubinstein, P., Wallenstein, S., and Davies, T. F. (1992) Genetics of autoimmune thyroid disease: lack of evidence for linkage to HLA within families. *J. Clin. Endocrinol. Metab.* **74,** 496–503.

42. O'Connor, G., Neufeld, D. S., Greenberg, D. A., Concepcion, E. S., Roman, S. H., and Davies, T. F. (1993). Lack of disease-associated HLA-DQ restriction-fragment-length-polymorphisms in families with autoimmune thyroid-disease. *Autoimmunity* **14,** 237–241.

43. Phillips, D. I. W., Shields, D. C., Dugoujon, J. M., Prentice, L., McGuffin, P., and Rees-Smith, B. (1993) Complex segregation analysis of thyroid autoantibodies: are they inherited as an autosomal dominant trait?. *Hum. Hered.* **43,** 141–146.

44. Badenhoop, K., Schwarz, G., Schleusener, H., Weetman, A. P., Recks, S., Peters, H., et al. (1992) Tumor necrosis factor-β polymorphisms in Graves' disease. *J. Clin. Endocrinol. Metab.* **74,** 287–291.

45. Cavan, D. A., Penny, M. A., Jacobs, K. H., Kelly, M. A., Jenkins, D., Mijovic, C. H., et al. (1994) Analysis of a Chinese population suggests that the TNFB gene is not a susceptibility gene for Graves' disease. *Hum. Immunol.* **40,** 135–137.

46. Dinarello, C. A. (1991) Interleukin-1 and interleukin-1 antagonism. *Blood* **77,** 1627–1652.

47. Tarlow, J. K., Clay, F. E., Cork, M. J., Blakemore, A. I. F., McDonagh, A. J. G., and Duff, G. W. (1994) Severity of alopecia areata is associated with a polymorphismin the interleukin-1 receptor antagonist gene. *J. Invest. Dermatol.* **103,** 387–390.

48. Blakemore, A. I. F., Watson, P. F., Weetman, A. P., and Duff, G. W. (1995) Association of Graves' disease with an allele of the interleukin-1 receptor antagonist gene. *J. Clin. Endocrinol. Metab.* **80,** 111–115.

49. Yanagawa, T., Hidaka, Y., Guimaraes, V., Soliman, M. and Degroot, L. J. (1995) CTLA-4 gene polymorphism associated with Graves' disease in a Caucasian population. *J. Clin. Endocrinol. Metab.* **80,** 41–45.

50. Kotsa, K., Watson, P., and Weetman, A. P. (1997) A CTLA-4 gene polymorphism is associated with both Graves' disease and Hashimoto's thyroiditis. *Clin. Endocrinol.* **46,** 551–554.

51. Davies, J. L., Kawaguchi, Y., Bennett, S. T. Copeman, J. B., Cordell, H. J., Pritchard, L. E., et al. (1994) A genome-wide search for human type 1 diabetes susceptibility genes. *Nature* **371,** 130–136.

52. Fong, S., Tsoukas, C. D., Frincke, L. A., Lawrence, S. K., Holbrook, T. L., and Carson, D. A. (1981) Age associated changes in Epstein-Barr virus induced human lymphocyte autoantibody production. *J. Immunol.* **25**, 479–485.

53. Weetman, A. P. (1996) Infection and endocrine autoimmunity, in *Microorganisms and Autoimmune Diseases* (Friedman, H., Rose, N.R., and Bendinelli, M., eds,), Plenum, NY, pp. 257–275.

54. Gripenberg, M., Miettinen, A., Kurki, P., and Linder, E. (1978) Humoral immune stimulation and anti-epithelial antibodies in Yersinial infections. *Arthritis Rheum.* **21**, 904–908.

55. Shenkman, L. and Bottone, E. J. (1976) Antibodies to *Yersinia enterocolitica* in thyroid disease. *Annals Int. Med.* **85**, 735–739.

56. Ebner, S., Alex, S., Klugnam, T., et al. (1991) Immunization with *Yersinia enterocolitica* purified outer membrane protein induces lymphocytic thyroiditis in the BB/WOR rat. *Thyroid* 1 (supplement), S-28 (abstract).

57. Ciampollilo, A., Mirakian, R., Schulz, T., Vittoria, M., Buscema, M., Pujol-Borrell, R., et al. (1989) Retrovirus-like sequences in Graves' disease: implications for human autoimmunity. *Lancet* **ii,** 1096–1099.

58. Lagaye, S., Vexiau, P., Morozov, V., Guenebaut-Claudet, V., Tobaly-Tapiero. J., Canivet, M., et al. (1992) Human spurmaretrovirus-related sequences in the DNA of leukocytes from patients with Graves' disease. *Proc. Natl. Acad. Sci. USA* **89**, 10,070–10,074.

59. Wick, G., Trieb, K., Aguzzi, A., Recheis, H., Anderl, H., and Grubeck-Loebenstein, B. (1993) Possible role of human foamy virus in Graves' disease. *Int. Virol.* **35**, 101–107.

60. Hidaka, Y, Masai, T., Sumizaki, H., Takeoka, K., Tada, H., and Amino, N. (1996) Onset of Graves' thyrotoxicosis after an attack of allergic rhinitis. *Thyroid* **6**, 349–351.

61. McGregor, A. M., Weetman, A. P., Ratanachaiyavong, S., Owen, G. M., Ibbertson, H. K., and Hall, R. (1985) Iodine: an influence on the development of thyroid autoimmune disease? in *Thyroid Disorders Associated with Iodine Deficiency and Excess* (Hall, R. and Kobberling, J., eds.), Raven, NY, pp. 209–216.

62. Boukis, I. A., Koutras, D. A., Souvantzoglou, A., Evangelopolou, A., Vrontakis, A., and Moulopoulos, S. D. (1983) Thyroid hormone and immunological studies in endemic goitre. *J. Clin. Endocrinol. Metab.* **57**, 859–862.

63. Jansson, R., Safwenberg, J., and Dahlberg, P. A. (1985) Influence of the HLA-DR4 antigen and iodide status on the development of autoimmune postpartum thyroiditis. *J. Clin. Endocrinol. Metab.* **60**, 168–173.

64. Bagchi, N., Brown, T. R., Urdanivia, E., and Sundick, R. S. (1985) Induction of autoimmune thyroiditis in chickens by dietary iodine. *Science* **230**, 325–327.

65. Cohen, S. B. and Weetman, A. P. (1988) The effect of iodine depletion and supplementation in the Buffalo strain rat. *J. Endocrinol. Invest.* **11**, 625–627.

66. Many, M. C., Maniratunga, S., Varis, I., Dardenne, M., Drexhage, H. A., and Denef, J. F. (1995) Two-step development of Hashimoto-like thyroiditis in genetically autoimmune prone non-obese diabetic mice: effects of iodine-induced cell necrosis. *J. Endocrinol.* **147**, 311–320.

67. Nagataki, S., Shibata, Y., Inoue, S., Yokoyama, N., Izumi, M., and Shimaoka, K. (1994) Thyroid-diseases among atomic-bomb survivors in Nagasaki. *J. Am. Med. Assoc.* **272**, 364–370.

68. Lazarus, J. H., John, R., Bennie, E. H., Chalmers, R. J., and Crockett, G. (1981) Lithium-therapy and thyroid-function—a long-term study. *Psychol. Med.* **11**, 85–92.
69. Wemeau, J. L., Lejeune, P., Devemy, F., et al. (1995) Mecanismes des dysfonctions thyroidiennes liees a l'amiodarone. implications sur leur pronostic et les choix therapeutiques. Mechanisms of amiodarone-induced thyroid dysfunctions. consequences in prognostic, and therapeutic choices. *Revue Francaise d'Endocrinologie Clinique - Nutrition et Metabolisme* **36**, 381–393.
70. Cappiello, E., Boldorini, R., Tosoni, A., Piraneo, S., Bernasconi, R., and Ragii, U. (1995) Ultrastructural evidence of thyroid damage in amiodarone-induced thyrotaxicosis. *J. Endocrinol. Invest.* **18**, 862–868.
71. Samaras, K. and Marel, G. M. (1996) Failure of plasmapheresis, corticosteroids and thionamids to ameliorate a case of protracted amiodarone-induced thyroiditis. *Clin. Endocrinol.* **45**, 365–368.
72. Burman, P., Karlsson, F. A., Oberg, K., et al., (1985) Autoimmune thyroid disease in interferon-treated patients. *Lancet* **2**, 100–101.
73. Vialettes, B., Guillerand, M. A., Viens, P., Stoppa, A. M., Baume, D., Sauvan, R., et al. (1993) Incidence rate and risk-factors for thyroid-dysfunction during recombinant interleukin-2 therapy in advanced malignancies. *Acta Endocrinol.* **129**, 31–38.
74. Winsa, B., Adami, H. O., Berstrom, R., Gamstedt, A., Dahlberg, P. A., Adamson, U., et al. (1991) Stressful life events and Graves' disease. *Lancet* **338**, 1475–1479.
75. Sonino, N., Girelli, M. E., Boscaro, M., Fallo, F., Busnardo, B., and Fava, G. A. (1993) Life events in the pathogenesis of Graves' disease. A controlled study. *Acta Endocrinol.* **128**, 293–296.
76. Radosavljevic, V. R., Jankovic, S. M., and Marinkovic, J. M. (1996) Stressful life events in pathogenesis of graves-disease. *Eur. J. Endocrinol.* **134**, 699–701.
77. Weetman, A. P. (1992) Autoimmune thyroiditis: predisposition and pathogenesis. *Clin. Endocrinol.* **36**, 307–323.
78. Ferrari, C., Boghen, M., Paracchi, A., Rampini, P., Raiteri, F., Benco, R., et al. (1983) Thyroid autoimmunity in hyperprolactinaemic disorders. *Acta Endocrinol. (Copenh.)* **104**, 35–41.
79. Weetman, A. P., Black, C. M., Cohen, S. B., Tomlinson, R., Banga, J. P., and Reimer, C. B. (1989) Affinity purification of IgG subclasses and the distribution of thyroid auto-antibody reactivity in Hashimoto's thyroiditis. *Scand. J. Immunol.* **30**, 73–82.
80. Prentice, L., Kiso, Y., Fukuma, N., Horimoto, M., Petersen, V., Grennan, F., et al. (1995) Monoclonal thyroglobulin autoantibodies: variable region analysis and epitope recognition. *J. Clin. Endocrinol. Metab.* **80**, 977–986.
81. McIntosh, R. S., Asghar, M. S., Watson, P. F., Kemp, E. H., and Weetman, A. P. (1996) Cloning and analysis of IgG-kappa and IgG-lambda antithyroglobulin autoantibodies from a patient with Hashimotos-thyroiditis - evidence for in vivo antigen-driven repertoire selection. *J. Immunol.* **157**, 927–935.
82. Bogner, U., Hegedus, L., Hansen, J. M., Finke, R., and Schleusener, H. (1995) Thyroid cytotoxic antibodies in atrophic and goitrous autoimmune thyroiditis. *Eur. J. Endocrinol.* **132**, 69–74.
83. Li, L., Paul, S., Tyutyulkova, S., Kazatchkine, M. D., and Kaveri, S. (1995) Catalytic activity of anti-thyroglobulin antibodies. *J. Immunol.* **154**, 3328–3332.

84. Bogner, U., Schleusener, H., and Wall, J. R. (1984) Antibody-dependent cell-mediated cytotoxicity against human thyroid cells in Hashimoto's thyroiditis but not Graves' disease. *J. Clin. Endocrinol. Metabol.* **59**, 734–738.

85. Chiovato, L., Bassi, P., Santini, F., Mammoli, C., Lapi, P., Carayon, P., et al. (1993) Antibodies producing complement-mediated thyroid cytotoxicity in patients with atrophic or goitrous autoimmune thyroiditis. *J. Clin. Endocrinol Metab.* **77**, 25–30.

86. Metcalfe, R. A., Oh, Y. S., Stroud, C., Arnold, K., and Weetman, A. P. (1997) Analysis of antibody-dependent cell-mediated cytotoxicity in autoimmune thyroid disease. *Autoimmunity* **25**, 65–72.

87. Song, Y. H., Li, Y. X., and MacLaren, N. K. (1996) The nature of autoantigens targeted in autoimmune endocrine diseases. *Immunol. Today* **17**, 232–238.

88. Ruf, J., Feldt-Rasmussen, U., Hegedus, L., Ferrand, M., and Carayon, P. (1994) Bispecific thyroglobulin and thyroperoxidase autoantibodies in patients with various thyroid and autoimmune diseases. *J. Clin. Endocrinol. Metab.* **79**, 1404–1409.

89. Wilson, B. E. and Netzloff, M. L. (1982) Congenital hypothyroidism and transient thyrotropin excess: differential diagnosis of abnormal newborn thyroid screening. *Ann. Clin. Lab. Sci.* **12**, 223–233.

90. Drexhage, H. A., Botazzo, G. F., Bitensky, L., Chayen, J., and Doniach, D. (1980) Evidence for thyroid growth-stimulating immunoglobulins in some goitrous thyroid diseases. *Lancet* **ii**, 287–292.

91. Drexhage, H. A., Botazzo, G. F., Doniach, D. Bitensky, L., and Chayen, J. (1981) Thyroid growth-blocking antibodies in primary myxoedema. *Nature* **287**, 594–596.

92. Davies, R., Lawry, J., Bhatia, V., and Weetman, A. P. (1995) Growth stimulating antibodies in endemic goitre: a reappraisal. *Clin. Endocrinol.* **43**, 189–195.

93. Matsui, I., Sakata, S., Ogawa, T., Takuno, H., Sarui, H., Komaki, T., et al. (1993) Biological-activities of rat antisera raised against synthetic peptides of human thyrotropin receptor. *Endoc. J.* **40**, 607–612.

94. Hirooka, Y., Mitsuma, T., Nogimori, T., Ishizuki, Y., Sakai, J., Naruse, M., et al. (1993) Production of bioactive rabbit antibodies against the mutated receptor peptide TSH-R-His17 and detection of hypertri-iodothyroninemia in the rabbit. *Biochem. Mol. Biol. Int.* **29**, 493–497.

95. Costagliola, S., Alcalde, L., Ruf, J., Vassart, G., and Ludgate, M. (1994) Over-expression of the extracellular domain of the thyrotrophin receptor in bacteria; production of thyrotrophin-binding inhibiting immunoglobulins. *J. Mol. Endocrinol.* **13**, 11–21.

96. Misrahi, M., Ghinea, N., Sar, S., Saunier, B., Jolivet, A., Loosfelt, H., et al. (1994) Processing of the precursors of the human thyroid-stimulating hormone-receptor in various eukaryotic cells (human thyrocytes, transfected cells and baculovirus-infected insect cells). *Eur. J. Biochem.* **222**, 711–719.

97. Rapoport, B., McLachlan, S. M., Kakinuma, A., and Chazenbalk, G. D. (1996) Critical relationship between autoantibody recognition and thyrotropin receptor maturation as reflected in the acquisition of complex carbohydrate. *J. Clin. Endocrinol. Metab.* **81**, 2525–2533.

98. Volpé, R. (1993) Suppressor T lymphocyte dysfunction is important in the pathogenesis of autoimmune thyroid disease: a perspective. *Thyroid* **3**, 345–352.

99. Martin, A. and Davies, T. F. (1992) T cells and human autoimmune thyroid disease: emerging data show lack of need to invoke suppressor T cell problems. *Thyroid* **2**, 247–261.
100. Volpé, R. (1994) Immunoregulation in autoimmune thyroid-disease. *Thyroid* **4**, 373–377.
101. Davies, T. F., Martin, A., Concepcion, E. S., Graves, P., Cohen, L., and Ben-Nun, A. (1991) Evidence of limited variability of antigen receptors on intrathyroidal T cells in autoimmune thyroid disease. *N. Engl. J. Med.* **325**, 238–244.
102. McIntosh, R. S., Watson, P. F., Pickerill, A. P., Davies, R., and Weetman, A. P. (1993) No restriction of intrathyroidal T cell receptor V-alpha families in the thyroid of Graves' disease. *Clin. Exp. Immunol.* **91**, 147–152.
103. Caso-Peláez, E., McGregor, A. M., and Banga, J. P. (1995) A polyclonal T cell repertoire of V-alpha and V-beta T cell receptor gene families in intrathyroidal lymphocytes of Graves' disease patients. *Scand. J. Immunol.* **41**, 141–147.
104. McIntosh, R. S., Watson, P. F., and Weetman, A. P. (1997) Analysis of the T cell receptor Vα repertoire in Hahsimoto's thyroiditis: evidence for the restricted accumulation of CD8+ T cells in the absence of CD4+ T cell restriction. *J. Clin. Endocrinol. Metab.* **82**, 1140–1146.
105. Wu, Z., Podack, E. R., Mckenzie, J. M., Olsen, K. J. and Zakarija, M. (1994) Perforin expression by thyroid-infiltrating T-cells in autoimmune thyroid-disease. *Clin. Exp. Immunol.* **98**, 470–477.
106. Canonica, G. W., Caria, M., Bagnasco, M., Cosulish, M. E., Giordana, G., and Moretta, L. (1985) Proliferation of T8-positive cytolytic T lymphocytes in response to thyroglobulin in human autoimmune thyroiditis: analysis of cell interactions and culture requirements. *Clin. Immunol. Immunopathol.* **65**, 323–331.
107. Del Prete, G. F., Vercelli, D., Tiri, A., Maggi, E., Mariotti, S., Pinchera, A., et al. (1986) In vivo activated cytotoxic T cells in the thyroid infiltrate of patients with Hashimoto's thyroiditis. *Clin. Exp. Immunol.* **65**, 140–147.
108. MacKenzie, W. A., Schwartz, A. E., Friedman, E. W., and Davies T. F. (1987) Intrathyroidal T cell clones from patients with autoimmune thyroid disease. *J. Clin. Endocrinol. Metab.* **64**, 818–824.
109. Mandrup-Poulsen, T., Nerup, J., Reimers, J. I., Pociot, F., Andersen, H. U., Karlsen, A., et al. (1996) Cytokine and the endocrine system. II. Roles in substrate metabolism, modulation of thyroidal and pancreatic endocrine cell functions and autoimmune endocrine disease. *Eur. J. Endocrinol.* **134**, 21–30.
110. Del Prete, G. F., Tiri, A., Mariotti, S., Pinchera, A., Ricci, M., and Romagnani, S. (1987) Enhanced production of γ-interferon by thyroid-derived T cell clones from patients with Hashimoto's thyroiditis. *Clin. Exp. Immunol.* **69**, 323–331.
111. Del Prete, G. F., Tiri, A, De Carli, M., Mariotti, S., Pinchera, A., Chretien, I., et al. (1989) High potential to tumour necrosis factor-production of thyroid infiltrating lymphocytes in Hashimoto's thyroiditis: a peculiar feature of thyroid autoimmunity. *Autoimmunity* **4**, 267–276.
112. Bagnasco, M., Ferini, S.,Venuti, D., Prigione, I., Torre, G., Biassoni, R., et al. (1987) Clonal analysis of T lymphocytes infiltrating the thyroid gland in Hashimoto's thyroiditis. *Int. Arch. Allerg. App. Immunol.* **82**, 141–146.
113. Mariotti, S., Del Prete, G. F., Chiovato, L., et al. (1992) Cytokines and thyroid autoimmunity. *Int. J. Immunopath. Pharmacol.* **5**, 103–113.

114. Sugihara, S., Fijuwara, H., and Shearer, G. M. (1993) Autoimmune thyroiditis induced in mice depleted of particular T cell subsets: characterization of thyroiditis-inducing T cell lines and clones derived from thyroid lesions. *J. Immunol.* **150,** 683–694.

115. Sugihara, S., Fujiwara, H., Niimi, H., and Shearer, G. M. (1995) Self-thyroid epithelial-cell (TEC)-reactive CD8+ T-cell clones derived from autoimmune-thyroiditis lesions: they recognize self-thyroid antigens directly on TEC to exhibit T-helper cell 1-type lymphokine production and cytotoxicity against TEC. *J. Immunol.* **155,** 1619–1628.

116. Grubeck-Loebenstein, B., Turner, M., Pirich, K., Kassal, H., Londei, M., and Feldmann, M. (1990) CD4⁺ T-cell clones from autoimmune thyroid tissue cannot be classified according to their lymphokine production. *Scand. J. Immunol.* **32,** 433–440.

117. Paschke, R., Schuppert, F., Taton, M., and Velu, T. (1994) Intrathyroidal cytokine gene expression profiles in autoimmune thyroiditis. *J. Endocrinol.* **141,** 309–315.

118. Ajjan, R. A., Watson, P. F., McIntosh, R. S., and Weetman, A. P. (1996) Intrathyroidal cytokine gene expression in Hashimoto's thyroiditis. *Clin. Exp. Immunol.* **105,** 523–528.

119. Heuer, M., Aust, G., Ode-Hakim, S., and Scherbaum, W.A. (1996) Different cytokine mRNA profile in Graves' disease, Hashimoto's thyroiditis, and nonautoimmune thyroid disorders determined by quantitative reverse transcriptase polymerase chain reaction (RT-PCR). *Thyroid* **6,** 97–105.

120. Fukuma, N., McLachlan, S. M., Rapoport, B., Goodacre, J., Middleton, S. L., Phillips, D. I., et al. (1990) Thyroid autoantigens and human T-cell responses. *Clin. Exp. Immunol.* **82,** 275–283.

121. Tandon, N., Freeman, M., and Weetman, A. P. (1991) T-cell responses to synthetic thyroid peroxidase peptides in autoimmune thyroid-disease. *Clin. Exp. Immunol.* **86,** 56–60.

122. Dayan, C. M., Londei, M., Corcoran, A. E., Grubeck-Loebenstein, B., James, R. F. L., Rapoport, B., et al. (1991) Autoantigen recognition by thyroid-infiltrating T cells in Graves' disease. *Proc. Natl. Acad. Sci. USA* **88,** 7415–7419.

123. Fisfalen, M. E., Soliman, M., Okamoto, Y., Soltani, K. and Degroot, L. J. (1995) Proliferative responses of T-cells to thyroid antigens and synthetic thyroid peroxidase peptides in autoimmune thyroid disease. *J. Clin. Endocrinol. Metab.* **80,** 1597–1604.

124. Lehman, P. V., Sercarz, E. E., Forsthuber, T., Dayan, C. M., and Gammon, G. (1993) Determinant spreading and the dynamics of the autoimmune T-cell repertoire. *Immunol. Today* **14,** 203–212.

125. Bottazzo, G. F., Pujol-Borrell, R., Hanafusa, T., and Feldmann, M. (1983) Role of aberrant HLA-DR expression and antigen presentation in induction of endocrine autoimmunity. *Lancet* **ii,** 1115–1119.

126. Sospedra, M., Obiols, G., Babi, L. F., Tolosa, E., Vargas, F., Roura-Mir, C., et al (1995) Hyperinducibility of HLA class-II expression of thyroid follicular cells from Graves' disease: a primary defect. *J. Immunol.* **154,** 4213–4222.

127. Lombardi, G., Arnold, K., Uren, J., Marelli-Berg, F., Hargreaves, R., Imami, N., et al. (1997) Antigen presentation by interferon-γ-treated thyroid follicular cells inhibits interleukin-2 (IL-2) and supports IL-4 production by B7-dependent human T-cells. *Eur. J. Immunol.* **27,** 62–71.

128. Weetman, A. P., Cohen, S. B., Makgoba, M. W., and Borysiewicz, L. K. (1989) Expression of an intercellular adhesion molecule, ICAM-1, by human thyroid cells. *J. Endocrinol.* **122,** 185–191.
129. Tandon, N., Makgoba, M. W., Gahmberg, C. G., and Weetman, A. P. (1992) The expression and role in T cell adhesion of LFA-3 and ICAM-2 on human thyroid cells. *Clin. Immunol. Immunopathol.* **64,** 30–35.
130. Fukazawa, H., Yoshida, K., Ichinohasama, R., Sawai, T., Hiromatsu, Y., Mori, K., et al. (1993) Expression of the Hermes-1 (CD44) and ICAM-1 (CD54) molecule on the surface of thyroid cells from patients with Graves' disease. *Thyroid* **3,** 285–289.
131. Vargas, F., Tolosa, E., Sospedra, M., Catalfamo, M., Lucas-Martin, A., Obiols, G., et al. (1994) Characterization of neural cell adhesion molecule (NCAM) expression in thyroid follicular cells: induction by cytokines and over-expression in autoimmune glands. *Clin. Exp. Immunol.* **98,** 478–488.
132. Weetman, A. P., Bright-Thomas, R., and Freeman, M. (1990) Regulation of interleukin-6 release by human thyrocytes. *J. Endocrinol.* **127,** 357–361.
133. Zheng, R. Q. H., Abney, E. R., Chu, C. Q., Field, M., Maini, R. N., Lamb, J. R., et al. (1992) Detection of in vivo production of tumour necrosis factor-alpha by human thyroid epithelial cells. *Immunology* **75,** 456–462.
134. Cowin, A. J. and Bidey, S. P. (1994) Transforming growth factor b_1 synthesis in human thyroid follicular cells. *J. Endocrinol.* **141,** 183–190.
135. Watson, P. F., Pickerill, A. P., Davies, R., and Weetman, A. P. (1995) Semi-quantitative analysis of interleukin-1, interleukin-6, and interleukin-8 mRNA expression by human thyrocytes. *J. Mol. Endocrinol.* **15,** 11–21.
136. Ajjan, R. A., Watson, P. F., and Weetman, A. P. (1997) Detection of IL-12, IL-13 and IL-15 in the thyroid of patients with autoimmune thyroid disease. *J. Clin. Endocrinol. Metab.* **82,** 666–669.
137. Tandon, N., Morgan, B. P., and Weetman, A. P. (1992) Expression and function of membrane attack complex inhibitory proteins on thyroid follicular cells. *Immunology* **75,** 372–377.
138. Tandon, N., Yan, S. L., Morgan, B. P., and Weetman, A. P. (1994) Expression and function of multiple regulators of complement activation in autoimmune thyroid disease. *Immunology* **81,** 643–647.
139. Weetman, A. P., Tandon, N., and Morgan, B. P. (1992) Antithyroid drugs and release of inflammatory mediators by complement-attacked thyroid cells. *Lancet* **340,** 633–636.
140. Bogner, U., Sigle, B., and Schleusener, H. (1988) Interferon-γ protects human thyroid epithelial cells against cell-mediated cytotoxicity. *Immunobiology* **176,** 423–431.
141. Bogner, U., Schneider, U., and Schleusener, H. (1989) Inhibitory effects of tumor necrosis factor-α and interferon-γ on cell mediated cytotoxicity against human thyroid cells. *Ann. Endocr.* **50,** 139.
142. Widder, J., Dorfinger, K., Wilfing, A., Trieb, K., Pirich, K., Loebenstein, R., et al (1991) The immunoregulatory influence of transforming growth factor-β (TGFβ) in thyroid autoimmunity: TGFβ inhibits autoreactivity in Graves' disease. *J. Autoimmun.* **4,** 689–701.
143. Kosugi, S. and Mori, T. (1995) TSH receptor and LH receptor. *Endocrinol. J.* **42,** 587–606.

144. Ohmori, M., Endo, T., Ikeda, M., and Onaya, T. (1991) Role of N-terminal region of the thyrotropin (TSH) receptor in signal transduction for TSH or thyroid stimulating antibody. *Biochem. Biophys. Res. Commun.* **178,** 733–738.
145. Endo, T., Ohmori, M., Ikeda, M., and Onaya, T. (1991) Rabbit antibodies toward extracellular loops of the membrane spanning region of human thyrotropin receptor possess thyroid stimulating activities. *Biochem. Biophys. Res. Commun.* **181,** 1035–1041.
146. Kosugi, S., Ban, T., Akamizu, T., and Kohn, L. D. (1991) Further characterization of a high affinity thyrotropin binding site on the rat thyrotropin receptor which is an epitope for blocking antibodies from idiopathic myxedema patients but not thyroid stimulating antibodies from Graves' patients. *Biochem. Biophys. Res. Commun.* **180,** 1118–1124.
147. Desai, R. K., Dallas, J. S., Gupta, M. K., Seetharamaiah, G. S., Fan, J. L., Tahara, K., et al. (1993) Dual mechanism of perturbation of thyrotropin-mediated activation of thyroid cells by antibodies to the thyrotropin receptor (TSHR) and TSH. *J. Clin. Endocrinol. Metab.* **77,** 658–663.
148. Zakarija, M. (1983) Immunochemical characterisation of the thyroid-stimulating antibody in Graves' disease: evidence for restricted heterogeneity. *J. Clin. Lab. Immunol.* **10,** 77–85.
149. Weetman, A. P., Byfield, P. G. H., Black, C., and Reimer, C. B. (1990) IgG heavy-chain subclass restriction of thyrotropin-binding inhibitory immunoglobulins in Graves' disease. *Eur. J. Clin. Invest.* **20,** 406–410.
150. Di Cerbo, A., Di Paola, R., Bonati, M., De Filippis, V., and Corda, D. (1995) Subgroups of Graves' patients identified on the basis of the biochemical activities of their immunoglobulins. *J. Clin. Endocrinol. Metab.* **80,** 2785–2790.
151. Takai, O., Desai, R. K., Seetharamaiah, G. S., Jones, C. A., Allaway, G. P., Akamizu, T., et al. (1991) Prokaryotic expression of the thyrotropin receptor and identification of an immunogenic region of the protein using synthetic peptides. *Biochem. Biophys. Res. Commun.* **179,** 319–326.
152. Kosugi, S., Akamizu, T., Takai, O., Prabhakar, B. S. and Kohn, L. D. (1991) The extracellular domain of the TSH receptor has an immunogenic epitope reactive with Graves' sera but unrelated to receptor function as well as epitopes having different roles for high affinity TSH binding and the activity of thyroid stimulating antibodies. *Thyroid* **1,** 321–330.
153. Mori, T., Sugawa, H., Piraphatdist, T., Inoue, D., Enomoto, T., and Imura, H. (1991) A synthetic oligopeptide derived from human thyrotropin receptor sequence binds to Graves' immunoglobulin and inhibits thyroid stimulating antibody-activity but lacks interactions with TSH. *Biochem. Biophys. Res. Commun.* **178,** 165–172.
154. Ueda, Y., Sugawa, H., Akamizu, T., Okuda, J., Kiho, Y. and Mori, T. (1993) Immunoglobulin-G that interferes with thyroid-stimulating antibody measurements can be eliminated specifically by incubation with synthetic peptides corresponding to partial sequences of the human thyrotropin receptor. *Thyroid* **3,** 111–117.
155. Ueda, Y., Sugawa, H., Akamizu, T., Okuda, J., Ueda, M., Kosugi, S., et al. (1995) Thyroid-stimulating antibodies in sera from patients with Graves' disease are heter-ogeneous in epitope recognition. *Eur. J. Endocrinol.* **132,** 62–68.
156. Ludgate, M. E. and Vassart, G. (1995) The thyrotropin receptor as a model to illustrate receptor and receptor antibody diseases. *Bailliere's Clin. Endocrinol. Metab.* **9,** 95–113.

157. Heufelder, A. E., Wenzel, B. E., and Scriba, P. C. (1996) Antigen receptor variable region repertoires expressed by T cells infiltrating thyroid, retroorbital, and pretibial tissue in graves' disease. *J. Clin. Endocrinol. Metab.* **81,** 3733–3739.
158. Catalfamo, M., Roura-Mir, C., Sospedra, M., Aparicio, P., Costagliola, S., Ludgate, M., et al. (1996) Self-reactive cytotoxic gamma-delta T-lymphocytes in Graves' disease specifically recognize thyroid epithelial-cells. *J. Immunol.* **156,** 804–811.
159. Mullins, R. J., Chernajovsky, Y., Dayan, C., Londei, M., and Feldmann, M. (1994) Transfection of thyroid autoantigens into EBV-transformed B cell lines: recognition by Graves' disease thyroid T cells. *J. Immunol.* **152,** 5572–5580.
160. Mullins, R. J., Cohen, S. B., Webb, L. M., Chernajovsky, Y., Dayan, C. M., Londei, M., et al. (1995) Identification of thyroid-stimulating hormone receptor-specific T cells in Graves' disease thyroid using autoantigen-transfected Epstein-Barr virus-transformed B cell lines. *J. Clin. Invest.* **96,** 30–37.
161. Watson, P. F., Pickerill, A. P., Davies, R., and Weetman, A. P. (1994) Analysis of cytokine gene expression in Graves' disease and multinodular goiter. *J. Clin. Endocrinol. Metab.* **79,** 355–360.
162. Soliman, M., Kaplan, E., Fisfalen, M. E., Okamoto, Y. and Degroot, L. J. (1995) T cell reactivity to recombinant human thyrotropin receptor extracellular domain and thyroglobulin in patients with autoimmune and nonautoimmune thyroid diseases. *J. Clin. Endocrinol. Metab.* **80,** 206–213.
163. Tandon, N., Freeman, M. A., and Weetman, A. P. (1992) T-cell responses to synthetic TSH receptor peptides in Graves' disease. *Clin. Exp. Immunol.* **89,** 468–473.
164. Akamizu, G., Ueda, Y., Hua, L., Okuda, J., and Mori, T. (1995) Establishment and characterization of an antihuman thyrotropin (TSH) receptor-specific CD4+ T cell line from a patient with Graves' disease: evidence for multiple T cell epitopes on the TSH receptor including the transmembrane domain. *Thyroid* **5,** 259–260.
165. Soliman, M., Kaplan, E., Yanagawa, T., Hidaka, Y., Fisfalen, M. E., and Degroot, L. J. (1995) T-cells recognize multiple epitopes in the human thyrotropin receptor extracellular domain. *J. Clin. Endocrinol. Metab.* **80,** 905–914.
166. Soliman, M., Kaplan, E., Straus, F., Fisfalen, M. E., Hidaka, Y., Guimaraes, V., et al. (1995) Graves' disease in severe combined immunodeficient mice. *J. Clin. Endocrinol. Metab.* **80,** 2846–2855.
167. Soliman, M., Kaplan, E., AbdelLatif, A., Scherberg, N. and Degroot, L. J. (1995) Does thyroidectomy, radioactive iodine therapy, or antithyroid drug treatment alter reactivity of patients' T cells to epitopes of thyrotropin receptor in autoimmune thyroid diseases? *J. Clin. Endocrinol. Metab.* **80,** 2312–2321.
168. Weetman, A. P. (1991) Thyroid-associated eye disease: pathophysiology. *Lancet* **338,** 25–28.
169. Bahn, R. S. and Heufelder, A. E. (1993) Pathogenesis of Graves' ophthalmopathy. *N. Engl. J. Med.* **329,** 1468–1475.
170. Heufelder, A. E. (1995) Pathogenesis of Graves' ophthalmopathy: recent controversies. *Eur. J. Endocrinol.* **132,** 532–541.
171. Paschke, R., Vassart, G., and Ludgate, M. (1995) Current evidence for and against the TSH receptor being the common antigen in Graves' disease and thyroid-associated ophthalmopathy. *Clin. Endocrinol.* **42,** 565–569.

172. Zhang, Z.-G., Wall, J. R., and Bernard, N. F. (1996) Tissue distribution and quantitation of a gene expressing a 64-kDa antigen associated with thyroid-associated ophthalmopathy. *Clin. Immunol. Immunopath.* **80**, 236–244.
173. Jansson, R., Karlsson, A., and Forsum, U. (1984) Intrathyroidal HLA-DR expression and T lymphocyte phenotypes in Grave's thyrotoxicosis, Hashimoto's thyroiditis and nodular colloid goitre. *Clin. Exp. Immunol.* **58**, 264–272.
174. Jansson, R., Thompson, P. M., Clark, F., and McLachlan, S. M. (1986) Association between thyroid microsomal antibodies of subclass IgG-1 and hypothyroidism in autoimmune postpartum thyroiditis. *Clin. Exp. Immunol.* 63, 80–86.
175. Hall, R., Fung, M., Kologlu, M., et al. (1987) Postpartum thyroid dysfunction, in *Thyroid Autoimmunity* (Pinchera, A., Ingbar, S. H., McKenzie, J. M., and Fenzi, G. F., eds.). Plenum, NY, pp. 211–219.
176. Briones-Urbina, R., Parkes, A. B., Bogner, U., Mariotti, S., and Walfish, P. G. (1990) Increase in antimicrosomal antibody related IgG1 and IgG4 and titres of antithyroid peroxidase antibodies, but not antibody dependent cell mediated cytotoxicity in post-partum thyroiditis with transient hypothyroidism. *J. Endocrinol. Invest.* **13**, 879–886.
177. McCullough, B., Hall, R., Morgan, B. P., Parkes, A. B. and Lazarus, J. H. (1994) Lack of terminal complement component in postpartum thyroiditis–A possible explanation for transient disease. *J. Endocrinol.* **140**, 251–254.
178. Parkes, A. B., Othman, S., Hall, R., John, R., and Lazarus, J. H. (1995) Role of complement in the pathogenesis of postpartum thyroiditis: relationship between complement activation and disease presentation and progression. *Eur. J. Endocrinol.* **133**, 210–215.
179. Parkes, A. B., Adams, H., Othman, S., Hall, R., John, R., and Lazarus, J. H. (1996) The role of complement in the pathogenesis of postpartum thyroiditis. Ultrasound echogeneity and the degree of complement induced thyroid damage. *Thyroid* **6**, 169–174.
180. Stagnaro-Green, A., Roman, S. H., Cobin, R. H., El-Harazy, E., Wallenstein, S., and Davies, T. F. (1992) A prospective study of lymphocyte-initiated immunosuppression in normal pregnancy: evidence of a T-cell etiology for postpartum thyroid dysfunction. *J. Clin. Endocrinol. Metab.* **74**, 645–653.
181. Faustman, D., Eisenbarth, G., Daley, G., and Breitmayer, J. (1989) Abnormal T-lymphocyte subsets in type I diabetes. *Diabetes* **38**, 1462–1468.

5

Autoantigens of Sjögren's Syndrome

Isao Nishimori and Michael A. Hollingsworth

1. CLINICAL FEATURES

Sjögren's syndrome (SS) is a chronic inflammatory disorder characterized by lymphocytic infiltration of lacrimal and salivary glands that results in dry eyes and dry mouth. As in other connective tissue diseases of autoimmune origin, there is a marked preponderance of the disorder in females; the ratio of disease occurrence in females to males is 9:1 *(1,2)*. Estimates of the prevalence range from one in 1250–2500 females *(3)*. The disease often becomes evident in the fourth and fifth decades *(2)*. SS presents as a primary disease with no other abnormalities (primary SS) or in association with other autoimmune disorders (secondary SS) including rheumatoid arthritis (RA), systemic lupus erythematosus (SLE), polymyositis, and progressive systemic sclerosis (PSS) *(4)*. The skin, kidney, liver, lung, pancreas, and nervous system are affected in SS patients *(4)*; hence, SS is thought to be a relatively systemic disease in the spectrum of connective tissue diseases. In a few cases, a lymphoproliferative syndrome develops that includes lymphadenopathy and an increased risk of lymphoma *(4–6)*.

2. AUTOIMMUNE NATURE OF SJÖGREN'S SYNDROME

The etiology of SS is unknown and has been the subject of much debate. It is believed that both genetic and environmental factors contribute to the development of SS. There is an increased association of HLA–DR3 with SS in caucasians *(7)*, and other alleles are associated with the disease in different ethnic groups *(8–10)*. An increased frequency of DR3 is also seen in patients with serum antibodies to SS–A/SS–B *(10,11)*. The results of studies on the haplotypes associated with antibodies to SS–A/SS–B showed that patients heterozygous for HLA–DQ1 and DQ2 had the highest anti-SS–A antibody levels *(8,10)*.

Evidence that autoimmunity plays a role in the pathogenesis of SS patients includes the following:

1. The intense focal infiltrates in the lacrimal and salivary glands contain predominantly CD4⁺ T-cells with Th-1-like activity (e.g., production of inflammatory cytokines such as IFN-γ) and to a lesser extent B-cells *(12)*.

Contemporary Immunology: Autoimmune Reactions
Edited by: S. Paul © Humana Press Inc., Totowa, NJ

2. Salivary epithelial cells aberrantly express high levels of HLA-DR *(13)*.
3. Various autoantibodies are detected in sera including antibodies against nuclear antigen (SS–A/Lo and SS–B/Ra) and the Fc region of IgG (rheumatoid factor); these antibodies, however, show no specificity for the salivary or lacrimal glands and are found in other autoimmune diseases *(7,14–16)*.
4. Hypergammaglobulinemia with occasional monoclonal gammopathy is observed is SS *(5,6)*, providing evidence for monoclonal or oligoclonal expansion of B-cells in affected salivary glands *(4)*.
5. Lymphocytes in focal lesions of salivary glands of patients with SS are blocked in their ability to undergo apoptosis, even though they express *Fas*, possibly due to *bcl*-2 expression (*bcl*-2 can inhibit *Fas*-mediated apoptosis) *(17)*.

3. T-CELL RECEPTOR USAGE

Some restriction of T-cell receptor (TCR) gene usage in patients with SS *(18–20)* has been observed. There is a predominance of Vβ2 use by T-cells infiltrating the salivary glands. Another study reported that several identical TCR Vβ genes were detected in lacrimal and labial salivary glands from individual patients with SS *(21)*. To date, studies of TCR families do not encourage the idea of an immune response to a single antigen or a superantigen in patients with SS. A recent study on somatically driven expansion of TCR families (including Vβ2) in SS found limited junctional diversity in the inflamed glands *(22,23)*. Thus, it is likely that specific T-cells undergoing expansion in the SS gland respond to a limited number of autoantigens, and not to superantigens, which might be anticipated to stimulate a more "global" TCR expansion.

4. TARGET ANTIGENS

Several candidate target antigens for SS have been proposed based on different lines of evidence, including evidence from studies on serum autoantibodies, T-cell responses, and animal models of the disease. Candidate autoantigens in SS are listed in Table 1. A discussion of the molecular nature of these antigens and immune responses in patients with SS is described in Subheading 4.1.

4.1. SS–A/Ro and SS–B/La

Antibodies against SS–A/Ro and SS–B/La are often found in the serum of patients with SS *(6,7,16,24)*. The reported prevalence of autoantibodies varies in different studies and it also varies when different detection methods are used. The presence of serum antibodies to SS–A/Ro and/or SS–B/La has been nominated as a diagnostic parameter in the California criteria and the preliminary European criteria for classification of SS; however, diagnosis with these reagents is not definitive because the antibodies are also found in patients with other autoimmune diseases *(25,26)*.

There is considerable circumstantial but no direct evidence that anti-SS–A/Ro and anti–SS–B/La antibodies play a role in the immunopathogenesis of some

Table 1
Candidate Autoantigens in Sjögren's Syndrome

Antigen name	MW (kDa)	Tissue distribution	Molecular function	Serum antibody			Addtional features
				SS	SLE	Controls	
SS-A/Ro 60	60	Most eukaryotic cells	Unknown	42–38%	39–65%	0%	—
SS-A/Ro 52	52	Most eukaryotic cells	Unknown	35–37%	11–47%	0%	—
SS-B/La 48	48	Most eukaryotic cells	Terminal transcription factor for RNA polymerase III	46–77%	12–21%	0%	Translocated to the cell membrane with some viiral infection
Fcγ receptor IIIb	50–70	Various blood cells[a]	Receptor for the Fc domain of Ig	25,66 (38%)	— (6%)	2/34	CD16
Fcγ receptor II	40	Various blood cells[b]	Receptor for the Fc domain of Ig	6/52 (12%)	13/55 (24%)	0/15 (0%)	CD32
Carbonic anhydrase II	31 31	Some cell types in virtually all tissues[c]	Catalyze the hydration of CO_2 to bicarbonate and a proton	0–62%	25–32%	0–5%	—
PDC-E2	74	Mitochondria	Critical enzyme in energy metabolism	22–27%	33%	1%	See[d]
α fodrin	240	Most eukaryotic cells	Self-assembly, binding to actin filaments	41–43 (95%)	0/21 (0%)	0/15 (0%)	120 kDa fragment is specifically observed in labial glands of SS patients
HuD	35–40	Brain	Neuron-specific RNA processing?	3/45 (7%)	— (0%)	0/70	Significant homology with the N-terminus of SS-A/Ro 52 kDa
HTLV-1 gag p19	19	Ductal epithelia in salivary glands of SS patients[e]	Core protein of HTLV-1	3/19 (16%)	4/31 (13%)	2/52 (4%)	—
HIV gag p24	24	Ductal epithelia in salivary glands of SS patients[f]	Core protein of HIV	5/15 (33%)	— (0%)	0/10	—
HRES-1	28?	Endogeneous retrovirus	Unknown	10–52%	3–21%	2–4%	HTLV-1 related endogeneous sequence

[a] Neutrophils, granular lymphocytes, and macrophages.

[b] Neutrophils, monocytes, eosinophils, platelets, and B-cells.

[c] Including osteoclasts in bone, tubules, and collecting ducts in kidney, acinar, and ductal cells in salivary glands, pancreatic duct cells, gastric parietal cells, endometrium of the uterus, oligodendrocytes in brain, tubules, endothelial cells, erythrocytes, and epithelial cells of duodenum, intestine, and colon.

[d] Monoclonal antibodies to PDC-E2 showed an apical staining on the salivary glands epithelial cells in 4 of 9 patients with coexisting SS and primary biliary cirrhosis.

[e] Reactivity of monoclonal anti-HTLV-1 gag p19 antibody with ductal epithelia in labial salivary glands was observed in 31% of 39 SS patients.

[f] Reactivity of monoclonal anti-HIV gag p24 antibody with ductal epithelia in labial salivary glands was observed in 47% of 15 SS patients.

autoimmune diseases. The best evidence is derived from an examination of neonatal lupus erythematosus. Newborns from mothers with anti-SS–A/Ro antibody are 200 times more likely to develop congenital heart block (one in 50–100) compared to the normal population (one in 20,000) (27). It has been postulated that these antibodies pass through the placenta and cause myocardial damage in fetus (27).

The molecular structures of the SS–A/Ro and SS–B/La antigens are currently under investigation. The SS–A/Ro antigen (SS–A/Ro RNP) is comprised of SS–A/Ro proteins complexed with a subset of SS–B/La-associated RNA molecules, known as the RNA polymerase III-transcribed Y RNAs (28). Both the protein and RNA components in this complex are polymorphic. In human cells, at least five kinds of RNA polymerase III-transcribed Y RNAs have been reported, hY1-hY5 RNA. These are short RNAs 84–112 bases in length. It has been proposed that each SS–A/Ro RNP complex contains only one of the five RNAs (28). The protein element contained in the SS–A/Ro RNP complex was initially reported to be a 60 kDa protein. Recently, a 52 kDa protein has also been detected in these complexes (29). Circulating anti-SS–A/Ro antibodies in patients with SS react differently with the 60 kDa and 52 kDa proteins (30,31). The SS–B/La antigen (SS–B/La RNP) is reported as being a complex of a 47 kDa polypeptide and hY1-hY5 RNA (32). Some SS–A/Ro RNP complexes contain the SS–B/La protein (33,34). Furthermore, an alternatively spliced transcript (45 kDa protein) of the 52 kDa SS–A/Ro has been reported (35).

There is currently considerable interest in the mechanism of intracellular transport of the SS–B/La molecule, particularly concerning the effects of environmental factors and the potential for exposing the antigens to extracellular immune system recognition phenomenon. Studies of SS–A/Ro translocation have been limited by the lack of monoclonal anti-SS–A/Ro antibodies. Baboonian et al. using monoclonal anti-SS–B/La antibodies, demonstrated that viral infection and cytokines (e.g., IFN-γ) can influence the intracellular movement of SS–B/La to varying degrees. Infection with adenovirus 2, in particular, induced the translocation of SS–B/La to the cell membrane (36). This phenomenon has been reproduced in cells infected with the herpes simplex virus (37). Recently, a dramatic accumulation of SS–B/La was found on the cell membranes in the salivary glands and the conjunctiva of SS patients (38,39). These observations led to the hypothesis that surface expression of normally cryptic antigens can be induced by factors such as viral infection, which, together with upregulation of HLA class II antigen expression, can serve as the a stimulus for producing specific autoimmune responses in SS.

4.2. Fcγ Receptor

Anti-neutrophil antibodies have been found the sera of patients with several autoimmune conditions associated with neutropenia, including SLE, Felty's syndrome, and primary biliary cirrhosis (40). One antigen recognized by an anti-neutrophil antibody is the Fc-gamma receptor (FcγR). Antibodies to two different classes of receptors (FcγRII and FcγRIIIb) were detected in the sera of patients with SLE, PSS, and RA *(41)*. Lamour et al. *(42)* reported that 10 of 66 SS patients (15%) have serum antibodies reactive with neutrophils, and 25 of 66 SS patients (38%) have serum antibodies to FcγRIIIb. The results of another study showed that six out of 52 SS patients (12%) had serum antibodies reactive with mouse FcγRII *(43)*. However, the anti-FcγR antibodies were not specific for SS *(41,43)*, and there was no correlation between the antibody titer and the peripheral neutrophil count (neutropenia) *(42)*, suggesting that the presence of the antibodies might be an epiphenomenon *(40)*. Thus, it is not clear whether the anti-FcγR antibodies play a primary role in the pathogenesis of SS.

4.3. Epithelial Antigen of the Duct Cells in Exocrine Glands

Patients with SS have serum antibodies reactive with salivary gland epithelial cells *(6,44,45)* and with pancreatic ductal cells *(46,47)*. Primary biliary cirrhosis (PBC) and chronic pancreatitis are well-known complications associated with SS *(48–50)*. Histologically, the initial lesion observed in the salivary glands of patients with SS is a focal accumulation of mononuclear cells around the ducts and, to a lesser extent, the acini *(51)*. A similar pathology is evident in patients with PBC *(52)* and idiopathic chronic pancreatitis (primary inflammatory sclerosis of the pancreas) *(53)*. Further, ductal epithelial cells in the liver and the pancreas express MHC class II antigens aberrantly in patients with PBC *(54)* and idiopathic chronic pancreatitis *(55,56)*, respectively. Based on these common clinical features, the existence of a disease entity designated "autoimmune exocrinopathy" *(57)*, "dry gland syndrome" *(58)*, or "autoimmune epithelitis" *(59)* has been proposed. It is hypothesized that a common epithelial target antigen exists in the ductal cells of several exocrine glands, including the salivary glands, liver (bile duct), pancreas, and kidney (renal tubule), and that the common antigen plays an important role in eliciting exocrine organ-specific autoreactivity in SS and other autoimmune diseases.

The molecular nature of the antigen recognized by the antibodies reactive with the ductal epithelial cells is not known. Several candidate molecules expressed on the ductal epithelia have been proposed recently, including carbonic anhydrase II *(60)* and the E2 subunit of the pyruvate dehydrogenase complex *(61)*.

4.4. Carbonic Anhydrase II

Nishimori et al. *(62)* partially purified a 60-kDa antigen from porcine and human pancreas extracts and showed its reactivity with three of 11 SS patients (27%) and six of 20 patients with idiopathic chronic pancreatitis (ICP) (30%). Peripheral cellular (CD4$^+$ T-cell) immune responses to the 60-kDa antigen were also observed in patients with SS and ICP *(63,64)*. A monoclonal antibody (MAb) against the 60-kDa antigen was shown to react with carbonic anhydrase II (CA II). CA II is an epithelial autoantigen that is expressed commonly by ductal cells of most exocrine glands *(65)*. Serum autoantibodies to CA II were detected in 13 of 21 patients with SS (62%) and 11 of 33 patients with ICP (33%) *(60)*. Serum antibodies to CA II have also been reported in patients with SLE *(66,67)* and autoimmune cholangitis (AIC), which is a subgroup of PBC with the clinical and pathological features of PBC, but without antimitochondrial antibody and with antinuclear antibody *(68)*. Recently, we detected serum antibody to CA II in twelve of 40 patients with PBC (30%) and seven of 23 patients with AIC (30%) (unpublished data). Further, immunization of mice with human CA II produced sialoadenitis in an MHC-restricted manner in H-2^s and H-2^u mouse strains, with lesions similar to those observed in the early stage of human SS *(65)*. These results suggest that CA II recognition is a candidate mechanism underlying the exocrinopathy commonly observed in SS, ICP, AIC, and PBC. Autoantibodies reactive with carbonic anhydrase I, an isoenzyme expressed in red blood cells, but not in epithelial cells of exocrine organs, have been observed in sera of patients with SLE and SS *(60)*. The presence of serum autoantibodies to CA I and CA II suggests that other CA isozymes known to be expressed by epithelial cells should be investigated for potential roles in the pathogenesis of exocrine autoimmune disease.

4.5. E2 Subunit of the Pyruvate Dehydrogenase Complex

Consistent with findings that patients with SS often display the complications of PBC, patients with PBC have a high incidence of SS *(49,69,70)*. Serum antimitochondrial antibody (AMA) is observed with high specificity and high sensitivity in patients with PBC. The major antigen recognized by AMA is the E2 subunit of the pyruvate dehydrogenase complex (PDC-E2) *(71)*. Serum antibodies to PDC-E2 are present in 22–27% of SS patients *(49,72)*. Most SS patients with anti-PDC-E2 antibodies showed liver function tests below the normal range and histological findings compatible with early stages of PBC (stage I). Some antibody positive patients, however, have no histological or clinical features of PBC even upon long term followup *(49,72)*.

Surh et al. produced a panel of monoclonal antibodies reactive with PDC-E2 *(73)*. One antibody reacted with mitochondria and with the apical region of biliary epithelium from patients with PBC, but not with tissues from patients with other liver diseases or normal controls *(73)*. Subsequently, an MAb reactive with both PDC-E2 and the biliary duct epithelial cells was found to bind the apical region of salivary gland epithelial cells from four of nine patients with coexisting PBC and SS. The antibody was unreactive, however, with the epithelial cells from 11 patients with primary SS *(61)*. These results suggest an abnormal expression of PDC-E2 or a structurally related molecule in the ductal epithelial cells in PBC and PBC/SS patients.

4.6. α-Fodrin

Hayashi et al. established an animal model of SS in NFS/*sld* mutant mice thymectomized three days after birth (3d-Tx) *(74)*. These mice showed preferential expression of the TCR Vβ8 gene in inflamed glands and high serum levels of an IgG antibody reactive with salivary ducts *(74)*. Affinity purified antibodies from the serum were used to purify a 120-kDa organ-specific antigen from the salivary gland of the mice *(75)*. Amino acid sequencing showed the 120-kDa molecule was to be an α-fodrin fragment. Interestingly, this molecule was expressed only in the salivary glands of 3d-Tx NFS/*sld* mice; there was no expression in other tissues, nor was the antigen expressed in the salivary glands of nonthymectomized NFS/*sld* mice. Forty one of 43 sera from SS patients showed binding to the 120-kDa molecule and to recombinant α-fodrin. Furthermore, peripheral blood mononuclear cells from the patients displayed proliferative responses to the 120-kDa molecule *(75)*.

Fodrin is a major component of the cortical cytoskeleton in most eukaryotic cells, present as a heterodimer of an α-subunit (240 kDa) and a β-subunit (235 kDa) *(76)*. It remains to be determined how the α-fodrin fragment appears specifically in the salivary glands in 3d-Tx NFS/*sld* mice, and how this molecule contributes to the pathogenesis of SS. Note that the level of specificity (95%) and sensitivity (100%) of serum antibodies to α-fodrin in SS are very high compared to other types of autoantibodies found in patients with connective tissue diseases (*see* Table 1), which should encourage further studies of the role of α-fodrin.

4.7. HuD

Recently, antineuronal antibodies were detected in SS patients with central and peripheral neurological disorders. Moll et al. *(77)* reported that antineuronal antibodies were present in 55% of SS patients with major neurological complications, mainly polyneuropathy. Some sera from these patients reacted with a 38-kDa neuronal protein, which was also bound by an anti-Hu antibody. Serum anti-Hu antibodies were originally reported in two patients with subacute sensory neuropathy arising as a complication of oat cell carcinoma *(78)*. Patients with neuroendocrine-related tumors and paraneoplastic encephalomyelitis or paraneoplastic sensory neuropathy develop high titers of anti-Hu antibodies in sera and cerebrospinal fluid, with concomitant deposition of anti-Hu IgG in the nervous system and the tumor *(79,80)*. The neuronal antigen, termed HuD, has been isolated and cloned *(80)*. The deduced amino acid sequence of HuD contains three potential RNA recognition motifs and is highly homologous to the Drosophila proteins Elav and Sex-lethal, and the HuD protein is suggested to play a role in the development of the human nervous system.

The 52-kDa SS–A/Ro antigen has one domain that exhibits homology to HuD *(81)*. Serum antibodies to 52 kDa SS–A/Ro were detected in approximately four percent of patients with paraneoplastic anti-Hu syndrome but were not associated with SS. In one report, patients with SS and associated neurological disease were found not to express serum or cerebrospinal fluid antibodies to neuronal antigens *(82)*. Sera from SS patients capable of binding the 38-kDa band in Western blots of rat cerebellar homogenate (resembling anti-Hu immunoreactivity) failed to react with the recombinant HuD protein *(83)*. These results, however, do not disprove the possible association between anti-HuD antibodies and SS-associated neurological disease. Natural autoantibodies do not necessarily react with recombinant proteins because of differences in their molecular structure compared to native proteins. It remains unresolved, therefore, whether the neurological syndromes associated with cancer and SS share an underlying cause.

4.8. Viral Antigens

Viral infection is suggested to be a potential cause of a wide variety of autoimmune diseases, including SS. No viruses have been conclusively identified as causes of SS. Several groups have demonstrated increased levels of DNA, RNA, and proteins encoded by viruses in salivary and lacrimal gland biopsy specimens from patients with SS, including Epstein-Barr virus (EBV), human immunodeficiency virus (HIV), human T-cell lymphotropic virus type I (HTLV-1), and hepatitis-C virus (HCV). EBV has gained attention as a potential cause of SS, because the salivary glands are a natural site for harboring the virus during its latency and reactivation phases *(84)*. EBV can stimulate production of polyclonal antibodies to viral proteins and autoantibodies such as rheumatoid factor *(85)*. These antibodies have been observed in patients with SS. Increased expression of EBV-associated antigens and EBV DNA have been reported in the ductal epithelial cells of salivary glands and in lacrimal glands from patients with SS *(86–89)*.

Viral antigens delivered resulting from an exogenous infection into the salivary and lacrimal glands are not autoantigens; hence, diseases caused by viral infection are not autoimmune diseases in the strict sense of the term. There are two possible ways that viruses can participate in the pathogenesis of SS. One is via "reactivation" of an endogenous retroviral protein (i.e., a retroposon) and another, via molecular mimicry between a viral protein and a native autoantigen.

An example of the former possibility is seen with the tax gene of HTLV-1, but not the *gag, pol,* or *env* genes. *Tax* expression was detected in salivary gland biopsies from SS patients negative for serum anti-HTLV-1 antibodies, suggesting that only a portion of the viral genome is retained in patients destined to develop autoimmune disease *(90,91)*. Brookes et al. *(92)* reported that 16% and 32% of SS patients had serum antibodies reactive with synthetic peptides of HTLV-1 *gag* p19 and the HTLV-related endogenous sequence (HRES-1), respectively. The two types of antibodies were cross reactive with their cognate antigens. Banki et al. *(93)* reported two of 19 (10%) SS patients were positive for serum antibodies reactive to HRES-1 peptide. Expression of the HRES-1 peptide by certain cells could potentially render these cells susceptible to the antibody response. Further, rabbit polyclonal antibodies to HRES-1/p28 were bound by the HTLV-1 *gag* p24 protein. Shattles et al. found monoclonal anti-HTLV-1 *gag* p19 antibody to bind the ductal epithelia in labial salivary glands in 31% of 39 SS patients *(94)*. Together with the finding that salivary glands in SS patients contain no HTLV-1 *gag* gene, these results indicate that an endogenous retroviral protein, HRES-1, may serve as the autoantigen responsible for eliciting autoantibodies that crossreact with HTLV-1 *gag* antigens.

A similar account was reported for HIV: 30–33% SS patients showed serum antibody to HIV *gag* p24 protein *(95,96)*. A MAb to HIV *gag* p24 showed reactivity with epithelia in the labial salivary gland from seven of 15 SS patients, but from none of 10 control subjects. The HIV *gag* gene was not detected in the salivary gland or the peripheral blood of SS patients *(96)*. These results also raise the possibility that an unknown retrovirus is present in salivary glands that may contribute to the pathogenesis of SS.

An example of molecular mimicry between a virus and a native autoantigen may apply to SS: a sequence homology exists between one of the major antigenic determinants of the SS–A/Ro 60 kDa protein (EYRKK) and a nucleocapsid protein of vesicular stomatitis virus (VSV) *(97)*. Twenty eight of 45 (62%) of anti-SS–A/Ro antibody-positive sera from patients with SS and rheumatic disease reacted with a fragment (13 kDa) of VSV *(98)*. A subsequent study using a synthetic peptide (EYRKKMDI) containing the common sequence indicated that the crossreactive antibodies account for only a minority of the anti-SS–A/Ro 60-kDa autoantibodies *(99)*. Another example is the SS–B/La protein, with which a feline sarcoma virus *gag* polyprotein has some homology *(100)*.

5. FUTURE DIRECTIONS

Taken together, the studies summarized in this review suggest that SS and related autoimmune diseases are characterized by multiple sequelae. The primary causes of the different diseases are probably multiple in nature. A variety of factors can potentially modify the pathogenesis of the autoimmune reaction. It is impossible at this time to identify single parameters or combinations of parameters that explain the pathogenesis of SS or permit its unequivocal diagnosis. Nonetheless, immune responses to autoantigen(s) clearly play an important role in SS pathogenesis. The identification of key autoantigens recognized by autoreactive T-cells and autoantibodies will be a critical step in understanding SS.

To date, seven continuous and discontinuous antigenic epitopes have been identified for the SS–A/Ro protein *(101)*. Four continuous and one discontinuous epitopes of the SS–B/La protein are described *(102,103)*. Sumida et al. *(104,105)* produced T-cell lines reactive with the 52-kDa SS–A/Ro from cells that infiltrate labial salivary glands of patients with SS, and showed that a restricted peptide region of this antigen can stimulate some T-cell lines. There are no reports concerning the T-cell epitopes of the SS–B/La protein. Further studies, especially of T-cell epitopes recognized by CD4+ T-cells infiltrating salivary glands or lacrimal glands in patients with SS, are needed.

One possible approach to define additional target antigens is to purify MHC class II molecules from the ductal epithelial cells in the inflamed glands of SS patients and to sequence the peptides bound to the class II molecules. Freed et al. successfully identified the tissue-specific self peptides bound to specific MHC class II molecules *(106)*. In the case of SS, this approach requires the use of pure ductal cells without contamination of antigen presenting cells (APC), which might be difficult to achieve. Other possible approaches include the screening of random peptide or phage display libraries for binding by a specific TCR (i.e., Vβ2) or MHC class II molecule (i.e., DR3) *(107)*, or the screening of cDNA expression libraries from the ductal cells transfected into APC for the ability to stimulate T-cells from SS patients.

Induction of oral tolerance to autoantigens has succeeded in animal models of T-cell-mediated autoimmune disease, including RA, multiple sclerosis, uveitis, and diabetes *(see* ref. *108)*. Further, clinical trials to evaluate the therapeutic use of orally administered type II collagen in patients with RA, and of myelin to patients with multiple sclerosis, has yielded some encouraging results *(109,110)*. These successes encourage further work towards identification and characterization of the autoantigens of SS, establishment of animal models for the disease, and investigation of therapeutic approaches, including the induction of tolerance by oral administration of autoantigens.

ACKNOWLEDGMENTS

The authors would like to thank Saburo Onishi for his advice and Kaoru Nishimori for editorial and other helpful assistance. This work was supported by Japan Rheumatism Foundation.

REFERENCES

1. Bloch, K. J., Buchanan, W. W., Wohl, M. J., and Bunim, J. J. (1965) Sjögren's syndrome: a clinical, pathological, and serological study of sixty-two cases. *Medicine* **44**, 187–231.
2. Pavlidis, N. A., Karsh, J., and Moutsopoulos, H. M. (1982) The clinical picture of primary Sjögren's syndrome: a retrospective study. *J. Rhuematol. 9*, 685–690.
3. Fox, R. I. and Kang, H. (1993) Sjögren's syndrome, in *Text Book of Rheumatology* (Kelley, W.N., Harris, E.D., Ruddy, S., and Sledge C.B., eds.), Saunders, Philadelphia, PA, pp. 931–942.
4. Fox, R. I., Howell, F. V., Bone, R. C., and Michelson, P. (1984) Primary Sjogren syndrome: clinical and immunopathologic features. *Semin. Arth. Rheum.* **14**, 77–105.
5. Cummings, N. A., Schall, G. L., Asofsky, R., Anderson, L. G., and Talal, N. (1971) Sjögren's syndrome: newer aspects of research, diagnosis, and therapy. *Ann. Intern. Med.* **75**, 937–950.
6. Moutsopoulos, H. M., Chused, T. M., Mann, D. L., Klippel, J. H., Fauci, A. S., Frank, M. M., et al. (1980) Sjögren's syndrome (Sicca syndrome): current issues. *Ann. Intern. Med.* **92**, 212–226.
7. Harley, J. B. (1989) Autoantibodies in Sjögren's syndrome. *J. Autoimmun.* **2**, 383–394.
8. Harley, J. B., Reichlin, M., Arnett, F. C., Alexander, E. L., Bias, W. B., and Provost, T. T. (1986) Gene interaction at HLA-DQ enhances autoantibody production in primary Sjögren's syndrome. *Science* **232**, 1145–1147.
9. Kang, H., Fei, H. M., Saito, I., Sawada, S., Chen, S., Yi, D., et al. (1993) Comparison of HLA class II genes in Caucasoid, Chinese, and Japanese patients with primary Sjögren's syndrome. *J. Immunol.* **150**, 3615–3623.

10. Arnett, F. C., Goldstein, R., Duvic, M., and Reveille, J. D. (1988) Major histocompatibility complex genes in systemic lupus erythematosus, Sjögren's syndrome, and polymyositis. *Am. J. Med.* **85,** 38–41.

11. Wilson, R. W., Provost, T. T., Bias, W. B., Alexander, E. L., Edlow, D. W., Hochberg, M. C., et al. (1984) Sjögren's syndrome. Influence of multiple HLA-D region alloantigens on clinical and serologic expression. *Arthritis Rheum.* **27,** 1245–1253.

12. Fox, R., Kang, H. I., Ando, D., Abrams, J., and Pisa, E. (1994) Cytokines mRNA expression in salivary gland biopsies of Sjögren's syndrome. *J. Immunol.* **152,** 5532–5539.

13. Fox, R. I., Bumol, T., Fantozzi, R., Bone, R., and Schireiber, R. (1986) Expression of histocompatibility antigen HLA-DR by salivary gland epithelial cells in Sjögren's syndrome. *Arthritis Rheum.* **29,** 1105–1111.

14. Tan, E. M. (1982) Autoantibodies to nuclear antigens (ANA): their immunobiology and medicine. *Adv. Immunol.* **33,** 167–240.

15. Fox, R. I., Chan, E. K., and Kang, H. (1992) Laboratory evaluation of patients with Sjögren's syndrome. *Clin. Biochem.* **25,** 213–222.

16. Alspaugh, M. A., Talal, N., and Tan, E. M. (1976) Differentiation and characterization of autoantibodies and their antigens in Sjögren's syndrome. *Arthritis Rheum.* **19,** 216–222.

17. Kong, L., Ogawa, N., Nakabayashi, T., Liu, G. T., D'Souza, E., McGuff, H. S., et al. (1997) *Fas* and *Fas* ligand expression in the salivary glands of patients with primary Sjögren's syndrome. *Arthritis Rheum.* **40,** 87–97.

18. Sumida, T., Yonaha, F., Maeda, T., Tanabe, E., Koike, T., Tomioka, H., et al. (1992) T cell receptor repertoire of infiltrating T cells in lips of Sjögren's syndrome patients. *J. Clin. Invest.* **89,** 681–685.

19. Smith, M. D., Lamour, A., Boylston, A., Lancaster, F. C., Pennec, Y. L., van Agthoven, A., et al. (1994) Selective expression of Vβ families by T cells in the blood and salivary gland infiltrate of patients with primary Sjögren's syndrome. *J. Rheumatol.* **21,** 1832–1837.

20. Sumida, T., Kita, Y., Yonaha, F., Maeda, T., Iwamoto, I. and Yoshida, S. (1994) T cell receptor V alpha repertoire of infiltrating T cells in labial salivary glands from patients with Sjögren's syndrome. *J. Rheumatol.* **21,** 1655–1661.

21. Matsumoto, I., Tsubota, K., Satake, Y., Kita, Y., Matsumura, R., Murata, H., et al. (1996) Common T cell receptor clonotype in lacrimal glands and labial salivary glands from patients with Sjögren's syndrome. *J. Clin. Invest.* **97,** 1969–1977.

22. Yonaha, Y., Sumida, T., Maeda, T., Tomioka, H., Koike, T. and Yoshida, S. (1992) Restricted junctional usage of T cell receptor Vβ2 and Vβ13 genes, which are overrepresented on infiltrating T cells in the lips of patients with Sjögren's syndrome. *Arthritis Rheum.* **35,** 1362–1367.

23. Sumida, T., Matsumoto, I., Murata, H., Namekawa, T., Matsumura, R., Tomioka, H., et al. (1997) TCR in Fas-sensitive T cells from labial salivary glands of patients with Sjögren's syndrome. *J. Immunol.* **158,** 1020–1025.

24. Alexander, E., Hirsch, T. J., Arnett, F. C., Provost, T. T., and Stevens, M. B. (1982) Ro(SSA) and La(SSB) antibodies in the clinical spectrum of Sjögren's syndrome. *J. Rheumatol.* **9,** 239–246.

25. Fox, R. I., Robinson, C. A., Curd, J. G., Kozin, F., and Howell, F. V. (1986) Sjögren's syndrome: proposed criteria for classification. *Arthritis Rheum.* **29,** 577–585.

26. Vitali, C., Bombardieri, S., Moutsopoulos, H. M., Balestrieri, G., Bencivelli, W., Bernstein, R. M., et al. (1993) Preliminary criteria for the classification of Sjögren's syndrome: results of a prospective concerted action supported by the European Community. *Arthritis Rheum.* **36,** 340–347.

27. Lee, L. A. (1993) Neonatal lupus erythematosus. *J. Invest. Dermatol.* **100,** 9S–13S.

28. Wolin, S. L. and Steitz, J. A. (1983) Genes for two small cytoplasmic Ro DNAs are adjacent and appear to be single-copy in the human genome. *Cell* **32,** 735–744.

29. Ben-Chetrit, E., Chan, E. K. L., Sullivan, K. F., and Tan, E. M. (1988) A 52-kDa protein is a novel component of the SS–A/Ro antigenic particle. *J. Exp. Med.* **167,** 1560–1571.

30. Ben-Chetrit, E., Fox, R. I., and Tan, E. M. (1990) Dissociation of immune responses to the SS–A (Ro) 52-kDa and 60-kDa polypeptides in systemic lupus erythematosus and Sjögren's syndrome. *Arthritis Rheum.* **33,** 349–355.

31. Slobbe, R. L., Pruijn, G. J. M., Damen, W. G. M., van der Kemp, J. W. C. M., and van Venrooij, W. J. (1991) Detection and occurrence of the 60- and 52-kDa Ro (SS–A) antigens and of autoantibodies against these proteins. *Clin. Exp. Immunol.* **86,** 99–105.

32. Rinke, J. and Steiz, J. A. (1982) Precursor molecules of both human 5S ribosomal RNA and transfer RNAs are bound by a cellular protein reactive with anti-La lupus antibodies. *Cell* **29,** 149–159.

33. Boire, G. and Craft, J. (1990) Human Ro ribonucleoprotein particles: characterization of native structure and stable association with the La polypeptide. *J. Clin. Invest.* **85,** 1182–1190.

34. Slobbe, R. L., Pluk, W., van Venrooij, W. J., and Pruijn, G. J. M. (1992) Ro ribonucleoprotein assembly *in vitro*: identification of RNA-protein and protein-protein interactions. *J. Mol. Biol.* **227,** 361–366.

35. Chan, E. K. L., di Donato, F., Hamel, J. C., Tseng, C., and Buyon, J. P. (1995) 52-kDa SS–A/Ro: genomic structure and identification of an alternatively spliced transcript encoding a novel leucine zipper-minus autoantigen expressed in fetal and adult heart. *J. Exp. Med.* **182,** 983–992.

36. Baboonian, C., Venables, P. J. W., Booth, J., Williams, D. G., Roffe, L. M., and Maini, R.N. (1989) Virus infection induces redistribution and membrane localization of the nuclear antigen La (SSB): a possible mechanism for autoimmunity. *Clin. Exp. Immunol.* **78,** 454–459.

37. Bachmann, M., Althoff, H., Tröster, H., Selenka, C., Falke, D., and Müller, W. E. G. (1992) Translocation of the nuclear autoantigen La to the cell surface of herpes simplex virus type I infected cells. *Autoimmunity* **12,** 37–45.

38. de Wilde, P. C. M., Kater, L., Bodeutsch, C., van den Hoogen, F. H., van de Putte, L. B. A., and van Venrooij, W. J. (1996) Aberrant expression pattern of the SS–B/La antigen in the labial salivary gland of patients with Sjögren's syndrome. *Arthritis Rheum.* **39,** 783–791.

39. Yannopoulos, D. I., Roncin, S., Lamour, A., Pennec, Y. L., Moutsopoulos, H. M., and Youinou, P. (1992) Conjunctival epithelial cells from patients with Sjögren's syndrome inappropriately express major histocompatibility complex molecules, La(SSB) antigen, and heat-shock proteins. *J. Clin. Immunol.* **12,** 259–265.

40. Shastri, K. A. and Logue, G. L. (1993) Autoimmune neutropenia. *Blood* **81,** 1984–1995.

41. Boros, P., Odin, J. A., Chen, J., and Unkeless, J. C. (1994) Specificity and class distribution of FcγR-specific autoantibodies in patients with autoimmune disease. *J. Immunol.* **152**, 302–306.
42. Lamour, A., Le Corre, R., Pennec, Y. L., Carton, J., and Youinou, P. (1995) Heterogeneity of neutrophil antibodies in patients with primary Sjögren's syndrome. *Blood* **86**, 3553–3559.
43. Boros, P., Muryoi, T., Spiera, H., Bona, C., and Unkeless, J. C. (1993) Autoantibodies directed against different classes of FcγR are found in sera of autoimmune patients. *J. Immunol.* **150**, 2018–2024.
44. Feltkamp, T. E. W. and van Rossum, A. L. (1968) Antibodies to salivary duct cells, and other autoantibodies, in patients with Sjögren's syndrome and other idiopathic autoimmune diseases. *Clin. Exp. Immunol.* **3**, 1–16.
45. Anderson, L. G., Tarpley, T. M., Talal, N., Cummings, N. A., Wolf, R. O., and Schall, G. L. (1973) Cellular-versus-humoral autoimmune responses to salivary gland in Sjögren's syndrome. *Clin. Exp. Immunol.* **13**, 335–342.
46. Ludwig, H., Schernthaner, G., Scherak, O., and Kolarz, G. (1977) Antibodies to pancreatic duct cells in Sjögren's syndrome and rheumatoid arthritis. *Gut* **18**, 311–315.
47. Sundkvist, G., Lindahl, G., Koskinen, P., and Bolinder, J. (1991) Pancreatic autoantibodies and pancreatic function in Sjögren's syndrome. *J. Intern. Med.* **229**, 61–66.
48. Sheikh, S. H. and Shaw-Stiffel, T. A. (1995) The gastrointestinal manifestations of Sjögren's syndrome. *Am. J. Gastroenterol.* **90**, 9–14.
49. Skopouli, F. N., Barbatis, C., and Moutsopoulos, H. M. (1994) Liver involvement in primary Sjögren's syndrome. *Brit. J. Rheumatol.* **33**, 745–748.
50. Nishimori, I., Morita, M., Kino, J., Onodera, M., Nakazawa, Y., Okazaki, K., et al. (1995) Pancreatic involvement in patients with Sjögren's syndrome and primary biliary cirrhosis. *Int. J. Pancreatol.* **17**, 47–54.
51. Price, E. J. and Venables, P. J. W. (1995) The etiopathogenesis of Sjögren's syndrome. *Semin. Arth. Rheum.* **25**, 117–133.
52. Nakanuma, Y. and Ohta, G. (1979) Histometric and serial section observations of the intrahepatic bile ducts in primary biliary cirrhosis. *Gastroenterology* **76**, 1326–1332.
53. Sarles, H., Sarles, J. C., Muratore, R., and Guien, C. (1961) Chronic inflammatory sclerosis of the pancreas: an autonomous pancreatic disease? *Am. J. Dig. Dis.* **6**, 688–698.
54. Ballardini, G., Mirakian, R., Bianchi, F. B., Pisi, E., Doniach, D., and Bottazzo, G. F. (1984) Aberrant expression of HLA-DR antigens on bile duct epithelium in primary biliary cirrhosis: relevance to pathogenesis. *Lancet* **2**, 1009–1013.
55. Bovo, P., Mirakian, R., Merigo, F., Angelini, G., Cavallini, G., Rizzini, P., et al. (1987) HLA molecule expression on chronic pancreatitis specimens: is there a role for autoimmunity? *Pancreas* **2**, 350–356.
56. Jalleh, R. P., Gilbertson, J. A., Williamson, R. C. N., Slater, S. D., and Foster, C. S. (1993) Expression of major histocompatibility antigens in human chronic pancreatitis. *Gut* **34**, 1452–1457.
57. Strand, V. and Talal, N. (1980) Advances in the diagnosis and concept of Sjögren's syndrome (autoimmune exocrinopahty). *Bull. Rheum. Dis.* **30**, 1046–1052.

58. Epstein, O., Chapman, R. W. G., Lake-Bakaar, G., Foo, A. Y., Rosalki, S. B., and Sherlock, S. (1982) The pancreas in primary biliary cirrhosis and primary sclerosing cholangitis. *Gastroenterology* **83,** 1177–1182.
59. Moutsopulos, H. M. (1994) Sjögren's syndrome: autoimmune epithelitis. *Clin. Immunol. Immunopathol.* **72,** 162–165.
60. Kino-Ohsaki, J., Nishimori, I., Morita, M., Okazaki, K., Yamamoto, Y., Onishi, S., et al. (1996) Serum antibodies to carbonic anhydrase I and II in patients with idiopathic chronic pancreatitis and Sjögren's syndrome. *Gastroenterology* **110,** 1579–1586.
61. Tsuneyama, K., Van deWater, J., Nakanuma, Y., Cha, S., Ansari, A., Coppel, R., et al. (1994) Human combinational autoantibodies and mouse monoclonal antibodies to PDC-E2 produce abnormal apical staining of salivary glands in patients with coexis-tent primary biliary cirrhosis and Sjögren's syndrome. *Hepatology* **20,** 893–898.
62. Nishimori, I., Yamamoto, Y., Okazaki, K., Morita, M., Onodera, M., Kino, J., et al. (1994) Identification of autoantibodies to a pancreatic antigen in patients with idiopathic chronic pancreatitis and Sjögren's syndrome. *Pancreas* **9,** 374–381.
63. Nishimori, I., Okazaki, K., Yamamoto, Y., Morita, M., Tamura, S., and Yamamoto, Y. (1992) Sensitization against pancreatic antigen in Sjögren's syndrome and chronic pancreatitis. *Digestion* **51,** 71–74.
64. Nishimori, I., Okazaki, K., Yamamoto, Y., Morita, M., Tamura, S., and Yamamoto, Y. (1993) Specific cellular immune responses to pancreatic antigen in chronic pancreatitis and Sjögren's syndrome. *J. Clin. Immunol.* **13,** 265–271.
65. Nishimori, I., Bratanova, T., Toshkov, I., Caffrey, T., Mogaki, M., Shibata, Y., et al. (1995) Induction of experimental autoimmune sialoadenitis by immunization of PL/J mice with carbonic anhydrase II. *J. Immunol.* **154,** 4865–4873.
66. Inagaki, Y., Jinno-Yoshida, Y., Hamasaki, Y., and Ueki, H. (1991) A novel autoantibody reactive with carbonic anhydrase in sera from patients with systemic lupus erythematosus and Sjögren's syndrome. *J. Dermatol. Sci.* **2,** 147–154.
67. Itoh, Y. and Reichlin, M. (1992) Antibodies to carbonic anhydrase in systemic lupus erythematosus and other rheumatic diseases. *Arthritis Rheum.* **35,** 73–82.
68. Gordon, S. G., Quattrociocchi-Longe, T. M., Khan, B. A., Kodali, V. P. Chen, J., Silverman, A. L., et al. (1995) Antibodies to carbonic anhydrase in patients with immune cholangitis. *Gastroenterology* **108,** 1802–1809.
69. Tsianos, E. V., Hoofnagle, J. H., Fox, P. C., Alspaugh, M., Jones, E. A., Schafer, D. F., et al. (1990) Sjögren's syndrome in patients with primary biliary cirrhosis. *Hepatology* **11,** 730–734.
70. Uddenfeldt, P., Danielsson, Å., Forssell, Å., Holm, M., and Östberg, Y. (1991) Features of Sjögren's syndrome in patients wtih primary biliary cirrhosis. *J. Intern. Med.* **230,** 443–448.
71. Teoh, K., Rowley, M. J., Zafirakis, H., Dickson, E. R., Wiesner, R. H., Gershwin, M. R., et al. (1994) Enzyme inhibitory autoantibodies to pyruvate dehydrogenase complex in primary biliary cirrhosis: applications of a semiautomatched assay. *Hepatology* **20,** 1220–1224.
72. Zurgil, N., Bakimer, R., Moutsopoulos, H. M., Tzioufas, A. G., Youinou, P., Isenberg, D. A., et al. (1992) Antimitochondrial (pyruvate dehydrogenase) auto-antibodies in autoimmune rheumatic diseases. *J. Clin. Immunol.* **12,** 201–209.
73. Surh, C. D., Ahmed-Ansari, A., and Gershwin, M. E. (1990) Comparative epitope mapping of murine monoclonal and human autoantibodies to human PDH-E2, the major mitochondrial autoantigen of primary biliary cirrhosis. *J. Immunol.* **144,** 2647–2652.

74. Haneji, N., Hamano, H., Yanagi, K., and Hayashi, Y. (1994) A new animal model for primary Sjögren's syndrome in NFS/*sld* mutant mice. *J. Immunol.* **153**, 2769–2777.
75. Haneji, N., Nakamura, T., Takio, K., Yanagi, K., Higashiyama, H., Saito, I., et al. (1997) Identification of α-fodrin as a candidate autoantigen in primary Sjögren's syndrome. *Science* **276**, 604–607.
76. Glenney, J. R., Glenney, P., and Weber, K. (1982) F-actin-binding and cross-linking properties of porcine brain fodrin, a spectrin-related molecule. *J. Biol. Chem.* **257**, 9781–9787.
77. Moll, J. W. B., Markusse, H. M., Pijnenburg, J. J. J. M., Vecht, Ch.J., and Henzen-Logmans, S. C. (1993) Antineuronal antibodies in patients with neurologic complications of primary Sjögren's syndrome. *Neurology* **43**, 2574–2581.
78. Graus, F., Cordon-Cardo, C., and Posner, J. B. (1985) Neuronal antinuclear antibody in sensory neuropathy from lung cancer. *Neurology* **35**, 538–543.
79. Dalmau, J., Furneaux, H. M., Gralla, R. J., Kris, M. G., and Posner, J. B. (1990) Detection of the anti-Hu antibody in the serum of patients with small cell lung cancer–a quantitative Western blot analysis. *Ann. Neurol.* **27**, 544–552.
80. Szabo, A., Dalmau, J., Manley, G., Rosenfeld, M., Wong, E., Henson, J., et al. (1991) HuD, a paraneoplastic encephalomyelitis antigen, contains RNA-binding domains and is homologous to Elav and Sex-lethal. *Cell* **67**, 325–333.
81. Manley, G., Wong, E., Dalmau, J., Elkon, K., Posner, J., and Furneaux, H. (1994) Sera from some patients with antibody-associated paraneoplastic encephalomyelitis/ sensory neuropathy recognize the Ro-52K antigen. *J. Neuro-Oncol.* **19**, 105–112.
82. Spezialetti, R., Bluestein, H. G., Peter, J. B., and Alexander, E. L. (1993) Neuropsychiatric disease in Sjögren's syndrome: anti-ribosomal P and anti-neuronal antibodies. *Am. J. Med.* **95**, 153–160.
83. Sillevis-Smitt, P., Manley, G., Moll, J. W. B., Dalmau, J., and Posner, J. B. (1996) Pitfalls in the diagnosis of autoantibodies associated with paraneoplastic neurologic disease. *Neurology* **46**, 1739–1741.
84. Wolf, H., Haus, M., and Wilmes, E. (1984) Persistence of Epstein–Barr virus in the parotid gland. *J. Virol.* **51**, 795–798.
85. Slaughter, L., Carson, D.A., Jensen, F. C., Holbrook, T. L. and Vaughan, J. H. (1978) In vitro effects of Epstein–Barr virus on peripheral blood mononuclear cells from patients with rheumatoid arthritis and normal subjects. *J. Exp. Med.* **148**, 1429–1434.
86. Fox, R. I., Pearson, G., and Vaughan, J. H. (1986) Detection of Epstein–Barr virus-associated antigens and DNA in salivary gland biopsies from patients with Sjögren's syndrome. *J. Immunol.* **137**, 3162–3168.
87. Saito, I., Servenius, B., Compton, T., and Fox, R. I. (1989) Detection of Epstein–Barr virus DNA by polymerase chain reaction in blood and tissue biopsies from patients with Sjogren's syndrome. *J. Exp. Med.* **169**, 2191–2198.
88. Mariette, X., Gozlan, J., Clerc, D., Bisson, M., and Morinet, F. (1991) Detection of Epstein–Barr virus DNA by in situ hybridization and polymerase chain reaction in salivary gland biopsy specimens from patients with Sjögren's syndrome. *Am. J. Med.* **90**, 286–294.
89. Pflugfelder, S. C., Crouse, C. A., Monroy, D., Yen, M., Rowe, M., and Atherton, S. S. (1993) Epstein-Barr virus and the lacrimal gland pathology of Sjögren's syndrome. *Am. J. Pathol.* **143**, 49–64.
90. Mariette, X., Agbalika, F., Daniel, M. T., Bisson, M., Lagrange, P., Brouet, J. C., et al. (1993) Detection of human T lymphotropic virus type I *tax* gene in salivary gland epithelium from two patients with Sjögren's syndrome. *Arthritis Rheum.* **36**, 1423–1428.

91. Sumida, T., Yonaha, F., Maeda, T., Kita, Y., Iwamoto, I., Koike, T., et al. (1994) Expression of sequences homologous to HTLV-1 *tax* gene in the labial salivary glands of Japanese patients with Sjögren's syndrome. *Arthritis Rheum.* **37,** 545–550.
92. Brookes, S. M., Pandolfino, Y. A., Mitchell, T. J., Venables, P. J. W., Shattles, W. G., Clark, D. A., et al. (1992) The immune response to and expression of cross-reactive retroviral gag sequences in autoimmune disease. *Br. J. Rheum.* **31,** 735–742.
93. Banki, K., Maceda, J., Hurley, E., Ablonczy, E., Mattson, D. H., Szegedy, L., Hung, C., and Perl, A. (1992) Human T-cell lymphotropic virus (HTLV)-related endogenous sequence, HRES-1, encodes a 28-kDa protein: a possible autoantigen for HTLV-1 *gag*-reactive autoantibodies. *Proc. Natl. Acad. Sci. USA* **89,** 1939–1943.
94. Shattles, W. G., Brookes, S. M., Venables, P. J. W., Clark, D. A., and Maini, R. N. (1992) Expression of antigen reactive with a monoclonal antibody to HTLV-1 p19 in salivary glands in Sjögren's syndrome. *Clin. Exp. Immunol.* **89,** 46–51.
95. Talal, N., Dauphinée, M. J., Dang, H., Alexander, S. S., Hart, D. J., and Garry, R. F. (1990) Detection of serum antibodies to retroviral proteins in patients with primary Sjögren's syndrome (autoimmune exocrinopathy). *Arthritis Rheum.* **33,** 774–781.
96. Yamano, S., Renard, J. N., Mizuno, F., Narita, Y., Uchida, Y., Higashiyama, H., et al. (1997) Retrovirus in salivary glands from patients with Sjögren's syndrome. *J. Clin. Pathol.* **50,** 223–230.
97. Scofield, R. H. and Harley, J. B. (1991) Autoantigenicity of Ro/SSA antigen is related to a nucleocapsid protein of vesicular stomatitis virus. *Proc. Natl. Acad. Sci. USA* **88,** 3343–3347.
98. Scofield, R. H., Dickey, W. D., Jackson, K. W., James, J. A., and Harley, J. B. (1991) A common autoepitope near the carboxyl terminus of the 60-kD Ro ribonucleoprotein: sequence similarity with a viral protein. *J. Clin. Immunol.* **11,** 378–388.
99. Routsias, J. G., Sakarellos-Daitsiotis, M., Detsikas, E., Tzioufas, A. G., Sakarellos, C., and Moutsopoulos, H. M. (1994) Antibodies to EYRKK vesicular stomatitis virus-related peptide account only for a minority of anti-Ro60kD antibodies. *Clin. Exp. Immunol.* **98,** 414–418.
100. Kohsaka, H., Yamamoto, K., Fujii, H., Miura, H., Miyasaka, N., Nishioka, K., et al. (1990) Fine epitope mapping of the human SS-B/La protein: identification of a distinct autoepitope homologous to a viral *gag* polyprotein. *J. Clin. Invest.* **85,** 1566–1574.
101. Saitta, M. R., Arnett, F. C., and Keene, J. D. (1994) 60-kDa Ro protein autoepitopes identified using recombinant polypeptides. *J. Immunol.* **152,** 4192–4202.
102. Tzioufas, A. G., Yiannaki, E., Sakarellos-Daitsiotis, M., Routsias, J. G., Sakarellos, C., and Moutsopoulos, H. M. (1997) Fine specificity of autoantibodies to La/SSB: epitope mapping, and characterization. *Clin. Exp. Immunol.* **108,** 191–198.
103. Rischmueller, M., McNeilage, L. J., McCluskey, J., and Gordon, T. (1995) Human autoantibodies directed against the RNA recognition motif of La (SS-B) bind to a conformational epitope present on the intact La (SS-B)/Ro (SS-A) ribonucleoprotein particle. *Clin. Exp. Immunol.* **101,** 39–44.
104. Namekawa, T., Kuroda, K., Kato, T., Yamamoto, K., Murata, H., Sakamaki, T., et al. (1995) Identification of Ro (SSA) 52 kDa reactive T cells in labial salivary glands from patients with Sjögren's syndrome. *J. Rheumatol.* **22,** 2092–2099.
105. Sumida, T., Namekawa, T., Maeda, T., and Nishioka, K. (1996) New T-cell epitope of Ro/SS-A 52 kDa protein in labial salivary glands from patients with Sjögren's syndrome. *Lancet* **348,** 1667.

106. Freed, J. H. and Marrack, P. (1993) Tissue-specific expression of self peptides bound by major histocompatibility complex class II molecules, in *Chemical Immunology: Naturally Processed Peptides* (Sette, A. ed.), Karger, Basel, Germany, pp. 88–112.
107. Fujisao, S., Matsushita, S., Nishi, T., and Nishimura, Y. (1996) Identification of HLA-DR9 (DRB*0901)-binding peptide motifs using a phage fUSE5 random peptide library. *Hum. Immunol.* **45,** 131–136.
108. Weiner, H. L., Friedman, A., Miller, A., Khoury, S. J., Al-Sabbagh, A., Santos, L., et al. (1994) Oral tolerance: immunologic mechanisms and treatment of animal and human organ-specific autoimmune diseases by oral administration of autoantigens. *Ann. Rev. Immunol.* **12,** 809–837.
109. Trentham, D. E., Dynesius-Trentham, R. A., Orav, E. J., Combitchi, D., Lorenzo, C., Sewell, K. L., et al. (1993) Effects of oral administration of type II collagen on rheumatoid arthritis. *Science* **261,** 1727–1730.
110. Weiner, H. L., Mackin, G. A., Matsui, M., Orav, E. J., Khoury, S. J., Dawson, D. M., et al. (1993) Double-blind pilot trial of oral tolerization with myelin antigens in multiple sclerosis. *Science* **259,** 1321–1324.

6

Autoimmunity in Patients with Essential Hypertension

Israel Rubinstein

1. INTRODUCTION

Essential hypertension remains a major cause of morbidity and mortality world-wide despite improvements in its detection and treatment *(1–4)*. In addition, the economic impact of essential hypertension on the community is enormous, consisting of days out of work and increase in medical expense. Diverse mechanisms may underlie the pathogenesis and evolution of essential hypertension in individual subgroups of patients *(2,3)*. It is important to unveil these processes so that appropriate therapy can be designed for essential hypertension.

2. IMMUNOLOGICAL ABNORMALITIES

There is growing evidence that cellular and humoral immunity may be involved in the pathogenesis and/or evolution of essential hypertension in human subjects *(5–7)*. For instance, genes located in the major histocompatibility complex, such as HLA-B8, HLA-B12 and HLA-B15, are thought to be predisposing factors towards the development of essential hypertension in individuals from different ethnic backgrounds *(8–13)*. Kristensen *(14)* showed that patients with essential hypertension who are positive for HLA-B15 are 3.4-fold times more prone to develop vascular complications than are hypertensive patients negative for HLA-B15.

Patients with essential hypertension are reported to display elevated serum immunoglobulin levels, enhanced secretion of immunoglobulins, increased amounts of autoantibodies to nuclear antigens and smooth muscle cells, increased activity of sensitized T-lymphocytes, and hyporesponsiveness of suppressor T-lymphocytes to mitogenic stimuli *(7,15–24)*. Caforio et al. *(25)* showed that among patients with autoimmune polyendocrinopathy without overt cardiac disease, the prevalence of systemic hypertension and a family history of hypertension was higher in individuals positive for cardiac autoantibodies than in the autoantibody negative subgroup.

Several investigators have reported that patients with essential hypertension display increased T-lymphocyte responses to human arterial wall antigens relative to patients with secondary hypertension or normotensive controls *(7,18,*

Contemporary Immunology: Autoimmune Reactions
Edited by: S. Paul © Humana Press Inc., Totowa, NJ

26,27). In addition, Rivera et al. *(28)* showed recently that peripheral blood lymphocytes from a subgroup of patients with essential hypertension have elevated levels of cytosolic calcium.

The functional significance of T-lymphocyte dysfunction and autoantibodies in patients with essential hypertension is uncertain. Kristensen et al. *(21,22,27)* showed that the presence of antinuclear and smooth muscle antibodies tripled the five-year risk of vascular events in patients with essential hypertension. Fu et al. *(29)* detected autoantibodies of the IgM class in subgroups of patients with essential hypertension directed against an epitope on the second extracellular loop of the human α_1-adrenergic receptor, which is thought to play a role in regulation of systemic arterial pressure *(30)*. These autoantibodies were found to interfere with the signal transducing function of the receptor. The response was specific because there was no reaction of the autoantibodies with an M_2-muscarinic receptor peptide, which is an unrelated target for autoantibodies in some patients with idiopathic dilated cardiomyopathy *(31)*. Interestingly, antiphospholipid antibodies have been previously shown to attenuate production of prostacyclin, a potent vasodilator, and to elicit hypertension *(32,33)*.

An association between the development of essential hypertension and two key components of the immune system, the complement cascade and circulating leukocytes, has been reported in human subjects *(34–36)*. The presence of the complement C3-F allele and an increase in the number of circulating leukocytes were independently associated with an increased risk of developing essential hypertension *(34,36)*. The mechanisms whereby these processes predispose to the development of essential hypertension are uncertain.

3. CONCLUSION

On balance, these data outlined above suggest that genetically governed autoimmune process(es), alone or in combination with other factors, may alter the function and/or structure of arteriolar wall in the peripheral vasculature, the anatomic site regulating peripheral vascular resistance, which could then predispose certain patients to hypertension.

This hypothesis notwithstanding, several key questions regarding the role of the immune system in the pathogenesis and/or evolution of essential hypertension in human subjects remain to be answered. Is the autoimmune process(es) specific for essential hypertension or is it merely an epiphenomenon caused by ongoing vascular damage and disease progression *(22)*? Is there an HLA-mediated genetic background(s) that predisposes patients to so-called autoimmune essential hypertension? What are the specific vascular and extravascular targets for the autoimmune attack? Do the salutary effects of antihypertensive agents such as angiotensin I-converting enzyme inhibitors *(37)*, derive, in part, from their ability to suppress autoimmune manifestations in patients with essential hypertension? Should patients with essential hypertension and autoimmune manifestations be treated with immunosuppressive medications when conventional antihypertensive therapy fails? These issues remain to be addressed in carefully designed clinical studies aimed at elucidating the role of autoimmunity in essential hypertension.

ACKNOWLEDGMENT

This study was supported, in part, by grants from the National Institutes of Health (DE10347), American Heart Association of Metropolitan Chicago, and Laerdal Foundation for Acute Medicine. Israel Rubinstein is a recipient of a Research Career Development Award from the National Institutes of Health (DE00386) and a University of Illinois Scholar Award.

REFERENCES

1. Kannel, W. B. (1996) Blood pressure as a cardiovascular risk factor: prevention and treatment. *JAMA* **275**, 1571–1576.
2. Menotti, A., Jacobs, D. R., Jr., Blackburn, H., Kromhout, D., Nissinen, A., Nedeljkovic, S., et al. (1996) Twenty-five-year prediction of stroke deaths in the seven countries study: the role of blood pressure and its changes. *Stroke* **27**, 381–387.
3. Gueyffier, F., Froment, A., and Gouton, M. (1996) New meta-analysis of treatment trials of hypertension: improving the estimate of therapeutic benefit. *J. Hypertens.* **10**, 1–8.
4. Rastenyte, D., Tuomilehto, J., Domarkiene, S., Cepaitis, Z., and Reklaitiene, R. (1996) Risk factors for death from stroke in middle-aged Lithuanian men: results from a 20-year prospective study. *Stroke* **27**, 672–676.
5. Dzielak, D. J. (1991) Immune mechanisms in experimental and essential hypertension. *Am. J. Physiol.* **260**, R459–R467.
6. Khraibi, A. A. (1991) Association between disturbances in the immune system and hypertension. *Am. J. Hypertens.* **4**, 635–641.
7. Gudbrandsson, T., Hansson, L., Herlitz, H., Lindholm, L. and Nilsson, L.-Å. (1981) Immunological changes in patients with previous malignant essential hypertension. *Lancet* **i**, 406–408.
8. Gerbase-Delima, M., De Lima, J. J. G., Persoli, L. B., Silfva, H. B., Marcondes, M., and Bellotti, G. (1989) Essential hypertension and histocompatibility antigens. A linkage study. *Hypertension* **14**, 604–609.
9. Kristensen, B. Ø., Andersen, P. L., Lamm, L. U., and Kissmeyer-Nielsen, F. (1977) HLA-antigens in essential hypertension. *Tissue Antigens* **10**, 70–74.
10. Gubrandsson, T., Herlitz, H., Hansson, L., and Rydberg, L. (1980) Human leucocyte antigens in patients with previous essential malignant hypertension. *Clin. Sci.* **59**, 431–434.
11. Gelsthorpe, K., Doughty, R. W., Bing, R. F., O'Malley, B. C., Smith, A. J., and Talbot, S. (1975) HLA-antigens in essential hypertension. *Lancet* **i**, 1039–1040.
12. Fernandez-Cruz, A., Otero, M. L., Perez, L. L., Pinilla, C. F., and Claros, N. M. (1981) HLA-antigens in Spanish patients with essential hypertension. *Clin. Sci.* **61**, 367–368.
13. Gaulde, N., Michel, J. P., and Safar, M. E. (1978) Immunogenetics and hypertension. *Lancet* **ii**, 897.

14. Kristensen, B. Ø. (1979) Autoantibodies in untreated and treated essential hypertension: relationship to histocompatibility leucocyte antigen-B15 and vascular complications. *Clin. Sci.* **57**(Suppl 5), 287s–290s.
15. Hilme, E., Herlitz, H., Söderström, T., and Hansson, L. (1989) Increased secretion of immunoglobulins in malignant hypertension. *J. Hypertens.* **7**, 91–95.
16. Wilson, J. D., Bullock, J. Y., and Booth, R. J. (1978) Autoantibodies in essential hypertension. *Lancet* **ii**, 996.
17. Kristensen, B. Ø. and Andersen, P. L. (1978) Autoantibodies in untreated and treated essential hypertension. *Acta Med. Scand.* **203**, 55–59.
18. Lefkos, N., Boura, P., Boudonas, G., Zacharioudaki, E., Efthimiadis, A., Tsougas, M., et al. (1995) Immunopathogenic mechanisms in hypertension. *Am. J. Hypertens.* **8**, 1141–1145.
19. Hilme, E., Hansson, L., Sandberg, L., Söderström, T., and Herlitz, H. (1993) Abnormal immune function in malignant hypertension. *J. Hypertens.* **11**, 989–994.
20. Amenos, M. A., Buendia, E., Carreras, I., Font, I., Mestre, M., Rama, H., et al. (1985) Humoral and cellular immunological abnormalities in hypertensive patients. *Am. J. Hypertens.* **2**, 153–160.
21. Kristensen, B. Ø., Andersen, P. L., and Wiik, A. (1984) Autoantibodies and vascular events in essential hypertension: a five-year longitudinal study. *J. Hypertens.* **2**, 19–24.
22. Kristensen, B. Ø. and Solling, K. (1983) Serum concentrations of immunoglobulins and free light chains before and after vascular events in essential hypertension. *Acta Med. Scand.* **213**, 15-20.
23. Kristensen, B. Ø. and Andersen, P. L. (1978) Autoantibodies in untreated and treated essential hypertension. *Acta Med. Scand.* **203**, 55–59.
24. Olsen, F., Hilden, M., and Ibsen, H. (1973) Raised levels of immunoglobulins in serum of hypertensive patients. *Acta Med. Scand.* **81**, 775–778.
25. Caforio, A. L., Wagner, R., Gill, J. S., Bonifacio, E., Bosi, E., Miles, A., et al. (1991) Organ-specific cardiac antibodies: serological markers for systemic hypertension in autoimmune polyendocrinopathy. *Lancet* **337**, 1111–1115.
26. Olsen, F. (1991) Hypersensitivity of delayed type in hypertensive patients. *APMIS* **99**, 65–68.
27. Kristensen, B. Ø. (1984) Aspects of immunology and immunogenetics in human essential hypertension with special reference to vascular events. *J. Hypertens.* **2**, 571–579.
28. Rivera, A., Conlin, P. R., Williams, G. H., and Canessa, M. L. (1996) Elevated lymphocyte cytosolic calcium in a subgroup of essential hypertensive subjects. *Hypertension* **28**, 213–218.
29. Fu, M. L. X., Herlitz, H., Wallakat, G., Hilme, E., Hedner, T., Hoebeke, J., et al. (1994) Functional autoimmune epitope in α_1-adrenergic receptors in patients with malignant hypertension. *Lancet* **344**, 1660–1663.
30. Martin, C., Brodde, O-E., and Insel, P. A. (1990) Peripheral adrenergic receptors in hypertension. *Hypertension* **16**, 107–120.
31. Fu, L. X., Magnusson, Y., Bergh, C-H., Waagstein F., Hjalmarson, Å., and Hoebeke, J. (1993) Localization of a functional autoimmune epitope on the second extracellular loop of the human muscarinic receptor in patients with idiopathic dilated cardiomyopathy. *J. Clin. Invest.* **91**, 1964–1968.

32. Carreras, L. and Vermylen, J. (1981) Lupus anticoagulant and prostacyclin. *Lancet* **i**, 665.
33. Dudley, D. J., Mitchell, M. D., and Branch, D. W. (1990) Pathophysiology of antiphospholipid antibodies: absence of prostaglandin-mediated effect on cultured endothelium. *Am. J. Obstet. Gynecol.* **162,** 953–959.
34. Schaadt, O., Sorensen, H., and Krogsgaard, A. R. (1981) Association between the C3-F gene and essential hypertension. *Clin. Sci.* **61**(Suppl 7), 363s–365s.
35. Kristensen, B. Ø. and Petersen, P. L. (1978) Association between coronary heart disease and the CF-3 gene in essential hypertension. *Circulation* **58,** 622–625.
36. Friedman, G. D., Selby, J. V., and Quesenberry, C. P., Jr. (1990) The leukocyte count: a predictor of hypertension. *J. Clin. Epidemiol.* **43,** 907–911.
37. Shasha, S. M., Nusam, D., Labin, L., Kristal, B., Steinberger, O., Barzilai, M., et al. (1992) Effect of converting enzyme inhibitor captopril on T cell functions in essential hypertension. *Nephron* **59,** 586–590.

7

Autoimmune Antigen Presentation Mechanisms

Edward Dwyer

1. ANTIGEN PRESENTATION AND PROCESSING

Cell-mediated immunity involves a process whereby specific T-lymphocytes recognize a particular antigenic peptide as foreign, and thereby initiate a response whose goal is the elimination of the microbial source of the recognized foreign antigen. The capacity to recognize a peptide antigen as "foreign" necessarily implies a complementary ability to also recognize host antigens as "self." Autoimmune disease results when this discriminatory process is disturbed and there ensues an immune response, the outcome of which is the elimination of "self."

1.1. Antigen Presentation

T-cells do not detect peptide antigens as isolated entities, but rather are recognized in association with membrane-bound heterodimeric molecules of the major histocompatibility complex (MHC). More specifically, CD8 T-cells recognize antigenic peptides in association with polymorphic MHC class I heterodimers (e.g., HLA-A,B,C), which are formed from a 43-kDa class I molecule complexed with the 12-kDa β-microglobulin molecule, and are expressed on the surface of all nucleated cells in the body. In contrast, CD4 T-cells recognize antigen in the context of polymorphic MHC class II heterodimers (e.g., HLA-DR, DQ,DP), which are composed of a 34-kDa α-chain and a 29-kDa β-chain. These molecules are expressed on the surface of professional antigen-presenting cells (APC), e.g., macrophages, dendritic cells, and B-lymphocytes. In general, peptides associated with MHC class I are 8–10 amino acids in length while those associated with MHC class II are 12–25 amino acids in length (see ref. 1).

1.2. Antigen Processing

The intracellular pathways responsible for the sensitization reaction to a specific peptide epitope expressed by a protein are quite distinct for the MHC class I and class II antigen presentation pathways (see ref. 2). For example (Fig. 1), intracellular cytoplasmic proteins derived from foreign microbes such

Contemporary Immunology: Autoimmune Reactions
Edited by: S. Paul © Humana Press Inc., Totowa, NJ

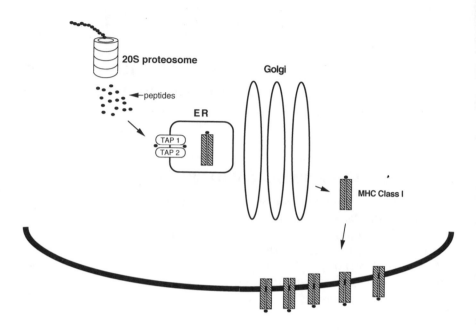

Fig. 1. MHC class I antigen processing pathway.

as viruses are initially processed by the 20S proteasome complex. The resultant peptides are transported from the cytosol to the endoplasmic reticulum (ER) by the TAP transporters, which traverse the ER membrane. In the ER, the peptide fragments combine with class I molecules and are transported to the trans-Golgi and eventually to the cell surface to be recognized by the αβT-cell receptor (TCR) of a CD8 T-cell. In contrast, the MHC class II pathway is responsible for the presentation of exogenous foreign antigens in the extracellular compartment (e.g., antigens expressed on the surface of microbes) (Fig. 2). The class II heterodimers are transported into the ER where they associate with the invariant chain (Ii). Proteolysis of the MHC-bound invariant chain results in a smaller CLIP (class II-associated Ii peptide) *(see* ref. *3).* The MHC class II-CLIP complex is transported from the ER to the trans-Golgi and eventually localizes to the endosomal compartment. In the endosomal compartment, HLA-DM facilitates the displacement of the MHC-bound CLIP by foreign antigenic peptides. The latter peptides are derived from the proteolysis of endocytosed foreign proteins in the lysosomal compartment *(4).* The MHC class II-peptide complexes are then transported to the cell surface where they are recognized by the αβTCR of CD4 T-cells. Although the pathways, as outlined above, emphasize the distinct origins of antigenic peptides presented by the class I and class II MHC complexes, it is slowly becoming clear that some overlap exists between

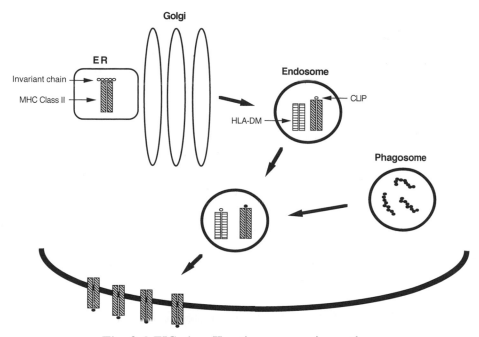

Fig. 2. MHC class II antigen processing pathway.

the two pathways. For example, it has been shown that CD8 cells can recognize exogenous antigens presented by MHC class II molecules *(5)*.

2. SELF-TOLERANCE

2.1. Positive and Negative Selection in the Thymus

Besides presenting foreign peptides to effector cells of the immune system, the MHC molecules have an equally important function in the maturation and differentiation of T-cells in the thymic microenvironment. The expression of MHC molecules by cortical thymic epithelial cells is critical to the process of positive selection, which helps shape the T-cell repertoire to exhibit the property of MHC restriction, i.e., a repertoire that is able to recognize foreign antigens specifically in the context of self-MHC recognition *(6)*. During the process of positive selection, CD4 and CD8 cells expressing αβTCRs capable of binding the self-MHC-peptide complexes are selected for further development. T-cells that do not display a sufficiently great binding affinity for the self-MHC-peptide complexes are allowed to undergo apoptosis and die. The surviving cells are then subjected to a process of negative selection in the thymic medulla, during which T-cells that exhibit too strong an affinity for the self-antigen complexes (i.e., the highly autoreactive cells) presented by monocyte-derived dendritic cells are actively destroyed. Approximately five percent of the positively selected population is killed by the negative selection process *(7)*. The summation of these two selection processes produces a peripheral T-cell repertoire capable of recognizing foreign antigen in the context of the self-MHC antigens, and yet, is discriminatory to the point that self-antigens complexed to the MHC molecules are not seen as immunogenic signals.

2.2. *Periperal Anergy*

The state of self-tolerance is thought to apply to all peptides expressed in the thymus. There are, however, many organ-specific proteins that are probably never expressed by thymic tissue. T-cells with reactivity towards these self-peptides can not be deleted by the thymic deletion mechanisms. These cells exit the thymus into the periphery with an intact potential to react against the tissue-specific self-proteins found in various organ microenvironments. One safeguard in the immune system against this eventuality is the requirement that the APC must deliver a second costimulatory signal coincident with the αβTCR antigen recognition signal for the T-cells to be activated in the periphery. This second signal is frequently provided by binding of the CD28 expressed on the responding T-cell with the B7 family of molecules expressed by the APC. A failure to deliver the second signal results in a state of anergy, in which the cell is not destroyed but is rendered incapable of responding to the antigenic stimulus *(8)*. The ability to deliver the second signal is restricted primarily to the professional class of APCs. Most organs are populated predominantly by nonprofessional APCs. The presentation of organ-specific self-antigens by such APCs, which lack the second signaling capability, results in anergy toward these antigens. Together, the processes of thymic deletion and peripheral anergy complement each other in an ongoing attempt to establish and maintain self-tolerance.

3. THE AUTOIMMUNE RESPONSE

The realization that antigen presentation mechanisms are important in the etiology and pathogenesis of autoimmune diseases is derived from two types of observations. First, it has been appreciated for several years that the autoimmune response is a truly antigen-driven response. This is supported by many studies that have examined both the functional and the structural elements of the autoantigen-recognition event. For example, the ongoing autoimmune response in disease states demonstrates both affinity maturation of the responding elements (e.g., the immunoglobulins) as well as determinant spreading within the targeted self macromolecular species (e.g., ribonucleoproteins). Second, it has been repeatedly observed for at least two decades that individuals with certain MHC class I or class II alleles are predisposed toward the development of specific autoimmune diseases. Examples are the associations between HLA-B27 and ankylosing spondylitis *(9)*, and, HLA-DR4 and rheumatoid arthritis *(10)*. The MHC gene products are highly polymorphic. Considerable effort is being invested towards examination of the structural variability of certain MHC alleles and their consequent ability to discriminate between various foreign and self peptides. The assumptions underlying these analyses have been the recognition by the T-cells of certain uniquely immunogenic MHC+foreign peptide combinations in the periphery engenders specific autoimmune consequences and/or the presence of certain MHC+self peptide combinations during thymic development favors the creation of a T-cell repertoire which retains certain self-reactive tendencies in the periphery, and allows the emergence of autoimmune disease.

4. MOLECULAR MIMICRY

4.1. Cryptic Epitopes

As noted in Subheading 2., maintenance of self-tolerance requires the presentation of self-peptides, which results in negative selection and deletion of T-cells in the thymus, and T-cell anergy in the periphery. Of all possible self peptides, only a finite set is generated and presented to T-cells. A hierarchical relationship among peptides derived from a single protein with regard to their "immunodominance" likely exists, but the full details of the relationship are yet to be worked out. The self-peptides that are actually presented to T-cells are influenced by several factors, including intracellular processing and proteolysis pathways of the protein antigens, as well as intrinsic structural requirements that allow only certain self-peptides to bind the MHC molecules. Each protein generates only a few self-peptides in sufficient quantity and possessing sufficiently high MHC antigen binding affinity to be effectively presented to the T-cells in the thymus. An obvious implication of the limited self peptide presentation is that there is a vast residual array of self-peptides that are not presented to T-cells in sufficient quantity to generate tolerance. These "cryptic" epitopes (11) are never recognized by potentially autoreactive T-cells under steady-state conditions, either because they are expressed in immunologically privileged anatomical sites (e.g., central nervous system) or they are not generated in sufficient quantity or in the appropriate context in the periphery (e.g., lack of costimulatory signals by APC) to generate an immune response (12). It is only during inflammatory conditions that disrupt this equilibrium, such as viral or bacterial infections, that the parameters of antigen-presentation are disturbed, and the potential for initiation of autoimmune responses against the cryptic epitopes is allowed. The disruption can be the result of a primary immune response directed against a viral peptide bearing sufficient structural similarity to a cryptic self-peptide that an autoimmune response by T-cells is initiated. Once the response against the self peptide is initiated and tolerance is disrupted, the resultant autoreactive T-cells permit sustenance and magnification of the antigen-driven response to additional immunological compartments, which would otherwise be unsustainable by naive T-cells. The phenomenon of molecular mimicry leading to T-cell activation is currently the favored hypothesis as the primary event in the pathogenesis of autoimmunity.

4.2. Degeneracy of T-Cell Recognition

It is important to emphasize that molecular mimicry does not imply molecular identity. The degeneracy with which the T-cells recognize different peptides allows for activation of the cells by nonidentical, yet structurally similar peptide antigens. For instance, activated T-cells responsive to a segment of myelin basic protein (amino acids 85 to 99, MBP 85-99) are present in patients with multiple sclerosis. The same T-cells have been shown to also be reactive with peptides derived from various viruses, such as herpes simplex, Epstein–Barr, influenza, and adenovirus *(13)*. Scrutiny of the structure of the peptides recognized by the T-cells reveals that in most cases the viral-derived peptides and the self MBP(85-99) peptide share only five or six common residues. These residues are, for the most part, the critical amino acids involved in binding within specific pockets of the MHC molecule, or in interactions with the αβTCR expressed by the responder cells.

5. ORGAN-SPECIFIC AUTOIMMUNE DISEASE

5.1. Multiple Sclerosis

The existence of peripheral T-cells with the potential for reactivity against MBP has long been thought to be a consequence of the sequestered, tissue-specific expression of MBP (i.e., in the central nervous system). According to this belief, T-cells capable of the MBP reactivity are not subjected to the negative selection mechanisms of the thymus. Recently, however, expression of MBP in the thymus has been described *(14)*. Presumably, thymocytes are tolerized through the process of negative selection to the dominant T-cell epitopes of MBP, the molecular structure of which is yet to be determined. Normal individuals possess "ignorant" *(15)* autoreactive T-cells directed against the same epitopes of MBP as multiple sclerosis patients *(16)*, supporting the hypothesis that these are cryptic, nondominant epitopes which, under normal conditions, are ignored by T-cells. Only during episodes of peripheral T-cell activation by crossreactive viral epitopes do these normally quiescent lymphocytes acquire the capacity to traverse the blood-brain barrier and initiate the immune response against myelin in the central nervous system.

5.2. Diabetes Mellitus

A similar mechanism may be responsible for induction of the most common autoimmune disease, i.e., insulin-dependent diabetes mellitus. The importance of antigen presentation mechanisms in initiating diabetes has been suspected for more than a decade. It was appreciated early on that a strong association exists between certain MHC class II alleles and susceptibility to diabetes. Specifically, the DQβ allele chains containing a negatively charged aspartic acid at position 57 appears to confer resistance to disease, whereas alleles containing uncharged amino acid (e.g., serine, alanine, or valine) at this position confers

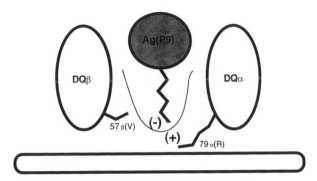

Fig. 3. Diabetes-susceptible DQ allele with nonpolar valine at position 57 of the β chain.

enhanced susceptibility to disease *(17)*. A similar situation holds for the murine NOD model of diabetes. This disease susceptible mouse strain expresses an uncharged residue at position 57 of the I-Aβ molecule, whereas resistant mouse strains express the aspartic acid at this position *(18)*. This structure-disease correlation is presumably reflected in the distinct peptide-binding profiles of the respective alleles (19–20). Susceptible alleles with an uncharged amino acid at position 57 exhibit a preference for binding peptides with a negative charge at the P9 position (Fig. 3). Presumably, such a complex is stabilized by a charge–charge interaction with arginine at position 79 in the DQα chain. Conversely, in resistant alleles, a negatively charged amino acid at position 57 of the DQβ chain would prohibit binding of peptides with a negative charge at the P9 position, since arginine in position 79 of DQα is neutralized by the charge–charge interaction with the aspartic acid of the DQβ chain (Fig. 4). These data predict that the distinguishing feature of disease-invoking self peptide(s) is the presence of a negatively charged amino acid at the P9 position.

In both human diabetes and animal models such as the NOD mouse, prediabetic individuals exhibit immune reactivity, including T-cell reactivity to the β-cell antigen glutamic acid decarboxylase (GAD) *(21–24)*. This enzyme is essential for the synthesis of γ-amino butyric acid, and is expressed only in the CNS, testis, fallopian tubes, and the β-cells of the islets of Langherans. The prediabetic T-cell reactivity to GAD is significant, in that it is directed towards a region of the molecule with considerable structural homology to the Coxsackie virus protein P2-C (25) (Fig. 5). A possible reason for the selective T-cell responsiveness is that a peptide derived from this GAD region binds with much greater affinity to susceptible DQ heterodimers (e.g., DQ3.2) than to resistant heterodimers (e.g., DQ3.1) *(26)*. A detailed analysis of the structural properties of this peptide has shown that only four of the nine residues are essential for DQ binding. The major difference in the peptide motifs capable of binding DQ3.1 and DQ3.2 is the requirement of a negatively charged glutamic acid at P9 for DQ3.2 binding, while the non-polar alanine is preferred for DQ3.1 binding

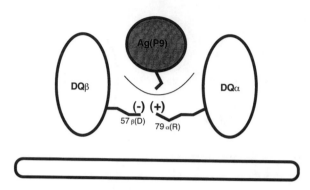

Fig. 4. Diabetes-resistant DQ allele with negatively charged aspartic acid at position 57 of the β chain.

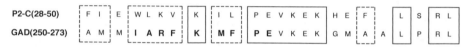

Fig. 5. Structural homology between Coxsackie virus protein P2-C(28–50) and human GAD(250–273). Amino acids enclosed with solid lines are identical and those enclosed with dashed lines represent nonidentical amino acids with similar charge *(see* ref. *25).* GAD peptide IARFKMFPE (in bold) selectively bind the diabetes-susceptible allele DQ3.2 *(see* Fig. 6).

(Fig. 6). These observations, taken together with the supporting clinical finding that Coxsackie infections often precede overt diabetes *(27),* has generated the hypothesis that an infectious episode of infection initiates the anti-islet T-cell immune response, owing to "mimicking" of the original immunogen, Coxsackie virus protein P2-C, by pancreatic GAD.

6. SECONDARY MECHANISMS

6.1. Th1 vs Th2 Effector Phenotypes

As the autoimmune response progresses, an amplification of reactivity to additional islet T-cell antigens is generated, e.g., insulin, carboxypeptidase H, peripherin, and HSP60 *(28).* This is termed determinant spreading, and represents the further breakdown of self tolerance. The underlying phenomena include tissue infiltration by CD4 cells of the Th1 phenotype. These cells produce γ-interferon (IFN-γ), which has the effect of upregulating MHC class II molecules on nonprofessional APCs (e.g., islet cells). In turn, the upregulated MHC expression allows the potential sensitization to novel self-peptides, to which tolerance does not exist. The differentiation of naive CD4 cells into the effector pathways of either Th1 or Th2 phenotypes is in part a result of which

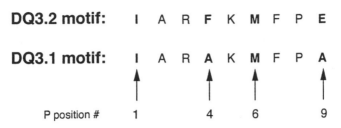

Fig. 6. Diabetes-susceptible DQ3.2 binding motif and diabetes-resistant DQ3.1 binding motif expressed by GAD(250–273) *(26)*. The only charge difference between the two motifs is the presence of a negatively charged glutamic acid (E) at position P9 of the DQ3.2 binding motif.

specific MHC class II allele is involved in antigen presentation *(29)*. For example, subtle structural differences between otherwise comparable peptide+MHC ligands can result in the differentiation of the responding CD4 cell into distinct effector phenotypes. The principle finding of one indepth study was that αβTCRs capable of binding a particular peptide+MHC ligand with high affinity will initiate a Th1 response, while αβTCRs that bind to the peptide+MHC ligand with weak affinity are more likely to initiate a Th2 effector response *(30)*. The Th1 response is generally regarded as possessing considerably greater autoreactive features. In the case of diabetes, it is possible that DQ heterodimers with a noncharged amino acid at the β57 position bind a specific immunogenic peptide (e.g., one derived from GAD) and engage the αβTCR with higher affinity, than alleles containing aspartic acid at the β57 position. The high-affinity interaction causes the responding CD4 cells in the pancreas to differentiate into IFN-γ producing Th1 cells, which serves to amplify the autoimmune response.

6.2. Alterations in Antigen Processing

The importance of the Th1 cytokine profile in the autoimmune response is due only in part to the ability of IFN-γ to upregulate MHC class II and other activation molecules on nonprofessional APCs. An additional factor is the effect of IFN-γ on the antigen processing pathways within APCs. IFN-γ induces the expression of various endopeptidases in the lysosomal compartment. The resultant patterns of proteolysis can be diverse and may ultimately allow for unique repertoires of self-peptides to become available for MHC class II binding. If tolerance to the self-peptides has not already been achieved during thymic selection, increased or altered self-peptide production has the potential to initiate a destructive autoimmune response. In a similar manner, IFN-γ also modifies the expression of various molecules associated with the 20s proteasome, which can influence the peptide population made available for MHC class I binding *(31)*. One such proteasome-associated molecular complex induced by IFN-γ, PA28, has recently been found to be essential for the generation of immunodominant MHC binding peptides *(32)*. In both of these instances, the novel peripheral antigen processing pathways induced by IFN-γ have the potential to generate self-peptide+MHC complexes not previously encountered by the immune system. Such complexes, if sufficiently immunogenic, will initiate an effector response against self.

7. FROM SYSTEMIC TO ORGAN-SPECIFIC AUTOIMMUNITY

In both diabetes mellitus and multiple sclerosis there is extensive evidence to support the hypothesis that an immune response directed against a tissue-specific self-antigen is responsible for initiating and maintaining an ongoing inflammatory response. Study of another common autoimmune disease, rheumatoid arthritis, has as yet failed to identify a joint-specific antigen responsible for the destructive inflammatory synovitis that is characteristic of this disease. That antigen-presentation is critical to the pathogenesis of rheumatoid arthritis is suggested by its very strong association with MHC class II molecules (e.g., DRB0401), which share common structural motifs in the third hypervariable region of the DRβ chain *(33)*. One explanation for this observation is that certain class II alleles are exclusively capable of binding a specific immunogenic peptide, perhaps expressed only by synovial tissue. Such a peptide, however, has eluded detection until now.

An alternative explanation for the allelic association of rheumatoid arthritis is suggested by a recently described murine model *(34)*. This model was generated serendipitously when a transgenic mouse strain that exclusively expressed an αβTCR specific for a peptide epitope of bovine RNase in the context of the MHC class II allele A^k was crossed with the NOD strain expressing a different allele, A^{g7}. Surprisingly, the hybrid strain rapidly developed severe and symmetric inflammatory and destructive polyarthritis. Further analysis revealed the disease activity to be exclusively correlated with the expression of the A^{g7} allele, and in vitro studies showed that the transgenic TCR to be alloreactive towards A^{g7}-expressing cells. An intact CD4 T-cell compartment as well as a functional B-cell population were essential to the development of disease. The alloreactive mechanism in this model is not unlike the features of human chronic graft vs host disease, in which the inflammatory reactions are preferentially targeted to specific organs (e.g., skin, liver, or intestine), even though the alloreactive response is usually considered to be directed against an array of different peptides. In both instances, a systemic autoimmune response apparently evolves into a tissue-specific inflammatory reaction, even though tissue-specific antigens do not appear to be the initiators of the autoimmune response. The molecular mechanisms of such a disease course remain obscure, but the pathogenesis is likely to involve the expression of unique cytokine profiles by the responding immune cells along with the cell-surface expression of various homing receptors (e.g., integrins), which may contribute to the final tissue destination of the responding cells. If this model is accepted, it seems that certain intrinsic and unidentified structural properties of the MHC molecule, rather than their peptide antigen binding characteristics, are responsible for generating the characteristic autoimmune response.

It is likely that continued research into the autoimmune response will reveal a multitude of pathways and mechanisms responsible for the breakdown of self-tolerance. The apparent critical role of antigen presentation in both initiating and sustaining the autoimmune response offers the opportunity to devise targeted interruptions of autoimmune recognition. Therapy remains a very formidable challenge, however, because the response is autoantigen driven and is not feasible to ever eradicate the autoantigen(s).

REFERENCES

1. Madden, D. R. (1995) The three-dimensional structure of peptide-MHC complexes. *Annu. Rev. Immunol.* **13,** 587–622.
2. Rammensee, H.-G. (1996) Antigen presentation-Recent developments. *Int. Arch. Allergy Immunol.* **110,** 299–307.
3. Cresswell, P. (1996) Invariant chain structure and MHC class II function. *Cell* **84,** 505–507.
4. Denzin, L. K. and Cresswell, P. (1995) HLA-DM induces CLIP dissociation from MHC class II alpha beta dimers and facilitates peptide loading. *Cell* **82,** 155–165.
5. Bevan, M. (1995) Antigen presentation to cytotoxic T lymphocytes in vivo. *J. Exp. Med.* **182,** 639–641.
6. Jameson, S. C., Hogquist, K. A., and Bevan, M. J. (1995) Positive selection of thymocytes. *Annu. Rev. Immunol.* **13,** 93–126.
7. Laufer, T. M., DeKoning J., Markowitz, J. S., Lo, D. and Glimcher, L. H. (1996) Unopposed positive selection and autoreactivity in mice expressing class II MHC only on thymic cortex. *Nature* **383,** 81–85.
8. Quill, H. (1996) Anergy as a mechanism of peripheral T-cell tolerance. *J. Immunol.* **156,** 1325–1327.
9. Brewerton, D. A., Hart, F. D., Nichols, A., Caffry, M., James, D. C., and Sturruck, R. D. (1973) Ankylosing spondylitis and HL-A 27. *Lancet* **1,** 904–907.
10. Stastny, P. (1978) Association of the B-cell alloantigen DRw4 with rheumatoid arthritis. *N. Engl. J. Med.* **298,** 869–871.
11. Sercarz, E. E., Lehmann, P. V., Ametani, A., Benichou, G., Miller, M., and Moudgil, K. (1993) Dominance and crypticity of T cell determinants. *Ann. Rev. Immunol.* **11,** 729–766.
12. Lanzavecchia, A. (1995) How can cryptic epitopes trigger autoimmunity. *J. Exp. Med.* **181,** 1945–1948.
13. Wucherpfennig, K. W., and Strominger, J. L. (1995) Molecular mimicry in T-cell mediated autoimmunity:viral peptides activate human T cell clones specific for myelin basic protein. *Cell* **80,** 695–705.
14. Pribyl, T. M., Campagnoni, C. W., Kampf, K., Kashima, T., Handley, V., McMahon, J., et al. (1993) The human myelin basic protein gene is included within a 179 kilobase transcription unit: expression within the immune and central nervous systems. *Proc. Natl. Acad. Sci. USA* **90,** 10,695–10,699.
15. Elson, C. J., Barker, R. N., Thompson, S. J., and Williams, N. A. (1995) Immunologically ignorant autoreactive T cells, epitope spreading and repertoire limitation. *Immunol. Today* **16,** 71–76.

16. Wucherpfennig, K., Zhang, J., Witek, C., Matsui, M., Modabber, Y., Ota, K., et al. (1994) Clonal expansion and persistence of human T cells specific for an immunodominant myelin basic protein peptide. *J. Immunol.* **152,** 5581–92.

17. Todd, J., Bell, J., and McDevitt, H. O. (1987) HLA DQb gene contributes to susceptibility and resistance to insulin-dependent diabetes mellitus. *Nature* **329,** 599–604.

18. Wicker, L. S., Todd, J. A., and Peterson, L. B. (1995) Genetic control of autoimmune diabetes in the NOD mouse. *Ann. Rev. Immunol.* **13,** 179–200.

19. Rammensee, H. C., Freide, T., and Stevanovic, S. (1995) MHC ligands and peptide motifs: first listing. *Immunogenetics* **41,** 178–228.

20. Reich, E. P., von Grafenstein, H., Barlow, A., Swenson, K. E., Williams, K., and Janeway, C. A. (1994) Self peptides isolated from MHC glycoproteins of non-obese diabetic mice. *J. Immunol.* **152,** 2279–2288.

21. Baekkeskov, S., Aanstoot, H. J., Christgau, S., Reetz, A., Solimena, M., Cascalho, M., et al. (1990) Identification of the 64K autoantigen in insulin dependent diabetes as the GABA-synthesizing enzyme glutamic acid decarboxylase. *Nature* **347,** 151–156.

22. Hogopian, W. A., Karlsen, A. E., Gottsater, A., Landin-Olsson, M., Grubin, C. E., Sundkvist, G., et al. (1993) Quantitative assay using recombinant human islet glutamic acid decarboxylase (GAD65) shows that 64K autoantibody positivity at onset predicts diabetes type I. *J. Clin. Invest.* **91,** 368–374.

23. Kaufman, D. L., Clare-Salzler, M., Tian, J., Forsthuber, T., Ting, G. S., Robinson, P., et al. (1993) Spontaneous loss of T cell tolerance to glutamic acid decarboxylase in murine insulin dependent diabetes. *Nature* **366,** 69–72.

24. Tisch, R., Yang, X. D., Singer, S. M., Liblau, R. S., Fogger, L., and McDevitt, H. O. (1993) Immune response to glutamic acid decarboxylase correlates with insulitis in nonobese diabetic mice. *Nature* **366,** 72–75.

25. Atkinson, M. A., Bowman, M. A., Campbell, L., Darrow, B. L., Kaufman, D. L., and Maclaren, N. K. (1994) Cellular immunity to a determinant common to glutamic acid decarboxylase and Coxsackie virus in insulin dependent diabetes. *J. Clin. Invest.* **94,** 2125–2129.

26. Kwok, W. W., Domeier, M. E., Raymond, F. C., Byers, P., and Nepom, G. T. (1996) Allele-specific motifs characterize HLA-DQ interactions with a diabetes-associated peptide derived from glutamic acid decarboxylase. *J. Immunol.* **156,** 2171–2177.

27. Barrett-Connor, E. (1985) Is insulin-dependent diabetes caused by Coxsackie virus B infection? A review of the epidemiologic evidence. *Rev. Infect. Dis.* **7,** 207–215.

28. Atkinson, M. A. and Maclaren, N. K. (1993) Islet cell autoantigens in insulin dependent diabetes. *J. Clin. Invest.* **92,** 1608–1616.

29. Murray, J. S., Madri, J., Tite, J., Carding, S. R. and Bottomly, K. (1989) MHC control of CD4+ T cell subset activation. *J. Exp. Med.* **170(6),** 2135–2140.

30. Pfeiffer, C., Stein, J., Southwood, S., Ketelaar, H., Sette, A., and Bottomly, K. (1995) Altered peptide ligands can control CD4 T lymphocyte differentiation in vivo. *J. Exp. Med.* **181,** 1569–1574.

31. Aki, M., Shimbara, M., Takashina, M., Akiyama, K., Kagawa, S., Tamura, T., et al. (1994) Interferon-gamma induces different subunit organizations and functional diversity of proteasomes. *J. Biochem.* **115,** 257–269.

32. Dick, T. P., Ruppert, T., Groettrup, M., Kloetzel, P. M., Kuehn, L., Koszinowski, U. H., et al. (1996) Coordinated dual cleavages induced by the proteasome regulator PA28 lead to dominant MHC ligands. *Cell* **86,** 253–262.
33. Gregersen, P. K., Silver, J., and Winchester, R. J. (1987) The shared epitope hypothesis. An approach to understanding the molecular genetics of susceptibility to rheumatoid arthritis. *Arthritis Rheum.* **30,** 1205–1213.
34. Kouskoff, V., Korganow, A.-S., Duchatelle, V., Degott, C., Benoist, C., and Mathis, D. (1996) Organ-specific disease provoked by systemic autoimmunity. *Cell* **87,** 811–822.

8

Induction of Pathogenic Autoimmune T-Cell and Autoantibody Responses Through T-Cell Epitope Mimicry

**Kenneth S. K. Tung,
Kristine M. Garza, and Ya-huan Lou**

1. INTRODUCTION

It has been proposed for some time that autoimmune responses and auto-immune disease may result from an immune response to foreign molecules that mimic self (*see* ref. *1*). Most past and recent studies have examined the molecular mimicry hypothesis constituents at the level of B-cell epitopes; an approach predicated on assumptions that autoimmune disease is triggered by foreign antigens recognized by B-cell receptors from diseased individuals, and that auto-antibodies are critical in the pathogenesis of autoimmune disease. However, both assumptions have been brought into question according to recent research findings.

Studies on experimental organ-specific autoimmune diseases have documented clearly that T-cell-mediated mechanisms, usually involving the CD4 T-cell subset, are both necessary and sufficient for obtaining tissue injury *(2–7)*. In contrast, actively induced or passively transferred autoantibodies alone rarely elicit autoimmune disease *(8–11)*. The notable exceptions to this statement are glomerulonephritis associated with glomerular basement membrane antibodies, and certain diseases induced by antibodies against cellular surface antigens and biologically functional cellular receptors *(8,12,13)*. Even in the experimental systemic lupus erythematosus (SLE) model, activation of pathogenic T-cells may be the initiating event *(14–22)*, and, as will be detailed in this chapter, autoantibody formation to various endogenous antigens may be elicited by immunization with structurally unrelated T-cell peptides.

This chapter will focus, therefore, on mimicry at the level of T-cell peptides. Our recent studies have documented the phenomenon of molecular mimicry of T-cell epitopes as a cause autoimmune disease. We will discuss the molecular basis for the crossreaction among T-cell peptides, and describe experiments that evaluate the frequency of T-cell mimicry occurrence. The second topic concerns an equally interesting observation, in which an autoreactive T-cell response alone leads rapidly to an autoantibody response against B-cell epitopes

Contemporary Immunology: Autoimmune Reactions
Edited by: S. Paul © Humana Press Inc., Totowa, NJ

distinct from the immunogenic peptide. This phenomenon can apparently occur through activation of primed B-cells by endogenous antigens. We will then briefly review recent literature that extrapolates this amplification (or epitope spreading) phenomenon to the pathogenesis of systemic autoimmunity, such as found in SLE, and discuss its relevance to self-tolerance mechanisms.

2. MURINE AUTOIMMUNE OOPHORITIS INDUCED BY A ZONA PELLUCIDA PEPTIDE (pZP3)

Molecular mimicry at the T-cell epitope was documented conclusively in a study on murine autoimmune ovarian disease, the model of a known cause of premature ovarian failure in women (*see* ref. *23*). These patients have inflamed ovaries (oophoritis) and serum antibodies to antigens that are unique to the ovary or are shared between ovary and placenta. Experimentally, ovarian failure has been observed in several animal species following immunization with heterologous zona pellucida (ZP) *(24–26)* or one of the ZP glycoproteins, ZP3 *(27)*. In 1992, an autoimmune mechanism was established as the basis of the ovarian failure in a new model of murine autoimmune oophoritis induced by a murine ZP3 peptide *(28)*.

ZP, an acellular matrix surrounding developing and ovulated oocytes, is also detected in the numerous atretic or degenerative follicles in the ovaries. ZP3 is a major ZP glycoprotein with 424 amino acids and an O-linked glycoconjugate that functions as the primary sperm receptor *(29,30)*. The murine pZP3 peptide residues 328–342), initially evaluated as an experimental contraceptive vaccine antigen *(31)*, was soon found to elicit a high incidence of severe murine auto-immune oophoritis when it was injected with complete Freund's adjuvant (CFA) or incomplete Freund's adjuvant (IFA) *(28)*. Ovarian autoimmune disease induction by pZP3 is MHC restricted: inbred and H-2 congenic mice of the k, a, u, and s haplotypes are responders whereas those of the b, d, and q haplo-types are nonresponders *(11)*. Most of our studies have used the highly responsive (C57BL/6xA/J)F1 (B6AF1) mice. They mount both peptide-specific T-cell responses and ZP autoantibodies, the latter detectable in serum and as bound IgG on the ovarian ZP. By studying the response to truncated ZP3 peptides (residues 328–342), at least two nested T-cell epitopes have been mapped, both overlapping with the known 7-mer native B-cell epitope (Table 1) *(32)*.

pZP3-specific CD4+ T-cells are sufficient to induce oophoritis. Thus the disease can be adoptively transferred by regional lymph node CD4+ (not CD8+) T-cells, and by pZP3-specific T-cell lines and T-cell clones *(28)*. The oophorito-genic CD4+ T-cell lines and T-cell clones produce IL-2, interferon-γ but not IL-4.

In contrast, passively transferred murine serum ZP3 antibody, which binds to ovarian ZP without C3 deposition, does not cause ovarian inflammation. In order to more vigorously evaluate the role of antibody in this disease, mice were immunized with a chimeric peptide consisting of a modified native ZP3 epitope (residues 337–342) linked to a bovine ribonuclease (bRNase) T-cell epitope (Table 1). Female mice hyperimmunized with the chimeric peptide

Table 1
Antigenic Peptides Used in the Murine Model for Autoimmune Oophoritis

Peptide	Amino acid sequence	Immunologic functions
pZP3 (330–342)	N S S S S Q F Q I H G P R	Self T epitopes + Self B epitope-1
pZP3 (330–338)	N S S S S Q F Q I[a]	Self T epitope-1
pAchR δ (120–128)	N N N D G S F Q I	Foreign T epitope mimics self epitope-1
pZP3 (332–340)	S S S Q F Q I H G	Self T epitope-2
phCD5 (482–492)	N S S D S D Y D L H G	Foreign T epitope mimics self epitope-2
pbCD5 (482–492)	N S S D S D Y E L H G	Foreign T epitope
pZP3 (335–342)	Q F Q I H G P R	Self B epitope-1
CP2	bRNase (94-104) -Q A Q I H G P R	Foreign T epitope + modified self B epitope-1
pZP3 (171–180)	F S L R L M E E N W	Self B epitope-2
pZP3 (301–310)	C S F N K T S N S W	Self B epitope-3

[a] Underlined letters indicate critical residues for T-cell epitope.

develop T-cell responses to the chimeric peptide that do not crossreact with pZP3. However, they produce high levels of circulating ZP antibodies that bound to ovarian ZP. Although the mice have reduced fertility, their ovaries are free of pathology *(11)*.

Murine autoimmune oophoritis as a model of peptide/adjuvant-induced autoimmune disease has certain unique features. First, the disease is readily induced. Pertussis toxin, an adjuvant essential for induction of murine autoimmune disease of the central nervous system and the testis *(33,34)*, is not required. Indeed, severe ovarian autoimmune disease of comparable incidence can be elicited by pZP3 in CFA or IFA. Second, pZP3 and MHC II positive macrophages and dendritic cells, potential targets of the CD4+ autoreactive T-cells, are present in normal ovaries accessible to the T-cells. In an adult cycling female mouse, a cohort of about 40 ovarian oocytes grow and mature from a primordial oocyte pool every four to five days; in the process, they synthesize and secrete ZP3 to construct the surrounding ZP. However, 80% of these ZP3-positive oocytes follow an apoptotic pathway and undergo atresia during development. The atretic follicles, located in the medulla of the ovary, are surrounded by numerous F4/80[+] macrophages that are MHC II positive. Indeed, it is to the atretic follicles that pZP3-specific T-cell clones invariably home upon adoptive transfer. The atretic follicles are the targets, therefore, for pZP3-specific T-cells *(11)*. Later, we will present evidence that ZP3 or processed pZP3 can leave the ovaries to reach the draining lymphoid tissues. The accessibility of pZP3 to the immune system, and the ease with which autoimmune oophoritis is induced may explain why molecular mimicry is so readily demonstrated in this model.

3. AUTOIMMUNE OOPHORITIS INDUCTION BY AN ACETYLCHOLINE RECEPTOR DELTA CHAIN T-CELL PEPTIDE BASED ON MOLECULAR MIMICRY WITH pZP3

Based on a search of the protein sequence library, the δ chain of murine acetylcholine receptor (AChR δ) was found to share four common amino acid residues with the ZP3 T-cell epitope 330–339 (Table 1). Direct evidence for mimicry between these peptides is evident from the following experiments *(35)*. First, in B6AF1 mice injected with the AChR δ 120–128 peptide, inflammatory infiltrates were noted in ovarian interfollicular space and within the Graafian follicles. The infiltrates contained macrophages, multinucleated giant cells and lymphocytes, of which many were CD3+. The nature and extent of ovarian histopathology of these mice resembled oophoritis in mice injected with pZP3(330–339). Second, crossreaction between pZP3 and the AChR δ peptides is evident from the observation of a proliferative response of an oophoritogenic, P3-specific T-cell clone to these peptides presented by a fibroblast cell line expressing a single murine MHC II ($A\alpha^k\beta^b$). Third, mice injected with the AChR δ peptide produced ZP antibodies detectable in the serum and bound to the ovarian ZP. As will be discussed later, the significance of these observations reaches beyond the molecular mimicry phenomenon.

The molecular mimicry at the level of T-cell epitopes observed by us in the zona pellucide system is by no means unprecedented or unique. It has also been described by others in various murine and human responses *(36–41)*.

4. MECHANISMS OF MOLECULAR MIMICRY AT THE LEVEL OF T-CELL PEPTIDES

Two mechanisms are considered important in T-cell epitope mimicry. The first is based on the sharing of critical residues required for pathogenic T-cell activation. By analysis of pZP3 analogs in which the AChR residues were substituted by an alanine, four residues in pZP3 were deduced to be critical for

1. Induction of autoimmune oophoritis.
2. Stimulation of the ZP3 specific T-cell clone.
3. Induction of ZP autoantibodies *(35)*.

These pZP3 residues are: Asn330, Gln335, Phe336 and Gln337. Importantly, three of the critical residues are shared between the pZP3 and the AChR δ peptide (Table 1). To seek direct evidence for T-cell mimicry, a polyalanine peptide containing the critical shared amino acid residues between the pZP3 and AChR δ peptides was studied. This peptide was found to be equally effective in eliciting oophoritis and ZP autoantibody, and in stimulating an oophoritogenic T-cell clone. A similar approach has been used to identify the functionally important residues in two encephalitogenic peptides of the myelin basic protein *(42,43)*.

T-cell peptide molecular mimicry may also occur in the absence of amino acid sequence homology, although the mechanism of the mimicry in these cases is less well understood. This phenomenon may be the result of a conformational similarity, i.e., a surface structure similarity between the unrelated peptides *(44–47)*, even though there is no primary structure homology.

5. THE FREQUENCY OF MOLECULAR MIMICRY AMONG T-CELL PEPTIDES

The two nested T-cell epitope of pZP3 had slightly different critical residue requirements for their biological activities (Table 1). We searched the protein sequence library for nonovarian peptides that shared complete or partial homology with the two critical residue motifs. Of 16 peptides studied, seven-induced ovarian inflammation and ovarian ZP autoantibodies (44%), in spite of the presence of only limited levels of homology *(32)*. The specificity of peptide recognition by the oophoritogenic T-cells remained exquisite, as demonstrated by the cellular response to bovine and human CD5 peptides (pbCD5 and phCD5, respectively). Administration of pbCD5 and phCD5 to mice showed that only the latter peptide was pathogenic, although the two peptides differ by only a single aspartic acid to glutamic acid substitution (Table 1, pbCD5 versus phCD5). Many peptides with amino acid homology comparable to that between phCD5 and pZP3 were nevertheless nonpathogenic. It is apparent, therefore, that the sharing of critical residue motif is not a sufficient condition for T-epitope mimicry.

The studies therefore document a rather high frequency of mimicry among peptides with limited sequence homology. Based on our current understanding that the peptide sequence requirements for MHC II anchor recognition and T-cell receptor recognition can be rather promiscuous, it is easy to rationalize the ability of the nonovarian peptides to stimulate pZP3-specific T-cells and induce ovarian autoimmune disease. More difficult to decipher was the observation that the T-cell peptide mimics can also induce autoantibody production. This unexpected finding was addressed by the experiments summarized in the next section.

6. T-CELL PEPTIDE OF A SELF PROTEIN ELICITS AUTOANTIBODY TO DISTANT SITES OF THE PROTEIN ANTIGEN: THE AMPLIFICATION (OR T-TO-B EPITOPE SPREADING) PHENOMENON

Mice injected with the human pCD5 and a papilloma viral peptide, pPVL2, produced serum antibodies to native murine ZP that did not crossreact with ZP3 *(32)*. In a competitive enzyme linked immunoassay (ELISA), the antibodies were removed by ovarian ZP but not by the immunizing peptides. This suggests that immunization with the nonovarian T-epitopes elicited autoantibodies against a ZP epitope(s) unrelated to the peptide immunogens. To further dissect this novel mechanism of autoantibody induction, we took advantage of the well-defined T- and B- epitopes present in pZP3 (Table 1).

Mice were injected with the pZP3 epitope composed of residues 330–340, which lacks the native B-cell stimulatory sequence 335–342. Serum antibodies from the mice did not recognize pZP3(335–342), but they recognized native ZP3 *(48)*. IgG eluted from the ovarian ZP of these mice was 200–400 times enriched in ZP antibody activity over serum IgG, supporting the conclusion that the pZP3(330–340) induces antibodies capable of binding the native ZP.

Evidence for autoantibody amplification was obtained by study of the reactivity of antibodies raised by immunization with pZP3(330–340) with 42 peptides that spanned the murine ZP3 sequence *(49)*. These were 20-mer overlapping peptides containing 10-mer common sequences. The serum IgG displayed preferential binding to four peptides: pZP3-17 and pZP2-18 with the shared sequence pZP3(171–180); pZP3-30 and pZP3-31 with the shared sequence pZP3(310–320); pZP3-34 (residues 331–350 containing the known native B epitope 335–342, Table 1); and pZP3-42 (residues 411–430). To prove that pZP3(171–180) and pZP3(310–320) were indeed native B-cell ZP3 epitopes, synthetic chimeric peptides containing these sequences and the bRNase T-epitope were prepared. Mice devoid of ovaries were injected with each of the chimeric peptides, and were observed to produce antibodies to native ZP detectable by indirect immunofluorescence and by immunoblotting against a ZP3 extract. Further, the antibody activity was completely absorbed by pretreatment with the respective peptide immunogen *(49)*. Thus, the amplification (or spreading) phenomenon was apparently not due to crossreactive antigenic B-cell peptides. As described in Subheading 7, the antigenic stimulus for the amplified ZP3 autoantibody response is actually provided by endogenous ovarian ZP3.

7. ENDOGENOUS OVARIAN ZP3 IS THE ANTIGENIC STIMULUS FOR THE AMPLIFIED AUTOANTIBODY RESPONSE AND OOPHORITIS IS NOT A PREREQUISITE

Autoantibodies reactive with ovarian ZP3 could be elicited by immunization with the pZP3 T-epitope only in the presence of ovaries. When the ovaries were removed two weeks prior to immunization, the antibody response was abrogated, despite a detectable T-cell response *(48,49)*. The possibility that the antibody response was simply a secondary response to ZP3 released from the inflamed ovaries is unlikely because of the following observation. When the endogenous ovarian stimulus was removed several days before the onset of ophoritis, or before a detectable T-cell response to pZP3 was evident, the mice still produced amplified autoantibodies to ZP3 (i.e., autoantibodies reactive with ZP residues 171–180 and 310–320) following immunization with the pZP3 T-epitope (residues 330–340) *(49)*. Insofar as oophoritis was not evident until day 7, and the T-cell response was first detected five days after immunization with the ZP3 T-epitope, the failure to block autoantibody induction by ovary removal on day two or day four indicates that ZP3 antigens present outside the ovaries have the capacity to stimulate the ZP antibody response *(49)*.

Our current hypothesis is ZP antigens or their processed T-cell epitopes are provided by atretic oocytes generated in the ovaries throughout the entire reproductive life, and the antigens egress from normal ovaries to reach the raining lymphoid tissue where they are recognized by ZP3-specific T- and B-cells. As the most straightforward scenario, we postulate that in the draining lymph node, ovarian ZP3 is processed by ZP3-specific B-cells. In the normal unimmunized mice, B-cell stimulation may occur but an autoantibody response is not mounted because T-cell help is lacking. We propose that activated pZP3-specific T-cells present in mice immunized with the pZP3 T-epitope recognize the pZP3 presented by B-cells, and they stimulate ZP3 antibody production through cognate T-cell help. Indeed, antibody to CD40 ligand and/or the CTLA4-Ig fusion protein can completely block the ZP3 autoantibody response, indicating the critical requirement for T-cell help *(53)*.

8. IMPLICATIONS OF AMPLIFIED AUTOANTIBODY RESPONSE FOR AUTOANTIBODY SPECIFICITY, SELF-TOLERANCE AND ANTIBODY FUNCTIONAL CAPACITY

The occurrence of the amplified autoantibody response indicates that autoantibody specificity need not be dictated by the structure of the immunogen that elicits the experimental autoimmune disease. A corollary of this conclusion is that the observed specificity of autoantibodies may not accurately predict the identity of the immunogen responsible for triggering the autoimmune disease. The latter proposition is also supported by the observed nature of the antibody responses in mice injected with T-cell epitopes of the murine AChR protein and murine cytochrome C *(50–52)*. A unique feature of our own studies is that the induction of the autoantibody spreading phenomenon to the new ZP3 B epitope does not require co-injection of the whole protein antigen.

The nature and kinetics of the amplified ZP3 autoantibody response following pZP3 T-epitope immunization are characteristic of a secondary immune response. Only antibodies of the IgG class are detected and the synthesis of the antibodies is mounted rapidly after immunization. The pZP3(330–340) T-cell epitope contains a B-cell epitope, antibodies to which do not crossreact with native ZP3. In mice injected with the pZP3(330–340) peptide, the amplified antibody reactive with native ZP3 was detected seven days after immunization, coincident with the onset of oophoritis. This was seven days before antibody to the B-cell epitope contained in pZP3(330–340) could be detected *(49)*. These findings further support the hypothesis that ZP3-specific B-cells are normally primed by endogenous ovarian ZP3, and they argue against some form of intrinsic B-cells tolerance to the ovarian ZP3 antigen, such as deletion of the B-cell clones. Instead, it is evident that ovarian autoimmunity is prevented under normal circumstances because of T-cell tolerance. Study of other models of autoimmune oophoritis, including a model involving thymectomy on day three or ones that followed the transfer of normal T-cell subsets to the athymic recipients, has also suggested that oophoritogenic T-cells are present in normal female mice, but their pathogenic expression is controlled by regulatory T-cell subsets *(54–57)*.

Most of the amplified autoantibodies in our studies react with conformational or carbohydrate antigenic determinants of ZP3. Thus, a pool of the overlapping ZP3 peptides spanning the entire sequence of ZP3 (*see* Subheading 6.) failed to absorb the serum ZP3 autoantibodies elicited by the pZP3 T-epitope peptide. Importantly, these autoantibodies are highly effective in reducing the fertility of female mice in vivo *(49)*. The relative concentration of the "amplified" antibody response in obtaining the contraceptive effect was tenfold less than of antibodies to the ZP3 B-cell epitope, i.e., residues 335–342. Moreover, the autoantibodies have been shown to effectively retarget T-cell-mediated inflammatory events from one part of the ovary to another *(58)*.

9. CAN SYSTEMIC AUTOIMMUNE DISEASE RESULT FROM CELL ACTIVATION AND AMPLIFIED AUTOANTIBODY RESPONSE?

Epitope spreading has been postulated as a potential mechanism for the autoantibody responses to multiple antigens found within a single macromolecular complex in human SLE *(20–22,59–63)*. Nucleosome peptide-specific T-cells have been shown to accelerate disease onset in SLE-prone mice and to stimulate production of antibodies to nucleosomes in vitro *(59)*. Rabbits immunized with a human Sm B/B' peptide, which shares over 90% homology between species, elicit an autoantibody response that spreads not only to distant Sm epitopes (i.e., epitopes not present in the immunogen), but also to native DNA with which the Sm is known to form a molecular complex. Some of the immunized rabbits were described to harbor glomerular immune complexes *(61)*. A cryptic T-cell peptide of the murine snRNP D-antigen has been observed to favor the production of autoantibody responses characteristic of lupus *(21)*. Mice immunized with a nuclear self-antigen, peptide La/SSB fragment, produced antibodies against other regions of La/SSB, as well as to Ro/SSA *(22)*. Conversely, mice immunized with a Ro/SSA fragment synthesized antibodies to La/SS B-antigen *(22,62)*.

The critical observation in these studies is that autoantibody responses were provoked in animals that were not injected with the whole self antigen molecule. In other words, autoantibody amplification or spreading has occurred. Based on the result of our pZP3 studies, we propose that the endogenous nuclear antigens may be responsible for stimulating the amplified autoantibody responses observed in SLE. Intracellular antigens, which normally become accessible to the immune system following cellular apoptosis, may provide the needed endogenous stimulus for antibody amplification *(63,64)*. It will be important to determine whether the nuclear immunogens in the SLE studies involving the Sm B/B', Ro/SSA and La/SSB antigens contain self-T-cell epitopes (or foreign T-cell epitopes) that mimic self epitopes. SLE is a complex autoimmune syndrome. Its etiopathogenesis is complex, likely dependent on multiple abnormal or dysregulated T- and B-cell responses to self antigens. The data reviewed here support the possibility that the disease process may be triggered by molecular mimicry leading to autoreactive T-cell activation, followed by T-epitope to B-epitope spreading (or autoantibody amplification).

10. SUMMARY

Human and experimental autoimmune diseases are often manifested as organ inflammation with loss of function, detectable autoreactive T-cell and autoantibody responses, and positive clinical response to immunosuppression. In this chapter, we show that in the proper genetic context, these parameters of autoimmunity can result from a single pivotal event: the induction of a strong and persistent T-cell response for a foreign or unrelated self-peptide that mimics the target self peptide (Fig. 1). This event may apply to organ-specific and systemic autoimmunity, regardless of whether the tissue inflammation results from T-cell mechanisms and/or antibodies. T-cell peptide mimicry, through sharing of critical residues or by less well-defined mechanisms, can result in autoimmune disease. Once triggered, the helper T-cell response leads rapidly to a concomitant autoantibody response spreading to distant B-cell determinants of the self protein antigen. In the presence of activated helper autoreactive T-cells, the endogenous antigens can stimulate B-cells to provoke a functional autoantibody response against conformational antigenic determinants. These findings are based on a novel autoimmune ovarian disease model induced by self-peptide with well-defined T- and B-cell epitopes. Studies on lupus models indicate that similar events can lead to systemic autoimmunity. Together, they support the proposition that effective immunotherapy is predicated on tolerance induction of autoantigen specific CD4+ T-cells.

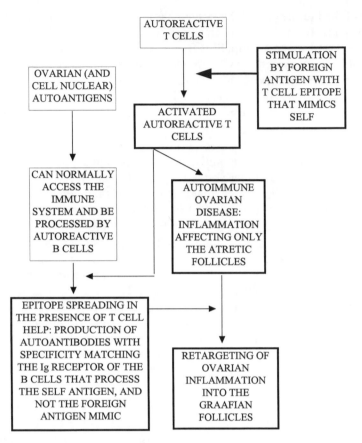

Fig. 1. Diagrammatic description of cellular events that may be responsible for the induction of pathogenic autoimmune T-cells, autoantibody responses and immunopathology through T-cell epitope mimicry.

ACKNOWLEDGMENTS

The authors would like to thank Marianne Volpe for preparation of this manuscript. This study was supported by a National Institutes of Health Grant AI-41236. Y.-H. Lou is supported by the Mellon Foundation. K. M. Garza is supported by a MARC Predoctoral Fellowship (1 F31 GM17853-02) awarded by the National Institute of General Medical Sciences.

REFERENCES

1. Oldstone, M. B. A. (1987) Molecular mimicry and autoimmune disease. *Cell* **50,** 819–820.
2. Rossini, A.A., Mordes, J. P., and Like, A. A. (1985) Immunology of insulin-dependent diabetes mellitus. *Ann. Rev. Immunol.* **3,** 289–320.

3. Miller, B. J., Appel, M. C., O'Neil, J. J., and Wicker, L. S. (1988) Both the Lyt-2 and L3T4+ T cell subsets are required for the transfer of diabetes in nonobese diabetic mice. *J. Immunol.* **140,** 52–58.
4. Haskins, K. and McDuffie, M. (1990) Acceleration of diabetes in young NOD mice with a CD4+ islet-specific T-cell clone. *Science* **249,** 1433–1436.
5. McCarron, R. M., Spatz, M. M., Kempski, O., Hogan, R. N., Muehl L., and McFarlin, D. E. (1986) Interaction between myelin basic protein-sensitized T lymphocytes and murine cerebral vascular endothelial cells. *J. Immunol.* **137,** 3428–3435.
6. van de Veen, R. C., Trotter, J. L., Hicky, W. F., and Kapp, J. A. (1990) The development and characterization of encephalitogenic cloned T cells specific for myelin proteolipid protein. *J. Neuroimmunol.* **26,** 139–145.
7. Yule, T. D. and Tung, K. S. K. (1993) Experimental autoimmune orchitis induced by testis and sperm antigen-specific T cell clones: an important pathogenic cytokine is tumor necrosis factor. *Endocrinology* **33,** 1098–1107.
8. Lindstrom, J. (1979) Autoimmune responses to acetylcholine receptors in myasthenia gravis and its animal model. *Adv. Immunol.* **27,** 1–50.
9. Weetman, A. P., Yatemen, M. E., Ealey, P. A., Black, C. M., Reimer, C. B., and Williams, R. C. (1990) Thyroid-stimulating antibody between different immunoglobulin G subclasses. *J. Clin. Invest.* **62,** 778–788.
10. Holmdahl, R., Vingsbo, C., Mo, J. A., Michaelsson, E., Malmstrom, V., Jansson, L., et al. (1995) Chronicity of tissue-specific experimental autoimmune disease: a role for B cells? *Immunol. Rev.* **144,** 109–135.
11. Lou, Y. H., Ang, J., Thai, H., McElveen, F., and Tung K. S. K. (1995) A ZP3 peptide vaccine induces antibody and reversible infertility without ovarian pathology. *J. Immunol.* **155,** 2715–2720.
12. Cohen, A. H. and Glassock, R. J. (1994) Anti-GBM glomerulonephritis including Goodpasture disease, in *Renal Pathology* (Tischer, C.G. and Brenner, B.M., eds.), J.B. Lippincott, Philadelphia, PA, pp. 524–552.
13. Engelfriet, C. P., Overbecke, M. A. M., and Vondemborne, A. E. G. K. (1992) Autoimmune hemolytic anemia. *Semin. Hematol.* **29,** 2–12.
14. Wofsy, D. J., Ledbetter, A., Hendler, P. L., and Seaman, W. E. (1985) Treatment of murine lupus with monoclonal anti-T cell antibody. *J. Immunol.* **134,** 852–857.
15. Santoro, T. J., Portanova, J. P., and Kotzin, B. L. (1987) The contribution of L3T4+ T cells to lymphoproliferation and autoantibody production in MRL-*lpr/lpr* mice. *J. Exp. Med.* **167,** 1713–1718.
16. Burlingame, R. W., Rubin, R. L., Balderas, R. S., and Theofilopoulos, A. N. (1993) Genesis and evolution of antichromatin autoantibodies in murine lupus implicates T-dependent immunization with self antigen. *J. Clin. Invest.* **91,** 1687–1695.
17. Singh, R. R., Kumar, V., Ebling, F. M., Southwood, S., Sette, A., Sercarz, E. E., et al. (1995) T cell determinants from autoantibodies to DNA can upregulate autoimmunity in murine systemic lupus erythematosus. *J. Exp. Med.* **181,** 2017– 2027.
18. Kaliyaperumal, A., Mohan, C., Wu, W., and Datta, S. K. (1995) Nucleosomal peptide epitopes for nephritis-inducing T helper cells of murine lupus. *J. Exp. Med.* **183,** 2459–2469.
19. Takeno, M. Nagafuchi, H., Kaneko, S., Wakisaka, S., Oneda, K., Takeba, Y., et al. (1997) Autoreactive T cell clone from patients with systemic erythematosus support polyclonal autoantibody production. *J. Immunol.* **158,** 3529–3538.

20. Mones, U., Seternes, O.-M., Hey, A. W., Silsand, Y., Traavik, T., Johansen, B., et al. (1995) In vivo expression of a single viral DNA-binding protein generates systemic lupus erythematosus-related autoimmunity to double-stranded DNA and histones. *Proc. Natl. Acad. Sci. USA* **92**, 12,393–12,397.
21. Bockenstedt, L., Gee, R. J., and Mamula, M. J. (1995) Self-peptides in the initiation of lupus autoimmunity. *J. Immunol.* **154**, 3516–3524.
22. Reynolds, P., Gordon, T. P., Purcell, A. W., Jackson, D. C., and McCluskey, J. (1996) Hierarchical self-tolerance to T cell determinants within the ubiquitous nuclear self-antigen La(SS-B) permits induction of systemic autoimmunity in normal mice. *J. Exp. Med.* **184**, 1857–1870.
23. Tung, K. S. K. and Lu, C. Y. (1991) Immunologic basis of reproductive failure, in *Pathology of Reproductive Failure* (Kraus, F.T., Damjanov, I., and Kaufman, N., eds.), Williams and Wilkins, New York, pp. 308–333.
24. Wood, D. M., Liu, C., and Dunbar, B. S. (1981) Effect of alloimmunization and heteroimmunization with zonae pellucidae on fertility in rabbits. *Eur. J. Immunol.* **25**, 439–450.
25. Mahi-Brown, C. A., Huang, T. T. F., and Yanagimachi, R. (1982) Infertility in bitches induced by active immunization with porcine zonae pellucidae. *J. Exp. Zool.* **222**, 89–95.
26. Sacco, A. G., Pierce, D. L., Subramanian, M. G., Yurewicz, E. C., and Dukelow, W. R. (1987) Ovaries remain functional in squirrel monkeys (Samiri sciureus) immunized with porcine zona pellucida 55,000 macromolecule. *Biol. Reprod.* **36**, 484–490.
27. Paterson, M., Wilson, M. R., Van Duin, M., and Aitken, R. J. (1996) Evaluation of zona pellucida antigens as potential candidate for immunocontraception. *J. Reprod. Fertil. Suppl.* **50**, 175–182.
28. Rhim, S. H., Millar, S. E., Robey, F., Dean, J., Allen, P., Tung, K. S. K., et al. (1992) Autoimmune disease of the ovary induced by a ZP3 peptide from the mouse zona pellucida. *J. Clin. Invest.* **89**, 28–35.
29. Bleil, J. D. and Wassarman, P. M. (1980) Structure and function of the zona pellucida: identification and characterization of the proteins of the mouse oocyte's zona pellucida. *Dev. Biol.* **76**, 185–202.
30. Dean, J. (1992) Biology of mammalian fertilization: role of the zona pellucida. *J. Clin. Invest.* **89**, 1055–1059.
31. Millar, S. E., Chamow, S. M., Baur, A. W., Oliver, C., Robey, F., and Dean, J. (1989) Vaccination with a synthetic zona pellucida peptide produces long-term contraception in female mice. *Science* **246**, 935–938.
32. Garza, K. and Tung, K. S. K. (1995) Frequency of T cell peptide crossreaction determined by experimental autoimmune disease and autoantibody induction. *J. Immunol.* **155**, 5444–5448.
33. Holoshitz, J., Naparstek, Y., Ben-Nun, A., Marquardt, P., and Cohen, I. R. (1984) T lymphocyte lines induce autoimmune encephalomyelitis, delayed hypersensitivity and bystander encephalitis or arthritis. *Eur. J. Immunol.* **14**, 729–734.
34. Mahi-Brown, C.A., Yule, T.D., and Tung, K. S. K. (1987) Adoptive transfer of murine autoimmune orchitis to naive recipients with immune lymphocytes. *Cell. Immunol.* **106**, 408–419.
35. Luo, A. M., Garza, K. M., Hunt, D., and Tung, K. S. K. (1993) Antigen mimicry in autoimmune disease: sharing of amino acid residues critical for pathogenic T cell activation. *J. Clin. Invest.* **92**, 2117–2123.

36. Singh, V. K., Yamaki, K., Abe, T., and Shinohara, T. (1989) Molecular mimicry between Uveitopathogenic site of retinal S-antigen and *Escherichia coli* protein: induction of experimental autoimmune uveitis and lymphocyte cross-reaction. *Cell. Immunol.* **122,** 262–273.
37. Atkinson, M. A., Bowman, M. A., Campbell, L., Darrow, B. L., Kaufman, D. L., and Maclaren, N. K. (1994) Cellular immunity to a determinant common to glutamate decarboxylase and coxsackie virus in insulin-dependent diabetes. *J. Clin. Invest.* **94,** 2125–2129.
38. Evavold, B. D., Sloan-Lancaster, J., Wilson, K. J., Rothbard, J. B., and Allen, P. M. (1995) Specific T cell recognition of minimally homologous peptides: evidence for multiple endogenous ligands. *Immunity* **2,** 655–664.
39. Harris, D. P., Vordemeier, H.-M., Singh, M., Moreno, C., Jurcevic, S., and Ivanyi, J. (1995) Cross-regulation by T cells of an epitope shared by two unrelated mycobacterial antigens. *Eur. J. Immunol.* **25,** 3173–3179.
40. Wucherpfennig, K. W. and Strominger, J. L. (1995) Molecular mimicry in T cell-mediated autoimmunity: viral peptides activate human T cell clones specific for myelin basic protein. *Cell* **80,** 695–705.
41. Avery, A. C., Zhao, Z. S., Rodriguez, A., Bikoff, E. K., Soheilian, M., Foster, C. S., et al. (1995) Resistance to herpes stromal keratitis conferred by an IgG2a-derived peptide. *Nature* **376,** 431–433.
42. Gautam, A. M., Pearson, C. I., Smilek, D. E., Steinman, L., and McDevitt, H. O. (1992) A polyalanine peptide with only five native myelin basic protein residues induces autoimmune encephalomyelitis. *J. Exp. Med.* **176,** 605–609.
43. Wraith, D. C., Bruun, B., and Fairchild, P. J. (1992) Cross-reactive antigen recognition by an encephalitogenic T cell receptor. *J. Immunol.* **149,** 3765–3770.
44. Bhardwaj, V., Kumar, V., Geysen, H. M., and Sercarz, E. E. (1993) Degenerate recognition of a dissimilar antigenic peptide by myelin basic protein-reactive T cells. *J. Immunol.* **151,** 5000–5010.
45. Quaratino, S., Thorpe, C. J., Travers, P. J., and Londei, M. (1995) Similar antigenic surfaces, rather than sequence homology, dictate T-cell epitope molecular mimicry. *Proc. Natl. Acad. Sci. USA* **92,** 10,398–10,402.
46. Brock, R., Wiesmuller, K.-H., Jung, G., and Walden, P. (1996) Molecular basis for the recognition of two structurally different major histocompatibility complex/peptide complexes by a single T-cell receptor. *Proc. Natl. Acad. Sci. USA* **93,** 13,108–13,113.
47. Vergelli, M., Hemmer, B., Kalbus, M., Vogt, A. B., Ling, N., Conlon, P., et al. (1997) Modifications of peptide ligands enhancing T cell responsiveness imply large numbers of stimulatory ligands for autoreactive T cells. *J. Immunol.* **158,** 3746–3752.
48. Lou, Y. H. and Tung, K. S. K. (1993) T cell peptide of a self protein elicits autoantibody to the protein antigen: implications for specificity and pathogenetic role of antibody in autoimmunity. *J. Immunol.* **151,** 5790–5799.
49. Lou, Y. H., McElveen, F., Garza, K., and Tung, K. S. K. (1996) Rapid induction of autoantibodies by endogenous ovarian antigens and activated T cells: implication in autoimmunity pathogenesis and B cell tolerance. *J. Immunol.* **156,** 3535–3540.
50. Yeh, T.-M. and Krolick, K. A. (1990) T cells reactive with a small synthetic peptide of the acetylcholine receptor can provide help for a clonotypically heterogeneous antibody response and subsequently impaired muscle function. *J. Immunol.* **144,** 1654–1660.

51. Lin, R.-H., Mamula, M. J., Hardin, J. A., and Janeway, Jr., C. A. (1991) Induction of autoreactive B cells allows priming of autoreactive T-cells. *J. Exp. Med.* **173**, 1433–1439.
52. Mamula, M. J. (1993) The inability to process a self-peptide allows autoreactive T cells to escape tolerance. *J. Exp. Med.* **177**, 567–571.
53. Griggs, N. D., Agersborg, S. S., Noelle, R. J., Ledbetter, J. A., Linsley, P. S., and Tung, K. S. K. (1996) The relative contribution of the CD28 and GP39 costimulatory pathways in the clonal expansion and pathogenic acquisition of self reactive T cells. *J. Exp. Med.* **183**, 801–810.
54. Sakaguchi, S., Fukuma, K., Kuribayashi, K., and Masuda, T. (1986) Organ-specific autoimmune diseases induced in mice by elimination of T-cell subsets. I. Evidence for the active participation of T cells in natural self-tolerance: deficit of a T-cell subset as a possible cause of autoimmune disease. *J. Exp. Med.* **161**, 72–87.
55. Smith, H., Sakamoto, Y., Kasai, K., and Tung, K. S. K. (1991) Effector and regulatory cells in autoimmune oophoritis elicited by neonatal thymectomy. *J. Immunol.* **147**, 2928–2933.
56. Smith, H., Lou, Y. H., Lacy, P., and Tung, K. S. K. (1992) Tolerance mechanism in ovarian and gastric autoimmune disease. *J. Immunol.* **149**, 2212–2218.
57. Sakaguchi, S., Sakaguchi, N., Asano, M., Itoh, M., and Toda, M. (1995). Immunologic self-tolerance maintained by activated T cells expressing IL-2 receptor a chains (CD25). Breakdown of a single mechanism of self-tolerance causes various autoimmune diseases. *J. Immunol.* **155**, 1151–1164.
58. Lou, Y. H., Park, K.-K., and Tung, K. S. K. (1996) Binding of autoantibody to the tissue antigen directs targeting of T cell-mediated autoimmune inflammation. Keystone Symposia on Lymphocyte Activation, Hilton Head, SC, Abst. 2051.
59. Mohan, C., Adams, S., Stanik, V., and Datta, S. K. (1993) Nucleosome: a major immunogen for pathogenic autoantibody-inducing T cells of lupus. *J. Exp. Med.* **177**, 1367–1381.
60. Fatenjad, S., Mamula, M. J., and Craft, J. (1993) Role of intermolecular/ intrastructural B- and T-cell determinants in the diversification of autoantibodies to ribonucleoprotein particles. *Proc. Natl. Acad. Sci. USA* **90**, 12,010–12,014.
61. James, J., Gross, T., Scofield, L. H., and Harley, J. B. (1995) Immunoglobulin epitope spreading and autoimmune disease after peptide immunization: Sm B/B'-derived PPPGMRPP and PPPGIRGP induce spliceosome autoimmunity. *J. Exp. Med.* **181**, 453–461.
62. Topfer, F. Gordon, T., and McCluskey, J. (1995) Intra- and intermolecular spreading of autoimmunity involving the nuclear self-antigens La(SS-B) and Ro(SS-A). *Proc. Natl. Acad. Sci. USA* **92**, 875–879.
63. Casciola-Rosen, L., Anhalt, G. J., and Rosen, A. (1995) DNA-dependent protein kinase is one of a subset of autoantigens specifically cleaved early during apoptosis. *J. Exp. Med.* **182**, 1625–1634.
64. Casciola-Rosen, L., Rosen, A., Petri, M., and Schlissel, M. (1996) Surface blebs on apoptotic cells are sites of enhanced procoagulant activity: implications for coagulation events and antigenic spreading in systemic lupus erythematosus. *Proc. Natl. Acad. Sci. USA* **93**, 1624–1629.

9

T-Cell Antigen Receptor
Repertoire in Rheumatoid Arthritis

James W. Edinger and David N. Posnett

1. INTRODUCTION

Rheumatoid arthritis (RA) is an organ-specific, but often also systemic auto-immune disease initiated and maintained by a chronic cell-mediated and humoral inflammatory response. T-cell response(s) to unknown antigen(s) are thought to be at the origin of RA, because early synovial histopathology resembles classic delayed type hypersensitivity and includes prominent infiltration consisting of antigen presenting dendritic cells clustered with CD4+ T-cells *(1–7)* in a perivascular location. Moreover, T-cell depleting therapy in RA, and in animal models of RA, can be beneficial. Finally, genetic susceptibility to RA is strikingly associated with certain MHC class II alleles which may either control peptide presentation to T-cells or influence T-cell repertoires during thymic maturation.

The following is a discussion of the still largely hypothetical pathogenesis of RA. The discussion is meant to highlight conclusions that can be drawn from the numerous T-cell receptor (TCR) repertoire studies in RA.

2. PATHOGENESIS OF RA

2.1. Genetics

Genetic analyses in families with RA suggest that many genes are involved in the pathogenesis of the disease *(8)* of which the MHC is one locus. A striking association with HLA DRB1 alleles 0101, 0401, 0404, and 1402 has been described *(9)*. In a recent American study, up to 96% of patients with RA had one of these alleles *(10)*, and in a similar Scandinavian study, the incidence of these allele was 93% *(11)*. However, in Greek patients only 43% had these alleles, and there was no association in this patient group with disease severity, as in other patient populations *(12,13)*. Thus, the RA susceptibility alleles may not be identical in different ethnic populations, as is often observed in studies of HLA associations with autoimmune disorders *(8)*.

The susceptibility alleles share a motif in the third hypervariable region of the DRβ chain: QKRAA. This led to the hypothesis that this "shared epitope"

Contemporary Immunology: Autoimmune Reactions
Edited by: S. Paul © Humana Press Inc., Totowa, NJ

was responsible for the disease association *(9)*. The charged R at position 71 is important in binding to the residue at position four or five of antigenic peptides bound in the MHC II groove. Thus, peptides that have a negative charge at position P4 and/or P5 bind 100–1000 fold more efficiently to a DR molecule with a positive charge at position 71, compared with alleles expressing a negative charge at position 71 such as DRB1*0402 *(14)*, which is not RA associated. Position 71 is also important in determining susceptibility to pemphigus vulgaris, in which case DRB1*0402 is associated with disease and the relevant peptides of the autoantigen desmoglein-3 have a positive charge at P4 *(15)*. Another example is provided by DQ alleles that differ at DQβ57 and are associated with either diabetes or pemphigus vulgaris perhaps because they determine the charge of residue P9 of the peptide in the groove. These data indicate a likely mechanism for the shared epitope hypothesis (Table 1, hypothesis 1). If the susceptibility alleles select a distinct array of peptides for presentation to T-cells, the idea is that one such peptide derived from a disease initiating microbe will stimulate T-cells that can crossreact with a similar autologous peptide, perhaps from an autoantigen such as cartilage proteoglycans, collagen type II, hsp 65, or fillagrin. Indeed, each one these proteins contains peptides that bind specifically to the susceptibility allele DR*0404 *(14)*.

An alternative hypothesis is that the selection of peptides by susceptibility alleles results in an altered TCR repertoire during thymic selection (Table 1, hypothesis 2). For instance, those T-cells with TCRs specific for DR*0404 molecules loaded with peptides containing a negative charge at P4 could be deleted by negative selection. It has been suggested that this would result in RA susceptibility because alternate TCRs used in a response to a RA-initiating microbe might be less efficient at clearing the initial pathogen, resulting in sustained inflammation. There is no good evidence for this possibility other than the observation that there is a group of patients with self-limited RA-like disease that lack DR*0404-like alleles *(16)*, i.e., it is implied that these patients are able to clear the disease initiating pathogen more efficiently. It could be speculated that DR*0404 specific T-cells that escape negative selection might have a greater potential for crossreactivity with autoantigens; such T-cells would not be present in the absence of susceptibility DR alleles. However, hypotheses based on negative selection are incompatible with the "dose-effect" of RA-associated alleles. Homozygosity, or a double dose, of the QKRAA shared epitope predicts severe RA *(10,17–19)*. Both a double dose and a single dose of a susceptibility allele are predicted to be sufficient to achieve negative selection, according to transgenic mouse models of thymic selection. However, as shown in transgenic mice by Berg et al. *(20)*, positive selection of T-cells specific for pigeon cytochrome C is twice as efficient with a double dose of the relevant IE^k class II molecule compared to a single dose in heterozygous animals. These authors hypothesize that heterozygous MHC alleles (found in the majority of subjects) favor selection of higher avidity TCRs because the higher avidity would be required in the setting of inefficient positive selection. The increased avidity

Table 1
Hypothetical Pathogenesis of RA and Expected Effects in the TCR Repertoire

Hypothesis	TCR repertoire pre-disease	TCR repertoire post-disease onset	Prediction
1. QKRAA of DRB1 allows binding of arthritogenic peptides	Repertoire differences do not affect susceptibility	Dependent on Ag stimulation—could be restricted due to similar peptides	Arthritogenic cells are DR*0401 restricted
2a. TCR repertoire selected by self peptides bound to susceptible DRB1 alleles	Repertoire differences affect susceptibility	Dependent on Ag stimulation—could be restricted due to similar peptides	Arthritogenic cells may or may not be DR*0401 restricted
2b. TCR repertoire selected by DRB1 HV3 peptides bound to DQ8	Repertoire differences affect susceptibility	Dependent on Ag stimulation—could be restricted due to similar peptides	Arthritogenic cells are DQ8 restricted

requirement could be provided by a higher affinity TCRαβ or it could be a result of higher levels of coreceptor expression (e.g., CD4 or CD8), known to affect thymic selection *(21)*. Thus, it is possible that the TCR repertoire selected in DR*0404 homozygous subjects might differ from the repertoire selected in heterozygous subjects.

A variation of this theme has been proposed by Chella David's group (Table 1, hypothesis 2b). They showed that peptides corresponding to HV3 (shared epitope region) are immunogenic in mice transgenic for human HLA DQ8, but only when they derive from non-RA associated alleles. The QKRAA containing peptides from DR*0401 and other RA-associated alleles were not immunogenic *(22)*. Indeed, humans that are either homozygous (DR*0401/*0401) or just heterozygous (DR*0401/*1501) seem to be tolerized to QKRAA peptides, but respond well to peptides from other DRB1 HV3 regions. These authors propose that DQ8 is the real susceptibility allele, not the DRB1 alleles like DR*0401. The latter are often in linkage disequilibrium with DQ8 *(23)*. In this hypothesis, the non-RA associated DRB1 alleles represent resistance genes, because they would lead to negative selection of reactive T-cells. The RA associated DRB1 alleles would be nonprotective because their HV3 derived peptides allow positive selection without inducing negative selection *(see* ref. *22*, Fig. 4). However, this hypothesis is also incompatible with the "dose-effect" of RA-associated DRB1 alleles, as both a single or a double dose of a protective DRB1 allele should exert an identical effect on negative selection.

This type of hypothesis (2a or 2b in Table 1) predicts minor alterations in the TCR repertoire, such that a few potentially arthritogenic T-cells are selected in a susceptible person. TCRs that are either DR 4 (or DQ8) restricted are the purported culprits. If such TCRs were homogeneous in terms of V gene usage they might be easily detectable, it is thought. It is likely that the T-cells with arthritogenic potential represent such a small population that differences in the overall TCR repertoire between normal DR4 homozygous and non-DR4 individuals would not be detectable by current methods, e.g., without prior in vitro stimulation with the yet unknown relevant antigen(s). Therefore, TCR repertoire studies have often focused on comparing T-cells from RA patients versus controls. In general, such studies give information on the repertoire of T-cells responding to either disease initiating antigens, antigens involved in disease maintenance or unrelated antigens. On the other hand, these studies do not help distinguish between the main hypotheses in Table 1. Transgenic mice expressing human DR and DQ alleles are becoming available *(24–29)*. It will be important to test the CD4[+] T-cells from RA patients for their arthritogenic potential in the transgenic mice.

2.2. Environment

Only 30–50% of identical twins are concordant for RA *(30)*. This simple fact proves unequivocally that environmental factors, such as microbial infections, are important in causing RA. When considering environmental factors, it is probably useful to distinguish between initiation and maintenance of the autoimmune inflammatory response. A good reason for assuming that these phases may differ is the analogy with Lyme disease due to the spirochete Borrelia Burgdorferii. In this disease, there is an acute infectious syndrome which can be successfully treated with antibiotics, and a postinfectious syndrome of autoimmune character which appears to be maintained by factors other than the initiating infection *(31)*. The histopathological changes in the synovia are strikingly similar to RA in Lyme disease.

It is possible that the initiating event in RA is quite nonspecific. Patients report trauma, surgery, or various infections as common preludes to RA *(32)*. But stress due to these conditions might also predispose to subclinical microbial infections. Various candidate microbes have been considered over the years. These include mycobacteria, mycoplasma, Lyme disease-like bacteria, herpesviruses (EBV), parvoviruses, lentiviruses, and rubella virus. In each case, there is no definitive data. Some of these microbes will be discussed in detail in Subheading 4.

2.3. Is RA Synovitis-Antigen Driven?

In considering microbial antigens as the source of immune activation in a disease like RA, it is useful to review some of the typical histopathological findings. The earliest inflammatory changes in RA synovial tissue are characterized by aggregates of dendritic cells and CD4$^+$ T-cells found in a perivascular distribution *(3,5,7,33–36)*. Typically, dendritic cells (DCs) function by capturing antigens in peripheral tissues, including the skin (where they are called Langerhans cells) and the mucous membranes (37). The DCs then travel to the draining lymph nodes and modulate their surface phenotype to acquire molecules needed for antigen presentation to T-cells, such as CD80 and CD86 (B7-1 and B7-2). DCs are approx 10–100-fold more efficient than other antigen presenting cells for presentation of the antigen to naive T-cells *(37)*. In animal models of EAE and thyroiditis, DCs have been shown to transfer the autoimmune disease to naive mice, which indicates that they can sequester the pathogenic autoantigens. The finding of clusters of DCs in early RA synovitis is a clear indication that antigens are being taken up for presentation to T-cells *(33)*.

Later changes include lymphoid aggregates with follicular structures similar to lymph nodes *(38)*. Sheets of CD4$^+$ CD45RO$^+$ memory T-cells have been described. These sheets are surrounded by heterogeneous cells, including macrophages, CD4$^+$, CD8$^+$, and plasma cells. T-cells make up over 50% of cells in the synovium while B-cells and plasma cells represent less than five percent *(1)*.

In spite of these findings, the conclusion that CD4$^+$ T-cells responding to an antigen are the basis of autoimmunity in RA is still debated. Two points are often made in questioning this conclusion. First, proliferation of CD4$^+$ T-cells within the synovium is apparently minimal *(30)*. The measured cellular proliferation in the synovium could be ascribed to other cell types like CD8$^+$ cells and type B synoviocytes *(30)*. However, there are powerful anti-inflammatory cytokines produced in abundance in the synovium, such as IL10, TGF-β, and IL1ra. Further, synovial CD4⁺ T-cells from RA patients can be readily cloned in vitro when taken out of the synovial cytokine milieu; which suggests that these cytokines may block proliferation. The second point is that the cytokine profiles show an abundance of monocyte/fibroblast derived cytokines but not T-cell cytokines. T-cell derived IL-2, IL-3, IL-4, and INF-γ are relatively scarce, but IL-1, IL-1ra, IL-6, IL-10, TNF-α, M-CSF, GM-CSF, TGF-β, INF-α, IL-8, MCP-1, and FGF, which are usually macrophage/fibroblast derived, are abundant. These findings have led to proposals that the synovial T-cell infiltration is not antigen-specific but is rather due to homing of T-cells to the joint. Perhaps homing occurs via expression of adhesion molecules such as VLA4 (α4β1), which mediates T-cell adhesion to VCAM-1 as well as the *CS1* sequence of fibronectin expressed by synovial endothelial cells (ECs). In patients with RA, 25% of synovial fluid T-cells express the α4β7 adhesion molecule compared with only seven percent of blood T-cells *(39)*. This adhesion molecule is involved in homing of cells to Peyer's patches. Moreover, the expression of the integrin α4β7, which is a specific marker for gut-associated T-lymphocytes, which is increased in synovial T-cells. The ligand for α4β7 is E-cadherin, which is abundantly expressed in the synovium *(40)*. Therefore, one might speculate that synovial T-cells may be activated in the gut before finding their way to the synovium.

These hypotheses can be tested by conducting TCR repertoire studies. A random infiltration of T-cells in synovia would yield a completely polyclonal repertoire equal to that in the blood, even when assayed by the most senstive PCR methods. This does not fit the data (see Subheading 3.) as oligoclonal expansions in RA synovial samples appear to be the rule, not the exception. However, synovial infiltration may be limited to T-cells that are preactivated. These T-cells might already be clonally expanded and might express a restricted TCR repertoire. For instance, it is known that intestinal immunoblasts have a dual binding specificity for mucosal and synovial endothelium, but not for lymph node endothelium *(41)*. It is also known that single expanded T-cell clones are widely disseminated over the entire surface of the gut mucosa, since the same TCR β-chain CDRIII sequences are found at distant sites in the small and large intestine *(42–44)*. Presumably, these clones exit into the circulation and return to the gut, rather than migrating laterally in the intestinal mucosa. Whether they could sometimes home to the synovium, instead of returning to the gut, could be tested by comparing the CDRIII sequences from the synovium, the blood and the gut in the same RA patient.

The findings on cytokines and the anergic state of T-cells in synovia are not atypical for what is observed in other chronic inflammatory disorders, even those that are clearly induced by antigenic stimulation of T-cells. For instance IL-1, TNFα, and IL-6 are prominent cytokines in inflammatory bowel disease (IBD), in Chagas disease and in chronic graft versus host disease (GVHD), while IL-2 and IL-4 are not increased *(45–48)*. Longitudinal analysis of cytokine profiles in GVHD has shown the evolution of the response, with high levels of IL-4, IL-2, IL-12, and IFNγ observed during the early but not later phases. If local synovial tissue cytokine profiles could be measured at very early time points in RA, a different cytokine profile from that seen in established RA patients might emerge.

These considerations serve as a warning for interpreting TCR repertoire studies. If a particular TCR is to indicate a disease-initiating antigen, it must derive from the earliest lesions. By comparison, in the EAE model induced in rats by immunizing with myelin basic protein (MBP), the pathogenic MBP-specific Vβ8 T-cells are seen infiltrating the CNS during the first week and are then rapidly diluted by influx of other T-cells *(49–52)*. This is owing in part to epitope spreading *(53–55)* or to nonspecific recruitment.

Although synovial pathology involves a heterogeneous mixture of cells *(see* Table 2), the maintenance phase of synovial inflammation in RA is also likely to be in part T-cell-dependent. Macroscopic changes in the RA joint point to proliferation of synovial tissue leading to pannus formation extending over cartilaginous surfaces. The synovial cell membrane is normally 1–2 cell layers deep, but 4–10 cells deep in RA. Both types of synoviocytes are increased in numbers. This abnormal synoviocyte proliferation is thought to be T-cell dependent. The synoviocyte proliferation also occurs in the MRL/lpr mouse strain, in which the basic defect is deficient apoptosis of T-lymphocytes *(56,57)*.

3. T-CELL RECEPTOR REPERTOIRE

There have been several reviews on the topic of TCR repertoires in RA and other diseases. Some focus on the methods for TCR repertoire analysis *(58–60)* and the relationship to genetic variations in the normal repertoire *(61,62)*. Mostly, the methods are based on RT-PCR, which measures RNA expression for a given TCR chain in a cell population, and the use of monoclonal antibodies (MAbs) specific for the various TCR chains and V gene elements, which measures protein expression on individual T-cells. There are disadvantages and advantages with either method *(59)*.

There were initial expectations of a simple result, e.g., usage of a particular TCR in the RA synovial immune response. However, the results varied from one study to another, and from one patient to the other, leaving the field in a state of confusion. A recent review by Struyk et al. *(63)* examines the evidence for involvement of T-cells in the pathology of RA based on TCR repertoire studies. The overall finding of the numerous published studies on this topic is that synovial T-cells in RA contain clonally expanded cell populations. It is easy to conclude that the T-cells are oligoclonal, based on the findings of TCR CDRIII sequences that are dominantly expressed in the synovium, while similar sequences are completely diverse in the blood of the same patient. The conclusion that individual T-cell clones are "expanded" in the synovium is often less well substantiated, as the cells themselves are usually not counted. However, normal synovial tissues contain very few lymphocytes compared with the inflamed synovium of an RA joint (Table 2), and thus, expansion is likely.

Table 2
Infiltrating Cell Types Found in RA Synovitis

Cell types	Early	ST/SF	Proposed role
Mature, functional DCs that can adoptively transmit disease	++	ST/SF	Efficient presentation of Ag to T cells
CD4 $\alpha\beta$ T-cells	++	ST>SF	Ag recognition ?
CD8 $\alpha\beta$ T-cells	++	SF>ST	Ag recognition ?
CD4 8 $\gamma\delta$ T-cells		SF>ST	Ag recognition ?
Monocytes/macrophages		ST/SF	Source of IL-10 and many prominent cytokines
Granulocytes		SF only!	Phagocytosis (ICs, Ig coated particles), attracted by chemokines, C5a, LTB4, PAF, source of fibronectin, IL-1ra
Proliferating synoviocyte A (macrophage-like)	++	ST	Source of cytokines
Proliferating synoviocyte B (fibroblastic)		ST	In vitro growth potential
B-cells & plasma cells		ST	Produce RF, collagen-II Ab; maintain synovitis because of immune complexes and complement activation, source of EBV
NK cells	++	ST	
Mast cells		ST	Stimulate synoviocytes ?
Endothelial cells (neovascularization)		ST	Expression of addressins ?

ST, synovial tissue; SF, synovial fluid; IC, immune complexes; RF, rheumatoid factor.

It is at least theoretically possible that the repertoire that is analyzed is derived from T-cells that survive (and have high TCRβ RNA content), rather than from apoptotic T-cells. But the latter might be the relevant disease-causing T-cells, having undergone TCR mediated activation induced cell death. This is a real concern, as synovial T-cells obtained ex vivo, of which 40–60% express Fas *(64)*, undergo rapid spontaneous apoptosis *(65)*. A recent paper directly addresses this point and finds that oligoclonal expansions are limited to the Fas+ T-cells (apoptosis sensitive cells) obtained ex vivo, while the Fas-resistant T-cells are completely polyclonal *(64)*. Apoptosis must be considered, therefore, in order to accurately evaluate the repertoire studies, specially when cells are expanded in vitro prior to repertoire analysis.

Studies that evaluate synovial T-cells after in vitro culture (with or without addition of IL-2) are indeed susceptible to artifactual skewing of the repertoire *(66)*. Although cell culture is frequently necessary to obtain sufficient numbers of cells or sufficient high-quality RNA for analysis, there should always be independent confirmation of the findings on fresh ex vivo tissues. For example, primers that anneal to CDRIII sequences can be used to detect the relevant expanded T-cell clone in biopsy material by PCR or other methods, and tissue sections can be stained with MAbs specific for TCR Vβ regions.

3.1. Clonal Expansions

In spite of these caveats, there are distinct conclusions that can be drawn from the cumulative repertoire studies. These conclusions are summarized in Table 3. With few exceptions *(67–72)*, most studies show evidence of T-cell clonal expansions (CE) in the inflamed RA joint (Table 3). These expansions are thought to be relevant because they are concentrated in either the synovial tissue or the synovial fluid compared with the patients' own peripheral blood lymphocytes (PBL). Moreover, if these cells are adoptively transferred to the joints of mice with severe combined immune deficiency disease (SCID), the mice develop synovial hyperplasia *(73)* and arthritis *(74)*. By contrast, synovial T-cells from RA that lack clonal expansions did not cause synovial hyperplasia in these mice *(73)*. The occurrence of clonal expansions in RA has been compared to unrelated disease controls or non-RA synovial controls *(75–77)*, or to controls that are matched for the DR4+ genotype *(78)*, or to unaffected siblings *(76)* or unaffected identical twins *(68,69)*. The clonal expansions can involve TCRαβ and/or TCRγδ T-cells. The latter are often Vγ9Vδ1 T-cells *(79–81)*. The clonal expansions can involve CD4+, CD8+, or double negative T-cells. A dominant phenotype seems to be the CD4+ CD57+ CD28− T-cell *(82)*, but clonally expanded CD8+ cells are also prevalent and also have a CD57+ CD28− phenotype (Table 3). CD4+ CD57+ CD28− T-cells were five times more prevalent in RA than in age-matched normal controls. Unlike CD28− cells from normal subjects, the CD4+ CD28− cells from RA proliferated in response to anti-CD3, responded in an autologous mixed lymphocyte reaction and were resistant to

Table 3
Findings of TCR Repertoire Studies in RA

Finding	References
TCR β clonal expansions (CE) in ST or SF	*(73,75-78,83,103,104,104, 132–151)*
TCR α–CE	*(72,77,79,142,145,152–154)*
TCR δγ CE	*(70,79–81,155-160)*
CE in CD4⁺	*(76,78,103,161)*
CE in CD8⁺	*(83,89,140)*
CE in CD4⁺ CD28⁻ (or CD57⁺)	*(82,138,162,163)*
CE in CD8⁺ CD28⁻ (or CD57⁺)	*(89,164)*
Microheterogeneity of CE in a single synovium	*(144,165)*
CE in symmetric joints	*(104,149,155,156)*
CE that persist over years	*(76,78,89,103,104,137,149,166)*
CE that are transient	*(167)*
CE in the blood (rather than synovium)	*(87,99,139,140,152)*
CE with CDRIII sequences or motifs shared between patients	*(63,82,89,140,147)*
CE are "auto"- reactive (DR4 restricted)	*(69,83,103,168)*
CE are reactive with EBV antigens	*(83,84)*

CE, clonal expansion.

apoptosis *(82)*. Longitudinal studies show that in some RA cases the clonal expansions can persist for many years, and in other cases they are transient. Interestingly, there is microheterogeneity within a single synovial tissue sample: some Vβ are found concentrated at one site but not at another site only a few millimeters distant. On the other hand, several papers describe clones that are present simultaneously in both affected knee joints of a given patient. Regarding the possible "auto"reactivity of the expanded clones, the data are still sparse. It is often difficult to distinguish true autoreactivity from reactivity with EBV encoded antigens, as the reactivities have usually been tested using EBV transformed autologous B-cell lines. Unambiguous studies showing reactivity with EBV antigens *(83,84)* have been carried out primarily with CD8 clones.

It is of interest that CD28⁻CD57⁺ populations (usually CD8⁺ or CD4⁻8⁻, but also CD4⁺) from normal individuals frequently contain clonal expansions *(85–89)* and these are often long-lived, persisting for many years in the blood *(67,87,90,91)*. Most of these cells are thought to represent cytotoxic effector cells, but they may also function as nonspecific suppressor cells *(92–95)*. The persistent clonal expansions imply that they are reactive with persistent antigens such as those of Herpes viruses *(96)*. Clonal expansions of CD8⁺CD57⁺CD28⁻ cells also occur in a number of other diseases, for example after bone marrow transplantation *(97)* or in HIV infection *(98)*. What then is unusual in RA, if clonal expansions are common in normal subjects? First, the frequency of the clonal expansions in the blood of RA patients appears to be higher than in normal subjects *(87,89,99)*. Second, the location of these cells in the synovial tissues in RA is unusual and perhaps implies that persistent antigens are located in this tissue. Third, the uncommon CD4$^+$CD57$^+$CD28$^-$ phenotype is considerably more prominent in RA than in normals *(82,138)*.

3.2. CDRIII Sequences

Great care should be taken in interpreting data on CDRIII sequences. While there have been many claims for CDRIII amino acid motifs characteristic for RA, each laboratory describes a different "motif" *(63)*. Usually, the motifs are particular to the patient and may be shared by various clones isolated from synovial tissues or blood. In rare cases, a motif shared between patients has been described, which indicates responses to the same antigen (Table 3).

For the TCRβ chain, the CDRIII region is defined as the sequences between the Vβ-CAS... and ...FGXG-Jβ segments *(100)*. There are distinct patterns of amino acid usage at each residue in the CDRIII region (Table 4) for both TCRβ and TCRα *(100–102)*. These are dictated by 1) the last few codons of the genomic V region (Fig. 1A), 2) the G rich sequences of the 2 Dβ segments which frequently encode glycine in any reading frame (Fig. 1B), and 3) the first few codons of the J segment. In addition, N region nucleotide preferences may exist *(100)*. The net effect is that CDRIII amino acids are not random at any given residue position and the bias probably differs for each combination of V and J gene segments *(100)*. Unfortunately, most CDRIII studies reported in RA do not take into account these important rules.

For instance, a Vβ17-CASS-**IGQxN**-Jβ2.1 CDRIII motif was described in four clones obtained from synovium of an RA patient *(103)*. However, the **I** represents the last codon of the genomic Vβ17, the **GQ** could be encoded by frame two of Dβ1, and the **N** is clearly encoded by Jβ2.1. The latter is known to be one of the most frequently used Jβ segments. Position three of CDRIII encodes a **G** in 20% of random Vβ sequences, although a **Q** at position four is less common (<10%) *(102)*. Thus, it is necessary to compare this sequence with a large number of Vβ17-Jβ2.1 sequences from the same patient's blood to identify it as a special "motif" characteristic of RA.

Another example is the paper by Alam et al. *(104)*. Here, the **TS** CDRIII motif represents mostly frame six of Dβ2.1 (Fig. 1) and is found mainly in association with Jβ2.1 or Jβ2.3. This may be due to an idiosyncrasy of recombinations between certain Vβ and certain Jβ segments, but it might also represent antigen driven selection. The same paper describes a **GxxG** motif in the CDRIII, but this is hardly surprising in view of the frequency of **G** found in random CDRIII sequences (Table 4 and Fig. 1). Therefore, the significance of this sequence can only be established after comparison with large numbers of carefully selected controls expressing the same Vβ and Jβ. Finally, this paper describes 14 clonal expansions encoding a valine in the CDRIII. Valine residues are frequently dispersed between CDRIII residues 1–8, and it is hard,

Table 4
Mouse Vβ17 CDRIII Sequences in CD4 T-Cells (100)

Amino acid position	Vβ			CDRIII (Vβ–N–Dβ–N–Jβ)				Jβ
	... CAS	1	2	3	4	5	6	... FGXG
Most freq. aa		S	L	G	G	G	.	
polar: QNTS[a]		93	9	20	38	31		
Hydrophobic: LIFMVA		1	63	11	14	15		
Acidic: DE		0	0	14	11	13		
Basic: RKH		4	6	5	8	3		
Tryptophane: W		0	1	1	2	0		
Glycine: G		1	1	33	31	36		
Proline: P		0	19	8	5	3		
Tyrosine: Y		0	0	10	2	4		

Human Vβ CDRIII Sequences in T-Cells (102)

Amino acid position	Vβ			CDRIII (Vβ–N–Dβ–N–Jβ)				Jβ
	... CAS	1	2	3	4	5	6	... FGXG
Most freq. CDRIII aa		S	L	G	G	G	.	
polar: QNTS[a]		27	26	22	33	36		
Hydrophobic: LIFMVA		33	23	21	15	14		
Acidic: DE		9	9	7	9	15		
Basic: RKH		12	13	10	9	8		
Tryptophane: W		2	1	1	0	1		
Glycine: G		8	20	33	27	18		
Proline: P		8	7	4	6	5		
Tyrosine: Y		0	0	2	1	3		

[a] The numbers indicate frequencies (%) at which an amino acid of the type listed in the left hand column are found at the

A

3' end of Vβ genomic sequences:

```
Vβ3           1   2   3 (position in CDR3)
  C    A    S    S    L
TGT GCC AGC AGT TTA TG 7mer-spacer-9mer
Vβ17
  C    A    S    S    I
TGT GCC AGT AGT ATA GA 7mer-spacer-9mer
Vβ5.5
  C    A    S    S    L
TGT GCC AGA AGC TTG G 7mer-spacer-9mer
Vβ8.1
  C    A    S    S    L
TGT GCC AGC AGT TTA GC 7mer-spacer-9mer
Vβ6.7
  C    A    S    S    L
TGT GCC AGC AGC TTA GC 7mer-spacer-9mer
Vβ5.1
  C    A    S    S    L
TGC GCC AGC AGC TTG G 7mer-spacer-9mer
```

B Dβ reading frames

```
Dβ1.1
GGGACAGGGGGC                                 usage (n=31)
  G   T   G   G          frame 1             5/31=16%
  - G   Q   G --          frame 2             4/31=13%
  -- D   R   G -          frame 3             6/31=19%
Dβ2.1
GGACTAGCGGGAGGCCACGA
  G   L   A   G   G   H --   frame 4          5/31=16%
  - D   X   R   E   G   T -   frame 5          2/31=6%
  -- T   S   G   R   A   R    frame 6          9/31=29%
```

Fig. 1. CDRIII sequences encoded in genomic V and D segments. (**A**) Most genomic sequences of Vβ genes encode a hydrophobic L after the CASS and 1 or 2 extra nucleotides that may form part of the next codon (i.e., codon 3 of the CDRIII). Genomic sequences for human Vβ genes can be accessed under Genbank accession # L36092. (**B**) The 3 reading frames of Dβ1 and Dβ2 are given and their usage was assessed based on 31 CDRIII sequences (Vβ5.2, Vβ5.3, Vβ6.7) *(86)* where Dβ segments could be unambiguously assigned. Note that frame 5 contains a stop codon and is rarely used.

therefore, to imagine that valines might be selected for by a single antigen. The Struyk review *(63)* contains a long list of similar putative motifs which are often difficult to interpret.

3.3. Conclusions

In all of the work summarized above, the main conclusion appears to be that clonal expansions of T-cells in RA are antigen driven and include both αβ and γδ T-cells and both CD4+ and CD8+ T-cells. The nature of the antigen(s) is unresolved. It is not clear whether the culprit antigen is an autoantigen or a foreign (microbial) antigen, whether one or multiple unrelated protein antigens are involved, whether the antigen(s) are located in the synovium or elsewhere (e.g., the gut), whether the antigenic stimulus changes over time, and whether the antigenic stimulus is important in disease initiation or in maintenance of the chronic inflammatory process. In a few cases, however, repertoire studies have led to identification of EBV antigens recognized by clonally expanded T-cells. These will be discussed below along with other evidence for a role of microbial antigens in RA.

4. MICROBIAL AGENTS

Many microbial agents have been suggested in the pathogenesis of RA, among them, mycoplasma, parvovirus B19, retroviruses, enteric bacteria, and EBV *(30)*. The putative mechanisms can be divided in two groups: either direct synovial infection or indirect immunopathogenic mechanisms.

An example of a viral infection that may be linked to an autoimmune disease is coxsackie virus, which was isolated from the pancreas of a fatal case of type I diabetes. Moreover, this virus caused diabetes in mice *(105,106)*. Like diabetes, RA has widespread prevalence. It is, therefore, attractive to consider a role for endemic virus(es) in these diseases.

4.1. Parvovirus B19

Antibodies have been detected against B19 in the blood of patients with early RA *(107)*. Viral DNA has also been detected by PCR in synovial tissue *(108)* and in RA patients' bone marrow *(109)*. These studies did not look for evidence of productive viral infection. Synoviocytes taken from the joint of a RA patient and cultured in vitro, produced another strain of parvovirus, RA-1 *(110)*. RA-1 is related to bovine parvovirus *(111)*. The epidemiology showing an association of parvovirus with RA has not yet been reported.

4.2. Human T-cell Leukemia Virus Type I (HTLV-I)

HTLV-1 is an endemic virus in southern Japan and in the West Indies. An extensive study in Japan has documented serological, histological, and PCR evidence indicating an association between the presence of the virus and a clinical disease indistinguishable from idiopathic RA *(112)*. Synoviocytes can be activated by the tax protein (HTLV-1 transactivator) as measured by increased mRNA levels of several cytokines, including IL-1β, IL-6, and TNF-α *(113)*. Importantly, HTLV-1 readily infects synovial cells in vitro. Since infection by this human virus is not possible in a mouse model, the investigators produced a transgenic mouse carrying the HTLV-1 tax gene under the control of the viral LTR. The transgenic mice develop RA-like disease with histopathology similar to that seen in the typical rheumatoid pannus *(114)*. Tax mRNA is easily found at relatively high levels in the synoviocytes of the transgenic mice. These contributions are instructive, in that an intact virus is not required for arthritis, but simply the expression of a viral transactivator protein.

A recent report from Britain failed to detect lentiviral DNA or RNA in the synovial tissue and the blood of British RA patients using a PCR method with a detection limit of 1 infected cell per 20,000 uninfected cells *(115)*. Thus, the role of HTLV-1 in RA may be limited to populations where the virus is endemic. In other populations, other viruses could provide transactivator genes that substitute for Tax in disease pathogenesis.

4.3. Cytomegalovirus

Among the most common endemic viruses worldwide are the herpesviruses. By analogy with HTLV-I, this family of viruses might participate in causing RA by transactivation of host cell genes without a requirement for the production of infectious virus in synovial tissues. Experiments to test the hypothetical role of herpesviruses are numerous. High titers of anti-cytomegalovirus (CMV) antibodies are associated with RA *(116–118)* which could indicate production of viral antigens. Examination of peripheral blood samples and synovial fluid for CMV DNA by PCR did not reveal any differences from normal controls *(119)*. However, these authors did not measure expression of viral mRNA. It should be noted that CMV is present in latent form in rare, bone marrow derived progenitors of the myelo-monocytic lineage of most normal adults *(120,121)*.

4.4. Epstein–Barr Virus (EBV)

Most adults have a controlled, latent infection by EBV. Approximately, 1/200,000 to 1/1,000,000 B-cells are infected *(122)*, as measured by the Gardella gel technique, in which DNA present in gel slices is amplified by PCR and detected by Southern blots. Contrary to the situation in normal adults, high titers of antibodies against EBV antigens have been found in patients with RA *(123)*. In addition, the frequency of B-cells infected by EBV in the peripheral blood of RA patients is high *(124,125)*. Despite these data, there is controversy over the role of EBV in RA. For example, the evidence for the presence of EBV in patients with RA was generated using PCR of genomic DNA from the lymphocytes found in synovial fluid and in peripheral blood *(126)*. In this study, the percentage of positive samples in RA synovial fluids was 19% versus 33% in reactive arthritis. Further, the prevalence of detectable EBV DNA in the peripheral blood was not very different in patients with RA (39%), reactive arthritis (39%), other arthropathies (27%) and normal controls (31%). One might expect to find larger differences among these populations of patients, if EBV were the causative agent of RA. Recently, EBV (EBER1) DNA was measured by *in situ* hybridization in synovial tissues and found in 23% of RA patients, but in no osteoarthritis patients (127). Antibody staining of synovial tissue also detected the EBV protein LMP1 in 12% of the RA patients. However, the transcription of EBV genes in the synovium was again not assessed.

It is clear that EBV infected B-cells do infiltrate the RA synovium as they can spontaneously transform into lymphoblastoid cell lines (128). One key question is whether the EBV infected B-cells are enriched in synovial tissues as compared with blood, for example.

Other herpes viruses commonly present in leukocytes, such as human herpes virus 6 (HHV6), the agent of roseola infantum, HHV7 and HHV8 (Kaposi's sarcoma associated virus), have not yet been rigorously examined in RA synovial tissue. HHV7 infects T-cells (129) and HHV8 infects B-cells (130). Recently, a PCR study showed that EBV and HHV6 DNA is present at a higher frequency in saliva (but not blood) of RA patients compared to normal individuals (131).

4.5. Clonal Expansions and EBV Antigens

To examine whether EBV might encode antigens that drive clonal expansions in RA, one needs to correlate the parameters of EBV infection with the appearance of clonal expansions. A recent paper addresses this point in three patients with acute infectious mononucleosis. Large clonal expansions are described, representing up to 30% of the circulating CD8$^+$ T-cells. The specific expansions detected with monoclonal antibodies and by PCR were

Patient 1:	Vβ3S1	Vβ13S1	Vβ14
Patient 2:	Vβ3S1	Vβ17S1	
Patient 3:	Vβ8	Vβ9	Vβ13S1

TCR repertoire analysis six months after recovery showed a normal Vβ repertoire without the previously observed expansions. This work illustrates that clonal expansions do occur in response to acute EBV infections. However, in a self-limited disease like infectious mononucleosis, the clonal expansions are transient, unlike the situation in RA (Table 3) or with HIV infection (98).

A recent comprehensive study of clonal expansions in RA has led to the identification and cloning of some of the involved antigens (83,84). In the first paper (83), a single patient with RA of six years duration was studied in detail. The Vβ repertoire of this patient was examined with Vβ-specific antibodies; the only expansions detected were in the CD8$^+$ T-cells of the synovium (Vβ2, Vβ14.1, aand Vβ22.1). No expansions were detected in the peripheral blood. The expansions were analyzed further by study of CDRIII length distribution (immunoscope analysis). There were alterations in the CDRIII length distribution in the synovial lymphocytes compared to peripheral blood. In this analysis, there were two sources of synovial lymphocytes: fluid and membrane. It is significant that many of the CDRIII lengths found in the synovial fluid were also present in the membrane, suggesting that the expanded clones not only accumulated in the fluid but also infiltrated the tissue. The size of the clonal expansions detected by CDRIII length analysis ranged from approximately one to 11% of the total synovial fluid lymphocytes. The clonal expansions were further characterized by sequencing the CDRIII region of the TCRβ chain. Seventy two IL-2 dependent T-cell clones were then obtained and were also sequenced across the TCR β CDRIII region, to identify clones that matched the ex vivo synovial clonal expansions. The T-cell clones were predominantly CD8+, and were frequently restricted by HLA-B*4002. The cells were cells reactive with autologous EBV-transformed B-lymphoblastoid cells. The reactivity toward autologous B-lymphoblastoid cells was also observed with clones from a second RA patient.

The second paper *(84)* addresses the antigenic specificity of the T-cells. The approach applied was to construct a cDNA expression library from the EBV+ B-lymphoblastoid cells of the original RA patient, transfect the library into COS cells that expressed the correct class I alleles, and screen for responses of cloned T-cells using a TNFα production assay. Several clones reactive with the EBV transactivator proteins BMLF1 and BZLF1, were identified representing approx 30% of the original set of 7Z T-cell clones. Both synovial membrane and synovial fluid, but not PBL T-cells, responded to stimulation with BMLF1 and BZLF1 in the TNFα assay. The responses were MHC-restricted and were present in five of 10 RA patients tested.

The results indicate that reactivation of latent EBV infection, with production of BZLF1 and BMLF1, might be responsible for clonal expansions in RA patients, possibly causing synovial inflammation. In addition, the transactivators might enhance synovial inflammation, by analogy to the HTLV-I tax transgenic mice (*see* Subheading 4.2.). Possibly, the transactivators activate various cytokine genes and cause nonspecific inflammation. Alternatively, the transactivators could induce expression of cryptic antigenic epitopes from self-antigens (e.g., collagen II), which may then serve as the antigenic stimuli for further clonal expansions (e.g., the CD4+ CD28- clonal expansions).

5. CONCLUSIONS

In this review, we discuss the evidence for antigen driven immune responses of RA synovial T-cells. The cumulative evidence from multiple repertoire studies strongly suggests that clonal expansions are driven by persistant microbial antigens. Candidate microbes are those that persist longterm, for example the herpes viruses. The most extensively studied herpes virus in RA is EBV. However, HHV-6, HHV-7, and HHV-8 have not been carefully evaluated in RA synovial tissues. TCR repertoire studies can lead to identification of novel antigens that could be relevant to autoimmunity, as exemplified by the elegant studies on EBV transactivators in RA.

REFERENCES

1. Van Boxel, J. A. and Paget, S. A. (1975) Predominantly T-cell infiltrate in rheumatoid synovial membranes. *N. Engl. J. Med.* **293,** 517–520.
2. Kurosaka, M. and Ziff, M. (1983) Immunoelectron microscopic study of the distribution of T cell subsets in rheumatoid synovium. *J. Exp. Med.* **158,** 1191–1210.

3. Randen, I., Mellbye, O. J., Forre, O., and Natvig, J. B. (1995) The identification of germinal centres and follicular dendritic cell networks in rheumatoid synovial tissue. *Scand. J. Immunol.* **41,** 481–486.
4. Thomas, R. and Quinn, C. (1996) Functional differentiation of dendritic cells in rheumatoid arthritis: role of CD86 in the synovium. *J. Immunol.* **156,** 3074–3086.
5. Thomas, R., Davis, L S., and Lipsky, P.E. (1994) Rheumatoid synovium is enriched in mature antigen-presenting dendritic cells. *J. Immunol.* **152,** 2613–2623.
6. Stagg, A. J., Harding, B., Hughes, R. A., Keat, A., and Knight, S. C. (1991) The distribution and functional properties of dendritic cells in patients with seronegative arthritis. *Clin. Exp. Immunol.* **84,** 66–71.
7. Waalen, K., Forre, O., Pahle, J., Natvig, J. B., and Burmester, G. R. (1987) Characteristics of human rheumatoid synovial and normal blood dendritic cells. Retention of class II major histocompatibility complex antigens and accessory function after short-term culture. *Scand. J. Immunol.* **26,** 525–533.
8. Vyse, T. J. and Todd, J. A. (1996) Genetic analysis of autoimmune disease. *Cell* **85,** 311–318.
9. Gregersen, P. K., Silver, J., and Winchester, R. J. (1987) The shared epitope hypothesis: an approach to understanding the molecular genetics of susceptibility to rheumatoid arthritis. *Arthritis Rheum.* **30,** 1205–1213.
10. Weyand, C. M., Hicok, K. C., Conn, D. L., and Goronzy, J. J. (1992) The influence of HLA-DRB1 genes on disease severity in rheumatoid arthritis (*see* comments). *Ann. Intern. Med.* **117,** 801–806.
11. Wallin, J., Hillert, J., Olerup, O., Carlsson, B., and Strom, H. (1991) Association of rheumatoid arthritis with a dominant DR1/Dw4/Dw14 sequence motif, but not with T cell receptor beta chain gene alleles or haplotypes (*see* comments). *Arthritis Rheum.* **34,** 1416–1424.
12. Boki, K. A., Panayi, G. S., Vaughan, R. W., Drosos, A. A., Moutsopoulos, H. M., and Lanchbury, J. S. (1992) HLA class II sequence polymorphisms and susceptibility to rheumatoid arthritis in Greeks. The HLA-DR beta shared-epitope hypothesis accounts for the disease in only a minority of Greek patients. *Arthritis Rheum.* **35,** 749–755.
13. Boki, K. A., Drosos, A. A., Tzioufas, A. G., Lanchbury, J. S., Panayi, G. S., and Moutsopoulos, H. M. (1993) Examination of HLA-DR4 as a severity marker for rheumatoid arthritis in Greek patients. *Ann. Rheum. Dis.* **52,** 517–519.
14. Hammer, J., Gallazzi, F., Bono, E., Karr, R. W., Guenot, J., Valsasnini, P., et al. (1995) Peptide binding specificity of HLA-DR4 molecules: correlation with rheumatoid arthritis association (*see* comments). *J. Exp. Med.* **181,** 1847–1855.
15. Wucherpfennig, K. W. and Strominger, J. L. (1995) Selective binding of self peptides to disease-associated major histocompatibility complex (MHC) molecules: a mechanism for MHC-linked susceptibility to human autoimmune diseases (comment). *J. Exp. Med.* **181,** 1597–1601.
16. Thomson, W., Pepper, L., Payton, A., Carthy, D., Scott, D., Ollier, W., et al. (1993) Absence of an association between HLA-DRB1*04 and rheumatoid arthritis in newly diagnosed cases from the community. *Ann. Rheum. Dis.* **52,** 539–541.
17. Weyand, C.M., Xie, C., and Goronzy, J. J. (1992) Homozygosity for the HLA-DRB1 allele selects for extraarticular manifestations in rheumatoid arthritis. *J. Clin. Invest.* **89,** 2033–2039.

18. Calin, A., Elswood, J., and Klouda, P. T. (1989) Destructive arthritis, rheumatoid factor, and HLA-DR4. Susceptibility versus severity, a case-control study (*see* comments). *Arthritis Rheum.* **32,** 1221–1225.

19. Jawaheer, D., Thomson, W., MacGregor, A. J., Carthy, D., Davidson, J., Dyer, P. A., et al. (1994) "Homozygosity" for the HLA-DR shared epitope contributes the highest risk for rheumatoid arthritis concordance in identical twins. *Arthritis Rheum.* **37,** 681–686.

20. Berg, L. J., Frank, G. D., and Davis, M. M. (1990) The effects of MHC gene dosage and allelic variation on T cell receptor selection. *Cell* **60,** 1043–1053.

21. Robey, E. A., Ramsdell, F., Kioussis, D., Sha, W., Loh, D., Axel, R., et al., (1992) The level of CD8 expression can determine the outcome of thymic selection. *Cell* **69,** 1089–1096.

22. Zanelli, E., Krco, C. J., Baisch, J. M., Cheng, S., and David, C. S. (1996) Immune response of HLA-DQ8 transgenic mice to peptides from the third hypervariable region of HLA-DRB1 correlates with predisposition to rheumatoid arthritis. *Proc. Natl. Acad. Sci. USA* **93,** 1814–1819.

23. Zanelli, E., Gonzalez-Gay, M. A., and David, C. A. (1995) Could HLA-DRB1 be the protective locus in rheumatoid arthritis? *Immunol. Today* **16,** 274–278.

24. Kong, Y. C., Lomo, L. C., Motte, R. W., Giraldo, A. A., Baisch, J., Strauss, G., et al. (1996) HLA-DRB1 polymorphism determines susceptibility to autoimmune thyroiditis in transgenic mice: definitive association with HLA-DRB1*0301 (DR3) gene. *J. Exp. Med.* **184,** 1167–1172.

25. Ito, K., Bian, H. J., Molina, M., Han, J., Magram, J., Saar, E., et al. (1996) HLA-DR4-IE chimeric class II transgenic, murine class II-deficient mice are susceptible to experimental allergic encephalomyelitis. *J. Exp. Med.* **183,** 2635–2644.

26. Schwartz, B. D. (1994) HLA class II transgenic mice: the chance to unravel the basis of HLA class II associations with disease (comment). *J. Exp. Med.* **180,** 11–13.

27. Altmann, D. M., Douek, D. C., Frater, A. J., Hetherington, C. M., Inoko, H., and Elliott, J. I. (1995) The T cell response of HLA-DR transgenic mice to human myelin basic protein and other antigens in the presence and absence of human CD4. *J. Exp. Med.* **181,** 867–875.

28. Rosloniec, E. F., Brand, D. D., Myers, L. K., Whittington, K. B., Gumanovskaya, M., Zaller, D. M., et al. (1997) An HLA-DR1 transgene confers susceptibility to collagen-induced arthritis elicited with human type II collagen. *J. Exp. Med.* **185,** 1113–1122.

29. Yeung, R. S., Penninger, J. M., Kundig, T. M., Law, Y., Yamamoto, K., Kamikawaji, N., et al. (1994) Human CD4-major histocompatibility complex class II (DQw6) transgenic mice in an endogenous CD4/CD8-deficient background: reconstitution of phenotype and human-restricted function. *J. Exp. Med.* **180,** 1911–1920.

30. Firestein, G. S. (1997) Etiology and pathogenesis of rheumatoid arthritis, in *Textbook of Rheumatology* (Kelley, W. N., Harris, E. D., Ruddy, S., and Sledge, C. R., eds.), WB Saunders, Philadelphia, PA, pp. 851–897.

31. Asch, E. S., Bujak, D. I., Weiss, M., Peterson, M. G., and Weinstein, A. (1994) Lyme disease: an infectious and postinfectious syndrome. *J. Rheumatol.* **21,** 454–461.

32. Harris, E. D., Jr. (1993) Etiology and pathogenesis of rheumatoid arthritis, in *Rheumatoid Arthritis* (Kelley, W. N., Jarris, E. D., Ruddy, S., and Sledge, C. R., eds.), WB Saunders, Philadelphia, PA, pp. 833–873.

33. Thomas, R. and Lipsky, P. E. (1996) Could endogenous self-peptides presented by dendritic cells initiate rheumatoid arthritis? *Immunol. Today* **17,** 559–564.
34. Tsai, V., Bergroth, V., and Zvaifler, N. J. (1988) Synovial dendritic cells and T cells in rheumatoid arthritis. *Scand. J. Rheumatol. Suppl.* **74,** 79–88.
35. Zvaifler, N. J., Steinman, R. M., Kaplan, G., Lau, L. L., and Rivelis, M. (1985) Identification of immunostimulatory dendritic cells in the synovial effusions of patients with rheumatoid arthritis. *J. Clin. Invest.* **76,** 789–800.
36. Wilkinson, L. S., Worrall, J. G., Sinclair, H. D., and Edwards, J. C. (1990) Immunohistological reassessment of accessory cell populations in normal and diseased human synovium. *Br. J. Rheumatol.* **29,** 259–263.
37. Steinman, R. M. (1991) The dendritic cell system and its role in immunogenicity. *Annu. Rev. Immunol.* **9,** 271–296.
38. Ziff, M. (1974) Relation of cellular infiltration of rheumatoid synovial membrane to its immune response. *Arthritis Rheum.* **17,** 313–319.
39. Jorgensen, C., Travaglio-Encinoza, A., Bologna, C., d'Angeac, A. D., Reme, T., and Sany, J. (1994) Human mucosyl lymphocyte marker expression in synovial fluid lymphocytes of patient with rheumatoid arthritis. *J. Rheumatol.* **21,** 1602–1607.
40. Trollmo, C., Nilsson, I. M., Sollerman, C., and Tarkowski, A. (1996) Expression of the mucosal lymphocyte integrin alpha E beta 7 and its ligand E-cadherin in the synovium of patients with rheumatoid arthritis. *Scand. J. Immunol.* **44,** 293–298.
41. Salmi, M., Andrew, D. P., Butcher, E. C., and Jalkanen, S. (1995) Dual binding capacity of mucosal immunoblasts to mucosal and synovial endothelium in humans: dissection of the molecular mechanisms. *J. Exp. Med.* **181,** 137–149.
42. Gross, G. G., Schwartz, V. L., Stevens, C., Ebert, E. C., Blumberg, R. S., and Balk, S. P. (1994) Distribution of dominant T cell receptor beta chains in human intestinal mucosa. *J. Exp. Med.* **180,** 1337–1344.
43. Regnault, A., Cumano, A., Vassalli, P., Guy-Grand, D., and Kourilsky, P. (1994) Oligoclonal repertoire of the CD8 alpha alpha and the CD8 alpha beta TCR-alpha/beta murine intestinal intraepithelial T lymphocytes: evidence for the random emergence of T cells. *J. Exp. Med.* **180,** 1345–1358.
44. Chowers, Y., Holtmeier, W., Harwood, J., Morzycka-Wroblewska, E., and Kagnoff, M.F. (1994). The Vδ1 T cell receptor repertoire in human small intestine and colon. *J. Exp. Med.* **180,** 183–190.
45. Gross, V., Andus, T., Leser, H.G., Roth, M., and Scholmerich, J. (1991) Inflammatory mediators in chronic inflammatory bowel diseases. *Klin. Wochenschr.* **69,** 981–987.
46. Zhang, L. and Tarleton, R. L. (1996) Persistent production of inflammatory and anti-inflammatory cytokines and associated MHC and adhesion molecule expression at the site of infection and disease in experimental Trypanosoma cruzi infections. *Exp. Parasitol.* **84,** 203–213.
47. Imamura, M., Hashino, S., Kobayashi, H., Kubayashi, S., Hirano, S., Minagawa, T., et al. (1994) Serum cytokine levels in bone marrow transplantation: synergistic interaction of interleukin-6, interferon-gamma, and tumor necrosis factor-alpha in graft-versus-host disease. *Bone Marrow Transp.* **13,** 745–751.
48. Rus, V., Svetic, A., Nguyen, P., Gause, W. C., and Via, C. S. (1995) Kinetics of Th1 and Th2 cytokine production during the early course of acute and chronic murine graft-versus-host disease. Regulatory role of donor CD8+ T cells. *J. Immunol.* **155,** 2396–2406.

49. Karin, N., Szafer, F., Mitchell, D., Gold, D. P., and Steinman, L. (1993) Selective and nonselective stages in homing of T lymphocytes to the central nervous system during experimental allergic encephalomyelitis. *J. Immunol.* **150,** 4116–4124.

50. Yu, M., Johnson, J. M., and Tuohy, V. K. (1996) A predictable sequential determinant spreading cascade invariably accompanies progression of experimental autoimmune encephalomyelitis: a basis for peptide-specific therapy after onset of clinical disease. *J. Exp. Med.* **183,** 1777–1788.

51. Lannes-Vieira, J., Gehrmann, J., Kreutzberg, G. W., and Wekerle, H. (1994) The inflammatory lesion of T cell line transferred experimental autoimmune encephalomyelitis of the Lewis rat: distinct nature of parenchymal and perivascular infiltrates. *Acta Neuropathol. (Berl.)* **87,** 435–442.

52. Tsuchida, M., Matsumoto, Y., Hirahara, H., Hanawa, H., Tomiyama, K., and Abo, T. (1993) Preferential distribution of V beta 8.2-positive T cells in the central nervous system of rats with myelin basic protein-induced autoimmune encephalomyelitis. *Eur. J. Immunol.* **23,** 2399–2406.

53. Jansson, L., Diener, P., Engstrom, A., Olsson, T., and Holmdahl, R. (1995) Spreading of the immune response to different myelin basic protein peptides in chronic experimental autoimmune encephalomyelitis in B10.RIII mice. *Eur. J. Immunol.* **25,** 2195–2200.

54. Lehmann, P. V., Forsthuber, T., Miller, A., and Sercarz, E. E. (1992) Spreading of T-cell autoimmunity to cryptic determinants of an autoantigen. *Nature* **358,** 155–157.

55. Lehmann, P. V., Sercarz, E. E., Forsthuber, T., Dayan, C. M., and Gammon, G. (1993) Determinant spreading and the dynamics of the autoimmune T-cell repertoire (*see* comments). *Immunol. Today* **14,** 203–208.

56. Tarkowski, A., Jonsson, R., Holmdahl, R., and Klareskog, L. (1987) Immunohistochemical characterization of synovial cells in arthritic MRL-lpr/lpr mice. *Arthritis Rheum.* **30,** 75–82.

57. Koopman, W. J., and Gay, S. (1988) The MRL-lpr/lpr mouse: a model for the study of rheumatoid arthritis. *Scand. J. Rheumatol. Suppl.* **75,** 284–289.

58. Westby, M., Manca, F., and Dalgleish, A.G. (1996) The role of host immune responses in determining the outcome of HIV infection. *Immunol. Today* **17,** 120–126.

59. Posnett, D. N., Romagne, F., Necker, A., Kotzin, B. L., and Sekaly, R. P. (1996) Summary: First human TCR monoclonal antibody workshop. *The Immunologist* **4,** 5–8.

60. Marguerie, C., Lunardi, C., and So, A. (1992) PCR-based analysis of the TCR repertoire in human autoimmune diseases (*see* comments). *Immunol. Today* **13,** 336–38.

61. Posnett, D. N. (1995) Environmental and genetic factors shape the human T-cell receptor repertoire. *Ann NY Acad. Sci.* **756,** 71–80.

62. Robinson, M. A. (1995) T-cell receptors in immune responses. *Adv. Exp. Med. Biol.* **386,** 121–132.

63. Struyk, L., Hawes, G. E., Chatila, M. K., Breedveld, F. C., Kurnick, J. T., and van den Elsen, P. J. (1995) T cell receptors in rheumatoid arthritis. *Arthritis Rheum.* **38,** 577–589.

64. Sumida, T., Hoa, T. T., Asahara, H., Hasunuma, T., and Nishioka, K. (1997) T cell receptor of Fas-sensitive T cells in rheumatoid synovium. *J. Immunol.* **158,** 1965–1970.

65. Salmon, M., Scheel-Toellner, D., Huissoon, A. P., Pilling, D., Shamsadeen, N., Hyde, H., et al. (1997) Inhibition of T cell apoptosis in the rheumatoid synovium. *J. Clin. Invest.* **99,** 439–446.

66. Karim, S. N., Murphy, E. A., Sturrock, R. D., and Goudie, R. B. (1995) T-cell clonality in synovial fluid from rheumatoid joints before and after culture in interleukin-2. *Br. J. Rheumatol.* **34,** 232–235.

67. Posnett, D. N., Gottlieb, A., Bussel, J. B., Friedman, S. M., Chiorazzi, N., Li, Y., et al. (1988). T cell antigen receptors in autoimmunity. *J. Immunol.* **141,** 1963–1969.

68. Kohsaka, H., Taniguchi, A., Chen, P. P., Ollier, W. E., and Carson, D. A. (1993) The expressed T cell receptor V gene repertoire of rheumatoid arthritis monozygotic twins: rapid analysis by anchored polymerase chain reaction and enzyme-linked immunosorbent assay. *Eur. J. Immunol.* **23,** 1895–1901.

69. Nanki, T., Kohsaka, H., Mizushima, N., Ollier, W. E., Carson, D. A., and Miyasaka, N. (1996) Genetic control of T cell receptor BJ gene expression in peripheral lymphocytes of normal and rheumatoid arthritis monozygotic twins. *J. Clin. Invest.* **98,** 1594–1601.

70. Kohsaka, H., Chen, P. P., Taniguchi, A., Ollier, W. E., and Carson, D. A. (1993) Divergent T cell receptor gamma repertoires in rheumatoid arthritis monozygotic twins. *Arthritis Rheum.* **36,** 213–221.

71. Uematsu, Y., Wege, H., Straus, A. L., Ott, M., Bannwarth, W., Lanchbury, J., et al. (1991) The T-cell receptor repertoire in the synovial fluid of a patient with rheumatoid arthritis is polyclonal. *Proc. Natl. Acad. Sci. USA* **88,** 8534–8538.

72. Pluschke, G., Ricken, G., Taube, H., Kroninger, S., Melchers, I., Peter, H. H., Eichman, K., and Grom, U. (1991) Biased T cell receptor Vα region repertoire in the synovial fluid of rheumatoid arthritis patients. *Eur. J. Immunol.* **21,** 2749–2754.

73. Mima, T., Saeki, Y., Ohshima, S., Nishimoto, N., Matsushita, M., Shimizu, M., et al. (1995) Transfer of rheumatoid arthritis into severe combined immunodeficient mice. The pathogenetic implications of T cell populations oligoclonally expanding in the rheumatoid joints. *J. Clin. Invest.* **96,** 1746–1758.

74. Sakata, A., Sakata, K., Ping, H., Ohmura, T., Tsukano, M., and Kakimoto, K. (1996) Successful induction of severe destructive arthritis by the transfer of in vitro-activated synovial fluid T cells from patients with rheumatoid arthritis (RA) in severe combined immunodeficient (SCID) mice. *Clin. Exp. Immunol.* **104,** 247–254.

75. Jenkins, R. N., Nikaein, A., Zimmermann, A., Meek, K., and Lipsky, P. E. (1993) T cell receptor V beta gene bias in rheumatoid arthritis. *J. Clin. Invest.* **92,** 2688–2701.

77. Waase, I., Kayser, C., Carlson, P. J., Goronzy, J. J., and Weyand, C. M. (1996) Oligoclonal T cell proliferation in patients with rheumatoid arthritis and their unaffected siblings. *Arthritis Rheum.* **39,** 904–913.

77. Williams, W. V., Fang, Q., Demarco, D., Von Feldt, J., Zurier, R. B., and Weiner, D. B. (1992) Restricted heterogeneity of T cell receptor transcripts in rheumatoid synovium. *J. Clin. Invest.* **90,** 326–333.

78. Goronzy, J. J., Bartz-Bazzanella, P., Hu, W., Jendro, M. C., Walser-Kuntz, D. R., and Weyand, C. M. (1994) Dominant clonotypes in the repertoire of peripheral CD4+ T cells in rheumatoid arthritis. *J. Clin. Invest.* **94,** 2068–2076.

79. Bucht, A., Soderstrom, K., Hultman, T., Uhlen, M., Nilsson, E., Kiessling, R., et al. (1992) T cell receptor diversity and activation markers in the Vδ1 subset of rheumatoid synovial fluid and peripheral blood T lymphocytes. *Eur. J. Immunol.* **22,** 567–574.

80. Olive, C., Gatenby, P. A., and Serjeantson, S. W. (1992) Variable gene usage of T cell receptor gamma- and delta-chain transcripts expressed in synovia and peripheral blood of patients with rheumatoid arthritis. *Clin. Exp. Immunol.* **87,** 172–177.

81. Meliconi, R., Pitzalis, C., Kingsley, G. H., and Panayi, G. S. (1991) Gamma/delta T cells and their subpopulations in blood and synovial fluid from rheumatoid arthritis and spondyloarthritis. *Clin. Immunol. Immunopathol.* **59,** 165–172.

82. Schmidt, D., Goronzy, J. J., and Weyand, C. M. (1996) CD4⁺ CD7⁻CD28⁻ T cells are expanded in rheumatoid arthritis and are characterized by autoreactivity. *J. Clin. Invest.* **97,** 2027–2037.

83. David-Ameline, J., Lim, A., Davodeau, F., Peyrat, M. A., Berthelot, J. M., Semama, G., et al. (1996) Selection of T cells reactive against autologous B lymphoblastoid cells during chronic rheumatoid arthritis. *J. Immunol.* **157,** 4697–4706.

84. Scotet, E., David-Ameline, J., Peyrat, M-A., Moreau-Aubry, A., Pinczon, D., Lim, A., et al. (1996) T cell response to Epstein-Barr virus transactivators in chronic rheumatoid arthritis. *J. Exp. Med.* **184,** 1791–1800.

85. Hingorani, R., Choi, I-H., Akolka, P., Gulwani-Akolkar, B., Pergolizzi, R., Silver, J., et al. (1993) Clonal predominance of T cell receptors within the CD8⁺ CD45RO⁺ subset in normal human subjects. *J. Immunol.* **151,** 5762–5769.

86. Posnett, D. N., Sinha, R., Kabak, S., and Russo, C. (1994) Clonal populations of T cells in normal elderly humans: the T cell equivalent to "Benign monoclonal gammapathy."*J. Exp. Med.* **179,** 609–618.

87. Fitzgerald, J. E., Ricalton, N. S., Meyer, A. C., West, S. G., Kaplan, H., Behrendt, C., et al. (1995) Analysis of clonal CD8⁺ T cell expansions in normal individuals and patients with rheumatoid arthritis. *J. Immunol.* **154,** 3538–3547.

88. Brooks, E. G., Balk, S. P., Aupeix, K., Colonna, M., Strominger, J. L., and Groh-Spies, V. (1993) Human T-cell receptor (TCR) alpha/beta⁺ CD4⁻CD8⁻ T cells express oligoclonal TCRs, share junctional motifs across TCR V beta-gene families, and phenotypically resemble memory T cells. *Proc. Natl. Acad. Sci. USA* **90,** 11,787–11,791.

89. Hingorani, R., Monteiro, J., Furie, R., Chartash, E., Navarrete, C., Pergolizzi, R., et al. (1996) Oligoclonality of V beta 3 TCR chains in the CD8⁺ T cell population of rheumatoid arthritis patients. *J. Immunol.* **156,** 852–858.

90. Grunewald, J., Jeddi-Tehrani, M., DerSimonian, H., Andersson, R., and Wigzell, H. (1992) A persistent expansion in the peripheral blood of a normal adult male: a new clinical entity? *Clin. Exp. Immunol.* **89,** 279–284.

91. Morley, J. K., Batliwalla, F. M., Hingorani, R., and Gregersen, P.K. (1995) Oligoclonal CD8⁺ T cells are preferentially expanded in the CD57⁺ subset. *J. Immunol.* **154,** 6182–6190.

92. Azuma, M., Phillips, J. H., and Lanier, L. L. (1993) CD28⁻ T lymphocytes. Antigenic and functional properties. *J. Immunol.* **150,** 1147–1159.

93. Hamann, D., Baars, P. A., Rep, M. H. G., Hooibrink, B., and Van Lier, R.A.W. (1997) Phenotypical and functional separation of memory and effector human CD8pos T cells. *J. Exp. Med.,* in press.

94. Autran, B., Leblond, V., Sadat-Sowti, B., Lefranc, E., Got, P., Sutton, L., et al. (1991) A soluble factor released by CD8⁺CD57⁺ lymphocytes from bone marrow transplanted patients inhibits cell-mediated cytolysis. *Blood* **77,** 2237–2241.

95. Wang, E. C., Lehner, P. J., Graham, S., and Borysiewicz, L. K. (1994) CD8ʰⁱᵍʰ (CD57⁺) T cells in normal, healthy individuals specifically suppress the genera-

tion of cytotoxic T lymphocytes to Epstein-Barr virus-transformed B cell lines. *Eur. J. Immunol.* **24,** 2903–2909.

96. Wang, E. C., Moss, P. A., Frodsham, P., Lehner, P. J., Bell, J. I., and Borysiewicz, L. K. (1995) CD8^highCD57+ T lymphocytes in normal, healthy individuals are oligoclonal and respond to human cytomegalovirus. *J. Immunol.* **155,** 5046–5056.

97. Gorochov, G., Debre, P., Leblond, V., Sadat-Sowti, B., Sigaux, F., and Autranj, B. (1994) Oligoclonal expansion of CD8+ CD57+ T cells with restricted T-cell receptor beta chain variability after bone marrow transplantation. *Blood* **83,** 587–595.

98. Prince, H. E. and Jensen, E. R. (1991) Three-color cytofluorometric analysis of CD8 cell subsets in HIV-1 infection. *J. Acquir. Immune Defic. Syndr.* **4,** 1227–1232.

99. DerSimonian, H., Band, H., and Brenner, B. M. (1991) Increased frequency of T cell receptor V-alpha 12.1 expression on CD8+ T cells: evidence that V-alpha participates in shaping the peripheral T cell repertoire. *J. Exp. Med.* **174,** 639–648.

100. Candeias, S., Waltzinger, C., Benoist, C., and Mathis, D. (1991) The V beta 17+ T cell repertoire: skewed J beta usage after thymic selection; dissimilar CDR3s in CD4+ versus CD8+ cells. *J. Exp. Med.* **174,** 989–1000.

101. Moss, P. A. and Bell, J. I. (1996) Comparative sequence analysis of the human T cell receptor TCRA and TCRB CDR3 regions. *Hum. Immunol.* **48,** 32–38.

102. Moss, P. A. and Bell, J. I. (1995) Sequence analysis of the human alpha beta T-cell receptor CDR3 region. *Immunogenetics* **42,** 10–18.

103. Li, Y., Sun, G. R., Tumang, J. R., Crow, M. K., and Friedman, S.M. (1994) CDR3 sequence motifs shared by oligoclonal rheumatoid arthritis synovial T cells. Evidence for an antigen-driven response. *J. Clin. Invest.* **94,** 2525–2531.

104. Alam, A., Lambert, N., Lule, J., Coppin, H., Mazieres, B., De Preval, C., et al. (1996) Persistence of dominant T cell clones in synovial tissues during rheumatoid arthritis. *J. Immunol.* **156,** 3480–3485.

105. Yoon, J. W., Austin, M., Onodera, T., and Notkins, A.L. (1979) Isolation of a virus from the pancreas of a child with diabetic ketoacidosis. *N. Engl. J. Med.* **300,** 1173–1179.

106. Eggers, H. J. and Mertens, T. (1986) Persistence of Coxsackie B virus-specific IgM [letter]. *Lancet* **2,** 284.

107. Kurtzman, G. J., Cohen, B., Meyers, P., Amunullah, A., and Young, N.S. (1988) Persistent B19 parvovirus infection as a cause of severe chronic anaemia in children with acute lymphocytic leukaemia. *Lancet* **2,** 1159–1162.

108. Saal, J. G., Steidle, M., Einsele, H., Muller, C. A., Fritz, P., and Zacher, J. (1992) Persistence of B19 parvovirus in synovial membranes of patients with rheumatoid arthritis. *Rheumatol. Int.* **12,** 147–151.

109. Foto, F., Saag, K. G., Scharosch, L. L., Howard, E. J., and Naides, S. J. (1993) Parvovirus B19-specific DNA in bone marrow from B19 arthropathy patients: evidence for B19 virus persistence. *J. Infect. Dis.* **167,** 744–748.

110. Simpson, R. W., McGinty, L., Simon, L., Smith, C. A., Godzeski, C. W., and Boyd, R. J. (1984) Association of parvoviruses with rheumatoid arthritis of humans. *Science* **223,** 1425–1428.

111. Simpson, R. W.,VanLeeuwen, D., Zazra, J. J., et al. (1985) Biological and molecular properties of the RA-1 parvoviruses. *Parvovirus Workshop, Bern, Switz.* (Abstract).

112. Hasunuma, T., Sumida, T., and Nishioka, K. (1997) Human T cell leukemia virus type-1 and rheumatoid arthritis. *Int. Rev. Immunol.,* in press.
113. Nakajima, T., Aono, H., Hasunuma, T., Yamamoto, K., Maruyama, I., Nosaka, T., et al. (1993) Overgrowth of human synovial cells driven by the human T cell leukemia virus type I tax gene. *J. Clin. Invest.* **92,** 186–193.
114. Iwakura, Y., Tosu, M., Yoshida, E., Takiguchi, M., Sato, K., Kitajima, I., et al. (1991) Induction of inflammatory arthropathy resembling rheumatoid arthritis in mice transgenic for HTLV-I. *Science* **253,** 1026–1028.
115. di Giovine, F.S., Bailly, S., Bootman, J., Almond, N., and Duff, G.W. (1994) Absence of lentiviral and human T cell leukemia viral sequences in patients with rheumatoid arthritis. *Arthritis Rheum.* **37,** 349–358.
116. Ferraro, A. S. and Newkirk, M. M. (1993) Correlative studies of rheumatoid factors and anti-viral antibodies in patients with rheumatoid arthritis. *Clin. Exp. Immunol.* **92,** 425–431.
117. Tsai, Y. T., Chiang, B. L., Kao, Y. F., and Hsieh, K. H. (1995) Detection of Epstein–Barr virus and cytomegalovirus genome in white blood cells from patients with juvenile rheumatoid arthritis and childhood systemic lupus erythematosus. *Int. Arch. Allergy. Immunol.* **106,** 235–240.
118. Tsuchiya, N., Murayama, T., Yoshinoya, S., Matsuta, K., Shiota, M., Furukawa, T., et al. (1993) Antibodies to human cytomegalovirus 65-kilodalton Fc binding protein in rheumatoid arthritis: idiotypic mimicry hypothesis of rheumatoid factor production. *Autoimmunity* **15,** 39–48.
119. Tamm, A., Ziegler, T., Lautenschlager, I., Nikkari, S., Mottonen, T., Luukkainen, R., et al. (1993) Detection of cytomegalovirus DNA in cells from synovial fluid and peripheral blood of patients with early rheumatoid arthritis. *J. Rheumatol.* **20,** 1489–1493.
120. Kondo, K., Kaneshima, H., and Mocarski, E. S. (1994) Human cytomegalovirus latent infection of granulocyte-macrophage progenitors. *Proc. Natl. Acad. Sci. USA* **91,** 11,879– 11,883.
121. Maciejewski, J. P., Bruening, E. E., Donahue, R. E., Mocarski, E. S., Young, N. S., and St Jeor, S. C. (1992) Infection of hematopoietic progenitor cells by human cytomegalovirus. *Blood* **80,** 170–178.
122. Decker, L. L., Klaman, L. D., and Thorley-Lawson, D. A. (1996) Detection of the latent form of Epstein–Barr virus DNA in the peripheral blood of healthy individuals. *J. Virol.* **70,** 3286–3289.
123. Inoue, N., Harada, S., Miyasaka, N., Oya, A., and Yanagi, K. (1991) Analysis of antibody titers to Epstein–Barr virus nuclear antigens in sera of patients with Sjogren's syndrome and with rheumatoid arthritis. *J. Infect. Dis.* **164,** 22–28.
124. Tosato, G., Steinberg, A. D., Yarchoan, R., Heilman, C. A., Pike, S. E., De Seau, V., et al. (1984) Abnormally elevated frequency of Epstein-Barr virus-infected B cells in the blood of patients with rheumatoid arthritis. *J. Clin. Invest.* **73,**1789–1795.
125. Yao, Q. Y., Rickinson, A. B., Gaston, J. S., and Epstein, M. A. (1986) Disturbance of the Epstein-Barr virus-host balance in rheumatoid arthritis patients: a quantitative study. *Clin. Exp. Immunol.* **64,** 302–310.
126. Zhang, L., Nikkari, S., Skurnik, M., Ziegler, T., Luukkainen, R., Mottonen, T., et al. (1993) Detection of herpesviruses by polymerase chain reaction in lymphocytes from patients with rheumatoid arthritis. *Arthritis Rheum.* **36,** 1080–1086.

127. Takei, M., Mitamura, K., Fujiwara, S., Horie, T., Ryu, J., Osaka, S., et al. (1997) Detection of Epstein–Barr virus-encoded small RNA 1 and latent membrane protein 1 in synovial lining cells from rheumatoid arthritis patients. *Intern. Immunol.* **9,** 739–743.
128. Koide, J., Takada, K., Sugiura, M., Sekine, H., Ito, T., Saito, K., et al. (1997) Spontaneous establishment of an Epstein–Barr virus infected fibroblast line from the synovial tissue of a rheumatoid arthritis patient. *J. Virol.* **71,** 2478–2481.
129. Berneman, Z. N., Ablashi, D. V., Li, G., Eger-Fletcher, M., Reitz, M. S. J., Hung, C-L., et al. (1992) Human herpesvirus 7 is a T-lymphotropic virus and is related to, but significantly different from, human herpesvirus 6 and human cytomegalovirus. *Proc. Natl. Acad. Sci. USA* **89,** 10,552–10,556.
130. Mesri, E. A., Cesarman, E., Arvanitkais, L., Rafii, S., Moore, M. A. S.. Posnett, D. N., et al. (1996) Human Herpesvirus-8/Kaposi's sarcoma associated herpes virus (HHV8/KSHV) is a new transmissible virus that infects B-cells. *J. Exp. Med.* **183,** 2385– 2390.
131. Newkirk, M. M., Watanabe Duffy, K. N., Leclerc, J., Lambert, N., and Shiroky, J. B. (1994) Detection of cytomegalovirus, Epstein–Barr virus and herpes virus-6 in patients with rheumatoid arthritis with or without Sjögren's syndrome. *Br. J. Rheumatol.* **33,** 317–322.
132. Walser-Kuntz, D. R., Weyand, C. M., Weaver, A. J., O'Fallon, W. M., and Goronzy, J. J. (1995) Mechanisms underlying the formation of T cell receptor repertoire in rheumatoid arthritis. *Immunity* **2,** 597–605.
133. Paliard, X., West, S. G., Lafferty, J. A., Clements, J. R., Kappler, J. W., Marrack, P., et al. (1991) Evidence for the effects of a superantigen in Rheumatoid Arthritis. *Science* **253,** 325–329.
134. Howell, M. D., Diveley, J. P., Lundeen, K. A., Esty, A., Winters, S. T., Carlo, D. J., et al. (1991) Limited T-cell receptor beta chain heterogeneity among interleukin 2 receptor-positive synovial T cells suggests a role for superantigen in rheumatoid arthritis. *Proc. Natl. Acad. Sci. USA* **88,** 10,921–10,925.
135. Williams, W. V., Kieber-Emmons, T., Fang, Q., Von Feldt, J., Wang, B., Ramanujam, T., et al. (1993) Conserved motifs in rheumatoid arthritis synovial tissue T-cell receptor beta chains. *DNA Cell Biol.* **12,** 425–434.
136. Sottini, A., Imberti, L., Gorla, R., Cattaneo, R., and Primi, D. (1991) Restricted expression of T cell receptor Vβ but not Vα genes in rheumatoid arthritis. *Eur. J. Immunol.* **21,** 461–466.
137. Grom, A. A., Thompson, S. D., Luyrink, L., Passo, M. Choi, E., and Glass, D. N. (1993) Dominant T-cell receptor beta chain variable region Vbeta 14[+] clones in juvenile rheumatoid arthritis. *Proc. Natl. Acad. Sci. USA.* **90,** 11,104–11,108.
138. Schmidt, D., Martens, P. B., Weyand, C. M., and Goronzy, J. J. (1996) The repertoire of CD4+ CD28- T cells in rheumatoid arthritis. *Mol. Med.* **2,** 608–618.
139. Monteiro, J., Hingorani, R., Choi, I. H., Pergolizzi, R., Silver, J., and Gregersen, P. K. (1995) Variability in CD8[+] T-cell oligoclonality patterns in monozygotic twins. *Ann. NY Acad. Sci.* **756,** 96–98.
140. Gonzalez-Quintial, R., Baccala, R., Pope, R. M., and Theofilopoulos, A.N. (1996) Identification of clonally expanded T cells in rheumatoid arthritis using a sequence enrichment nuclease assay. *J. Clin. Invest.* **97,** 1335–1343.
141. Sottini, A., Imberti, L., Bettinardi, A., Mazza, C., Gorla, R., and Primi, D. (1993) Selection of T lymphocytes in two rheumatoid arthritis patients defines different

T-cell receptor V beta repertoires in CD4+ and CD8+ T-cell subsets. *J. Autoimmun.* **6,** 621–637.

142. Lunardi, C., Marguerie, C., and So, A. K. (1992) An altered repertoire of T cell receptor V gene expression by rheumatoid synovial fluid T lymphocytes. *Clin. Exp. Immunol.* **90,** 440–446.

143. Pluschke, G., Ginter, A., Taube, H., Melchers, I., Peter, H. H., and Krawinkel, U. (1993) Analysis of T cell receptor V beta regions expressed by rheumatoid synovial T lymphocytes. *Immunobiology* **188,** 330–339.

144. Struyk, L., Hawes, G. E., Mikkers, H. M., Tak, P. P., Breedveld, F. C., and van den Elsen, P. J. (1996) Molecular analysis of the T-cell receptor beta-chain repertoire in early rheumatoid arthritis: heterogeneous TCRBV gene usage with shared amino acid profiles in CDR3 regions of T lymphocytes in multiple synovial tissue needle biopsies from the same joint. *Eur. J. Clin. Invest.* **26,** 1092–1102.

145. Struyk, L., Kurnick, J. T., Hawes, J. E., van Laar, J. M., Schipper, R., Oksenberg, J. R., et al. (1993) T-cell receptor V-gene usage in synovial fluid lymphocytes of patients with chronic arthritis. *Hum. Immunol.* **37,** 237–251.

146. Yamamoto, K., Sakoda, H., Nakajima, T., Kato, T., Okubo, M., Dohi, M., et al. (1992) Accumulation of multiple T cell clonotypes in the synovial lesions of patients with rheumatoid arthritis revealed by a novel clonality analysis. *Int. Immunol.* **4,** 1219–1223.

147. Ikeda, Y., Masuko, K., Nakai, Y., Kato, T., Hasanuma, T., Yoshino, S.I., et al. (1996) High frequencies of identical T cell clonotypes in synovial tissues of rheumatoid arthritis patients suggest the occurrence of common antigen-driven immune responses. *Arthritis Rheum.* **39,** 446–453.

148. Zagon, G., Tumang, J. R., Li, Y., Friedman, S. M., and Crow, M. K. (1994) Increased frequency of Vβ17-positive T cells in patients with rheumatoid arthritis. *Arthritis Rheum..* **37,** 1431–1440.

149. Alam, A., Lule, J., Coppin, H., Lambert, N., Mazieres, B., De Preval, C., et al. (1995) T-cell receptor variable region of the beta-chain gene use in peripheral blood and multiple synovial membranes during rheumatoid arthritis. *Hum. Immunol.* **42,** 331–339.

150. Maruyama, T., Saito, I., Miyake, S., Hashimoto, H., Sato, K., Yagita, H., et al. (1993) A possible role of two hydrophobic amino acids in antigen recognition by synovial T cells in rheumatoid arthritis. *Eur. J. Immunol.* **23,** 2059–2065.

151. Broker, B. M., Korthauer, U., Heppt, P., Weseloh, G., de la Camp, R., Kroczek, R. A., et al. (1993) Biased T cell receptor V gene usage in rheumatoid arthritis. Oligoclonal expansion of T cells expressing V alpha 2 genes in synovial fluid but not in peripheral blood. *Arthritis Rheum.* **36,** 1234–1243.

152. DerSimonian, H., Sugita, M., Glass, D.N., Maier, A. L., Weinblatt, M. E., Reme, T., et al. (1993) Clonal Vα12.1 T cell expansions in the peripheral blood of rheumatoid arthritis patients. *J. Exp. Med.* **177,** 1623–1631.

153. Pluschke, G., Ricken, G., Taube, H., Kroninger, S., Melchers, I., Peter, H. H., et al. (1991) Biased T cell receptor V alpha region repertoire in the synovial fluid of rheumatoid arthritis patients. *Eur. J. Immunol.* **21,** 2749–2754.

154. Bucht, A., Oksenberg, J. R., Lindblad, S., Gronberg, A., Steinman, L., and Klareskog, L. (1992) Characterization of T-cell receptor alpha beta repertoire in synovial tissue from different temporal phases of rheumatoid arthritis. *Scand. J. Immunol.* **35,** 159–165.

155. Doherty, P. J., Inman, R. D., Laxer, R. M., Silverman, E. D., Yang, S. X., Suurmann, I., et al. (1996) Analysis of T cell receptor gamma transcripts in right and left knee synovial fluids of patients with rheumatoid arthritis. *J. Rheumatol.* **23,** 1143–1150.

156. Reme, T., Portier, M., Frayssinoux, F., Combe, B., Miossec, P., Favier, F., et al. (1990) T cell receptor expression and activation of synovial lymphocyte subsets in patients with rheumatoid arthritis: phenotyping of multiple synovial sites. *Arthritis Rheum.* **33,** 485–492.

157. Jacobs, M. R. and Haynes, B. F. (1992) Increase in TCR gamma delta T lymphocytes in synovia from rheumatoid arthritis patients with active synovitis. *J. Clin. Immunol.* **12,** 130–138.

158. Meliconi, R., Uguccioni, M., D'Errico, A., Cassisa, A., Frizziero, L., and Facchini, A. (1992) T-cell receptor gamma-delta positive lymphocytes in synovial membrane. *Br. J. Rheumatol.* **31,** 59–61.

159. Olive, C., Gatenby, P. A., and Serjeantson, S. W. (1992) Molecular characterization of the V gamma 9 T cell receptor repertoire expressed in patients with rheumatoid arthritis. *Eur. J. Immunol.* **22,** 2901–2906.

160. Olive, C., Gatenby, P. A., and Serjeantson, S. W. (1992) Evidence for oligoclonality of T cell receptor delta chain transcripts expressed in rheumatoid arthritis patients. *Eur. J. Immunol.* **22,** 2587–2593.

161. Struyk, L., Hawes, G. E., Dolhain, R.J., van Scherpenzeel, A., Godthelp, B., Breedveld, F. C., et al. (1994) Evidence for selective in vivo expansion of synovial tissue-infiltrating CD4+ CD45RO+ T lymphocytes on the basis of CDR3 diversity. *Int. Immunol.* **6,** 897– 907.

162. Imberti, L., Sottini, A., Signorini, S., Gorla, R., and Primi D. (1997) Oligoclonal CD4+ CD57+ T-cell expansions contribute to the imbalanced T-cell receptor repertoire of rheumatoid arthritis patients. *Blood* **89,** 2822–2832.

163. Dupuy, A., Monier, S., Jorgensen, C., Gao, Q., Travaglio-Encinoza, A., Bologna, C., et al. (1993) Increased percentage of CD3+, CD57+ lymphocytes in patients with rheumatoid arthritis. Correlation with duration of disease [see comments]. *Arthritis Rheum.* **36,** 608–612.

164. Burns, C. M., Tsai,V., and Zvaifler, N. J. (1992) High percentage of CD8+, Leu7+ cells in rheumatoid arthritis synovial fluid. *Arthritis Rheum.* **35,** 865–873.

165. Travaglio-Encinoza, A., Chaouni, I., DerSimonian, H., Jorgensen, C., Simony-Lafontaine, J., Romagne, F., et al. (1995) T cell receptor distribution in rheumatoid synovial follicles. *J. Rheumatol.* **22,** 394–399.

166. Olive, C., Gatenby, P. A., and Serjeantson, S. W. (1994) Persistence of gamma/delta T cell oligoclonality in the peripheral blood of rheumatoid arthritis patients. *Immunol. Cell Biol.* **72,** 7–11.

167. Khazaei, H. A., Lunardi, C., and So, A. K. (1995) CD4 T cells in the rheumatoid joint are oligoclonally activated and change during the course of disease. *Ann. Rheum. Dis.* **54,** 314–317.

168. Maurice, M. M., Res, P. C., Leow, A., van Hall, T., Daha, M. R., Struyk, L., et al. (1995) Joint-derived T cells in rheumatoid arthritis proliferate to antigens present in autologous synovial fluid. *Scand. J. Rheumatol. Suppl.* **101,** 169–177.

10

The Role of Exogenous Stimulation in Pathogenesis of Autoimmune Diseases

Constantin Bona, Chihiro Murai, and Takeshi Sasaki

1. INTRODUCTION

A properly operating immune system enables the body to maintain a healthy status quo by distinguishing between the antigens associated with the organism itself, which are allowed to persist, and the antigens borne by foreign molecules, which are disposed. Burnet *(1)*. proposed that the ability of immune system to distinguish "self and nonself" antigens results from the elimination of self-reactive lymphocytes during ontogenic development. This concept is supported by recent data originating from studies carried out in transgenic mice demonstrating that self-reactive T- and B- lymphocytes are deleted from the repertoire. In the thymus, a process known as negative selection appears to result in deletion of T-cells bearing receptors with high affinity for self-antigens *(2,3)*. In the fetal liver and bone marrow, a similar process deletes the emerging B-cells bearing an Ig receptor specific for cellular antigens *(4)*.

Burnet *(1)* proposed that autoimmune disease result from somatic mutations which occur in the V-genes encoding antibodies to nonself-antigens, which once mutated, can recognize the self-antigens and mount a response against them. Ensuing years have seen this concept vanishing, because countless observations have demonstrated that self-reactive lymphocytes are an important components of the immune repertoire of healthy individuals. In certain conditions, self-reactive lymphoctye clones are activated subsequent to exposure of an organism to foreign antigens. In other conditions, the clones are rendered anergic by continuous contact with soluble antigens. Thus, it was shown that rheumatoid factors (RFs) are found not only in autoimmune diseases but also after vaccination of humans with tetanus toxoid *(5)*. On the other hand, it has been shown that the B-cells of transgenic mice expressing a gene encoding a soluble foreign antigens (hen white lysozyme) are anergic rather deleted *(4)*.

All these observations led to the unequivocal conclusion that autoimmunity results from the breaking of self-tolerance. In spite of recent progress in understanding the mechanisms of self-tolerance, however, the mechanistic understanding

Contemporary Immunology: Autoimmune Reactions
Edited by: S. Paul © Humana Press Inc., Totowa, NJ

of the pathogenesis of autoimmune diseases, particularly of the initiating autoimmune response, is still fragmentary, incomplete and speculative. The difficulties are related to the variety of factors that may lead to the activation of pathogenic self reactive clones. Roughly, these factors can be divided into exogenous and endogenous factors.

The purpose of this chapter is to review the observations trying to demonstrate that there is a link between exogenous stimulation and initiation of the autoimmune response, leading to an autoimmune disease. According to the "modified self" hypothesis, certain self antigens become immunogenic subsequent to interaction with foreign molecules (e.g., drugs, chemicals) by creation of neoself determinants. These will not be included in the discussion here, since the neoself determinants are not created frequently in cells infected with microbes or parasites, although they can be reproducibly created by well-defined inorganic or organic chemicals.

2. ASSOCIATION OF AUTOIMMUNE DISEASE WITH INFECTIONS

Exogenous agents that may be involved in triggering immunopathological phenomena are represented either by environmental macromolecules or microbes. Environmental macromolecules which are inhaled or ingurgitated may cause immediate hypersensitivity reactions leading to allergic diseases. Microbes or parasites have been often considered as agents involved in the onset of autoimmune diseases. It is noteworthy that in spite of the large body of evidence indicating the occurrence of autoimmune diseases following microbial infections (Table 1), there are only a few examples demonstrating that the injection of microbes causes an autoimmune disease. The best known example is adjuvant arthritis caused in animals by injection of Mycobacteria or Nocardia in mineral oil, a phenomenon associated with production of rheumatoid factors. As we mentioned above, self-reactive B-cell clones producing RFs were activated in healthy subjects subsequent to vaccination with tetanus toxoid (5). Production of RFs in normal animals was also induced by injecting T-dependent hapten carrier conjugates (36), bacterial TI_1 or TI_2 antigens (37) or anti-Id antibodies carrying the internal image of foreign antigens (38). Furthermore, in animals prone to produce RFs spontaneously, such as 129/Sv or MRL/lpr mice (39,40), the injection of foreign antigens increased the serum RF levels considerably (41). There is also a wealth of information demonstrating the presence of autoantibodies in the sera of people afflicted by various infectious agents (Table 2).

Despite these countless observations, there is no statistically or mechanistically compelling evidence demonstrating a cause-effect relationship between a microbe and an autoimmune disease. The lack of the cause-effect evidence is related to the following.

Table 1
Autoimmune Diseases Occurring after Microbial Infections

Microbe	Autoimmune disease	Ref.
Hepatitis A virus	Cryoglobulinemia	*6*
Hepatitis B virus	Autoimmune hepatitis	*7*
Hepatitis C virus	Behcet's syndrome	*8*
CMV	Guillain-Barre syndrome	*9–10*
EBV	SLE	*11*
	Rheumatoid arthritis	*12–16*
	Idiopathic aplastic anemia	*17*
	Sjogren's syndrome	*18–21*
HSV type 6	Sjogren's syndrome	22
Coxsackie virus	Myocarditis	*23–26*
Parvovirus B19	Rheumatoid arthritis	27
	Polyarteritis nodosa	28
Rubella, mumps, measles	Diabetes	*29–32*
HTLV-1	Rheumatoid arthritis	*32*
	Sjogren's syndrome	*33–34*
	Uveitis	*35*

Table 2
Microbial Infections Associated
with Occurrence of Autoantibodies

Hepatitis A virus
Hepatitis B virus
Mumps
Measles
Rubella
HIV
Influenza virus
EBV
Coxsackie B virus
Chickenpox
Trypanosoma cruzi
HTLV-1

See ref. 33.

1. The inability to determine that a single microbe is involved in a single autoimmune disease. This is not to say that we expect the occurrence of a given autoimmune disease to be obligatory after an infection caused by a single agent. It is possible that multiple infectious agents contribute to the onset of a single disease.

2. The inability to reproducibly isolate the microbe purported to be the cause of the autoimmune disease from the affected target tissue or organ. For example, the HTLV-1 virus has been implicated in the pathogenesis of multiple sclerosis (MS) because of the presence of anti-HTLV-1 antibodies in the blood and cerebrospinal fluid. A great deal of work to isolate the virus from brain lesions was carried out. However, no direct evidence has been presented to support the notion that HTLV-1 virus is associated with MS *(34)*.

Stronger evidence has been provided on the association of rheumatoid arthritis with parvovirus B19 and HTLV-1 virus infections. Reid et al. *(27)* were among the first to observe that acute febrile disease caused by parvovirus B19 is often associated with polyarthritis and vasculitis. Futo et al. *(44)* detected viral DNA in the bone marrow of B19 infected patients with prolonged arthritis. Sasaki et al. *(45)* reported an individual with persistent parvovirus B19 infection who began to exhibit detectable serum RFs 2 months after infection and developed joint pain six years later. Viral DNA was detected in the bone marrow by PCR at the time of appearance of polyarthritis. Murai et al. *(46)* found viral DNA and IgM class of anti-B19 antibodies in 11 of 67 patients showing inflammatory arthritis. Three of the 11 patients developed active polyarthritis with destructive lesions in the joints. RFs were present in the sera of these three patients two to four months after onset of the disease. These observations convincingly show that some patients with persistent parvovirus B19 infection and positive for anti-B-19 antibodies developed rheumatoid arthritis.

Occurrence of destructive arthropathy associated with T-cell leukemia caused by HTLV-1 virus was also reported by Japanese physicians *(33)*. In Kyushu island, which is highly endemic for HTLV-1 with 26.7% of the inhabitants infected with the virus, 111 of 7000 subjects studied developed rheumatoid arthritis. The prevalence of rheumatoid arthritis among HTLV-1 sero-positive patients was 0.56% compared to 0.31% in seronegative patients *(42)*. Proviral DNA was detected by PCR in the synovial tissue of the patients. Taken together, these observations demonstrate a direct association between the occurrence of rheumatoid arthritis and infections with human parvovirus B19 or HTLV-1. It is likely, however, that other factors also contribute to the occurrence of auto-immune disease, because the frequency of arthritis in patients infected with the two viruses, although significant, is still quite low.

3. POSSIBLE MECHANISMS OF INDUCTION OF AUTOIMMUNE DISEASE BY EXOGENOUS AGENTS

Because of the legion of circumstantial evidence associating autoimmune diseases and exogenous stimulation, several mechanisms were entertained to explain the role of exogenous agents in the pathogenesis of autoimmune diseases. The mechanisms are as follows:

1. Polyclonal activation.
2. Alteration of host cellular immunity.
3. Cryptic self epitopes.
4. Molecular mimicry.

3.1. Polyclonal Activation

A characteristic of certain autoimmune diseases, particularly systemic diseases such as systemic lupus erthymatosus (SLE) and rheumatoid arthritis, is the polyclonal activation of B-cells. This is clearly exemplified in lupus, which is associated with autoantibodies produced against a myriad of self-antigens. It is well known that a large number of molecules of microbial origin are endowed with the ability to induce polyclonal activation of B-cells and T-cells. Izui et al. *(48)* showed that mice injected with bacterial lipopolysaccharides produce IgM RFs. In the case of T-cells, such polyclonal activators were called superantigens, since they can induce the proliferation of clones expressing TCR encoded by certain Vβ family genes regardless of their antigenic specificity. Polyclonal activation of B-cells, resulting in the production of a large variety of autoantibodies, has also been observed in graft-versus-host disease *(49)*. A direct role for polyclonal activation in autoimmune disease was demonstrated in transgenic mice expressing an autoantibody specific for murine erythrocyte antigen. This autoantibody causes hemolytic anemia leading to death only after injection of lipopolysaccharide, a polyclonal activator of B-cells *(50)*.

The role of polyclonal activators of microbial origin in the onset of autoimmune disease. is questionable, however, for the following reasons.

1. Autoantibodies produced subsequent to injection of polyclonal activators are predominantly of the IgM class and they exhibit low affinity for antigens. This contrasts with the majority of pathogenic autoantibodies, which are of the IgG class and exhibit high affinity for autoantigens, acquired by antigen-driven affinity maturation of their V domains.
2. In spite of the fact that the parenteral injection of polyclonal activators can accelerate the onset of autoimmune disease in susceptible animals *(50)*, the polyclonal activators do not cause disease in normal animals.

In summary, macromolecules of bacterial origin endowed with mitogenic properties do not appear to contribute importantly to the onset of autoimmune disease. Apparently, polyclonal activation of B-cells observed in systemic autoimmune diseases is the effect rather the cause of the disease.

3.2. Alteration of Host Cellular Immunity

Host immunological responses to antigenic challenge are frequently altered upon the occurrence of infectious diseases. Often, infections lead to detectable alterations in individual T-cell subsets, which could play a role in the development of autoimmune diseases. For example, the depletion of RT.6.1$^+$ T-cells from the diabetes-resistent BB rats increases the susceptibility to disease, and the depletion of CD8$^+$ T-cells suppresses the occurrence of myasthenia gravis in rats *(51)*.

Targeted gene mutations in mice defective in lymphokine production showed that the lack of production of certain lymphokines, or alterations in the relative amounts of individual lymphokines in the cytokine network, can lead to formation of autoantibodies and even overt autoimmune disease. Inflammatory lymphokines such as IL-1, IL-6, and TNFα may play an important role in the occurrence of destructive lesions in rheumatoid arthritis. It is noteworthy that certain gene products of parvovirus B- and HTLV-1 viruses which are reported to contribute to the pathogenesis of rheumatoid arthritis associated with these infections, may be capable of directly activating the production of inflammatory lymphokines. Moffatt et al. *(52)* showed that hematopoietic and endothelial cells secreted IL-6 after transfection with the gene for the non-structural protein NS1 of parvovirus B19.

The NS-1 effect was mediated by an NF-κB binding site in the IL-6 promoter, suggesting that NS-1 functions as a transactivating transcriptional factor for the IL-6 promoter. This observation is pertinent to findings that high amounts of IL-6 are present in the fluid from joints of patients with rheumatoid arthritis *(53)*. The deregulated expression of IL-6 may be involved in polyclonal activation and synovial proliferation in the joints of these patients *(55,56)*. Studies of synovial cell clones from HTLV-1 virus infected patients who developed rheumatoid arthritis showed an overexpression of the viral *Tax* protein in synovicytes, which was directly associated with increased expression of IL-6, TNFα, and IL-1β mRNA, as well as the expression of several protooncogenes *(57)*. The Tax protein may function as a transactivator of synovicytes. This notion is supported by two important observations. First, HTLV-1 *Tax* transgenic mice exhibit histopathological lesions similar to those present in rheumatoid arthritis *(58)*. Second, normal synovicytes transfected with the HTLV-1 *Tax* gene exhibit alterations similar to those found in synovicyte clones isolated from HTLV-1 infected patients with rheumatoid arthritis, i.e., upregulation of DNA synthesis and of protooncogene and cytokine gene expression *(47)*. These data strongly suggest that alterations of cytokine production subsequent to viral infections can be mediated by viral genes with transactivating transcriptional activities, and that this phenomenon may play a role in the pathogenesis of autoimmune diseases.

3.3. Cryptic Self-Epitopes

The concept of the role of cryptic self epitopes in the induction and activation of self reactive lymphocytes derives from experiments carried out in normal undiseased animals. There is little direct evidence that cryptic epitopes are involved in triggering an autoimmune disease. The concept of cryptic self-epitopes resides in two major ideas: each protein molecule, including each self-protein, displays only a few immunodominant peptides which generally are responsible for the negative selection, i.e., deletion of autoreactive T-cells from the repertoire and subdominant or cryptic epitopes unable to induce toler-ance, permitting the persistence of autoreactive T-cell clones in the repertoire *(59)*. Available data provided by studies on pathogenic T-cells demonstrate that these cells are actually specific for immunodominant epitopes rather cryp-tic epitopes. It remains a mystery how the cryptic epitopes can be generated before the onset of autoimmune diseases. One may argue that infectious agents contribute to the generation of cryptic epitopes, but no direct evidence have been provided to support this mechanism.

3.4. Molecular Mimicry

The term molecular mimicry is used to define shared amino acid sequences of foreign and self-peptides. The implication of this concept is straightforward; the foreign molecules sharing epitopes with self molecules can break the self tolerance and can induce, therefore, an autoimmune response. This concept roots in the classical experiments of Witebsky *(60)*, who induced autoimmune thyroiditis subsequent to injection of heterologous thyroglobulin in Freund's complete adjuvant (FCA). Current interest in this concept has strengthened following studies showing the cross reactivity between Streptococcal antigens and proteins in the target tissues damaged in patients afflicted by rheumatoid fever, Sydenham's chorea and acute poststreptococcal glomerulonephritis.

In rheumatic fever, Kaplan and Svec *(61)* demonstrated that group A Strepto-cocci were crossreactive with heart tissue. Later it was shown that anti-Strepto-coccal antibodies obtained by immunization of experimental animals with the bacteria were crossreactive with human heart tissue. The role of antigen mimi-cry in the pathogenesis of rheumatic fever has seen support by several other findings including:

1. Isolation antibodies which bind the human heart from the serum of patients with rheumatic fever and acute poststreptococcal carditis *(61,62)*.
2. Demonstration of shared antigenic epitopes between human heart sarco-lemma proteins and streptococcal M protein from type 5 group A strepto-cocci *(63,64)*.
3. Isolation of monoclonal antibodies that bind muscle myosin and the Strep-tococcus pyogenes M protein *(65)*.

In the case of Sydenham's chorea, which is clinical manifestation of acute rheumatic fever involving the subthalamic and caudate nuclei in the brain, serum antibodies that bind to a neuronal cytoplasmic antigen(s) as well as group A streptococci have been identified *(66)*. In acute poststreptococcal glomerulo-nephritis, anti-heparan sulfate antibodies crossreactive with human and strep-tococcal hyalursonate have been identified *(67)*.

These observations have lead to the idea that antibodies specific for various bacterial components elicited subsequent to streptococcal infection can cross-react with human proteins, and may cause tissue damage leading to rheumatic fever, chorea, or glomerulonephritis. These observations motivated many investigators to search for sequence homologies between the proteins of infectious agents and mammalian tissues. Without claiming to review all of the reported data, we will present some pertinent examples.

3.4.1. Experimental Acute Encephalitis (EAE)

EAE is an experimental model for multiple sclerosis induced by injection of myelin basic protein (MBP) in adjuvants. The disease is mediated by T-cells. Fujinami et al. *(68)* reported a shared hexapeptide by bovine MBP and HeB virus polymerase.

MBP	TTHYGSLPQL
HeB virus polymerase	IGCYGSLPQE

Injection with bovine MBP in FCA in rabbits induced EAE. No evidence was provided in this study that the MBP-reactive T-cells recognize the decapeptide corresponding to 66–75 aminoacid residues of bovine MBP. Subsequently, homologies were also found between human MBP and various viruses such as EBV, measles, influenza A and B *(69)*. It is noteworthy that T-cells capable of responding to MBP were isolated from patients following infections with varicella and measles *(70,71)*.

3.4.2. Myasthenia Gravis

This is an organ specific autoimmune disease mediated by autoantibodies specific for the acetylcholine receptor (AcR). Production of anti-AcR antibodies is a T-cell dependent phenomenon, and the T-cells involved are specific for a peptide derived from the a chain of AcR. Homologies between AcR and viral protein sequences were reported as shown below. The functional significance of the homology of the viral peptides and AchR has not been elucidated.

AchR	TVIKESRGTK	*(72)*
poliovirus VP2	TTKERRGTT	*(52)*
and,		
AchR	PESDQPDL	*(73)*
HSVgpD	PNATQPEL	
Parvovirus H1WP2	TETNQPDT	
Polyoma virus-middle T antigen	PESDQDQL	

4.3. Experimental Autoimmune Uveitis (EAU)

EAU is considered as an experimental model for human uveitis. The disease can be induced by immunization with minute amount of a soluble retinal protein, designated S-antigen. A striking homology was reported between human S-antigen and an *E. coli* protein *(74)*.

S-antigen	TNLASSTI
E. coli protein	ANLASSTQ

EAU and pinelatis were induced in rats by injection of the *E. coli* peptide homologous to S-antigen. Furthermore, it was shown that lymph nodes from rats immunized with the peptide exhibited significant in vitro proliferation in the presence of both the S-antigen peptide and the *E. coli* peptide *(74)*.

3.4.4. Scleroderma

This is a clinically heterogenous disease represented by three major syndromes: progressive systemic sclerosis (PSS), CREST syndrome and morphea. The syndromes are associated with the presence of autoantibodies specific for nuclear antigens, such as topoisomerase I, RNA polymerase I and III, fibrillarin, nuclear organizer antigen. The CREST syndrome is more specifically associated with anti-centromere autoantibodies. Shared sequences between viral proteins and topoisomerase I, fibrillarin and centromere proteins (CENP-B) have been reported.

Topo 1	PIEKIYNKTQRE	*(75)*
Moloney murine leukemia virus (MOMLV)	EAEKVYNKRETT	
Feline Sarcoma virus (FSV)	EAEKIYNKRETP	
Topo 1	KDEPEDDGYFVPPK	*(76)*
Cytomegalovirus (CMV) UL70 protein	YKMDQDDGYFMHRR	
Fibrillarin	NRGRSRGGKRGN	*(77)*
Epstein–Barr virus (EBV) -NP protein	SGGRGRGGSGGR	
Fibrillarin	GVYRPPPKUKN	*(77)*
Herpes simplex virus (HSV) -p40 protein	AVYRPPPHSAP	

Homologies have been identified in the N and C terminal portions of CENP-B, the target of anticentromere autoantibodies in CREST syndrome, and various viral proteins *(78)* Thus, pentapeptides or hexapeptides located in N-terminal region of CENP-B are homologous to the HSV–1 DNA binding protein and gpD protein, gagp27 and protease of SRV-1, gag of HIV-1, $12p^{gag}$, and $30p^{gag}$ of Felv, and the 93 kDa protein of EBV.

From the experiments cited above, it becomes conceivable that infectious agents may participate in the induction of autoimmune disease through the process of antigen mimicry. Assessment of the involvement of molecular mimicry in the onset of an autoimmune disease should fill certain requirements as follows:

1. A statistically significant correlation should exist between the occurrence of the autoimmune disease and the presence of the infectious agent bearing structural similarity to the target antigen in a given autoimmune disease.
2. The disease should be preceded by an infection caused by the microbe crossreactive with the self antigens.

3. There should be a lag period between the infection and the onset autoimmune disease, indicative of stimulation of lymphocytes by the cross-
reactive microbial epitopes.

Except in the case of rheumatic fever, evidence based on above criteria that
antigen mimicry is involved in the pathogenesis of autoimmune diseases is
quite incomplete.

The concept of a break in self-tolerance induced by cross reactive microbial
epitopes is supported by findings demonstrating induction of autoimmune diseases by injection of heterologous proteins. The best example is the induction of myasthenia gravis in mammals injected with AchR prepared from
Torpedo star fish. Second, the microbial crossreactive epitopes should elicit a
strong autoimmune response. Long lasting persistence of such crossreactive
antigens, either because of a persistent infection or a defect in clearing foreign
macromolecules, can perpetuate the autoimmune response, which could ultimately
cause damage to cells expressing the crossreactive self epitopes. This mechanism is supported by the well-known example of appearance of neuroparalytic
disease in humans vaccinated with the rabies vaccine (78). This vaccine is prepared from rabies-infected animals and is contaminated with heterologous
MBP, which cross-reacts with human MBP. The MBP initiates an autoimmune
response, resulting in a neurological disease (79).

In strict terms, molecular mimicry has been defined by homology of linear
sequences shared between microbial and self-antigens. If efficient stimulation
of autoreactive T-cells is to be obtained, the microbial crossreactive epitope
and the self-epitope should share the same anchor residues responsible for binding to MHC molecules, as well as the critical amino acid residues capable of
interacting with the TCR. It can be predicted, therefore, that major involvements of antigen mimicry in the activation of pathogenic autoreactive CD8
T-cells may require homologies spanning nonapeptides sequences, and of CD4
T-cells, deca to dodeca peptide sequences.

Most studies on antigen mimicry deal with the crossreactivity of autoantibodies to microbial antigens sharing linear sequences with self antigens. This
represents a major problem in understanding how crossreactive epitopes of
microbial proteins can be recognized by the Ig receptor of pathogenic B cells,
since the majority of antigenic epitopes recognized by pathogenic B cell are
conformational rather sequential (80).

4. CONCLUSIONS

During the past decades, a big effort has been made to understand the pathogenesis of autoimmune diseases by characterizing the phenotypic and genetic
properties of human autoreactive lymphocytes, the immunochemical and molecular properties of V genes encoding the autoantibodies, and the utilization of
animal models developing spontaneous or induced autoimmune diseases. Despite
this effort, however, little progress was made in the understanding of the mecha-

nisms responsible for the primary injury leading to the onset of disease. Autoimmune diseases are clearly not due to monogenic defects. It remains a solid working hypothesis, therefore, that exogenous factors can be a cause of primary injury leading to the onset of autoimmune diseases. The data reviewed herein show that further work should be undertaken to establish a cause-effect relationship between exogenous agents and the onset of autoimmune disease. This effort should be aimed at determining: whether the association of a given autoimmune disease with the exogenous microbial agent is statistically significant, whether the exogenous agent can be isolated from the target tissue affected by the autoimmune phenomenon and can induce either autoantibodies or activate T-cells specific for pathogenic self epitopes, whether the infection precedes the onset of autoimmune disease, and whether there is a lag period between the infection and the onset of the disease, permitting the stimulation of autoreactive lymphocytes by exogenous antigen to reach the threshold required for the occurrence of autoimmunity. Well-programmed studies will be needed to provide definitive evidence on the causal role of exogenous factors in autoimmune diseases.

REFERENCES

1. Burnett M. (1959) *The Clonal Selection Theory of Acquired Immunity,* Vanderbilt University Press, Nashville, TN.
2. Jacobs, H., von Boehmer, H., Melief, C. J., and Berns, A. (1990) Mutations in the major histocompatibility complex class I antigen presenting groove affect both negative positive selection of T cells. *Eur. J. Immunol.* **20,** 2333–2337.
3. Hogguist, K. A., Jameson, S. C., Heath, W. R., Howard, J. L., Bevan, M. J., and Carbone, F. R. (1994) T cell receptor antagonist peptides induce positive selection. *Cell* **76,** 229,230.
4. Hartly, S. B., Croslic, R., Brink, R., Kantor, A. B., Basten, A., and Goodnow, C. C. (1991) Elimination from peripheral lymphoid tissues of self-reactive B lymphocytes recognizing membrane-bound antigens. *Nature* **353,** 765–769.
5. Welch, M. J., Fong, S., Vaugham, J. H., and Carson, D. A. (1983) Increased frequency of rheumatoid factor precursor B lymphocytes after immunization of normal adults with tetanus toxoid. *Clin. Exp. Immunol.* **51,** 299.
6. Inman, R. D., Hodge, M., and Johnston, M. E. A. (1986) Arthritis, vasculitis and cryoglobulinemia associated with relapsing hepatitis A virus infection. *Ann. Intern. Med.* **105,** 700–703.
7. Czaja, A. J., Carpenter, H. A., and Santrach, P. J. (1993) Evidence against hepatitis viruses as important causes of severe autoimmune hepatitis in the United States. *J. Hepatol.* **18,** 342–352.
8. Munke, H. F., Stockmann, F., and Ramdori, G. (1995) Possible association between Bechet's syndrome and chronic hepatitis C virus infection. *N. Engl. J. Med.* **332,** 400–401.
9. Anonymous. (1988) Guillian–Barre syndrome. *Lancet* **2,** 659–661.
10. Hart, I. K. and Kennedy, P. G. E. (1988) Guillain–Barre syndrome associated with cytomegalovirus infection. *Quart. J. Med.* **253,** 425–430.

11. Marchini, B. Dolcher, M. P., and Sabbatini, A. (1994) Immune response to different sequences of the EBNA I molecule in Epstein-Barr virus-related disorders and in autoimmune diseases. *J. Autoimmun.* **7,** 179–191.
12. Tosato, G., Steinber, A. D., and Blaesc, R. M. (1981) Defective EBV-specific suppressor T-cell function in rheumatoid arthritis. *N. Engl. J. Med.* **305,** 1238–1243.
13. Silverman, S. L. and Schmacher, H. R. (1981) Antibodies to Epstein-Barr viral antigens in early rheumatoid arthritis. *Arthritis Rheum.* **24,** 1465–1468.
14. Tosato, G., Steinberg, D., and Yarchoan R. (1984) Abnormally elevated frequency of Epstein–Barr virus-infected B cells in the blood of patients with rheumatoid arthritis. *J. Clin. Invest.* **73,** 1789–1795.
15. Roudier, J. G., Rhodes, J., Petersen, F., et. al. (1988) The Epstein-Barr virus glycoprotein gp110, a molecular between HLA DR4, HLA DR1 and rheumatoid arthritis. *Scand. J. Immunol.* **27,** 367–371.
16. Wilder, R. L. (1994) Hypothesis for retorviral causation of rheumatoid arthritis. *Curr. Opin. Rheumatol.* **6,** 295–299.
17. Baranski, B., Armstrong, G., and Truman, J. T. (1988) Epstein–Barr virus in the bone marrow of patients with aplastic anemia. *Ann. Intern. Med.* **109,** 695–704.
18. Whittingham, S. M., McNeilage, J., and Mackay, I. R. (1985) Primary Sjogren's syndrome after infectious mononucleosis. *Ann. Intern. Med.* **102,** 490–493.
19. Fox, R. I., Luppi, M., Kang, H. I., and Pisa, P. (1991) Reactivation of Epstein–Barr virus in Sjögren's syndrome. *Springer Semin. Immunopathol.* **13,** 217–231.
20. Deacon, I. M., Shattles, W. G., and Mathews, J. B. (1992) Frequency of EBV DNA detection in Sjögren's syndrome. *Am. J. Med.* **92,** 453–454.
21. Fox, R. I., Luppi, M., and Pisa, P. (1992) Potential role of EBV in Sjögren's syndrome and rheumatoid arthritis. *J. Rheumatol.* **19,** 18–24.
22. Baboonian, C., Benables, P. J. W., and Maini, R. N. (1990) Antibodies to human herpesvirus-6 in Sjogren's syndrome. *Arthritis Rheum.* **33,** 1749,1750.
23. Huber, S. A. and Lodge, P. A. (1984) Coxsackie B-3 myocarditis in BALB/c mice. *Am. J. Pathol.* **116,** 21–29.
24. Wolfgram, L. J., Beisel, K. W., and Rose, N. R. (1985) Heart-specific autoantibodies following murine coxsackievirus B3 myocarditis. *J. Exp. Med.* **161,** 1112–1121.
25. Beisel, K. W., Srinivasappa, J., and Prabhakar, B. S. (1991) Identification of a putative shared epitope between Coxsackie virus B4 and alpha cardiac myosin heavy chain. *Clin. Exp. Immunol.* **86,** 49–55.
26. Neumann, D. A., Rose, N. R., and Ansari, A. A. (1994) Induction of multiple heart autoantibodies in mice with coxsackievirus B3 and cardiac myosin-induced autoimmune myocarditis. *J. Immunol.* **152,** 343–350.
27. Reid, D. M., Reid, T. M., and Brown, T. (1985) Human parvovirus-associated arthritis: a clinical and laboratory description. *Lancet* **1,** 422–425.
28. Corman, L. C. and Dolson, D. J. (1992) Polyarteritis nodosa and parvovirus B19 infection. *Lancet* **339,** 491.
29. Secry, J. P. (1990) The link between viral infection and autoimmunity. *Rev. Infect. Dis.* **12,** 1202.
30. Bodansky, H. J., Liitlewood, J. M., Bottazzo, G. F. Dean, B. M., and Hambling, M. H. (1984) Which virus causes the initial islet lesion in type 1 diabetes? *Lancet* **1,** 401,402.

31. Oldstone, M. B., Nerenberg, M., and Southern, P. (1991) Virus infection triggers insulin-dependent diabetes mellitus in a transgenic model: role of anti-self (virus) immune response. *Cell* **65**, 319–331.

32. Taniguchi, A., Takenaka, Y., Noda, Y., Ueno, Y., Shichikawa, K., Sato, K., et al. (1988) Adult T cell leukemia presenting with proliferative synovitis. *Arthritis Rheum.* **31**, 1076,1077.

33. Banki, K., Maceda, J., Hurley, E., Ablonczy, E., Mattson, D. H., Szegedy, L., et al. (1992) HTLV-related endogenous sequence, HRES-1 encodes a 28KD protein: a possible autoantigen for HTLV-1 gag reactive autoantibodies. *Proc. Natl. Acad. Sci. USA* **89**, 1939–1943.

34. Matsumoto, Y., Hibino, N., Kamimura, M., and Nishioka, K. (1990) *Jpn. J. Int. Med.* **79**, 1589–1590.

35. Sagawa, K., Moochizuki, M., Masuoka, K., Katagiri, K., Katayama, T., Maeda, T., et al. (1995) Immunopathological mechanisms of HTLV-1 uveilts. *J. Clin. Invest.* **95**, 852–858.

36. Nemazee, D. A. and Sato, V. L. (1983) Induction of rheumatoid antibody in the mouse: regulated production of autoantibody in the secondary humoral response. *J. Exp. Med.* **158**, 545.

37. Manheimer, A. and Bona, C. (1985) Anti-immunoglobulin antibodies VI. Age-dependent isotype and autoimmunoglobulin variation during secondary immune response in 129 mice. *Mech. Ageing Dev.* **30**, 187–199.

38. Bailey, N. C., Fidanza, V., Mayer, R., Mazza, G., Fougereau, M., and Bona, C. (1989) Activation of clones producing self-reactive antibodies by foreign antigen and antiidiotype antibody carrying the internal image of the antigen. *J. Clin. Invest.* **84**, 744–756.

39. Coutelier, J. P., van der Logt, J. J. M., Hessen, F. W. A., Warmier, G., and van Snick, J. (1986) Rheumatoid factor production in 129/Sv mice: involvement of an intestinal infectious agent. *J. Immunol.* **137**, 337.

40. Theophilopoulos, A. N., Balderas, R. S., Hand, L., and Dixon, F. J. (1983) Monoclonal IgM Rheumatoid factors derived from arthritic MRL/MP-1pr/1pr mice. *J. Exp. Med.* **158**, 901.

41. Manhcimcr, A. J., Victor-Kobrin, C., Stein, K. E., and Bona, C. A. (1984) Anti-immunoglobulin antibodies V. Age-dependent variation of clones stimulated by polysaccharide T1-2 antigens in 129 and MRL mice spontaneously producing anti-γ globulin antibodies. *J. Immunol.* **133**, 562.

42. Cohen, A. D. and Shoenfeld, Y. (1995) The viral autoimmunity relationship. *Viral Immunol.* **8**, 1–9.

43. Newmark, P. (1995) Multiple sclerosis and viruses. *Nature* **318**, 101.

44. Futo, F., Saag, K. G., and Scharosch, L. L. (1993) Parvovirus B19-specific DVH in bone marrow from B19 arthropathy patients: evidence for B19 virus persistence. *J. Infect. Dis.* **167**, 744–748.

45. Sasaki, T., Murai, C., Muryoi, T. Takahashi, Y., Munakata, Y., Sugamura, M., et al. (1995) Persistent infection of human parvovirus B19 in a normal subject. *Lancet* **346**, 851.

46. Murai, C., Munakata, Y., Takahashi, Y., Ishii, T., Muryoi, T., Abe, K., et al. Rheumatoid arthritis after humanparvovirus B19 infection (submitted).

47. Hasunuma, T., Sumida, T., and Nishioka, K. (1997) Human T cell leukemia virus type 1 and rheumatoid arthritis. *Int. Rev. Immunol.,* in press.

48. Izui, S., Eisenberg, R. A., and Dixon, F. J. (1979) IgM rheumatoid factors in mice injected with bacterial lipopolysaccharides. *J. Immunol.* **122,** 2096.
49. Theophilpoulos, A. (1995) The basis of autoimmunity. *Immunol. Today* **16,** 90–98.
50. Murakami, M., Tsubata, T., Okamoto, M., Shimizu, A., Kumagai, S., Imura, H., et al. (1992) Antigen-induced apoptotic death of Ly-1 B cells that are responsible for autoimmune disease in transgenic mice. *Nature* 357, 77–80.
51. Zang, G.-X., Ma, C.-G., Xiao, B.-G., Bakhiet, M., Link, H. and Olson, T. (1995) Depletion of CD8+ T cells suppresses the development of myasthenia gravis in Lewis rats. *Eur. J. Immunol.* **25,** 1191–1198.
52. Moffatt, S., Tanaka, N., Tada, K., Nose, M., Nakamura, M., Muraoka, O., et al. (1996) A cytotoxic non structural protein, NS1, of human parvovirus B19. *J. Virol.* **70,** 8485–8491.
53. Hirano, T. T., Matsuda, M., Turner, N., Miyasaka, G., Buchan, B., Tang, K., et al. (1988) Excessive production of interleukin 6/B cell stimulatory factor-2 in rheumatoid arthritis. *Eur. J. Immunol.* **18,** 1797–1801.
54. Hirano, T., Akira, S., Taga, T., and Kishimoto, T. (1990) Biological and clinical aspects of interleukin 6. *Immunol. Today* **11,** 443–449.
55. Jorgensen, C., Angel, J., and Fournier, C. (1991) Regulation of synovial cell proliferation and prostaglandin E2 production by combined action of cytokines. *Eur. Cytokine Netw.* **2,** 207–215.
56. Mihara, M., Moriya, Y., Kishimoto, T., and Ohsugi, Y. (1995) Interleukin-6 (IL-6) induces the proliferation of synovial fibroblastic cells in the presence of soluble IL-6 receptor. *Br. J. Rheum.* **34,** 321–325.
57. Nakajima, T., Aono, H., Hasunuma, T., Yamamoto, K., Maruyama, I., Nosaka, T., et al. (1993) Overgrowth of human synovial cells driven by HTLV-1 virus Tax gene. *J. Clin. Invest.* **92,** 186–193.
58. Iwakura, Y., Saijo, S., Kioka, Y., Nakayama-Yamada, J., Itagaki, K., Tosu, M., et al. (1995) Autoimmunity induction by HTLV-1 virus in transgene mice that develop chronic flammatory arthropathy resembling rheumatoid arthritis in humans. *J. Immunol.* **155,** 1588–1598.
59. Gamow, G., Sercarz, E. E., and Benichou, G. (1991) The dominant self and the cryptic self: shaping the autoreactive T-cell repertoire. *Immunol. Today* **12,**193–195.
60. Witebsky, E., Rose, N. R., Terplan, K., Paine, J. R., and Egan, R. W. (1957) Chronic thyroiditis and autoimmunization. *J. Am. Med. Assoc.* **164,** 1439–1447.
61. Kaplan, M. H. and Sevc, K. H. (1964) Immunologic relations of streptococcal and tissue antigens. III. Presence in human sera of streptococcal antibody crossreactive with heart tissue. Association with streptococcal infection, rheumatic fever and glomerulonephritis. *J. Exp. Med.* **119,** 651–666.
62. Zabriskie, J. B., Hsu, K. C., and Seegal, B. C. (1970) Heart-reactive antibody associated with rheumatic fever: characterization and diagnostic significance. *Clin. Exp. Immunol.* **7,** 147–159.
63. Krisher, K. and Cunningham, M. W. (1985) Myosin: a link between streptococci and heart. *Science* **227,** 413–415.
64. Cunningham, M. W., Hall, N. K., and Krisher, K. K. (1986) A study of anti-group A streptococcal monoclonal antibodies cross-reactive with myosin. *J. Immunol.* **136,** 293–298.
65. Dale, J. B. and Beachey, E. H. (1986) Epitopes of streptococcal M proteins shared with cardiac myosin. *J. Exp. Med.* **162,** 583–591.

66. Husby, G., van de Rijn, I., Zabriskie, J. B., Abdin, Z. H. and Williams, R. C., Jr. (1976) Antibodies reacting with cytoplasm of subthalamic and caudate nuclei neutrons in chorea and acute rheumatic fever. *J. Exp. Med.* **144**, 1094–1110.

67. Fillit, H., Damle, S. P., and Gregory, J. D. (1985) Sera from patients with poststreptococcal glomerulonephritis contain antibodies to glomerular heparan sulfate proteoglycan J. *Exp. Med.* **161**, 277–289.

68. Fujinami, R. S. and Oldstone, M. B. A. (1985) Amino acid homology between the encephalitogenic site of myelin basic protein and virus: mechanism for autoimmunity. *Science* **230**, 1043–1045.

69. Jahnke, U., Fischer, E. H., and Alvord, E. C., Jr. (1985) Sequence homology between certain viral proteins and proteins related to encephalomyelitis and neuritis. *Science* **229**, 282–284.

70. Johnson, R. T., Griffin, D. E., Hirsch, R. L., Wolinsky, J. W., Roedenbeck, S., Lindo de Sorian, I., et al. (1984) Measles encephalomyelitis: clinical and immunological studies. *N. Engl. J. Med.* **310**, 137–141.

71. Johnson, R. I. and Griffin, E. D. (1996) Virus-induced autoimmune demyelinating disease of the central nervous system, in *Concepts in Viral Pathogenesis, Vol. II* (Notkins, A.L. and Oldstone, M.B.A., eds), Springer-Verlag, New York, pp. 203–209.

72. Oldstone, M. B. A. (1987) Molecular mimicry and autoimmune disease. *Cell* **50**, 819–820.

73. Dyrberg, T. and Oldstone, M. B. A. (1986) Peptides as probes to study molecular mimicry and virus induced autoimmunity. *Curr. Top. Microbiol. Immunol.* **130**, 25–37.

74. Singh, V. K., Yamaki, K., Abe, T., and Shinohara, T. (1989) Molecular mimicry between uveitopathogenic site of retinal S-antigen and Escherichia coli protein: induction of experimental autoimmune Uveitis and lymphocyte Cross-reaction. *Cell. Immunol.* **122**, 262–273.

75. Maul, G. G., Jimenez, S. A., Riggs, E., and Ziemnicka-Kotula, D. (1989) Determination of an epitope of the diffuse systemic sclerosis marker antigen DNA topoisomerase I: sequence similarity with retroviral p30gag protein suggest a possible cause for autoimmunity in systemic sclerosis. *Proc. Natl. Acad. Sci. USA* **86**, 8492–8496.

76. Muryoi, T., Kasturi, K., Kafina, M. J., Cram, D. S., Harrison, L. C., Sasaki, T., et al. (1993) Antitoposiomerase I monoclonal autoantibodies from scleroderma patients and tight skin mouse interact with similar epitopes. *J. Exp. Med.* **175**, 1103–1109.

77. Kasturi, K., Hatakeyama, A., Spiera, H., and Bona, C. (1985) Antifibrillarin autoantibodies present in systemic sclerosis and other connective tissue diseases interact with similar epitopes. *J. Exp. Med.* **181**, 1027–1036.

78. Douvas, A. and Sobelman, S. (1991) Multiple overlapping homologies between two rheumatoid antigens and immunosuppressive viruses. *Proc. Natl. Acad. Sci. USA* **88**, 6328–6332.

79. Hemachudha, T., Griffin, D. E., and Giffels, J. J. (1987) Myelin basic protein as an encephalitogen in encephalomyelitis and polyneuritis following rabies vaccination. *N. Engl. J. Med.* **316**, 369–374.

80. Bona, C. (1991) Postulates defining pathogenic autoantibodies and T-cells. *Autoimmunity* **10**, 169–172.

11

Dysregulation of the Idiotype Network in Autoimmune Diseases

Haraldine A. Stafford and Morris Reichlin

1. INTRODUCTION

The hallmark of autoimmune disorders is the presence of serologically detectable autoantibodies. The appearance of autoantibodies in patients is tacitly assumed to reflect the acquisition of new antibody activities. However, it is now well recognized that some autoantibodies are also present in healthy individuals *(1)*. Recent evidence suggests that their expression may be regulated by an idiotype network *(2)*.

The idiotype network consists of a series of antibodies that arise during the development of a specific immune response. Ab1 is the initial antibody that develops in response to a nominal antigen, i.e., the antigen that triggered the immune response. Since each antibody has unique antigenic sites within its variable region, it can elicit an autoantibody response. Consequently, Ab1 can elicit an autoantibody response (an anti-idiotype or Ab2), then Ab2 can elicit an autoantibody response (an anti-anti-idiotype or Ab3), and potentially a cascade of anti-immunoglobulin responses could develop. A single antigenic site within the antibody variable region is termed an idiotope. A set of idiotopes on one antibody molecule is termed an idiotype. Idiotopes can be located within the antigen-combining site (paratope) or in the framework region. There are three common categories of anti-idiotypes, which are classified by antigen competition for their binding to idiotype and by antigen mimicability. Antibodies that arise to idiotopes within the paratope are antigen inhibitable, and either are or are not the internal image of the nominal antigen (Ab2β and Ab2γ). In contrast, antibodies to the idiotopes within the framework region (Ab2α) are not antigen inhibitable. The autoantibody repertoire generated in response to a given antibody is termed its anti-idiotype. These anti-idiotypes are capable of influencing the outcome of an immune response. Initially, it was postulated that this network was responsible for suppression of the nominal antigen-driven immune response. Later, it became evident that this network can also promote the nominal antigen-specific immune response.

Contemporary Immunology: Autoimmune Reactions
Edited by: S. Paul © Humana Press Inc., Totowa, NJ

This chapter provides an overview of the idiotype network in health and disease. It is not an exhaustive review of the literature, but rather a logical perspective on how this network functions to maintain immune homeostasis. Evidence is presented that supports the hypothesis that dysregulation of the idiotype network may contribute to autoimmunity. Initial discussion is aimed at supporting a role for anti-idiotypes in normal immune regulation. This is followed by a discussion of how anti-idiotypes may be protective against auto-immune disease in healthy individuals by masking autoantibodies. Finally, a discussion on anti-idiotypes in autoimmune disease is presented.

2. ANTI-IMMUNOGLOBULINS IN HEALTHY INDIVIDUALS

Nasu et al. were the first to describe naturally occurring human antibodies to the F(ab')$_2$ of IgG *(3)*. These antibodies belonged to both the IgG and IgM isotypes and were identified in serum by their ability to bind and precipitate radiolabeled, heat-aggregated F(ab')$_2$ fragments. Anti-F(ab')$_2$ antibodies were predominantly identified in patients with rheumatologic diseases, especially rheumatoid arthritis, but were also found in a small proportion of normals. These antibodies that were later termed generic anti-idiotypes *(4)* are distinct from other "serum agglutinators" *(5,6)* including the well-studied pepsin agglutinator *(7)*. These "agglutinators" are antibodies that react to enzymatically cleaved fragments of IgG. Neoantigens on the F(ab')$_2$ fragments arise from enzymatic digestion of IgG and are distinct from idiotopes.

Determination of the epitope(s) that reacted with these generic anti-F(ab')$_2$ followed. Initial efforts localized the sites of antibody activity to antigenic determinants within the Fv portion of the antibody *(8)*, principally on the λ light chain *(9)*. (The Fv portion of the antibody is encoded by the variable region genes). Through the use of a prototype human λ light chain and the linear epitope mapping technique, a profile of reactive epitopes on the constant and variable regions of the λ light chain was identified, with several invariant epitopes identified among all individuals *(10)*. These epitopes were found predominantly in the complementarity-determining regions (CDRs, or hypervariable regions), were on the surface of the λ chain and were highly solvent accessible. The authors also showed that IgG generic anti-idiotypes from some normals react with the concordant (or corresponding) CDRs on the VH and VL of several anti-DNA and antirabies monoclonal antibodies *(11)*. These findings emphasize the universality of the idiotype-anti-idiotype network. To our knowledge, no other human anti-idiotype has been studied to this extent.

3. ANTI-IDIOTYPES IN NORMAL IMMUNOREGULATION

The exogenous administration of anti-idiotypes to experimental animals has emphasized the importance of idiotypic-anti-idiotypic interactions in the regulation of immune responses *(12–16)*. These interactions also appear to be important during the normal immune response. Their presence has been well described during immunizations and during the course of natural infection. Certain immunologic dyscrasias elicit an anti-idiotypic response. Anti-idiotypes have also been described during transplantation, allergic challenge and desensitization, and during pregnancy and fertility. Examples in each of these categories will now follow.

Anti-idiotypes can arise as a consequence of immunization. They were recognized initially in animals immunized with a wide range of antigens. Some examples include mice immunized with TNP-Ficoll *(17)* and rabbits immunized with sheep red cells *(18)*. Geha was the first to demonstrate their presence in humans after immunization. Humans immunized with tetanus toxoid develop an anti-idiotypic response that correlates with lower anti-tetanus toxoid antibody levels *(19,20)*. Four of eleven seroconverters after hepatitis B vaccination developed idiotype-specific B lymphocytes to anti-hepatitis B surface antibody one month after their last immunization *(21)*. Anti-idiotypes to poliovirus antibodies arising after poliovirus vaccination have been demonstrated in commercial immunoglobulin preparations, human serum, colostrum, and milk of vaccinated females *(22)*. These authors also showed that newborn infants had specific secretory IgA and IgM antibodies to poliovirus in their saliva, meconium, and amniotic fluid in the absence of poliovirus exposure *(23)*. Taken together, their data suggest that anti-idiotypes to poliovirus antibodies actively induce a specific immune response in the fetus. Clearly, anti-idiotypes develop after immunization. Their functional role in promoting or suppressing the immune response, however, cannot be predicted clearly.

Exogenously administered drugs can also elicit anti-idiotypes. The titers of anti-insulin antibodies and their presumed anti-idiotypes were reciprocally related in insulin-requiring diabetics *(24)*. Anti-insulin antibodies frequently arise during insulin therapy in diabetics. In some patients, anti-idiotypes develop, which are associated with a decrease in anti-insulin antibodies.

Anti-idiotypes can arise as a consequence of infection. BALB/c mice infected with trypanosomes develop both antiphosphocholine antibodies and their anti-idiotypes *(25)*. Antibodies to the Fab portion of IgG were identified in a large proportion of patients with infectious mononucleosis and in patients with cystic fibrosis with concurrent bacterial infections *(26)*. Anti-idiotypes to antibodies specific for hepatitis B surface antigen arise in patients with acute *(27)* and chronic hepatitis B infections *(27,28)*. Moreover, some IgM cryoglobulins that develop as a consequence of hepatitis B infection are probably anti-idiotypes to anti-HBs antibodies *(29)*. Children with lyme arthritis have anti-idiotypes to antibodies specific for most *Borrelia burgdorferi* antigens. In this system, antibodies to the antigens OSP-A and OSP-B do not evoke an anti-idiotype response, and these antibodies are postulated to be pathogenic *(30)*. This study suggests that not all immune responses generate an anti-idiotype response. Perhaps, the structure or dose of the antigen is important in determining if anti-idiotypes will arise. These observations indicate that anti-idiotypic responses may serve an integral, but as yet incompletely defined role in regulating the immune system.

Anti-idiotypes have been found to arise as a consequence of lymphoproliferative disorders. Peripheral blood lymphocytes from patients with multiple
myeloma and monoclonal gammapathy of undetermined significance produce
anti-idiotypic antibodies directed against the autologous monoclonal immunoglobulin *(31)*. Similarly, the development of putative anti-idiotypes to the paraprotein has been suggested in Waldenstrom's macroglobulinemia *(32)*. It seems
likely that these anti-idiotypes develop as a consequence of the extensive antibody burden. On the other hand, the anti-idiotypes do not seem capable of
suppressing the production of the idiotype (the paraprotein).

Anti-idiotype synthesis associated with the immune responses to various
allergens has been documented. Circulating anti-IgE autoantibodies have been
described in individuals with atopy at levels corresponding to their serum IgE
levels *(33,34)*. The anti-IgE antibodies are often difficult to detect as they form
immune complexes with the IgE *(34)*. Some of these autoantibodies, in particular those of the IgM and IgA classes, display restricted specificity for individual IgE myeloma proteins, suggesting that they may be idiotype-specific
and not isotype-specific *(35)*. Detailed epitope analysis has suggested that some
of the IgM antibodies react with epitopes within the hinge region of IgE. In
contrast, the IgA antibodies react only with the Fab portion of the specific IgE
myeloma *(36)*. The IgA antibodies to IgE are present in non-atopic individuals,
but they are found at higher levels in atopic individuals and patients with proto-
zoal infections. Children, both nonatopic and atopic, had low levels of these
antibodies, which the authors attributed to the low IgA concentration in childhood. The low affinity of the IgA antibodies for IgE prompted the authors to
suggest that the binding is to carbohydrate determinants, as opposed to peptidic
epitopes. Other authors have been unable to corroborate these findings. Hebert
and Castracane have identified the highest levels of anti-idiotypes to IgE in
normal donors, suggesting that the high levels of IgE in atopic individuals could
result from deficiencies in anti-idiotypic regulation *(37,38)*. Moreover, specific immunotherapy in atopic individuals increases the levels of anti-idiotypes
to IgE. This finding has been confirmed by others *(39)*, suggesting that the
anti-idiotype response to IgE is beneficial in suppressing atopy. Note that the
conflicting studies cited above may be owing, in part, to the heterogeneity of
the anti-IgE antibody response, and additional studies may be necessary to
delineate the anti-idiotypic component of the response.

Anti-idiotypes can develop as a consequence of HLA incompatibilities.
Anti-HLA antibodies and anti-anti-HLA antibodies frequently arise in this setting. Moreover, there is strong evidence that the putative anti-idiotypes to anti-
HLA antibodies may play a role in allograft survival. The development of the
anti-idiotypes to anti-HLA in renal transplant recipients receiving blood trans-
fusions is associated with allograft survival, whereas the absence of the anti-
idiotypes is associated with early allograft loss *(40)*. Patients who received heart
or kidney allografts may develop anti-HLA antibodies which are suggested to

lead to graft rejection *(41)*. Nine of ten liver allograft recipients in one study developed the putative anti-idiotypes to anti-donor HLA *(42)*. All nine recipients had prolonged graft survival. The authors imply that the antibodies to anti-HLA antibodies are anti-idiotypes, but this was not proven rigorously. The antibodies were identified functionally, based on their ability to inhibit HLA-dependent lymphocytotoxicity. Ideally, immunochemical confirmation of the idiotype restriction is necessary to qualify the antibodies as anti-idiotypes. Several additional studies have suggested that anti-IgG antibodies of undetermined isotype and fine specificity are associated with kidney graft survival *(43–45)*. Patients with high titers of pretransplant IgA anti-F(ab')$_{2g}$ display significantly better kidney graft survival as compared to patients with low titers of these antibodies *(46)*. The F(ab')$_{2g}$ epitope reactive with the IgA anti-immunoglobulins has recently been mapped to the hinge rather than the variable region *(47)*. Thus, these antibodies are not anti-idiotypes. Whether the antibodies to anti-HLA antibodies discussed above are this type of anti-F(ab')$_{2g}$ or are actually anti-idiotypes remains to be determined.

Anti-idiotype synthesis may also be a component of the maternal immune responses to the fetus. Using an HLA-dependent inhibition assay, putative anti-idiotypes to maternal antibodies directed against paternal HLA antigens are purported to be responsible for fetal survival in multiparous females *(48)*. It has been suggested that anti-idiotypes to antisperm antibodies may play a role in maintenance of fertility *(49)*. Antibodies to a sperm-specific glycoprotein, the fertilization antigen, are present in infertile woman but are undetectable in fertile or virgin females. Antibodies that react with Fab' fragments of a murine monoclonal antibody specific for the fertilization antigen are detectable in a large proportion of fertile females, minimally in infertile females, and not at all in virgin females. These antibodies were also capable of neutralizing the anti-sperm antibodies in infertile females. Thus, these anti-idiotypes are suggested to be important in promoting conception.

4. REGULATED AUTOANTIBODIES IN HEALTHY INDIVIDUALS

Healthy individuals appear to regulate their autoantibody levels. While rheumatoid factors and antinuclear antibodies are occasionally found in low titers in young healthy adults, the titer and prevalence of these autoantibodies increased in elderly subjects who otherwise display signs of decreased immunity *(50–52)*. Autoantibodies associated with organ-specific autoimmune diseases, such as anti-actin or anti-thyroglobulin, are detectable in healthy individuals, but only after their sera have been treated by certain procedures that could potentially remove inhibitory anti-idiotypes *(53,54)*. High affinity C3 nephritic factors (autoantibodies to the alternate pathway C3 convertase present in patients with glomerulonephritis) and their anti-idiotypes have been identified in newborns and normal adults *(55,56)*. Moreover, anti-idiotypes to C3 nephritic factor have been purified from normal and patient sera *(57)*. Pooled intravenous immunoglobulin (IVIg), especially from aged donors and multiparous females contains neutralizing antibodies to anti-Factor VIII, an autoantibody associated with auto-immune hemophilia A *(58)*. The anti-Factor VIII antibodies were only identifiable in healthy adults in another study after immunoadsorption with insolubilized Factor VIII *(59)*. The unbound IgG fractions from the immunoabsorbent expressed anti-idiotypic antibody activity to the anti-Factor VIII antibodies. Antibodies with specificity for the F(ab')$_2$ fragments of anti-single-stranded DNA (anti-ssDNA) antibodies have been identified in sera from healthy adults *(60)*. Such antibodies are found at greater levels in healthy relatives of SLE patients than in normal control families *(61)*. The anti-idiotype antibodies in the unaffected relatives had relatively high specificity towards the anti-ssDNA antibodies of the SLE proband as compared to the anti-ssDNA antibodies from unrelated SLE patients. Normal cord blood B lymphocytes can produce high affinity IgG anti-double-stranded (ds) DNA autoantibodies and Igm anti-idiotypes to anti-ds DNA, suggesting that this idiotype-anti-idiotype network exists early in development *(62)*. These examples suggest that certain autoantibodies exist in normal subjects, but their presence may be masked by the anti-idiotypes.

Support for the beneficial regulatory role of anti-idiotypes to autoantibodies in healthy individuals has been adduced from the observation that IVIg has clinical utility in some autoimmune diseases *(63)*. Studies in patients with acquired hemophilia A support this view *(64)*. IVIg can terminate bleeding in patients who have developed antibodies to factor VIII. This property has been accredited to the presence of naturally occurring anti-idiotypes to anti-factor VIII antibodies in IVIg. Anti-idiotypic antibody activities to a variety of human antibodies have been described in IVIg, including antibodies to thyroglobulin *(65,66)*, microsomal antigens *(67)*, intrinsic factor *(66)*, DNA *(66)*, platelet glycoprotein IIb/IIIa *(68)*, neutrophil cytoplasmic antigen *(69)*, myeloperoxidase *(70)*, peripheral nerve antigens *(71)*, acetylcholine receptor *(72)*, and phospholipids *(73)*. The evidence for anti-idiotypes in IVIg includes observations that F(ab')$_2$ fragments of IVIg neutralize antigen binding by the F(ab')$_2$ fragments of autoantibodies; auto-antibodies can be affinity purified on immobilized F(ab')$_2$ fragments of IVIg; the IVIg lacks anti-allotypic activity against the commonest allotypes expressed in the F(ab')$_2$ region of human IgG; and anti-idiotypes against idiotypic determinants expressed on autoantibodies defined by heterologous anti-idiotypes are present in IVIg *(65,66)*. For some autoantibodies, the type of anti-idiotypes present in IVIg has been characterized. For example, anti-idiotypes to anti-thyroglobulin antibodies are directed towards a cross-reactive idiotype, T44 *(65)*. This idiotype is immunodominant, disease-associated, and was defined using heterologous anti-idiotypic antibodies. Consequently, these anti-idiotypes are of the Ab2α type. These findings suggest that regulatory factors, i.e., anti-idiotype antibodies, exist in healthy individuals, and may interfere with the expression and/or detection of autoantibodies in these individuals.

We have identified a hidden SLE-specific autoantibody, anti-ribosomal P, in the sera of virtually all healthy adults *(74)*. These autoantibodies are quantitatively and qualitatively similar to those identified in patient sera. They can only be identified after sera from the healthy individuals have been immunoabsorbed on immobilized ribosomes or ribosomal P antigens *(75)*. Sera from these individuals contain IgG antibodies that bind the autoantibodies to ribosomal P antigens, and inhibit the binding of the latter autoantibodies to the ribosomal P antigens. Because these IgG antibodies were identified by their ability to inhibit the autoantibody binding to the immunodominant epitope of ribosomal P antigens, we assume that the inhibitory antibodies are anti-idiotypes. Ribosomal P antigens, either free or complexed to IgG, are not responsible for this inhibition. IgG-depleted fractions of sera did not inhibit autologous anti-ribosomal P binding to the antigen, whereas acid-treated and rechromatographed IgG inhibited the reaction as potently as untreated IgG. Further experiments are in progress using affinity-purified inhibitory antibodies to verify that they are genuine anti-idiotypes.

According to Jerne's theory of the idiotype network, anti-idiotypes suppress the antibody response to the nominal antigen. We have so far discussed evidence in this chapter that anti-idiotypes can decrease the effective concentrations of autoantibodies by masking the autoantibodies. Do the anti-idiotypes have any additional suppressive functions at the cellular level? Autologous IgG anti-F(ab')$_2$ antibodies of the IgG class have been reported to inhibit the synthesis of anti-erythrocyte antibodies by B cells from normal donors *(76)*. Anti-DNA-producing B cells from patients with SLE were inhibited by autologous anti-F(ab')$_2$ *(77)* and by F(ab')$_2$ fragments of anti-idiotypes to anti-DNA *(78)*. These studies suggest that anti-idiotypes can suppress the synthesis of idiotypes, which could potentially be important in regulation of the concentration of autoantibodies.

5. OTHER POTENTIAL ANTIBODY INHIBITORS IN HEALTHY INDIVIDUALS

Other components in human serum have been described that potentially could inhibit the activity of autoantibodies. Kra-Oz et al. *(79)* investigated the presence of inhibitors to anti-cardiolipin (ACL) autoantibodies in the sera of eight healthy adults. ACL were not serologically detected in any of these sera. Purification of their IgG fractions allowed the detection of ACL antibodies that were indistinguishable from those identified in patients with anti-phospholipid syndrome. Both unfractionated human and animal sera, as well as β_2-glycoprotein I, inhibited the binding of the autoantibodies to cardiolipin, suggesting that β_2-glycoprotein I is an inhibitor of ACL antibodies in normal human sera. In contrast, β_2-glycoprotein I did not inhibit the activity of ACL antibodies from the patients, suggesting that there are differences in the reactivity patterns of the antibodies in normals and patients *(80)*. Analogous experiments were done with anti-histone antibodies in normal individuals *(81)*. The inhibitor in serum was found to be a histone-binding protein(s), the identity of which is as yet unknown. Therefore, non-antibody components of serum are capable of inhibiting autoantibody activities. It is advisable to eliminate such non-immunoglobulin inhibitors before constructing the hypotheses that the inhibitory activity is due to antibodies.

6. ANTI-IDIOTYPES IN AUTOIMMUNE DISEASE

Naturally occurring anti-idiotypes also appear to develop against autoanti-bodies in autoimmune diseases. Autoantibodies directed to the $F(ab')_2$ portion of lgG occur at high titer in rheumatoid arthritis and various other autoimmune diseases *(3)*. Presumed anti-idiotypes to a variety of autoantibodies associated with organ-specific autoimmunity have been reported. Such reports have often lacked definitive experiments, but circumstantial evidence has been presented to implicate anti-idiotypic antibodies. Inhibitory IgG antibodies that blocked the binding of anti-insulin antibodies to insulin (presumed anti-idiotypes to anti-insulin antibodies) may also be capable of insulin receptor binding, and the presence of such receptor binding antibodies has been described in an insulin-treated diabetic patient *(82)*. Antibodies that bind specifically to anti-acetylcholine receptor antibodies in patients with myasthenia gravis are putative anti-idiotypes *(83)*. Putative anti-thyroglobulin anti-idiotypic antibodies have been identified in sera of patients with Hashimoto's thyroiditis and Graves' disease *(84,85)*. Presumed IgM anti-idiotypic antibodies against anti-microsomal antibodies in patients with thyroid autoimmunity have been identified by inhibition studies *(67)*. The IgM fraction from sera of patients with primary biliary cirrhosis contained anti-bodies that bound to murine monoclonal anti-mitochondrial antibodies, and inhibited binding of the latter antibodies to the cognate antigen *(86)*. Putative anti-idiotypes to anti-phosphotyrosine antibodies have been identified in SLE sera *(87)*. In most studies the anti-idiotype antibodies have been detected mainly based on the capacity of serum or its immunoglobulin fraction to inhibit auto-antibody binding to the cognate antigen. Mackworth-Young and Schwartz were the first to affinity purify anti-idiotypes to a specific cross-reactive idiotype, LL, on anti-DNA antibodies *(88)*. Taken together, these studies support the notion that anti-idiotypes arise as part of the autoimmune response.

As is the case for normal subjects, it is often necessary to purify the anti-bodies before certain autoantibody activities can be detected in diseased individuals. Hidden 19S lgM rheumatoid factors are present in patients with juvenile and adult rheumatoid arthritis, and are detectable only after the serum has been subjected to certain specific treatments *(89)*. Anti-Jo-1 autoantibodies stain HEp-2 cells in some individuals only after antibody purification *(90)*. Some anti-Ro/SSA, anti-La/SSB, and anti-U_1RNP autoantibodies are anti-idiotypes to anti-dsDNA. In exploring the isolation and unmasking of autoantibodies to DNA from SLE sera with no measurable anti-DNA activity, anti-idiotype activity was found in the affinity-purified anti-Ro/SSA, and anti-La/SSB antibody fractions. Moreover, the interaction of anti-DNA with anti-Ro/SSA or anti-La/SSB was inhibited by their cognate antigens (DNA and Ro/SSA but not RNA and La/SSB for anti-Ro/SSA; DNA and La/SSB but not RNA and Ro/SSA for anti-La/SSB) *(91)*. Similar experiments have been carried out for anti-U_1RNP antibodies *(92)*. These studies suggest that the low prevalence of anti-dsDNA antibody and nephritis in subsets of SLE patients producing anti-idiotypes (such as anti-Ro/SSA, anti-La/SSB, and anti-U$_1$RNP) may be due to the masking of the anti-dsDNA by anti-idiotypes. Further, the anti-idiotypes might down-regulate the synthesis of anti-dsDNA antibodies. The nature of the antigenic stimuli for the synthesis of these anti-idiotypes remains obscure. Broadly crossreactive anti-idiotypes to anti-dsDNA have been isolated on anti-dsDNA F(ab')$_2$ columns from each of the anti-idiotype specificities cited above as well as from normal persons *(93)*. It may be hypothesized that such anti-idiotypes to anti-dsDNA have the therapeutic potential of down-regulating anti-dsDNA levels in SLE patients.

7. DYSREGULATION BY ANTI-IDIOTYPES IN AUTOIMMUNE DISEASES

Dysregulation of the idiotype network leading to autoimmune disease could occur by two opposing mechanisms. There could be loss of anti-idiotypic regulation leading to unregulated autoantibody production. Alternatively, there could be augmentation of autoimmune diseases by the presence of anti-idiotypes. This apparent paradox may be understandable in the light of the likely heterogeneity inherent to the anti-idiotype response. If anti-idiotypes arise as internal images of the antigen-combining sites (Ab2β), these antibodies may behave like the nominal antigen, i.e., bind to antigen receptors and stimulate or block them. In contrast, if anti-idiotypes arise to other idiotopes in the framework region (Ab2α) or paratope (Ab2γ), they can not mimic antigen, but instead, may suppress the antigen-specific immune response. We postulate that non-Ab2β anti-idiotypes are the missing components resulting in upregulated autoantibody production. Examples of both types of dysregulation follow.

7.1. Loss of Anti-idiotype Regulation

Studies in experimental animals yielded the first clues that anti-idiotypes may control autoimmune disease processes by regulating potentially pathogenic autoantibodies. In the PL/J mouse model of experimental allergic encephalomyelitis, administration of monoclonal anti-idiotypes to anti-myelin basic protein alleviates the disease process *(94)*. In the NZB mouse model of SLE, the F1 hybrids have higher titers of anti-idiotypes to anti-erythrocyte antibodies and milder hemolytic disease as compared to their NZB parents *(95)*. Moreover, administration of a syngeneic monoclonal antibody to anti-DNA suppresses nephri-itis in autoimmune NZB/NZW mice *(96)*. These studies support the hypothesis that anti-idiotypes can serve to down-regulate autoimmunity.

The role of anti-idiotypes in the regulation of autoantibodies can not be as readily determined in human autoimmune disease. Instead, their functions can only be surmised indirectly, by comparing the levels of anti-idiotypes and their corresponding autoantibody idiotypes at different stages of disease activity, and following therapeutic maneuvers.

Anti-idiotype analysis in human SLE has been limited to generic anti-idiotypes (broadly cross-reactive) and to anti-idiotypes to anti-DNA. The levels of IgG antibodies capable of binding $F(ab')_2$ vary inversely with disease activity. Negligible levels of these generic anti-idiotypes are present when the disease is active, whereas the levels are comparable to those seen in normal individuals when the disease is inactive (4,97). Autologous anti-$F(ab')_2$ antibodies inhibit the synthesis of anti-DNA but not anti-tetanus toxoid antibodies by pokeweed mitogen-stimulated peripheral blood lymphocytes from patients in remission (77). When present, therefore, these generic anti-idiotypes may suppress anti-DNA antibody synthesis. By linear epitope mapping studies, Williams et al. (98) showed that patients with active SLE had no detectable antibody to the complementarity determining regions (CDRs), whereas those in remission showed strong concordant anti-CDR reactivity comparable to that seen in normal individuals (see Subheading 2.). These findings suggest that the resolution of active disease is associated with the development of concordant anti-CDR and improved anti-idiotypic responsiveness. Some of the generic anti-$F(ab')_2$ species are antibodies to anti-DNA (99), and their levels during disease remission are inversely related to those of the anti-DNA autoantibodies (4). Others have reported that some SLE patients develop anti-idiotypes to anti-DNA coincident with decreased disease activity (100), and decreased levels of anti-DNA (101). Treatment with affinity-purified anti-idiotypes to anti-DNA isolated from IVIg has been described to substantially reduce the disease activity in two SLE patients with active nephritis (defined as proteinuria greater than 2 gm/d) (102). The reduced disease activity was measured as decreased proteinuria (in one of the two patients), decreased anti-DNA levels, increased C4 and decreased prednisone requirements. Less striking improvement was seen in a control group of three nephritis patients treated with unfractionated IVIg. These studies suggest that when anti-idiotypes are present, they are capable of suppressing the disease activity.

In patients with p-ANCA-associated systemic vasculitis, natural or therapeutic anti-idiotypes to anti-myeloperoxidase (an ANCA-defined autoantigen reactivity) regulate the detection and function of the anti-myeloperoxidase. ANCA-negative sera from patients in the remission stage of ANCA-associated vasculitis contain IgG and IgM antibodies which neutralize the ANCA activity present in autologous sera collected during the acute disease stage (69). A reciprocal relationship was demonstrated between the levels of the putative anti-idiotypes to anti-myeloperoxidase and the anti-myeloperoxidase in paired acute and remission sera, and in serial samples collected from patients with systemic vasculitis (103). In an open study of IVIg in 14 patients with ANCA-associated vasculitis, a reduction in disease activity was observed in 13, which resulted in clinical remission in eight (104). Sustained decreases in ANCA levels occurred in all patients suggesting that these putative anti-idiotypes suppressed the ANCA production. The $F(ab')_2$ fragments of IVIg are described to bind the $F(ab')_2$ fragments of anti-myeloperoxidase, and to prevent the binding of the latter $F(ab')_2$

species to the antigen *(70)*. A regulatory role for anti-idiotypes to ANCA-associated antigens in autoimmune responses, therefore, appears likely.

Therapeutic interventions in autoimmune diseases can also lead to *de novo* anti-idiotype responses. Two patients undergoing desensitization with high doses of Factor VIII for hemophilia A displayed a transition from anti-Factor VIII antibody positivity to negativity during this procedure *(105)*. Affinity chromatography of the post-desensitization sera on immobilized Factor VIII showed that the anti-Factor VIII antibodies were present at levels indistinguishable from those detected in the pretreatment samples, suggesting an inhibitory phenomenon induced by the Factor VIII administration. Putative anti-idiotypes were identified in the non-retained sera fractions and, as expected, these did not bind the immobilized Factor VIII. Inhibitory IgGs (presumed anti-idiotypes) were identified in remission sera from patients with Graves' disease treated with Methimazole *(106)*. These antibodies and their $F(ab')_2$ fragments were mixed in vitro with sera from patients with active disease, which contained anti-TSH receptor antibodies, and were found to suppress the activity of the anti-TSH receptor antibodies by forming immune complexes. The results of these studies suggest that active disease is correlated with disappearance of anti-idiotypes, which might be the cause of unregulated autoantibody activity, and perhaps also the cause of the clinical symptoms of the disease.

Little information is available regarding the mechanism underlying loss of the anti-idiotypes in active disease. Are these anti-idiotypes not synthesized, or are they synthesized at adequate levels, but dysfunctional, or are they rapidly cleared from the circulation? Evidence from Williams et al. *(107)* suggests that some of the generic anti-idiotypes may be consumed during active disease by the process of immune complex formation. Kidney biopsies from 26 patients with glomerulonephritis, the majority of which showed diffuse proliferative glomerulonephritis, were treated with low pH buffer to remove bound immunoglobulins. The acid eluates contained high levels of IgG and IgG anti-DNA antibodies, and lower but detectable levels of IgG anti-$F(ab')_2$ antibodies. Both types of autoantibody specificities were relatively enriched in the renal eluates compared to the corresponding sera. This study suggests that the serum levels of generic anti-idiotypes may be low as a consequence of their sequestration in the kidney as components of immune complexes. Sequestration of immune complexes composed of anti-idiotypes and their corresponding idiotypes could occur in other organs as well, especially those with an active reticuloendothelial system. Currently, there is no direct experimental evidence to support this theory. It is also possible that the anti-idiotype response generated in autoimmune disease is no longer effective in controlling the autoantibody response owing to a change in epitope binding specificity. Generic anti-idiotypes present in patients with SLE have a different antigen-reactivity profile compared to those from normals, as defined by their reactivity with a panel of V λ-related peptides *(10)*. A decrease in reactivity towards certain immunodominant residues in the V λ CDRs in SLE was noted, suggesting a failure of anti-idiotypic control. In the case of other autoantibodies, anti-idiotypes may not be synthesized at all, although this issue is yet to be addressed experimentally.

7.2. Augmentation of Autoimmunity with Anti-idiotypes

The experimental or spontaneous generation of anti-idiotypes in selected cases has led to enhanced autoimmunity. Administration of anti-idiotypes in the spontaneously occurring models of murine lupus has occasionally led to increased autoimmunity (108,109). One model to explain these findings postulates that anti-idiotypes can induce the production of antibodies (Ab3) with antigen binding properties shared by the original autoantibody. The Ab3 antibodies possess the potential to cause autoimmune disease (see ref. 110). Alternatively, some anti-idiotypes can bind to both the stimulating idiotype and the nominal antigen of the idiotype. Immunization of normal rabbits with human and murine anti-DNA antibodies led to the production of anti-idiotypes with autoantigen-binding properties shared with the original immunizing autoantibody (111). This type of anti-idiotype is termed epibody (112). Binding to the autoantigen by these epibodies could amplify the Ab1 autoantibody response and/or promote tissue injury.

Internal image anti-idiotypes (Ab2β) have the potential to behave like the physiologic autoantigen. Anti-idiotypes to anti-Bis Q (an acetylcholine analog) produced in rabbits caused the development of myasthenia gravis in these animals (113). One patient with Graves' disease had documented anti-idiotypes to anti-TSH capable of binding the TSH receptor (114), which were postulated to be responsible for unregulated thyroxine production and clinical hyperthyroidism. Thus, antibodies specific for autoantibodies to natural ligands can and do behave as anti-receptor antibodies. They can either inhibit the receptor (in the case of the acetylcholine receptor causing myasthenia gravis) or stimulate the receptor (as in the case of Graves' disease). In principle, then, immunization with antibodies to a ligand should generate anti-receptor antibodies in the immunized animal. Monoclonal antibodies (MAbs) to the adenosine receptor have been prepared by immunization with antibodies to adenosine. Additionally, a hybridoma cell line isolated from an animal immunized with a conjugate of triamcinolone-thyroglobulin reacted specifically both with polyclonal rabbit anti-triamcinolone and with cytosolic glucocorticoid receptor (115).

An interesting aspect of the internal image concept is the development of autoantibodies with enzymatic activity. Thus, human autoantibodies to vasoactive intestinal peptide (VIP) have proteolytic activity to VIP (116). Human autoantibodies to DNA have DNase activity (117). Murine MAbs elicited by antibodies to the active site of acetylcholinesterase exhibited cholinesterase activity (118). It will be interesting to determine whether the catalytic antibodies subset plays a role in the disease process (119).

8. SUMMARY

We have summarized the literature supporting the role of the idiotype network in health and disease. Natural anti-idiotypes arise in the normal immune response and in the autoimmune response. In many cases, the anti-idiotype response appears to control the level of Ab1. However, this does not always appear to be the case in autoimmunity. Examples are cited suggesting that the anti-idiotypes can promote or suppress the autoimmune response and the resultant disease. As discussed, this paradox arises from the inherent complexity of the idiotype network. The heterogeneity of the immune response and the presence of multiple idiotopes within a single antibody molecule contribute to the complexity. Moreover, genetics and environmental factors, e.g., antigen dose, route of administration, etc., are also probably important factors in determining which type of anti-idiotype response is elicited. Further studies will be needed to delineate the precise circumstances under which dysregulation of idiotype-anti-idiotype interactions is a crucial factor in disease expression.

REFERENCES

1. Avrameas, S. (1991) Natural autoantibodies: from 'horror autotoxicus' to 'gnothi seauton.' *Immunol. Today* **12**, 154 159.
2. Jerne, N. K. (1974) Towards a network theory of the immune system. *Ann. Immunol.* **125C**, 373
3. Nasu, H., Chia, D. S., Knutson, D. W., and Barnett, E. V. (1980) Naturally occurring human antibodies to the F(ab')$_2$ portion of IgG. *Clin. Exp. Immunol.* **42**, 378–386.
4. Silvestris, F., Bankhurst, A. D., Searles, R. P., and Williams, R. C., Jr. (1984) Studies of anti-F(ab')$_2$ antibodies and possible immunologic control mechanisms in systemic lupus erythematosus. *Arthritis Rheum.* **27**, 1387–1396.
5. Osterland, C. K., Harboe, M., and Kunkel, H. G. (1963) Anti-γ-globulin factors in human sera revealed by enzymatic splitting of anti-Rh antibodies. *Vox Sanguinis* **8**, 133–152.
6. Harboe, M., Rau, B., and Aho, K. (1965) Properties of various anti-γ-globulin factors in human sera. *J. Exp. Med.* **121**, 503–519.
7. Natvig, J. B. (1966) Heterogeneity of anti-gamma-globulin factors detected by pepsin-digested human gamma G-globulin. *Acta. Pathol. Microbiol. Scand.* **66**, 369–382.
8. Silvestris, F., Williams, R. C., Jr., and Searles, R. P. F (1986) Human anti-F(ab')$_2$ antibodies and pepsin agglutinators react with Fv determinants. *Scand J. Immunol.* **23**, 499–508.
9. Yancey, W. B., Jr., Silvestris, F., Conlon, M., Rodriguez, M., Malone, C., and Williams, R. C., Jr. (1992) Human anti-F(ab')$_2$ antibodies show preferential reactivity for F(ab')$_2$ molecules bearing lambda light chains. *Clin. Immunol. Immunopath.* **65**, 176–182.
10. Williams, R. C., Jr., Malone, C. C., Silvestris, F., and Solomon, A. (1995) Molecular localization of human IgG anti-F(ab')$_2$ reactivity with variable- and constant-region lambda light-chain epitopes. *J. Clin. Immunol.* **15**, 349–362.

11. Williams, R. C., Jr., Malone, C. C., and Silvestris, F. (1996) Shared V-region antigens and cross-reacting specificities of human IgG anti-F(ab')$_2$ and anti-DNA antibodies. *Clin. Immunol. Immunopath.* **80,**194–203.

12. Weinberger, J. Z., Germain, R. N., Ju, S. T., Greene, M. I., Benacerraf, B., and Dorf, M. E. (1979) Hapten-specific T-cell responses to 4-hydroxy-3-nitrophenyl acetyl. II. Demonstration of idiotypic determinants on suppressor T cells. *J. Exp. Med.* **150,** 761–776.

13. Bona, C. and Paul, W.E. (1979) Cellular basis of regulation of expression of idio-type. I. T-suppressor cells specific for MOPC 460 idiotype regulate the expression of cells secreting anti-TNP antibodies bearing 460 idiotype. *J. Exp. Med.* **149,** 592–600.

14. Binz, H. and Wigzell, H. (1976) Shared idiotypic determinants on B and T lymphocytes reactive against the same antigenic determinants. V. Biochemical and serological characteristics of naturally occurring, soluble antigen-binding T-lymphocyte-derived molecules. *Scand. J. Immunol.* **5,** 559–571.

15. Robertson, M. (1977) Immunoglobulin genes and the immune response. *Nature* **269,** 648–650.

16. Woodland, R. and Cantor, H. (1978) Idiotype-specific T helper cells are required to induce idiotype-positive B memory cells to secrete antibody. *Eur. J. Immunol.* **8,** 600–606.

17. Schrater, A. F., Goidl, E. A., Thorbecke, G. J., Siskind, G. W. (1979) Production of auto-anti-idiotypic antibody during the normal immune response to TNP-ficoll. I. Occurrence in AKR/J and BALB/c mice of hapten-augmentable, anti-TNP plaque-forming cells and their accelerated appearance in recipients of immune spleen cells. *J. Exp. Med.* **150,** 138–153.

18. Bankert, R. B. and Pressman D. (1976) Receptor-blocking factor present in immune serum resembling auto-anti-idiotype antibody. *J. Immunol.* **117,** 457–462.

19. Geha, R. S. (1982) Presence of auto-anti-idiotypic antibody during the normal human immune response to tetanus toxoid antigen. *J. Immunol.* **129,** 139–144.

20. Arreaza, E. E., Gibbons, J. J., Jr., Siskind, G. W., and Weksler, M. E. (1993) Lower antibody response to tetanus toxoid associated with higher auto-anti-idio-typic antibody in old compared with young humans. *Clin. Exp. Immunol.* **92,** 169–173.

21. Kobayashi, K., Ueno, Y., Suzuki, H., Miura, M., Nagatomi, R., Ishii, M., et al. (1994) Anti-idiotypic antibody production in hepatitis B vaccine recipients. *J. Gastroenterol.* **29,** 740–744.

22. Hahn-Zoric, M., Carlsson, B., Jeansson, S., Ekre, H. P., Osterhaus, A. D., Roberton, D., et al. (1993) Anti-idiotypic antibodies to poliovirus antibodies in commercial immunoglobulin preparations, human serum, and milk. *Ped. Res.* **33,** 475–480.

23. Mellander, L., Carlsson, B., and Hanson, L.A. (1986) Secretory IgA and IgM antibodies to E. coli O and poliovirus type I antigens occur in amniotic fluid, meconium and saliva from newborns. A neonatal immune response without antigenic exposure: a result of anti-idiotypic induction? *Clin. Exp. Immunol.* **63,** 555–561.

24. Casiglia, D., Triolo, G., and Giardina, E. (1991) IgG auto-anti-idiotype antibodies against antibody to insulin in insulin-dependent (type 1) diabetes mellitus. Detection by capture enzyme linked immunosorbent assay (ELISA) and relationship with anti-insulin antibody levels. *Diabetes Res.* **16,** 181–184.

25. Rose, L. M., Goldman, M., and Lambert, P. H. (1982) Simultaneous induction of an idiotype, corresponding anti-idiotypic antibodies, and immune complexes during African trypanosomiasis in mice. *J. Immunol.* **128**, 79–85.

26. Hassan, J., Feighery, C., Bresnihan, B., and Whelan, A. (1992) Prevalence of anti-Fab antibodies in patients with autoimmune and infectious diseases. *Clin. Exp. Immunol.* **89**, 423–426.

27. Troisi, C. L. and Hollinger, F. B. (1985) Detection of an IgM antiidiotype directed against anti-HBs in hepatitis B patients. *Hepatology* **5**, 758–762.

28. Kobayashi, K., Suzuki, H., Ueno, Y., Nagatomi, R., Kanno, A., Otsuki, M., et al. (1990) Anti-idiotypic antibodies directed against anti-HBs among the patients with chronic hepatitis B. *Tohoku J. Exp. Med.* **161**, 261–271.

29. Geltner, D., Franklin, E. C., and Frangione, B. (1980) Antiidiotypic activity in the IgM fractions of mixed cryoglobulins. *J. Immunol.* **125**, 1530–1535.

30. Lebo, D. B., Ilowite, N. T., Sood, S., et al. (1993) Anti-idiotypic antibodies (ab2) are present in pediatric lyme arthritis (LA) sera for all Borrelia burgdorferi (BB) antigens except OSP-A and OSP-B. (Abstract) *Arthritis Rheum.* **36**, S152.

31. Bergenbrant, S., Yi, Q., Osby, E., Osterborg, A., Ostman, R., Bjorkholm, M., et al., (1994) Anti-idiotypic B lymphocytes in patients with monoclonal gammopathies. *Scand J. Immunol.* **40**, 216–220.

32. Keshgegian, A. A. and Sevin, P. (1979) Waldenstrom's macroglobulinemia associated with a mixed cryoglobulin. Report of a case with partial precipitation in vitro at 37 degrees C. *Arch. Path. Lab. Med.* **103**, 270–273.

33. Carini, C. and Brostoff, J. (1983) An antiglobulin: IgG anti-IgE. Occurrence and specificity. *Ann. Allergy* **51**, 251–254.

34. Vassella, C. C., dè Weck, A. L., and Stadler, B. M. (1990) Natural anti-IgE autoantibodies interfere with diagnostic IgE determination. *Clin. Exp. Allergy* **20**, 295–303.

35. Magnusson, C. G. and Vaerman, J. P. (1986) Autoantibodies of the IgM class against a human myeloma protein IgE(DES). II. Specificity. *Int. Arch. Allergy Applied Immunol.* **79**, 157–163.

36. Magnusson, C. G. (1994) Naturally occurring human IgA autoantibodies against IgE-DES mycloma protein. Prevalence and specificity. *Allergy* **49**, 820–826.

37. Hebert, J., Bernier, D., and Mourad, W. (1990) Detection of auto-anti-idiotypic antibodies to Lol p I (rye I) IgE antibodies in human sera by the use of murine idiotypes: levels in atopic and non-atopic subjects and effects of immunotherapy. *Clin. Exp. Immunol.* **80**, 413–419.

38. Castracane, J. M. and Rocklin, R. E. (1988) Detection of human auto-anti-idiotypic antibodies (Ab2). II. Generation of Ab2 in atopic patients undergoing allergen immunotherapy. *Int. Arch. Allergy Appl. Immunol.* **86**, 295–302.

39. Khan, R. H., Szewczuck, M. R., and Day, J. H. (1991) Bee venom anti-idiotypic antibody is associated with the protection in beekeepers and bee sting-sensitive patients receiving immunotherapy against allergic reaction. *J. Allergy Clin. Immunol.* **88**, 199–208.

40. Reed, E., Hardy, M., Benvenisty, A., Lattes, C., Brensilver, J., McCabe, R., et al. (1987) Effect of antiidiotypic antibodies to HLA on graft survival in renal-allograft recipients. *N. Engl. J. Med.* **316**, 1450–1455.

41. Reed, E., Cohen, D. J., Barr, M. L., Ho, E., Marboe, C. C., Rose, E. A., et al. (1992) Effect of anti-HLA and anti-idiotypic antibodies on the long-term survival of heart and kidney allografts. *Transplant. Proc.* **24,** 2494–2495.
42. Chauhan, B., Phelan, D. L., Marsh, J. W., and Mohanakumar, T. (1993) Characterization of antiidiotypic antibodies to donor HLA that develop after liver transplantation. *Transplantation* **56,** 443–448.
43. Chia, D., Horimi, T., Terasaki, P. I., and Hermes, M. (1982) Association of anti-Fab and anti-IgG antibodies with high kidney transplant survival. *Transplant. Proc.* **14,** 322–324.
44. Horimi, T., Chia, D., Terasaki, P. I., Ayoub, G., and Iwaki, Y. (1982) Association of anti-F(ab')$_2$ antibodies with higher kidney transplant survival rates. *Transplantation* **33,** 603–605.
45. Feduska, N. J., Jr., Chia, D., Terasaki, P. I., and Sugich, L. (1991) Effect of anti-Fab antibodies on renal allografts. *Transplant. Proc.* **23,** 1277–1278.
46. Susal, C., Groth, J., Tanzi-Fetta, R. F., Kirste, G., Doerr, C., Terness, P., et al. (1992) Characterization of protective anti-Fab autoantibodies in kidney graft recipients. *Transplant. Proc.* **24,** 2523–2526.
47. Terness, P., Navolan, D., Moroder, L., Siedler, F., Weyher, E., Kohl, I., et al. (1996) A natural IgA-anti-F(ab')$_{2\gamma}$ autoantibody occurring in healthy individuals and kidney graft recipients recognizes an IgG1 hinge region epitope. *J. Immunol.* **157,** 4251–4257.
48. Agrawal, S., Sharma, R. K., Kishore, R., and Agarwal, S. S. (1994) Development of anti-idiotypic antibodies to HLA antigens during pregnancy. *Indian J. Med. Res.* **99,** 42–46.
49. Naz, R. K., Ahmad, K., and Menge, A. C. (1993) Antiidiotypic antibodies to sperm in sera of fertile women that neutralize antisperm antibodies. *J. Clin. Invest.* **92,** 2331–2338.
50. Bartfeld, H. (1969) Distribution of rheumatoid factor activity in nonrheumatoid states. *Ann. NY Acad. Sci.* **168,** 30–40.
51. Svec, K. H. and Veit, B. C. (1967) Age-related antinuclear factors: immunologic characteristics and associated clinical aspects. *Arthritis Rheum.* **10,** 509–516.
52. Silvestris, F., Anderson, W., Goodwin, J. S., and Williams, R. C., Jr. (1985) Discrepancy in the expression of autoantibodies in healthy aged individuals. *Clin. Immunol. Immunopath.* **35,** 234–244.
53. Lutz, H. U. and Wipf, G. (1982) Naturally occurring autoantibodies to skeletal proteins from human red blood cells. *J. Immunol.* **128,** 1695-1699.
54. Guilbert, B., Dighiero, G., and Avrameas, S. (1982) Naturally occurring antibodies against nine common antigens in human sera I. detection, isolation, and characterization. *J. Immunol.* **128,** 2779–2787.
55. Spitzer, R. E., Stitzel, A. E., and Tsokos, G. C. (1990) Human anti-idiotypic antibody responses to autoantibody against the alternative pathway C3 convertase. *Clin. Immunol. Immunopath.* **57,** 19–31.
56. Spitzer, R. E., Stitzel, A. E., and Tsokos, G. C. (1992) Autoantibody to the alternative pathway C3/C5 convertase and its anti-idiotypic response. A study in affinity. *J. Immunol.* **148,** 137–141.
57. Tsokos, G. C., Stitzel, A. E., Patel, A. D., Hiramatsu, M., Balow, J. E., and Spitzer, R. E. (1989) Human polyclonal and monoclonal IgG and IgM complement 3

nephritic factors: evidence for idiotypic commonality. *Clin. Immunol. Immunopath.* **53**, 113–122.

58. Dietrich, G., Algiman, M., Sultan, Y., Nydegger, U. E., and Kazatchkine, M. D. (1992) Origin of anti-idiotypic activity against anti-factor VIII autoantibodies in pools of normal human immunoglobulin G (IVIg). *Blood* **79**, 2946–2951.

59. Gilles, J. G. and Saint-Remy, J. M. (1994) Healthy subjects produce both anti-factor VIII and specific anti-idiotypic antibodies. *J. Clin. Invest.* **94**, 1496–1505.

60. Zouali, M. and Eyquem, A. (1983) Expression of anti-idiotypic clones against auto-anti-DNA antibodies in normal individuals. *Cell. Immunol.* **76**, 137–147.

61. Silvestris, F., Searles, R. P., Bankhurst, A. D., and Williams, R. C. (1985) Family distribution of anti-F(ab')$_2$ antibodies in relatives of patients with systemic lupus erythematosus. *Clin. Exp. Immunol.* **60**, 329–338.

62. Warrington, R. J., Wong, S. K., Ramdahin, S., and Rutherford, W. J. (1995) Normal human cord blood B cells can produce high affinity IgG antibodies to dsDNA that are recognized by cord blood-derived anti-idiotypic antibodies. *Scand J. Immunol.* **42**, 397–406.

63. Buskila, D. and Shoenfeld, Y. (1992) From the practical viewpoint–immunomodulation with natural auto-anti-idiotypic antibodies: the role of treatment with intravenous immunoglobulins (IVIg) in *Natural Autoantibodies: Their Physiological Role and Regulatory Significance* (Shoenfeld, Y. and Isenberg, D. A., eds.), CRC, Boca Raton, FL, pp. 303–336.

64. Sultan, Y., Kazatchkine, M. D., Maisonneuve, P., and Nydegger, U. E. (1984) Anti-idiotypic suppression of autoantibodies to factor VIII (antihaemophilic factor) by high-dose intravenous gammaglobulin. *Lancet* **2**, 765–768.

65. Dietrich, G. and Kazatchkine, M. D. (1990) Normal immunoglobulin G (IgG) for therapeutic use (intravenous Ig) contain antiidiotypic specificities against an immunodominant, disease-associated, cross-reactive idiotype of human anti-thyroglobulin autoantibodies. *J. Clin. Invest.* **85**, 620–625.

66. Rossi, F. and Kazatchkine, M. D. (1989) Antiidiotypes against autoantibodies in pooled normal human polyspecific Ig. *J. Immunol.* **143**, 4104–4109.

67. Tandon, N., Jayne, D. R., McGregor, A. M., and Weetman, A. P. (1992) Analysis of anti-idiotypic antibodies against anti-microsomal antibodies in patients with thyroid autoimmunity. *J. Autoimmun.* **5**, 557–570.

68. Berchtold, P., Dalc, G. L., Tani, P., and McMillan, R. (1989) Inhibition of auto-antibody inding to platelet glycoprotein IIb/IIIa by anti-idiotypic antibodies in intravenous gammaglobulin. *Blood* **74**, 2414–2417.

69. Rossi, F., Jayne, D. R., Lockwood, C. M., and Kazatchkine, M. D. (1991) Anti-idiotypes against anti-neutrophil cytoplasmic antigen autoantibodies in normal human polyspecific IgG for therapeutic use and in the remission sera of patients with systemic vasculitis. *Clin. Exp. Immunol.* **83**, 298–303.

70. Pall, A. A., Varagunam, M., Adu, D., Smith, N., Richards, N. T., Taylor, C. M., et al. (1994) Anti-idiotypic activity against anti-myeloperoxidase antibodies in pooled human immunoglobulin. *Clin. Exp. Immunol.* **95**, 257–262.

71. van Doorn, P. A., Rossi, F., Brand, A., van Lint, M., Vermeulen, M., and Kazatchkine, M. D. (1990) On the mechanism of high-dose intravenous immunoglobulin treatment of patients with chronic inflammatory demyelinating polyneuropathy. *J. Neuroimmunol.* **29**, 57–64.

72. Liblau, R., Gajdos, P., Bustarret, F. A., el Habib, R., Bach, J. F., and Morel, E. (1991) Intravenous gamma-globulin in myasthenia gravis: interaction with anti-acetylcholine receptor autoantibodies. *J. Clin. Immunol.* **11,** 128–131.
73. Caccavo, D., Vaccaro, F., Ferri, G. M., Amoroso, A., and Bonomo, L. (1994) Anti-idiotypes against antiphospholipid antibodies are present in normal polyspecific immunoglobulins for therapeutic use. *J. Autoimmun.* **7,** 537–548.
74. Stafford, H. A., Anderson, C. J., Reichlin, M. (1995) Unmasking of anti-ribosomal P autoantibodies in healthy individuals. *J. Immunol.* **155,** 2754–2761.
75. Pan, Z. J. and Stafford, H. A. (1996) Recombinant ribosomal P2 protein can unmask anti-ribosomal P autoantibodies from healthy adults. *J. Lab. Clin. Med.* **127,** 333–339.
76. Terness, P., Marx, U., Sandilands, G., Roelcke, D., Welschof, M., and Opelz, G. (1993) Suppression of anti-erythrocyte autoantibody-producing B cells by a physiological IgG-anti-F(ab')₂ antibody and escape from suppression by tumour transformation; a model relevant for the pathogenesis of autoimmune haemolytic anaemia. *Clin. Exp. Immunol.* **93,** 253–258.
77. Silvestris, F., Williams, R. C., Jr., Frassanito, M. A. and Dammacco, F. (1987) In vitro inhibition of anti-DNA producing cells from systemic lupus erythematosus patients by autologous anti-F(ab')₂ antibodies. *Clin. Immunol. Immunopath.* **42,** 50–62.
78. Evans, M. and Abdou, N. I. (1993) In vitro modulation of anti-DNA secreting peripheral blood mononuclear cells of lupus patients by anti-idiotypic antibody of pooled human intravenous immune globulin. *Lupus* **2,** 371–375.
79. Kra-Oz, Z., Lorber, M., Shoenfeld, Y., and Scharff, Y. (1993) Inhibitor(s) of natural anti-cardiolipin autoantibodies. *Clin. Exp. Immunol.* **93,** 265–268.
80. Lorber, M., Kra-Oz, Z., Guilbrud, B., and Shoenfeld, Y. (1995) Natural (antiphospholipid-PDH,-DNA) autoantibodies and their physiologic serum inhibitors. (Review). *Isr. J. Med. Sci.* **31,** 31–35.
81. Bustos, A., Boimorto, R., Subiza, J. L., Pereira, L. F., Marco, M., Figueredo, M. A., et al. (1994) Inhibition of histone/anti-histone reactivity by histone-binding serum components; differential effect on anti-H1 versus anti-H2B antibodies. *Clin. Exp. Immunol.* **95,** 408–414.
82. Shoelson, S. E., Marshall, S., Horikoshi, H., Kolterman, O. G., Rubenstein, A. H., and Okefsky, J. M. (1985) Antiinsulin receptor antibodies in an insulin-dependent diabetic may rise as autoantiidiotypes. *J. Clin. Endocrinol. Metab.* **63,** 56–60.
83. Dwyer, D. S., Bradley, R. J., Urquhart, C. K., and Kearney, J. F. (1983) Naturally occurring anti-idiotypic antibodies in myasthenia gravis patients. *Nature* **301,** 611–614.
84. Sikorska, H. M. (1986) Anti-thyroglobulin anti-idiotypic antibodies in sera of patients with Hashimoto's thyroiditis and Graves' disease. *J. Immunol.* **137,** 3786–3795.
85. Xiu, L. L. (1994). Studies on autoimmune mechanisms of thyroglobulin autoantibody in autoimmune thyroid disease. *Hiroshima J. Med. Sci.* **43,** 1–11.
86. Zhang, L., Jayne, D. R., and Oliveira, D. B. (1993) Anti-idiotype antibodies to anti-mitochondrial antibodies in the sera of patients with primary biliary cirrhosis. *J. Autoimmun.* **6,** 93–105.
87. Stefanescu, M., Matache, C., Onu, A., Cristescu, C., Cremer, L., and Szegli, G. (1993) Identification of anti-idiotypic antibodies to anti-phosphotyrosine antibodies in human sera. *Autoimmunity* **15,** 181–186.

88. Mackworth-Young, C. G., and Schwartz, R. S. (1988) An idiotope-specific autoantibody in SLE. *Clin. Exp. Immunol.* **71,** 56–61.

89. Moore, T. L., Dorner, R. W., Alexander, R. L., and Osborn, T. G. (1988) Enzyme linked (ELISA) immunoabsorbent assay for the detection of hidden 19S IgM rheumatoid factors in juvenile rheumatoid arthritis. *J. Rheumatol.* **15,** 87–90.

90. Targoff, I. N. and Reichlin, M. (1985) Unmasking of cytoplasmic fluorescence of anti-Jo-1 by purification of antibody. *Arthritis Rheum.* **28,** S74.

91. Zhang, W. and Reichlin, M. (1996) Some autoantibodies to Ro/SSA and La/SSB are antiidiotypes to antidouble-stranded DNA. *Arthritis Rheum.* **39,** 522–531.

92. Zhang, W. and Reichlin, M. (1996) Some autoantibodies to U1RNP are idiotypes to anti-dsDNA. (Abstract) *Arthritis Rheum.* **39,** S178.

93. Zhang, W., Reichlin, M., Wasson, C., et al. (1996) Broad cross-reaction of an anti-id reagent with anti-dsDNA from several patients with systemic lupus erythematosus (SLE). (Abstract) *Arthritis Rheum.* **39,** S178.

94. Zhou, S-R. and Whitaker, J. N. (1993) Specific modulation of T cells and murine experimental allergic encephalomyelitis by monoclonal anti-idiotypic antibodies. *J. Immunol.* **150,** 1629–1642.

95. Cohen, P. L. (1982) Anti-idiotypic antibodies to the Coombs antibody in NZB F1 mice. *J. Exp. Med.* **156,** 173–180.

96. Hahn, B. H. and Ebling, F. M. (1983) Suppression of NZB/NZW murine nephritis by administration of a syngeneic monoclonal antibody to DNA. Possible role of anti-idiotypic antibodies. *J. Clin. Invest.* **71,** 1728–1736.

97. Silvestris, F., Bankhurst, A. D., Searles, R. A., et al. (1983) Anti-F(ab')$_2$ antibodies and possible auto-idiotypic control mechanism in systemic lupus erythematosus. (Abstract) *Clin. Res.* **31,** 785A.

98. Williams, R. C., Jr., Malone, C. C., and Silvestris, F. (1995) CDR molecular localization of possible anti-idiotypic anti-DNA antibodies in normal subjects, patients with SLE, and SLE first-degree relatives. *J. Lab. Clin. Med.* **126,** 44–56.

99. Nasu, H., Chia, D.S., Taniguchi, O., and Barnett, E. V. (1982) Characterization of anti-F(ab')$_2$ antibodies in SLE patients. Evidence for cross-reacting auto-anti-idiotypic antibodies. *Clin. Immunol. Immunopath.* **25,** 80–90.

100. Abdou, N. I., Wall, H., Lindsley, H. B., Halsey, J. F., and Suzuki, T. (1981) Network theory in autoimmunity: in vitro suppression of serum anti-DNA antibody binding to DNA by anti-idiotypic antibody in systemic lupus erythematosus. *J. Clin. Invest.* **67,** 1297–1304.

101. Zouali, M. and Eyquem, A. (1983) Idiotypic/antiidiotypic interactions in systemic lupus erythematosus: demonstration of oscillary levels of anti-DNA autoantibodies and reciprocal antiidiotypic activity in a single patient. *Ann. Immunol.* **134c,** 377–391.

102. Silvestris, F., D'Amore, O., Cafforio, P., Savino, L., and Dammacco, F. (1996) Intravenous immune globulin therapy of lupus nephritis: use of pathogenic anti-DNA-reactive IgG. *Clin. Exp. Immunol.* **1,** 91–97.

103. Jayne, D. R., Esnault, V. L., and Lockwood, C. M. (1993) Anti-idiotype antibodies to anti-myeloperoxidase autoantibodies in patients with systemic vasculitis. *J. Autoimmun.* **6,** 221–226.

104. Jayne, D. R., Esnault, V. L., and Lockwood, C. M. (1993) ANCA anti-idiotype antibodies and the treatment of systemic vasculitis with intravenous immunoglobulin. (Review). *J. Autoimmun.* **6,** 207–219.

105. Gilles, J. G., Desqueper, B., Lenk, H., Vermylen, J., and Saint-Remy, J. M. (1996) Neutralizing antiidiotypic antibodies to factor VIII inhibitors after desensitization in patients with hemophilia A. *J. Clin. Invest.* **97,** 1382–1388.
106. Balazs, C. and Molnar, I. (1995) In vitro suppression of anti-TSH receptor antibody by autologous anti-idiotypic antibody in patients with Graves' disease. *Acta Microbiologica et Immunologica Hungarica* **42,** 163–169.
107. Williams, R. C., Jr., Malone, C. C., Huffman, G. R., Silvestris, F., Croker, B. P., Ayoub, E. M., et al. (1995) Active systemic lupus erythematosus is associated with depletion of the natural generic anti-idiotype (anti-F(ab')$_2$) system. *J. Rheumatol.* **22,** 1075–1085.
108. Teitelbaum, D., Rauch, J., Stollar, B. D., and Schwartz, R. S. (1984) In vivo effects of antibodies against a high frequency idiotype of anti-DNA antibodies in MRL mice. *J. Immunol.* **132,** 1282–1285.
109. Carteron, N. L., Schimenti, C. L., and Wofsy, D. (1989) Treatment of murine lupus with F(ab')$_2$ fragments of monoclonal antibodies. *Eur. J. Immunol.* **17,** 541.
110. Shoenfeld, Y. (1994) The significance of experimental models of systemic lupus erythematosus and antiphospholipid syndrome induced by idiotypic manipulation. *Isr. J. Med. Sci.* **30,** 10–18.
111. Puccetti, A., Migliorini, P., Sabbaga, J., and Madaio, M. P. (1990) Human and murine anti-DNA antibodies induce the production of anti-idiotypic antibodies with autoantigen-binding properties (epibodies) through immune-network interactions. *J. Immunol.* **145,** 4229–4237.
112. Bona, C. A., Finley, S., Waters, S., and Kunkel, H. G. (1982) Anti-immunoglobulin antibodies. III. Properties of sequential anti-idiotypic antibodies to heterologous anti-gamma globulins. Detection of reactivity of anti-idiotype antibodies with epitopes of Fc fragments (homobodies) and with epitopes and idiotopes (epibodies). *J. Exp. Med.* **156,** 986–999.
113. Wassermann, N. H., Penn, A. S., Freimuth, P. I., Treptow, N., Wentzel, S., Cleveland, W. L., et al. (1982) Anti-idiotypic route to anti-acetylcholine receptor antibodies and experimental myasthenia gravis. *Proc. Natl. Acad. Sci. USA* **79,** 4810–4814.
114. Bako, G., Islam, M. N., and Farid, N. R. (1985) Photoaffinity labelling of the porcine thyrotropin receptor—effect of Graves' immunoglobulin G and anti-TSH anti-idiotypic antibodies. *Clin. Invest. Med. - Medecine Clinique et Experimentale* **8,** 152–159.
115. Erlanger, B. F., Cleveland, W. L., Wasserman, N. H., Ku, N. H., Hill, B. L., Sarangarajan, R., et al. (1986) The auto-anti-idiotypic route to anti-receptor antibodies, in *Idiotypes* (Erlanger, B. F., Cleveland, W. L., Wasserman, N. H., Reichlin, M., Capra, J. D., et al., eds.), Academic, Orlando, FL, pp. 157–178.
116. Paul, S., Volle, D. J., Beach, C. M., Johnson, D. R., Powell, M. J., and Massey, M. J. (1989) Catalytic hydrolysis of vasoactive intestinal peptide by human autoantibody. *Science* **224,** 1158–1162.
117. Shuster, A. M., Gololobov, G. V., Kvashuk, O. A., Bogomolova, A. E., Smirnov, I.V., and Gabibov, A.G. (1992) DNA hydrolyzing autoantibodies. *Science* **256,** 665–667.
118. Izadyar, L., Friboulet, A., Remy, M. H., Roseto, A., and Thomas, D. (1993) Monoclonal anti-idiotypic antibodies as functional internal images of enzyme active sites: Production of a catalytic antibody with a cholinesterase activity. *Proc. Natl. Acad. Sci. USA* **90,** 8876–8880.
119. Mayfurth, R. D. and Quintans, J. (1990) Designer and catalytic antibodies. *N. Engl. J. Med.* **323,** 173–178.

12

The Role of Variable Region Gene Rearrangements in the Generation of Autoantibodies

Anne Davidson

1. INTRODUCTION

The diversity of the preimmune antibody repertoire is generated during B-cell ontogeny by several mechanisms that depend on the assembly of complete immunoglobulin coding sequences from multiple gene segments (VDJC and VJC for the heavy and light chains respectively). Combinatorial diversity—the random joining of different V, D, and J heavy chain segments or V and J light chain segments—leads to the production of a large number of immunoglobulin heavy and light chains from a much smaller number of germline V, D, and J genes. Imprecise joining of the various gene segments, together with random association of the heavy and light chains, generate further diversity in the preimmune repertoire. Theoretically, there are about 10^{11} different immunoglobulin molecules that can be derived by these mechanisms from the gene segments in the murine germline. Formation of the preimmune repertoire is, however, not completely random. The repertoire is influenced by preferred V region usage, preferred VH/VL combinations, deletion of B-cells bearing highly autoreactive immunoglobulin, mechanisms to avoid autoreactivity by secondary heavy and light chain gene rearrangements, and possibly, by selection for and against particular antigenic specificities in the periphery. The study of monoclonal autoantibodies and of transgenic animals bearing autoreactive immunoglobulin genes has contributed much information about the regulation of the immunoglobulin repertoire. This review will discuss the role of VDJ and VJ immunoglobulin gene rearrangement in the generation of autoreactive specificities and the possible mechanisms of regulation of autoantibodies, with particular focus on rheumatoid factors.

2. VDJ RECOMBINATION

Immunoglobulin gene rearrangement is developmentally regulated in the bone marrow during B-cell ontogeny *(1,2)*. The first genetic rearrangement to

Contemporary Immunology: Autoimmune Reactions
Edited by: S. Paul © Humana Press Inc., Totowa, NJ

occur, usually on both chromosomes, is DH–JH joining. Subsequently, VH to DJH joining occurs. Expression of an intact heavy chain with the surrogate light chain complex on the B-cell surface triggers light chain gene rearrangement. Expression of a complete immunoglobulin molecule on the cell surface then results in inactivation of the recombinase machinery. This ensures that each B-cell produces only a single immunoglobulin species (allelic exclusion).

The mechanisms of VDJ and VJ recombination have been the subject of several recent reviews (1,2). Immunoglobulin genes and T-cell receptors (TCR) both undergo similar recombination events that are regulated by the same recombinase gene products acting on recombination signal sequences flanking each immunoglobulin or TCR gene segment. The recombination signal sequences (RSS) are conserved palindromic heptamer and nonamer sequences separated from each other by a spacer of either 12(±1) or 23±1) nucleotides in length. These signal sequences are sufficient for recombination to occur regardless of the nature of the coding gene segment. One signal sequence of each type is required, and the recombination is the result of deletion or inversion of the intervening nucleotides. The joining of the coding ends of the rearranged gene segments is imprecise due to base additions, base losses and out of frame joining. Base additions can occur by addition of copies of the last nucleotides of the coding region (templated or "P" additions) or by random nucleotide additions by the enzyme terminal deoxynucleotidyl transferase (TdT, "N" additions). This imprecision of joining generates "junctional" diversity. There is also marked junctional diversity generated in the heavy chain D region due to the use of multiple gene segments from long atypical D region genes (DIR genes), D–D joining and D inversion (3). Thus, the CDR3 region contributes the greatest diversity to the immunoglobulin molecule.

The components of the VDJ recombination machinery are partly understood. RAG-1 and RAG-2 are two essential genes required for recombination (RAG, recombination activating gene), but their precise function is still unknown. Other important elements have been identified by gene complementation studies in CHO cells transfected with the *RAG*1 and *RAG*2 genes and a recombination substrate (i.e., the gene undergoing rearrangement). The regulatory elements include DNA–PK, which is a trimolecular complex containing a catalytic subunit and the heterodimeric KU antigen. This complex is important for repair of double stranded DNA breaks that initiate recombination, as evaluated from its defective function in mice with the SCID mutation (4). At least one other complementation group has been identified, but it is not yet well characterized (2). Defects in the enzyme TdT do not interfere with recombination per se, but they result in VDJ joins without N region additions. TdT, therefore, can influence the immunoglobulin repertoire profoundly. Activation of the recombinase machinery is likely to involve cis-regulatory elements, some of which lie within the immunoglobulin intronic enhancer. There is evidence for the existence of certain differences in the way the recombinase machinery of the B- and T-cells is regulated (1,2).

3. SELECTION AND REGULATION
OF REARRANGED V REGIONS IN THE BONE MARROW

Autoreactivity in the preimmune repertoire can be generated in three ways. First, some germline encoded V regions could be intrinsically autoreactive. The usage of different V regions is biased, and only a fraction of the potential repertoire is expressed *(5)*. In addition to negative selection, the factors influencing biased V region usage could include those that are intrinsic to the genes themselves, such as the chromosomal position of the genes, the gene copy number, the presence of transcriptional enhancers and the sequence of the RSS itself. The immunoglobulin gene repertoires of pre-B-cells have been shown to display biased VH use, and it appears that some V regions are not used because they are autoreactive. The second mechanism for generating autoreactivity in the preimmune repertoire is by pairing particular heavy and light chain combinations that form an autoreactive antigen binding site, even though the same heavy and light chains in a different pair do not. This has been shown by Radic and colleagues for anti-DNA antibodies that use the same heavy chain and different light chains *(6)*, and by us for rheumatoid factors *(7)*. Finally, autoreactive antibody specificities can be produced via junctional diversification of either or both of the antibody subunits (heavy and light chains). We have shown the feasibility of this mechanism in studies of rheumatoid factors *(7)*.

Under normal circumstances, most immature B-cells in the bone marrow that express high affinity autoreactive specificities are eliminated or inactivated. The factors that contribute to this outcome have been extensively reviewed by Goodnow and colleagues *(8)*. A critical concentration of antigen, a threshold level of antibody affinity and the ability to crosslink antigen receptors is thought to be required for elimination or inactivation of B-cell in the bone marrow. Self-reactive cells in the bone marrow can also edit their antigen binding receptor (the antibody molecule) to generate a nonautoreactive specificity, as shown in certain transgenic mouse systems. This involves reactivation of the recombinase machinery, perhaps as a result of signals mediated by the interaction of self-antigen with surface immunoglobulin, allowing an upstream V gene to recombine with a downstream J and form a new light chain *(6,9)*. Recently, receptor editing of heavy chains has also been described, a phenomenon involving a signal sequence embedded in the 3' end of many VH genes *(10)*. In addition, it appears that further editing of the antigen binding specificity can occur in the germinal centers, rescuing B-cells otherwise destined for apoptosis *(11,12)*. Transgenic systems have demonstrated the failure of allelic exclusion in autoreactive B-cells, perhaps because of the downregulation of transgene expression due to coexpression of an endogenous heavy chain *(13)*.

4. SELECTION AND REGULATION
OF REARRANGED V REGIONS IN THE PERIPHERY

Not all potentially pathogenic B-cells are eliminated in the bone marrow. Studies of transgenic animals have shown that in some models, B-cells producing autoantibodies can escape into the periphery (8,13,14). Even in normal individuals, not all autoreactive B-cells are eliminated in the bone marrow. Likely features allowing the escape of certain autoreactive B-cells from the marrow are related to the lack of the self-antigen in the bone marrow, and a relatively low avidity of antigen binding, which could result from the limited ability of soluble self-antigens to crosslink surface immunoglobulin compared to membrane-bound antigens. Some B-cells in the marrow undergo biochemical changes that render them anergic, while other cells probably express low avidity autoreactivities (8). The absence of pathogenic effects, even in animal models where the escaping B-cells produce potentially pathogenic antibodies, suggests that there are additional peripheral mechanisms to avoid autoreactivity (8,14). One mechanism has recently been described by Cyster et al. (15), in which the proliferation of autoreactive cells is regulated in the periphery in the course of antigenic selection events. In this model system, autoreactive B-cells with a high affinity for self-antigen can enter the T-cell zone of the germinal center, but they are unable to migrate into primary follicles if there are sufficient numbers of competing nonautoreactive B-cells. Because the autoreactive cells do not enter into the follicular regions where the microenvironment favors their survival, they are unable to expand and they undergo premature cell death. Interestingly, the cause of B-cell autoreactivity in immunodeficient animals is proposed to be an insufficient number of normal B-cells capable of competing with autoreactive B-cells for follicular entry (8). The molecular basis for competitive entry is unknown, but could be related to a differential expression of cell surface markers important in cell trafficking pathways, perhaps as a result of partial activation by continuous exposure to the self antigen.

Three strains of mice transgenic for rheumatoid factor (RF) have been described, none of which can mutate the transgenic RF construct. In the first model, a RF with high affinity for human Fc was expressed in a normal mouse. Only a low-level expression of RF is encountered in the mouse. This suggests that the RF affinity for soluble mouse immunoglobulins is too low to obtain B-cell deletion in the bone marrow, but the B-cells fail to compete successfully for follicular entry and thereby fail to expand. When the mouse is infused with soluble human IgG, for which the transgenic RF has a high affinity, B-cells expressing the transgene are deleted (16,17). In the second model, transgenic mice expressing a moderate affinity, near germline-sequence RF with specificity for either a self or non-self IgG allotype were generated. In the self background, the transgenic B-cells are not deleted. Furthermore, the transgenic cells can be activated by immune complexes containing the IgG of the self-allotype, showing that they are not anergized. Once activated, these cells can go on to become memory cells, just as in the nonself background. These data do not support the existence of a follicular exclusion mechanism regulating the synthesis of this antibody. It is suggested that the affinity of an antibody for the self-antigen plays an important role in determining the mechanism by which each individual autoreactive specificity is regulated (18). The third model is similar to the second, but this time the RF expresses high affinity for IgG binding. In this model, deletion of autoreactive B-cells occurs in the bone marrow. Interestingly, however, there is a time window during neonatal development of transgenic mice in which the level of circulating IgG (self-antigen) declines (as a result of decreased maternal antibody levels). At this time, animals that contract a viral infection and generate increased immune complexes can lose the tolerance to self-IgG. This model illustrates the importance of continued central exposure to self-antigen for the maintenance of tolerance (M. Shlomchik, personal communication).

5. IMMUNOGLOBULIN STRUCTURE AND THE ROLE OF THE CDR3 REGION IN THE GENERATION OF ANTIGENIC SPECIFICITY

The V region of immunoglobulin heavy and light chains includes four conserved framework regions and three hypervariable or complementarity determining regions (CDRs). CDR3 encompasses the 3' end of the V region gene and the VJ junction for light chains; and the V–D junction, the D region and the D–J junction for heavy chains *(19)*. The general three dimensional structure of immunoglobulin molecules is now well known from X-ray crystallographic studies *(20)*. The antigen binding region is formed by proper apposition of the VH and VL domains. The framework regions of each V region form a beta sheet that provides a structural framework, while the CDR regions form the loops that make up the antigen binding site. Studies of antigen-antibody complexes have shown that these loops form a cleft into which small antigens can fit. The binding of protein antigens is mediated by noncovalent forces and usually involves all six CDRs, although in some cases amino acids outside the CDRs can also contribute. The sequence of the CDRs and the way in which the heavy and light chain CDRs interact determine the size, shape, hydrophobicity, and charge of the antigen binding cleft *(19)*.

The contribution of each of the heavy and light chain CDRs to antigenic specificity has been studied by Kabat and Wu, who, based on an analysis of a large number of antibody sequences, have suggested that CDR3 of the heavy chain is the predominant determinant of antibody specificity *(21)*. When the same VL gene is used in certain antibodies with differing specificity, substitutions at the VJ junction are often present *(21)*. Together, these findings suggest that the CDR3 of the heavy and light chains contribute disproportionately to antigenic fine specificity.

Studies of low affinity polyreactive "natural autoantibodies," which are thought to be products of B-cells that escape negative selection in the bone marrow, have also suggested that the heavy chain CDR3 is a major contributor to the antigenic specificity. This has led to a revision in the thinking regarding polyreactive autoantibodies. Rather than being dependent on the germline sequence of the VH and VL regions, the polyreactivity has been suggested to arise from the somatic junctional diversity generated during the shaping of the preimmune repertoire *(22,23)*. In a recent study *(22)*, the introduction of individual mutations into a heavy chain CDR3 caused the loss of polyreactivity, suggesting that the antigenic reactivity for multiple autoantigens is dependent on the CDR3 structure.

6. STRUCTURE OF HUMAN RHEUMATOID FACTORS

6.1. The Heavy Chain

Human rheumatoid factors were among the first autoantibodies to be studied in detail because of their overrepresentation in the paraproteins found in myeloma proteins. The light chains of these RFs have a restricted V gene repertoire, but their V_H gene usage is more diverse, and includes members of the VH1, VH3 and VH4 families *(24)*. Interestingly, the pairing of heavy and light chains in these antibodies is also restricted. VkIIIa family light chains are usually paired with members of the VH3 and VH4 gene families, and the VkIIIb family light chains are usually paired with the VH1 family. Further understanding of the structural basis for RF specificity has been obtained by molecular analysis of the heavy and light chains of human monoclonal RFs generated from the peripheral blood lymphocytes and the synovial tissue of RA patients. The first significant finding was that the VH and VL gene usage in RFs from RA patients is considerably broader than in myeloma RFs. Second, most of the RA-derived RFs contain some somatic mutations. In one instance, analysis of two clonally related cell lines showed that the somatic mutations resulted in a superior affinity for the antigen binding *(25)*. Compared to RFs from B-cell dyscrasias, the monoclonal RFs from RA patients generally express higher affinities for Fc and exhibit more extensive binding site heterogeneity, including the ability to bind the Fc region of IgG3 *(26)*.

Our laboratory has generated a large panel of monoclonal RF producing cell lines from several patients with RA. The heavy and light chain genes used by the RFs were cloned and sequenced *(27,28)*. The structural requirements for binding the Fc were studied using a gene expression system that allows us to generate various combinations of the wild-type or mutant heavy and light chains of the RFs. The V region of interest is cloned into an expression cassette that already contains constant region sequence of the IgA or the κ light chain. The heavy and light chain constructs are then cotransfected into a nonsecreting mouse myeloma cell line *(7)*. We studied four related B-cell lines in considerable detail (Table 1). Two of the lines (B19 and B'20) secrete RF, and 2 (MF8 and B9601) produce antibodies without RF activity but express RF-related idiotypes. To determine the contribution of the heavy chain to RF specificity, the heavy chains of the MF8, B19 and B'20 cell lines were recombined with various light chains and light chain mutants. Initial studies of the recombined RFs and their mutants suggests that the Fc binding specificity is highly dependent on the heavy chain. For example, the MF8 heavy chain paired with any of the light chains was always RF negative. The B20 heavy chain paired with various light chains was always RF positive, and expressed varying binding

Table 1
Characteristics of Rheumatoid Factor Secreting Cell Lines

Cell line	Reaction with anti-Ids 4C9	6B6.6	Affinity for nonaggregated IgG (K_D mol/l)	Vk family	VK mutations, numbers	Jk	VH family	JH
MF8	+++	++	NEG	328	0	1	4.22	4
B9601	++	++	NEG	Vg	0	2	3	3
B'20	+++	+++	1.8×10^{-7}	328	2	1	3	4
B19	EG	NEG	1.3×10^{-6}	328	2	5	1	5

NEG, negative.

```
          *                                     *       *           *
          FR1                                   CDR1   FR2          CDR2

B'20H     EVQLLESGGGLVQPGGSLRLSCAASGFTFSSYAMSWVRQAPGKGLEWVSAISGSGGGTYYADS
9601H     ----V----------------S-----------H-----------Y-----SN--S------
B'20Hgl   ----V--------------------------------------------------S------
B9601gl   ----V----------------S-----------H-----------Y-----SN--S------

          *                                 *
          FR3                               CDR3

B'20H     VKGRFTISRDNSKNTLYLQMNSLRAEDTAVYYCAK   DRAPYSSS   FDYWGQGTLVTVSSRSAS
9601H     --------------------S------------V-   --VLEWL-TGYA --I-----M-----G---
B'20Hgl   -----------------------------------
B9601gl   -----------------V--S------------V-
```

Fig. 1. Amino acid sequences of the rheumatoid factor B'20 and B9601 heavy chains compared with the most homologous published germline gene (gl). B'20 has only two replacement mutations, while B9601 has one mutation.

affinities depending on its light chain partner. The B19 heavy chain, in contrast, was RF positive only with its own light chain *(7)*.

As discussed above, the heavy chain CDR3 is quite influential in determining autoantibody polyreactivity, including the RF reactivity *(22,23,29)*. Since these studies were performed with low affinity natural autoantibodies, we wished to determine whether a similar structural correlation is found in the higher affinity RFs derived from RA patients. To this end, the B'20 antibody was chosen for several reasons. First, when paired with the germline encoded MF8 light chain, which contains a VJ junction identical to the B'20 light chain, the B'20 heavy chain retains a high affinity for the Fc fragment. Second, the B'20 heavy chain has only two replacement mutations compared to the most homologous germline gene, one located in FR1 and another in CDR2. Third, the B'20 heavy chain is highly homologous to the germline-encoded B9601 heavy chain that is present in a RF-negative antibody. The sequences of the VH3 encoded heavy chains of B'20 and B9601 and their germline gene counterparts are shown in Fig. 1. Both B'20 V region mutations result in substitutions that are part of the germline B9601 sequence, suggesting that these are not important in conferring

RF specificity. Using chimeras of B'20 and B9601, we observed that the B'20 D region is instrumental in conferring the RF specificity to the B'20 heavy chain, a conclusion smiliar to that reached using natural autoantibodies. Further examination of the B'20 D region shows that it is formed by a D-D fusion between a 5' unknown D region and the 3' DN1 gene in the germline configuration *(28)*. Since the unknown D region contributes only 2 amino acids that are different from the 5' end of the B9601 D region, it is tempting to speculate that the B20 autoantibody has acquired its high affinity for Fc because of the junctional diversity generated in the preimmune repertoire. Due to the marked heterogeneity of the human D region, however, it is not possible to be certain whether somatic mutations may have occurred in this region. For this reason, we chose to direct further attention to the light chain contributions in RF specificity, since the VJ junction is less complex than the V-D-J junction.

6.2. The Light Chain

Monoclonal rheumatoid factors (RF) isolated from patients with B-cell dyscrasias express highly restricted idiotypic specificities, with 60–80% expressing either the 17.109 or 6B6.6 idiotype (Ids). These Ids serve as markers for the human VkIIIb subgroup gene Humkv 325 and the VkIIIa subgroup gene Humkv 328, respectively *(30,31)*. The Ids are expressed on only a small fraction of the polyclonal RFs from RA patients *(32)*, even though a majority (approximately, 60%) of the known monoclonal rheumatoid factors derived from RA patients use VkIII encoded genes. We described an anti-idiotypic antibody (anti-Id), 4C9, that recognizes a light chain determinant in serum RFs of approximately 80% of seropositive patients with RA *(33)*. An overlap in the RFs recognized by the 6B6.6 and 4C9 anti-Ids was evident, but the 4C9 recognized a broader range of RFs than 6B6.6, and its Id was expressed by a higher percentage of polyclonal RF from RA sera *(28)*.

The 17.109 idiotype appears to be dependent on the presence of the germline CDR2 region of light chains encoded by the VkIIIb subgroup. Expression of this Id can be lost via somatic mutations in CDR2 *(27)*. It has been generally assumed that expression of the 6B6.6 Id is similarly dependent on the germline sequence of VkIIIa genes, and that idiotypic reactivity may be lost as a result of somatic mutations. Our findings using a panel of 4C9/6B6.6 positive light chains and their mutants suggests that the structural basis for expression of these Ids is more complex. For these studies, we used the same cell lines as described in Table 1. The sequences of the light chains and the informative mutants, along with the Humkv328 and Vg germline sequences, are shown in Fig. 2. The B9601FR1-3/MF8CDR3 is a chimeric light chain in which the CDR3 of MF8 was switched into the B9601 light chain.

The observations on idiotypic specificity are as follows (*see* Table 2): the expression of the 6B6.6 and 4C9 Ids was relatively independent of heavy/light chain pairing when the Id-positive light chain (MF8 and B19) originated from the Humkv328 gene, but was highly dependent on heavy/light chain pairing

```
                    *                            *         *                   *
                    FR1                          CDR1      FR2                 CDR2

Humkv 328           EIVMTQSPATLSVSPGERATLSCRASQSVSSNLAWYQQKPGQAPRLLIYGASTRAT

MF8                 -------------------------------------------------------
B19                 ---------------------------I---------------------------
B'20                -------------------------------------------------------
B19g                --------------------^----------------------------------
Vg                  ---L--------L-------------------Y----------------D--N---
B9601               ---L--------L-------------------Y----------------D--N---
B9601FR1-3/MF8CDR3  ---L--------L-------------------Y----------------D--N---


                    *                            *         *
                    FR3                          CDR3      FR4

Humkv 328           GIPARFSGSGSGTEFTLTISSLQSEDFAVYYCQQYNNWP

MF8                 -------------------------------------- PW TFGQGTKVEIKR
B19                 ---------------------------------D--    ------RL----
B'20                -M----R------------------------------- PW -----------
B19g                --------------------------------^..    ------RL----
Vg                  ------------D--------EP----------RS---
B9601               ------------D--------EP----------RS--- PY -------L----
B9601FR1-3/MF8CDR3  ------------D--------EP#-------------- PW -----------
```

^ indicates sites of mutation back to germline
# indicates switch site of the chimera

Fig. 2. Amino acid sequences of the rheumatoid factor light chains and light chain mutants compared with the germline Humkv328 and Vg sequences.

when the light chain originated from the Vg gene (B9601). Thus, the same Vg derived light chain was Id-positive in association with one heavy chain but not with a highly homologous heavy chain. Further, the same germline-encoded VL gave rise to an Id-positive and an Id-negative light chain when paired with different heavy chains, a phenomenon that appears to depend on the sequence and length of the CDR3 region formed by VJ joining (Table 2). For example, the MF8 germline encoded light chain was positive for both Ids, but the B19g light chain that used the same *V* gene but contained a different VJ junction was negative. Similarly, 6B6.6 reactivity of the germline-encoded B9601 light chain could be restored by switching its CDR3 with the MF8 CDR3 *(7)*.

These observations suggest that the reactivity with the 4C9 and 6B6.6 anti-Ids requires a structural feature(s) encoded by the VkIIIa light chain gene. The combinatorial diversity at the VJ junction dictates that only sometimes will a CDR3 be generated that is permissive for expression of 4C9 and 6B6.6 Ids. In addition, combinatorial diversity at the level of heavy–light chain pairing will only sometimes be permissive for idiotype expression. The higher level of expression of the 4C9 Id in RA sera compared with the 6B6.6 Id may reflect the less stringent requirements for proper heavy–chain pairing permissive for the 4C9 Id specificity. It is of interest that the 6B6.6 Id is highly expressed among the Humkv 328 gene-encoded RFs from B-cell dyscrasias, suggesting that these

Table 2
Idiotypic and Rheumatoid Factor Activity
of Heavy and Light Chain Combinations [a]

Heavy chain	Light chain	Reaction with anti-Ids 4C9[c]	6B6.6[c]	RFb activity Aggregated	IgG[c] Fc[c]
MF8	MF8	+++	+++	−	−
MF8	B19	−	−	−	
MF8	B9601	+++	−	−	−
MF8	B19g	−	−		−
MF8	B9601FR1-3/MF8CDR3	++	++	−	−
B19	B19	−	−	++	−
B19	B19g	−	−	+++	−
B19	MF8	+++	+++	−	−
B19	B9601	+	−	−	−
B19	B9601FR1-3/MF8CDR3	+++	+++	−	−
B'20	B'20	+++	+++	+++	+++
B'20	MF8	+++	+++	+++	+++
B'20	B9601	+	−	++	+
B'20	B19g	−	−	++	+
B'20	B9601FR1-3/MF8CDR3	++	++	+++	+++

[a] See Figs. 1 and 2 for sequences of the heavy and light chains.

[b] High affinity binding is demonstrated by binding to isolated Fc fragment and low affinity by binding to aggregated IgG.

[c] Values in OD Units: − < 0.200; + 0.200-0.500; ++ 0.500-1.000; +++ >1.000.

B-cells have a highly restricted repertoire, not only in terms of light chain V region usage, but also the associated heavy chain and the VJ junctions. The fact that this Id is expressed only at very low levels in normal sera suggests that the corresponding B-cells never exit from the marrow or are anergized peripherally, perhaps because they express a high affinity for the Fc fragment.

The light chain structural correlates of RF reactivity were examined using a panel of recombinant antibodies and mutants (Table 2). Although the heavy chain exercised a strong influence on RF specificity, in recombinants containing the same heavy chain, different light chains altered the affinity of Fc binding substantially. For example, the B'20 heavy chain combined with the MF8 light chain, which is the germline counterpart of the B'20 light chain, yielded an antibody with slightly higher affinity for Fc than the B'20/B'20 construct. When the B'20 heavy chain was recombined with the B19g light chain or the B9601 light chain, however, the constructs displayed considerably lower affinity for the Fc, and they were able to bind only the aggregated immunoglobulin (Table 2). Similar observations have been reported for anti-DNA antibodies, in which the heavy chain was shown to contribute essential determinants for DNA binding, but the light chains modulated the fine specificity and binding affinity, and in certain cases prevented the binding altogether *(6)*. Association of the same heavy chain with different light chains can also alter the fine specificity for carbohydrate antigens, some of which are autoantigens *(34)*. Sudies of anti-bodies to a foreign antigen (arsonate) have also shown that the generation of anti-arsonate specificity is dependent on the structure of the heavy chain VDJ junction and the light chain VJ junction *(35)*. As discussed in Section 2, a possible mechanism to avoid the continued synthesis of self-reactive light chains is receptor editing. In studies of anti-DNA antibodies, Radic et al. have shown that light chain editing in the bone marrow is applied towards avoiding self-reactivity, but a potentially pathogenic heavy chain continues to be used for antibody synthesis *(36)*.

Analysis of our panel of light chain mutants suggested that the effect of the light chain on affinity for Fc was again dependent on the structure of the VJ junction. This is illustrated by comparing the RF activity of the B19g and MF8 light chains, which differ from each other at the VJ junctions. The MF8 light chain has a CDR3 of 10 amino acids while the B19g has a CDR3 of 8 amino acids. Recombination of the B19 heavy chain with the MF8 light chain resulted in loss of the RF activity. Similarly, recombination of the B'20 heavy chain with the B19 or B9601 light chains resulted in a significant loss of affinity for Fc. Further evidence for the importance of the light chain CDR3 in RF specificity came from the B9601/MF8 light chain chimera, in which switching of the MF8 CDR3 into the B9601 light chain resulted in complete restoration of affinity for Fc as well as restoration of idiotype expression, provided the light chain was paired with the permissive B'20 heavy chain.

It has been suggested recently that the length of the light chain CDR3 generated by VJ junctional diversity is increased preferentially in antibodies derived from the rheumatoid synovium compared to those from normal individuals, and that patients with RA might select for or might not select against the long CDR3 *(37,38)*. In our own studies, the effect of CDR3 length on antigen binding specificity was variable and it was highly dependent on the associated heavy chain. Further study is required to clarify the significance of a long light chain CDR3 in RA.

SUMMARY

It is highly likely that VDJ and VJ gene rearrangements and combinatorial diversity mechanisms can generate autoantibody specificities. Most of the B-cells expressing the autospecificities encounter self-antigens in the bone marrow and are censored by deletion, anergy or further gene rearrangements. Cells that escape this process and exit to the periphery may not compete effectively for follicular entry into germinal centers. The studies of mice transgenic for rheumatoid factor have illustrated the important role of various checkpoints in the regulation of autoreactivity along the path of B-cell development and prior to B-cell entry into the germinal centers. Failure of bone marrow censoring, or the failure to exclude self-reactive B-cells from the germinal centers might allow expansion of these cells in the periphery. Under normal circumstances, the remaining autoreactive cells generated in the preimmune repertoire express too low an affinity to be activated by self-antigen, and are not pathogenic. Such cells can synthesize high affinity pathogenic autoantibodies via the somatic mutation process if peripheral tolerance mechanisms fail. Unfortunately, the available transgenic models of autoantibody production do not allow unambiguous study of the role of somatic mutations as a means to generate self-reactivity. The somatic mutation process represents, of course, another dangerous mechanism whereby self-reactivity can be generated, i.e., by elaboration of an autoreactive specificity from a non-autoreactive antibody.

Studies of RFs derived from human patients with RA have shown that the heavy chain makes a major contribution to RF specificity, to which the somatically generated CDR3 region makes a disproportionate contribution. The heavy chain contribution is somewhat variable and depends on the particular heavy chain used for the RF assembly. VkIII-encoded light chains are present in a substantial proportion of monoclonal RFs both from patients with B-cell tumors and from RA patients. Studies of a highly related set of VkIIIa encoded RFs show that provided the heavy/light chain pairing is permissive for autoreactivity, both RF specificity and 6B6.6 and 4C9 idiotypic specificity are highly dependent on the CDR3 structure formed by the VJ joint. Our studies suggest that RFs of moderately high affinity might be generated in the preimmune repertoire via combinatorial and junctional diversity, and cells making such RFs might escape to the periphery. Abnormal release, activation, expansion or mutation of these B-cells might contribute to the generation of a high titer RF response in patients with RA.

REFERENCES

1. Schatz, D. G., Oettinger, M. A., and Schlissel, M. S. (1992) V(D)J Recombination: molecular biology and regulation. *Ann. Rev. Immunol.* **10,** 359–383.
2. Schwartz, K. and Bartram, C. R. (1996) V(D)J recombination pathology. *Adv. Immunol.* **61,** 285–326.
3. Sanz, I., Wang, S. S., Meneses, G., and Fischbach, M. (1994) Molecular characterization of human Ig heavy chain DIR genes. *J. Immunol.* **152,** 3958–3969.
4. Weaver, D. T. (1995) What to do at an end: DNA double-strand-break repair. *Trends Genet.* **11,** 388–392.
5. Fanning, L. J., Connor, A. M., and Wu, G. E. (1996) Development of the immunoglobulin repertoire. *Clin. Immunol. Immunopath.* **79,** 1–14.
6. Radic, M. Z., Mascelli, M.A., Erikson, J., Shan, H., and Weigert, M. (1991) Ig H and L contributions to autoimmune specificities. *J. Immunol.* **146,** 176–182.
7. Zhang, M., Spey, D., Ackerman, S., Majid, A., and Davidson, A. (1996) Rheumatoid factor idiotypic and antigenic specificity is strongly influenced by the light chain VJ junction. *J. Immunol.* **156,** 3570–3575.
8. Goodnow, C. C., Cyster, J. G., Hartley, S. B., Bell, S. E., Cooke, M. P., Healy, J. I., et al. (1995) Self-tolerance checkpoints in B lymphocyte development. *Adv. Immunol.* **59,** 279–368.
9. Radic, M. Z. and Zouali, M. (1996) Receptor editing, immune diversification, and self-tolerance. *Immunity* **5,** 505–511.

10. Chen, C., Nagy, Z., Prak, E. L., and Weigert, M. (1995) Immunoglobulin heavy chain gene replacement: a mechanism of receptor editing. *Immunity* **3**, 747–755.
11. Hikida, J., Mori, M., Takai, R., Tomochika, K., Hamatani, K., and Ohmori, H. (1996) Reexpression of RAG-1 and RAG-2 genes in activated mature mouse B cells. *Science* **274**, 2092–2097.
12. Han, S., Dillon, S. R., Zheng, B., Shimoda, M., Schlissel, M. S., and Kelsoe, G. (1997) V(D)J recombinase activity in a subset of germinal center B lymphocytes. *Science* **278**, 301–305.
13. Iliev, A., Spatz, L., Ray, S., and Diamond, B. (1994) Lack of allelic exclusion permits autoreactive B cells to escape deletion. *J. Immunol.* **153**, 3551–3556.
14. Tsao, B. P., Chow, A., Cheroutre, H., Song, Y. W., McGrath, M. E., and Kronenberg, M. (1993) B cells are anergic in transgenic mice that express IgM and DNA antibodies. *Eur. J. Immunol.* **23**, 2332–2339.
15. Cyster, J. G., Hartley, S. B., and Goodnow, C. C. (1994) Competition for follicular niches excludes self-reactive cells from the recirculating B-cell repertoire. *Nature* **371**, 389–395.
16. Tighe, J., Chen, P. P., Tucher, R., Kipps, T. J., Roudier, J., Jirik, F. R., et al. (1993) Function of B cells expressing a human immunoglobulin M rheumatoid factor autoantibody in transgenic mice. *J. Exp. Med.* **177**, 109–118.
17. Tighe, H., Heaphy, P., Baird, S., Weigle, W. O., and Carson, D. A. (1995) Human immunoglobulin (IgG) induced deletion of IgM rheumatoid factor B cells in transgenic mice. *J. Exp. Med.* **181**, 599–606.
18. Hannum, L. G., Ni, D., Haberman, A. M., Weigert, M. G., and Shlomchik, M. J. (1996) A disease-related rheumatoid factor autoantibody is not tolerized in a normal mouse: implications for the origins of autoantibodies in autoimmune disease. *J. Exp. Med.* **184**, 1269–1278.
19. Janeway, C. and Travers, P. (1997) Structure of the antibody molecule and immunoglobulin genes, in *Immunobiology: The Immune System in Health and Disease* (Janeway, C. and Travers, P., eds.), *Curr. Biol.*
20. Alzari, P. M., Lascombe, M., and Poljak, R. J. (1988) Three dimensional structure of antibodies. *Ann. Rev. Immunol.* **6**, 555–580.
21. Kabat E. A. and Wu, T. T. (1991) Identical V region amino acid sequences and segments of sequences in antibodies of different specificities. *J. Immunol.* **147**, 1709–1719.
22. Martin, T. R. Crouzier, R., Weber, J. C., Kipps, T. J., and Pasquali, J. L. (1994). Structure function studies on a polyreactive antibody. *J. Immunol.* **152**, 5988–5993.
23. Ichiyoshi, Y. and Casali, P. (1994) Analysis of the structural correlates for antibody polyreactivity by multiple reassortments of chimeric human imunoglobulin heavy and light chain V segments. *J. Exp. Med.* **180**, 885–895.
24. Sasso, E. H. (1992) Immunoglobulin V region genes in rheumatoid arthritis. *Rheum. Dis. Clin. N. Am.* **18**, 809–836.
25. Randen I., Brown, D., Thompsen, K. M., Hughes-Jones, N., Pascual, V., Victor, K., et al. (1992) Clonally related IgM rheumatoid factors undergo affinity maturation in the rheumatoid synovial tissue. *J. Immunol.* **148**, 3296–3301.
26. Bonagura, V., Artandi, S., Davidson, A., Agostino, N., Randen, I., Thompsen, K., et al. (1993) Mapping studies reveal unique epitopes on IgG recognized by rheumatoid arthritis-derived monoclonal rheumatoid factors. *J. Immunol.* **151**, 3840–3848.

27. Youngblood, K., Fruchter, L., Ding, G., Lopez, J., Bonagura, V., and Davidson, A. (1994) Rheumatoid factors from the peripheral blood of patients with rheumatoid arthritis are genetically heterogeneous and somatically mutated. *J. Clin. Invest.* **93**, 852–861.

28. Davidson, A., Schrohenloher, R., and Koopman, W. J. (1995) Molecular characterization of B cell lines bearing the 4C9 rheumatoid factor associated idiotype. *Autoimmunity* **20**, 171–183.

29. Martin, T., Duffy, S., Carson, D. A., and Kipps, T. J. (1992). Evidence for somatic selection of natural autoantibodies. *J. Exp. Med.* **175**, 983–987.

30. Chen P. P., Silverman, G. J., Liu, M. F., and Carson , D. A. (1990) Idiotypic and molecular characterization of human rheumatoid factors. *Chem. Immunol.* **48**, 63–81.

31. Schrohenloher, R. E., Accavitti, M. A., Bhown, A. S., and Koopman, W. J. (1990) Monoclonal antibody 6B6.6 defines a cross-reactive kappa light chain idiotype on human monoclonal and polyclonal rheumatoid factors. *Arthritis Rheum.* **33**, 187–198.

32. Chen P. P., Silverman, G. J., Liu, M. F., and Carson, D. A. (1990). Idiotypic and molecular characterization of human rheumatoid factors. *Chem. Immunol.* **48**, 63–81.

33. Davidson A., Lopez, J., Sun, D., and Prus, D. (1992). A monoclonal anti-idiotype specific for human polyclonal IgM rheumatoid factor. *J. Immunol.* **148**, 3873–3878.

34. Kao C. Y. and Sharon, J. (1993) Chimeric antibodies with anti-dextran derived complementarity determining regions and anti-p azophenylarsonate derived framework regions. *J. Immunol.* **151**, 1968–1979.

35. Hasemann, C. A. and Capra, J. D. (1991) Mutational analysis of arsonate binding by a CRIA+ antibody. *J. Biol.Chem.* **266**, 7626–7632.

36. Radic, M. Z., Erikson, J., Litwin, S., and Weigert, M. (1993) B lymphocytes may escape tolerance by revising their antigen receptors. *J. Exp. Med.* **177**, 1165–1173.

37. Bridges, S. L., Jr., Lee, S. K., Johnson, M., Lavelle, J. C., Fowler, P. G., Koopman, W. J. et al. (1995) Somatic mutation and CDR3 lengths of immunoglobulin k light chains expressed in patients with rheumatoid arthritis and in normal individuals. *J. Clin. Invest.* **96**, 831–841.

38. Martin, T., Blaison, G., Levallois, H., and Pasquali, J. L. (1992) Molecular analysis of the VkIII junctional diversity of polyclonal rheumatoid factors during rheumatoid arthritis frequently reveals N addition. *Eur. J. Immunol.* **22**, 1773–1779.

13
Autoantibodies Against Ig Immunoglobulin Framework Epitopes

Heinz Kohler and Sybille Müller

1. INTRODUCTION

The concept of antibodies against antibodies is now more than 40 years old. In 1955 Slater et al. *(1)* reported that a rabbit antiserum against a human myeloma protein continued to react with the immunizing myeloma protein after extensive absorption on normal human immunoglobulins (Igs). This experiment showed for the first time that it is possible to induce antibodies specific for unique epitopes (idiotopes) on another antibody. It was not clear, however, that such antiantibodies were present or could be induced in the same species and individual which served as the source of the immunogenic Ig. In 1957, Milgrom and Dubiski *(2)* concluded from experiments in rabbits that the immunoglobulins of an individuals own body may become antigenic. Ten years later, the concept of antiantibodies blossomed, as many laboratories began work on idiotypes and anti-idiotypes, including auto-anti-idiotypic immune responses, which provided the experimental support for Niels Jerne's network theory (*see* rcf. *3*).

Antiantibodies are divided into two broad categories according to their antigenic specificity: 1) antibodies against the Fc portion of Ig are typically called rheumatoid factors and are the oldest known kind of antiantibodies and 2) antibodies against epitopes located in the Fab segment, which can be further divided into anti-idiotypic antibodies and antiframework residue antibodies. In the present discussion, we will focus on antiframework autoantibodies, which we detected in normal sera and sera from HIV-1 infected individuals.

The structure of the variable Ig domains involves two types of elements: 1) the complementarity determining regions (CDRs) and 2) the framework regions (FRs). Each Ig subunit, i.e., the H chain and the L chain, contributes three CDRs and four FRs to the Fv, which is the minimal Ig fragment capable of simulating the high affinity antigen binding activity of intact antibodies. The sequence of the CDRs is highly variable, and the structure of the CDRs is adapted during antigen selection and affinity maturation to make high affinity contacts with the antigen. The FRs maintain the overall structure of the antigen binding site as a seven beta-sheeted scaffold. Similarities and structural homologies among FR

Contemporary Immunology: Autoimmune Reactions
Edited by: S. Paul © Humana Press Inc., Totowa, NJ

sequences reveal the heritage of variable domain genes from socalled V-gene families. The size of these gene families varies in different species from 2 to 100 genes.

Besides being important for the structure of Igs, the FRs are endowed with certain biological functions. FR residues often contribute in antigen contacts either directly or indirectly, by correctly positioning the antigen contacting CDR loops. Recently, another biological role of FR residues has been discovered, i.e., they serve as important contacts in the binding of the so-called B-cell superantigens by antibodies (*see* ref. *4*). The B-cell superantigens have an analogous biological function as the T-cell superantigens, in that both are polyclonal stimulators. In the case of the B-cell superantigens, selective expansion of cells expressing certain V-gene families occurs *(5,6)*. The epitopes located in the FRs can serve as targets for autoantibodies, as mentioned above. Whether these autoantibodies play a biological role is not established, but their existence allows us to conceive such functions. We encountered autoantibodies against the FR epitopes over the course of work with synthetic FR peptide implicated in certain unrelated antibody functions, i.e., the self-binding site and the idiotopes expressed by antibodies.

2. SELF-BINDING ANTIBODIES IN RODENTS AND HUMANS

2.1. Characterization of the Self-Binding Site

Self-binding of certain antibodies involving the variable domain regions was discovered using a monoclonal murine antibody from the S107/T15 VH family *(7)*. This type of self-binding is different from the Fc–Fc mediated aggregation seen with certain antibody isotypes. An IgM antibody, 11E7, was obtained from a nude BALB/c hybridoma fusion experiment which exhibited self-binding in solid phase ELISA and RIA systems. The antigen binding site of 11E7 recognizes phosphorylcholine (PC) which is also the major antigenic epitope for antibodies of the S107/T15 family. The self-binding phenomenon observed using 11E7 is efficiently inhibited by the free hapten, PC. Interestingly, 11E7 can also bind members of the S107/T15 V gene family which carry different isotypes, i.e., have a different constant region structure. As the concentration of the insolubilized T15 was increased, the self-binding of 11E7 was reduced, suggesting that T15 might compete with 11E7 self-binding.

The structural requirements for the self-binding phenomenon were delineated by immunochemical and structural studies *(9)*. Fab fragments of T15, but not the free H or L chains, were potent inhibitors of the 11E7 self-binding reaction, indicating that an intact V-domain structure is required for self-binding. The amino acid sequence for 11E7 was deduced from the cloned and sequenced VL and VH genes and shown to be identical to germline sequence of S107. The self-binding reaction is governed, therefore, by germline encoded structural elements, as opposed to somatically derived elements. Self-binding is highly dependent on the polymerization state of the Ig structure *(10)*, as monomeric T15 only showed marginal self-binding, dimeric T15 showed greater self-binding and pentameric IgM 11E7 showed the strongest self-binding when compared at equivalent molar concentrations.

The amino acid sequences of S107 and M603, two antibodies with different self-binding strengths, were analyzed for hydropathic complementarities as defined previously *(11)*. This parameter is a useful predictor of peptide-peptide binding potential. Two peptide sequences in the VH domain revealed strong hydropathic complementarity: VH50-60 was complementary to VH63-74 *(9)*. The differences in the hydropathic scores of T15 and M603 complementarities are in agreement with the differences in their self-binding strength. A 24-mer peptide was synthesized covering the sequence VH50-73 and tested as an inhibitor of the self-binding phenomenon. The self-binding reactions observed in T15 and M603 antibody preparations were inhibited at micromolar concentration of this peptide but not by control peptides. The peptide segment VH50-60 is located in CDR2 while the complementary sequence, VH63-74 is located in FR3. These peptide determinants (VH50-60 and VH63-74) can be seen as the receptor-ligand pair mediating the self-binding reaction.

2.2. Biological Implications

Solution phase immune complex formation plays important roles in immune defense and autoimmune pathology. Thus, it was of interest to see if the self-binding antibodies exist as complexes in solution. This question was studied using radiolabeled self-binding antibodies from the S107/T15 family *(12)*. Complexes of T15 and U4 [a DNA binding mutant of S107 *(13)*] could be demonstrated by size-exclusion and by PEG facilitated precipitation. The free hapten recognized by the antigen binding site inhibited formation of the self-binding complex.

Interestingly, the presence of the VH50-73 peptide enhanced the PEG facilitated complex formation of T15. At face value, the enhancement conflicts with our earlier finding indicating that this peptide inhibits solid-phase self-binding. Further reflection has revealed, however, a way to reconcile the observations. Since the VH50-73 peptide has complementary surfaces for both CDR2 and FR3, it may crosslink antibodies containing the self-binding sites consisting of one end of the synthetic peptide bound to one antibody and the second end of the peptide bound to another antibody. The peptide may facilitate formation of a three-dimensional (3-D) lattice in this manner. Such a peptide-mediated lattice formation in solution might compete with the solid-phase self-binding reaction, causing the inhibition by the VH50-73 peptide described previously.

Immune complexes can cause tissue damage by various mechanisms in autoimmune disease, including activation of the complement system. It is not known whether the self-binding phenomenon is involved in pathological autoimmune processes. As pointed out by us *(10)* and later by Chapman and colleagues *(14)*, the self-binding potential can increase the deposition of antibodies on target cells. The increased antibody density due to self-binding can be expected to result in increased avidity of antigen binding. This effect might be particularly important for T-independent antibody responses such as against carbohydrate antigens, and possibly certain anti-DNA responses, where self-binding antibodies might compensate for the lack of affinity driven maturation of the V regions *(14)*.

2.3. Self-Binding as an Autoantibody Phenomenon

Another biologically interesting aspect of the self-binding antibodies was the discovery that autoantibodies are capable of binding the self-binding VH50-73 peptide *(15)*.

Certain strains of mice contain readily detectable levels of S107/T15 positive Ig which binds to the hapten PC. Since the S107/T15 monoclonal antibodies are the protype of self-binding Igs it was expected that these natural T15-positive Ig in mouse sera may be capable of a) self-binding and b) binding to the VH(50-73) self-binding peptide. Three strains of mice differing in their expression levels of natural S107/T15 antibodies were tested for binding to T15. Anti-T15 antibodies were detected corresponding to concentration of circulating T15-positive Ig. Furthermore, self-binding antibodies could be isolated by affinity chromatography on the immobilized VH(50-73) peptide column. The affinity-isolated antibodies displayed specific binding to the VH(50-73) peptide and to each other.

Similar self-binding and peptide-binding antibodies were isolated from normal human donors and from pooled human Ig (IVIg). These studies demonstrated the existence of a population of natural antibodies specific for a CDR/FR epitope which are self-binding.

In a follow-up study *(16)*, we isolated anti-phosphorylcholine (PC) antibodies from human sera and demonstrated that a subpopulation of the anti-PC antibodies were self-binding, i.e., the T15 Id-positive subpopulation. Self-binding by these human anti-PC antibodies was effectively inhibited by the VH(50–73) self-binding peptide in a fashion similar to the mouse anti-PC antibodies.

Antibodies which associate via the self-binding site are not classical autoantibodies. Nonetheless, binding of an antibody to another autologous antibody via the self-binding site can be legitimately held to be an example of an autoimmune phenomenon, which could potentially produce changes in the functional role of the antibodies. From the structural standpoint, the involvement of CDR2, which is part of the classical antigen binding site, justifies the antibody association phenomenon via the self-binding site as an autoantibody interaction. The binding of CDR2 to a conserved framework site in self-binding is analogous to the rheumatoid factor autoantibody binding to a conserved Fc region.

2.4. Conclusion

The studies with mouse and human self-binding antibodies have established several points. Self-binding antibodies are evolutionarily conserved and their activity is dependent, in part, on a conserved framework structure of the VH domain, and, in part, a CDR2 site and certain self-binding Igs are directed against the PC epitope, which is an important constituent of a biologically relevant antigen, the C-polysaccharide antigen. The self-binding activity of certain antibodies might result in augmentation of the avidity of antigen binding. Whether autoantibodies against conserved FR epitopes play a role in autoimmune diseases can be the subject of speculation within the context of anti-idiotype:idiotype regulation of the immune response *(17)*.

3. AUTOANTIBODIES AGAINST 1F7 EPITOPE IN HIV-1 INFECTED INDIVIDUALS

3.1. Generation of Anti-Clonotype Antibody

A panel of monoclonal anti-idiotypic-antibodies was made in BALB/c mice immunized with the Ig fraction prepared from a pool of 17 HIV-seropositive subjects *(18,19)*. Hybridoma fusions were screened by sandwich ELISA for binding to idiotopes expressed by HIV-specific Ig. Plates were coated with recombinant gp120 or p24 and reacted with the pooled serum from HIV-1 infected donors. The captured anti-HIV-1 antibodies were then incubated with primary hybridoma fusion wells, and the reaction detected with a secondary anti-mouse antibody. The so-selected and anti-idiotypic antibodies reacted with antibodies in pools of HIV seropositive sera but not with normal human Ig, or with antibodies to other antigens in the HIV sera and HIV seronegative sera. One of the anti-Ids, designated 1F7, was an IgM antibody that recognized an idiotype present on a variety of anti-HIV-1 antibodies, including antibodies directed to gp120, p24, precursor env and gag proteins, as well as reverse transcriptase *(19)*. Approximately 70% of HIV-infected individuals express the 1F7-reactive epitope in their serum IgG *(19)*. The 1F7-idiotope positive antibodies were present at considerably lower levels in healthy individuals, HIV seronegative patients with lupus, B-cell lymphoma patients *(18)* and immune deficient transplantation patients (unpublished data). Studies with sera from seronegative volunteers vaccinated with recombinant gp120IIIB and gp120MN as well as from chimpanzees experimentally infected with HIV-IIIB showed that the 1F7 idiotope is predominantly expressed on antibodies generated to the envelope of HIV strain used for primary vaccination *(20)*. The 1F7 idiotope was also observed in antibodies directed against gp120IIIB developing in macaques infected with Human/ Simian Immunodeficiency Chimera Virus (SHIVIIIB) *(21)* and SIV *(22)*.

The crossreactive idiotope (1F7) described above is expressed by antibodies found in a majority of HIV-infected individuals, the idiotope is expressed at all disease stages of AIDS at an equivalent level, and its expression is only decreased in the terminal, lymphopenic stages of AIDS. Since the 1F7 idiotope is associated with serum antibodies and monoclonal antibodies specific to several different HIV-antigens (*env, gag, pol*), it is considered to be a disease marker for HIV-infection.

It was suggested that the shared idiotope bound by 1F7 was actually a clonotypic marker characteristic for a particular VH family. We found, however, that 1F7 reactivity was expressed on human monoclonal anti-gp120 and anti-p24 antibodies derived from the VH_1 and VH_4 gene families, respectively *(19)*, and on Fab fragments derived from various VH families cloned from the B cells of an HIV-infected individual (D. Burton, J. Binley, S. Müller, 1994, unpublished). Preliminary data from "panning" of the phage-displayed Fab library indicated that 1F7 is expressed in three Fab constructs derived from the VH_1 gene family, five constructs from the VH_4 family and one from the VH_3 family.

Analogous observations have been made by other authors. It has been demonstrated that idiotopes expressed by human monoclonal rheumatoid factors are crossreactive and are shared by H chain from different VH families, e.g., the VH_3 and VH_1 families (23). The 1F7 idiotope is not associated with any particular light chain isotype (unpublished data).

Therefore, the 1F7 idiotope is not a marker for a particular VH family. The 1F7 idiotope does not appear to reside in the antigen-binding site of the antibodies, since the 1F7 anti-idiotypic antibody did not inhibit the binding of the 1F7 idiotope positive antibodies to HIV antigens (19). Most idiotopes are thought to be associated partially or entirely with the complementary-determining regions (CDRs). Some idiotopes, however, can span parts of the CDRs combined with parts of the framework region (24). This produces either unique idiotopes that are found only in an antibody of a given epitope specificity and residing in the antigen binding site (private Ids), or shared idiotopes found in antibodies with different specificities and residing in the framework region (crossreactive or nonparatopic Ids).

3.2. Characterization of the Self-Idiotope-Peptide

To determine the idiotope:anti-idiotope contacts in anti-HIV antibodies, we used a computer algorithm based on recognition of inverse hydropathy between the variable domain sequences of 1F7 antibody and human monoclonal anti-gp120 or anti-p24 antibodies (25). For this, the VH and VL cDNAs of the 1F7 antibody were cloned and sequenced. The region predicted by inverse hydropathy as being favorable for interaction with the variable regions of 1F7 are located in the framework 3 and the CDR3 (FR3-CDR3) of the heavy chains of the anti-gp120 and anti-p24 antibodies (26).

To test the prediction of contacts at the FR3-CDR3 site, a peptide corresponding to the contact residues (p422) was synthesized. p422 was bound by the 1F7 anti-idiotype antibody in ELISA. Further, p422 inhibited the binding of the 1F7 antibody to human anti-HIV-1 antibodies expressing the 1F7 idiotope, and the 1F7 antibody inhibited the binding of rabbit anti-p422-peptide antibodies to p422 (25).

Because of the broad reactivity and association of 1F7 with HIV infection, it is conceivable that the 1F7 idiotope is also the target for self-recognition in infected individuals. We hypothesized that autoantibodies capable of recognizing the 1F7 idiotope might exist in HIV infected individuals. A survey of sera derived from normal and HIV-infected individuals revealed the presence of antibodies that bind to p422 in HIV-1 but not normal sera (25, Table 1). These results show that an autoanti-idiotypic activity, i.e., a 1F7-like activity, is correlated with the expression of the corresponding 1F7 idiotope in the HIV-infected patients.

While the idiotope target for 1F7 on human monoclonal anti-HIV antibodies can be mimicked by the p422 peptide, synthetic peptides corresponding to the CDRs of the 1F7 antibody (anti-Id) failed to bind the anti-HIV antibodies. This suggested that the binding site of the 1F7 anti-Id is a conformational determinant composed of more than one CDR, as opposed to a linear CDR peptide. This model is compatible with our current understanding of antibody structure. In contrast, the idiotope structure in anti-HIV antibodies appears to consist predominantly of a linear region which covers sequences spanning FR3 and CDR3. The combined involvement of FR and hypervariable regions in forming the idiotope is consistent with our previously described model of idiotope determining regions (IDR) in antibodies *(27)*.

In the strictest sense, these anti-p422 antibodies are not autoantibodies since the p422 peptide was not derived from polyclonal antibodies in the HIV$^+$ sera studied here. However, since the 1F7 anti-Id binds human monoclonal anti-gp120 and anti-p24 antibodies, and the p422 peptide sequence was based on the structures of the latter antibodies *(19,25,26)*, the human anti-p422 peptide antibodies qualify as examples of autoantibodies.

3.3. Biological Implications of Clonotypic Autoantibodies

The biological significance of the 1F7-like autoantibodies in the disease pathogenesis of AIDS is not known fully. Our data indicate that the 1F7-Id positive antibodies in HIV sera can modulate the level of apoptosis of peripheral blood CD4$^+$ and CD8$^+$ T-cells induced by the addition of 1F7 monoclonal antibodies (mAbs) in vitro *(28)*. Thus, the presence of 1F7-like autoantibodies can potentially modulate the T-cell functional status in HIV-infected individuals. It remains to be seen whether in vivo application of 1F7 antibody modulates the immune response in AIDS in a way that is beneficial. Recent data indicate that the antibody response to gp120 and non-HIV related antigens in monkeys infected with a HIVIIIB/SIV chimera was broadened after immunization with 1F7 monoclonal antibody in vivo *(29)*.

Autoantibodies involved in the pathological disease manifestation of AIDS-related immunologic thrombocytopenic purpura (ITP) have been demonstrated by Karpatkin et al. *(30,31)*. The authors found that immune complexes containing anti-HIV–1 antibody are present on the platelets of HIV-1 infected individuals. Further analysis showed that HIV+ patients with ITP have autoantibodies to CD4 which are the internal image of the CD4-binding site on gp120. Apparently, the complexes of anti-CD4 antibodies bound to anti-gp120 antibodies were associated with the platelets. The authors conclude that this phenomenon represents an idiotype:anti-idiotype complexation that may potentially influence the number or function of CD4$^+$ cells by inhibiting HIV-1 binding to the CD4$^+$ cells or by contributing to the HIV-1 associated thrombocytopenia *(31)*. It remains to be seen whether HIV antibody peptides, such as the peptide p422 reactive with 1F7 anti-idiotypic antibody, can be used to counteract the pathological immune complex formation between anti-gp120 antibodies and auto-antibodies to CD4.

REFERENCES

1. Slater, R. J., Ward, S. M., and Kunkel, H. G. (1955) Immunologic relationship among the myeloma proteins. *J. Exp. Med.* **101,** 85–108.
2. Milgrom, F. and Dubiski, S. (1957) Antigenicity of antibodies in the same species. *Nature* **17,** 1351–1352.
3. Kohler, H., Kaveri, S., Kieber-Emmons, T., Morrow, W. J. W., Müller, S., and Raychaudhuri, S. (1989) Overview of idiotypic networks and the nature of molecular mimicry. *Methods in Enzymol.* **178,** 3.
4. Tramontano, A. (1997) Framework structures of immunoglobulin variable domains: implications for antigen and superantigen binding, in *Human B Cell Superantigens* (Zouali, M. and Landes, R. G., eds.), R. G. Landes, Georgetown, TX; Springer Verlag, Heidelberg, Germany, pp. 11–23.
5. Berberian, L. Goodglick L. Kipps, T. J., and Braun J. (1993) Immunoglobulin VH3 gene products: natural ligands for HIV gp120. *Science* **261,** 1588.
6. Müller, S., Wang, H., Silverman, G. J., Bramlet, G., Haigwood, N., and Kohler, H. (1993) B-cell abnormalities in AIDS: stable and clonally-restricted antibody response in HIV-1 infection. *Scand. J. Immunol.* **38,** 327–334.
7. Kang, C.-Y., Cheng, H.-L., Rudikoff, S., and Kohler, H. (1987) Idiotypic self- binding of a dominant germline idiotype (T15): autobody activity is affected by antibody valency. *J. Exp. Med.* **165,** 1332.
8. Greenspan, N. S., Dacek, D. A., and Cooper, L. J. (1989) Cooperative binding of two antibodies to independent antigens by an Fc-dependent mechanism. *FASEB J.* **10,** 2203–2207.
9. Kang, C.-Y., Brunck, T. K., Kieber-Emmons, T., Blalock, J. E., and Kohler, H. (1988) Inhibition of self-binding antibodies (autobodies) by a VH-derived peptide. *Science* **240,** 1034–1036.
10. Kang, C.-Y., Cheng, H.-L., Rudikoff, S., and Kohler, H. (1987) Idiotypic self-binding of a dominant germline idiotype (T15): autobody activity is affected by antibody valency. *J. Exp. Med.* **165,** 1332.
11. Blalock, J. E. (1990) Complementary peptides specified by "sense" and "antisense" strands of DNA. *Trends Biotechnol.* **8,** 140–144.
12. Kaveri, S.-V., Halpern, R., Kang, C.-Y., and Kohler, H. (1990) Self-binding antibodies (autobodies) from specific complexes in solution. *J. Immunol.* **145,** 2533–2538.
13. Kaveri, S., Halpern, R., Kang, C.-Y., and Kohler, H. (1991) Antibodies of different specificities are self-binding: implication for antibody diversity. *Mol. Immunol.* **2,** 733–778.
14. Xiyun, Y., Evans, S.V., Kaminki, M. J., Gillies, S. D., Reisfeld, R. A., Noughton, A. N., et al. (1996) Characterization of an Ig Vh idiotype that results in specific homophilic binding and increased avidity for antigen. *J. Immunol.* **157,** 1582–1588.
15. Kaveri, S., Kang, C.-Y., and Kohler, H. (1990) Natural mouse and human antibodies bind to a peptide derived from a germline variable heavy chain: evidence for evolutionary conserved self-binding locus, *J. Immunol.* **145,** 4207–4213.
16. Halpern, R., Kaveri, S., and Kohler, H. (1991) Human anti-PC antibodies share idiotopes and are self-binding. *J. Clin. Inv.* **8,** 476–482.
17. Kohler, H. Paul, S., and Marchalonis, J. J. (1997) Multifunctional variable domains. *The Immunologist* **513,** 98–103.

18. Müller, S., Wang, H.-T., Kaveri, S.-V., Chattopadhyay, S. and Kohler, H. (1991) Generation and specificity of monoclonal anti-idiotypic antibodies against human HIV-specific antibodies. *J. Immunol.* **147**, 933–941.

19. Wang, H.-T., Müller, S., Zolla-Pazner, S., and Kohler, H. (1992) Human monoclonal and polyclonal anti-human immunodeficiency virus-1 antibodies share a common clonotypic specificity. *Eur. J. Immunol.* **22**, 1749–1755.

20. Müller, S. , Schwartz, D. , Wang, H.-T., Wang, Q., Kohler, H., Pahwa, S., et al. (1995) Expression of an HIV-1 Infection related idiotype/clonotype in antibodies directed to envelope glycoprotein gp120 of HIV-1: early and concomitant idiotype increase in antibodies against the homologous vaccine strain. *Vaccine Res.* **4**, 71–85.

21. Müller, S. Margolin, D. H., and Min, G. (1997) An HIV-1 infection related idiotype/ Clonotype (1F7) Is expressed on antibodies directed to envelope glycoprotein in simian immunodeficiency virus- and chimeric simian/human immunodeficiency virus-infected rhesus monkeys. *Hybridoma* **16**, 17–21.

22. Grant, M. D., Whaley, M. D., Mayne, A., Hoffmann, G. W., and Ansari, A. A. (1996) Similar abnormalities of idiotype and immunoglobulin light chain expression and of cell-mediated cytotoxicity in HIV-infected humans and simian immunodeficiency virus (SIV)-infected macaques. *Immunol. Cell. Biol.* **74**, 38–44.

23. Knight, G. B., Agnello, V., Bonagura, V., Barnes, J. L., Panka, D. J., and Zhang, Q. X. (1993) Human rheumatoid factor cross-idiotypes. IV. Studies on WA XId-positive IgM without rheumatoid factor activity provide evidence that the WA Xid is not unique to rheumatoid factors and is distinct from the 17.109 and G6 Xids. *J. Exp. Med.* **178**, 1903–1911.

24. Poljak, R. J. (1994) An idiotope-anti-idiotope complex and the structural basis of molecular mimicking. *Proc. Natl. Acad. Sci. USA* **91**, 1599–1600.

25. Wang, Q. L., Wang, H. T., Blalock, E., Müller, S., and Kohler, H. (1995) identification of an idiotypic peptide recognized by autoantibodies in HIV-1 infected individuals. *J. Clin. Invest.* **96**, 775–780.

26. Andris, J. S., Johnson, S., Zolla-Pazner, S., and Capra, D. (1991) Molecular characterization of five human anti-human immunodeficiency virus type 1 antibody heavy chains reveals extensive somatic mutation typical of an antigen-driven immune response. *Proc. Natl. Acad. Sci. USA* **88**, 7783–7787.

27. Kieber-Emmons, T., Getzoff, E., and Kohler, H. (1987) Perspectives on antigenicity and idiotypy. *Int. Rev. Immunol.* **2**, 339.

28. Müller, S., Brams, P., Collins, H., Dorigo, O., Wang, H.-T., and Kohler, H. (1995) Apoptosis of CD4⁺ and CD8⁺ cells from HIV-1 infected individuals: role of anti-idiotypic antibodies. *Vaccine Research* **4**, 229–238.

29. Müller, S., Margolin, D. H., Min, G., Alvord, W. G., Nara, P., and Kohler, H. (1998) Clonotypic suppression broadens antiviral antibody responses in SHIV-infected rhesus macaques. *Proc. Natl. Acad. Sci. USA* **95**, 276–281.

30. Karpatkin, S., Nardi, M. A., Lennette, E. T., Byrne, B. and Poiesz, B. (1988) Anti-human immunodeficiency virus type 1 antibody complexes on platelets of sero-positive thrombocytopenic homosexuals and narcotic addicts. *Proc. Natl. Acad. Sci. USA* **85**, 9763–9767.

31. Karpatkin, S., Nardi, M. A., and Kouri, Y. H. (1992) Internal-image anti-idiotype HIV-1gp120 antibody in human immunodeficiency virus 1 (HIV-1)-seropositive individuals with thrombocytopenia. *Proc. Natl. Acad. Sci. USA* **89**, 1487–1491.

14

Autoantibodies to T-Cell Receptors

John J. Marchalonis,
Samuel F. Schluter, and David E. Yocum

1. INTRODUCTION

It is well documented that humans *(1)* and experimental animals *(2)* can produce autoantibodies directed against autologous immunoglobulins in infections and in autoimmune diseases; most notably, rheumatoid arthritis, in which the rheumatoid factors (Rfs) are autoantibodies, usually but not always of the IgM isotype, that bind to conformational determinants on the Fc fragments of autologous γ chains *(3,4)*. In addition, autoantibodies directed against the Fab fragments of human immunoglobulins occur frequently in individuals infected with HIV *(5,6)*. Both types of autoantibodies may be regulatory in initial disease emergence, but may become involved in disease pathogenesis at later stages. Using comprehensive peptide synthesis methods *(7)* to map epitopes of T-cell receptor (TCR) β chains *(8–11)*, we found that purified polyclonal human IgG immunoglobulin (IVIG) contains low levels of autoantibodies directed against Vβ epitopes in CDR1, FR3, and a loop in the constant domain. The latter can be expected to be glycosylated in the cell-expressed TCR (Fig. 1). Further studies showed the existence of autoantibodies directed against recombinant single chain TCRs containing the complete Vα and Vβ domains *(11–13)* and the shared peptide-epitope specificities of these antibodies and those reactive with the T-cell expressed TCR *(11–13)*. The titers and isotypes of these autoantibodies vary with normal physiological conditions such as aging *(9,10)* and pregnancy *(14)*, with allograft transplantation *(15)*, with autoimmune diseases *(9–11)* and with retroviral infections in humans (16,17) and in mice *(18–22)*. Monoclonal human *(23–25)* and murine *(26,27)* autoantibodies to TCR Vβ CDR1 epitopes have been generated to analyze the binding specificities and possible functions of these molecules. Moreover, the tendency of humans and mice to respond to retroviral infections by generating autoantibodies with similar specificities has allowed the development of a peptide-based immunotherapy for retrovirally induced immunodeficiency in mice *(19–22)*, with implications for human AIDS *(28)*.

Contemporary Immunology: Autoimmune Reactions
Edited by: S. Paul © Humana Press Inc., Totowa, NJ

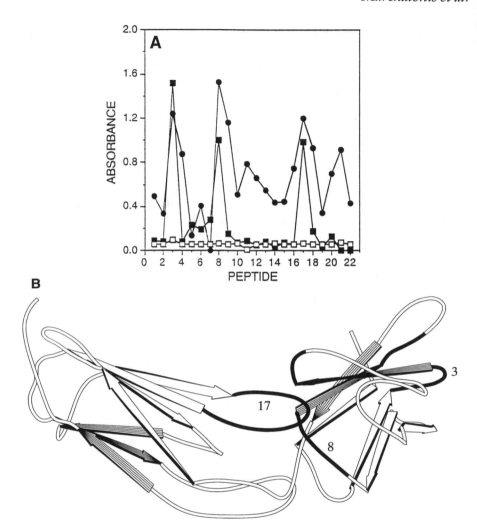

Fig. 1. (A) Localization of peptide epitopes bound by autoantibody subsets in human intravenous immunoglobulin (IVIG) preparations. A set of 22 hexadecameric peptides (overlapping by 5 residues) was used to model the complete covalent structure of the human β chain of the JURKAT cell line. The molecule incorporates Vβ8.1, Jβ1.2, and Cβ1 sequences. Peptides 1 through 11 correspond to the complete variable segments and peptides 12–22 model the Cβ segment. (■), Gammagard; (●) Sandoglobulin; (□), conjugate control. Enzyme linked immunosorbent assay was performed as described in ref. *8*. **(B)** Localization of peptides recognized by IgG autoantibodies in a model for the 3-D structure of the complete immunoglobulin domains of the TCRβ chain. Peptide number 3 corresponds to the CDR1 segment; peptide number 8 is contained in the FR3 of the Vβ and peptide number 17 corresponds to a large forward projecting loop in the Cβ domain. The model was first presented in *(8)*.

2. ANTI-TCR AUTOANTIBODIES IN NORMAL PHYSIOLOGICAL PROCESSES

2.1. Aging

The cross-over age at which a pronounced decline in IgM and increase in IgG autoantibody concentrations in humans occurs is the sixth decade of life. We carried out studies in C57Bl/6 mice and found that the titers of autoantibodies to the TCR at age 16 mo were significantly higher than in younger individuals at four months *(29)*. The mouse observations are consistent with previous studies documenting a rise in IgG autoantibodies to immunoglobulins and TCR epitopes as a function of age *(9–11)*.

2.2. Pregnancy

The fetus is a natural allograft protected from immunological rejection by a complex set of structural and regulatory mechanisms *(30)*. Wang et al. *(14)* determined whether healthy pregnant women differed significantly from healthy nonpregnant controls in their capacity to produce autoantibodies to defined antigenic determinants of the α/β TCR. Although the two groups of women expressed comparable levels of autoantibodies against the intact recombinant TCR containing the complete Vα/Vβ structures, analysis of their comparative reactivity against individual peptide segments of the TCR indicated enhanced reactivity to regions corresponding to the CDR1 of the TCR α chain and to the FR3 of the variable region of the β chain in the pregnant women. The increased reactivity of IgG autoantibodies in the pregnant women was particularly marked in the case of peptide epitopes corresponding to the "switch" region joining the variable and constant domains. This region corresponds to peptides 10 and 11 of the β chain set in Fig. 1. The phenomenon of reactivity against the CDR3/J segment was noted with both the TCR α and β chains, and the reactivity was found to be directed against highly conserved determinants in these molecules. Antibodies to this region of the TCR are lacking in nonpregnant controls. It is possible, thus, that autoantibodies directed against conserved regions of the TCR might suppress the T-cell reactivity against fetal determinants.

3. APPEARANCE OF ANTI-TCR AUTOANTIBODIES IN HUMAN ALLOTRANSPLANTATION

Autoantibodies against TCRs have previously been found in two alloimmunization situations in humans: renal transplantation *(31)* and pregnancy, as described above. More recently, we *(15)* carried out longitudinal studies of human heart transplant recipients in which autoantibody production to the following antigens was monitored: a recombinant single chain TCR Vα/Vβ construct; a set of nested, overlapping peptides spanning the complete covalent structure of an individual TCR β chain; and a set of peptides spanning the first complementarity determining (CDR) segments of 24 distinct human Vβ gene products. The goals were to define the time course, epitope specificity and recognition heterogeneity of the autoantibody response. Autoantibodies against intact and peptide-defined Vβ and Cβ determinants were found to be generated following human heart allotransplantation. The responses generally showed an increase following transplantation and a subsequent decrease with time, a result analogous to the antibody response observed upon a single immunization with an experimental antigen. However, some patients showed elevated responses for as long as 12 mo following the transplant. Analyses of the anti-CDR1 auto-antibody spectrotype disclosed individualized differences among the patients, but five of the eight patients characterized in detail consistently showed elevated IgG binding to CDR1 peptide epitopes of the Vβ6.1, 21.1, and 22.1 gene families. Autoantibodies to CDR1 epitopes of Vβ7.1 and 8.1 were elevated in pre-trans-plant sera and remained high after transplantation. Similarly, the increase in levels of certain other autoantibodies that are usually present in low quantity, e.g., the anti-Vβ2.1, 3.1 and anti-24.1 antibodies, was not impressive. Since allografting often involves restricted T-cell responses to MHC antigens *(32,33)*, it would be expected that autoantibodies complementary to epitopes on these molecules would arise following the allograft response. The generation of clono-typic autoantibodies to TCR has been described in human renal transplantation *(31)*, consistent with our own results on autoantibody binding to the intact Vα/Vβ construct. In our experiments, there was a great disparity between the MHC haplotypes of the donors and recipients, and substantial individual differences among the patients. The degree of restriction in the autoantibody response was surprising, therefore, and suggests a common step in recognition and regula-tion of the response to allografts. Figure 2 illustrates the time course of IgG autoantibody binding to autoantigens and to the control protein ovalbumin for two patients followed over one year following transplantation. The antigens here were the recombinant single chain TCR containing Vα and Vβ domains isolated from the monoclonal T-cell line JURKAT *(12)*, the irrelevant protein antigen ovalbumin, and CDR1 and FR3 peptides duplicating the segments of individual Vβ gene products chosen on the basis of their reactivity with the autoantibodies. Patient 13 showed minimal binding to the irrelevant antigen and slightly elevated binding to the recombinant Vα/Vβ construct. The sera of this patient, however, contained substantial levels of autoantibodies to the CDR1 epitope of the human Vβ21.1 gene product and the Vβ22.1 gene prod-uct. Elevated autoantibody activity against FR3 epitopes of the human Vβ8.1 and 17.1 gene products was also noted. The individual nature of the transplant recipient responses to distinct Vβ products is illustrated by the comparison of patient 14 and patient 13. None of the titers in patient 14 reached the magnitude achieved against the Vβ21.1 gene product by patient 13. However, patient 14 showed an overall increase in autoantibody binding to the intact single chain TCR, and a decrease in binding to the irrelevant antigen ovalbumin over the time period studied. Autoantibody binding to the CDR1 peptide of Vβ7.1 showed a transient elevation at four months followed by a decline in patient 14, whereas binding to the CDR1 of Vβ21.1 showed an elevation at five months

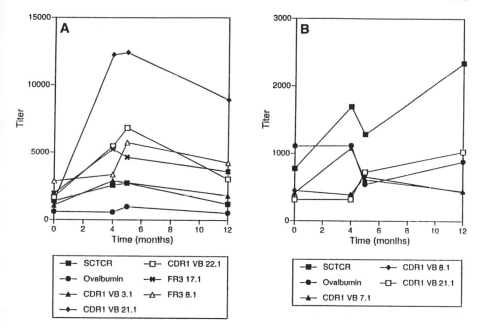

Fig. 2. Time course of autoantibody binding in two transplant patients to the recombinant single chain TCR, the irrelevant protein ovalbumin and a set of TCR epitopes to which the respective sera showed significant binding. (**A**) Patient number 13; (**B**) Patient number 14. (Taken from ref. *15*).

and a slow increase by 12 months. We chose ovalbumin as a useful irrelevant antigen because approx 70% of healthy individuals in Tucson *(9,11)* and elsewhere *(34)* have high levels of natural IgG antibodies to this common dietary protein, and the levels of such antibodies might be taken as an indicator of the capacity of the different individuals to mount secondary immune responses. Fig. 2 illustrates two key points. First, each patient has an individual profile of reactivities. Second, the process of autoimmunization is not uniform, in that the time course of the responses to both the recombinant Vα/Vβ constructs and the individual peptide segments of autologous TCRs can show different kinetics. Thus, even though the anti-TCR response to allografting displays kinetics superficially resembling that of a response to a single immunization, the mechanism of processing the autologous TCRs in different individuals might be disparate.

4. ANTI-TCR AUTOANTIBODIES IN AUTOIMMUNE DISEASES

4.1. Rheumatoid Arthritis

Because autoantibodies to immunoglobulins and other autoantigens have been observed in rheumatoid arthritis (RA) and systemic lupus erythematosus (SLE), we carried out studies to determine whether autoantibodies to TCRs were also apparent in patients with these diseases. Table 1 gives the geometric means of the titers for IgM autoantibodies displaying binding to TCR Vβ

Table 1
Geometric Mean Titers of Igm Autoantibodies to TCR Vβ Peptide Epitopes

		Titer		
Group	Number of individuals	Blank (No antigen)	pep CDR1	pep FR3
Asymptomatic	32	24	95	200
RA	14	66[a]	708[a]	324
SLE	8	23	36[b]	194
OA	10	20	39[b]	47[b]

[a] Significance of $p < 0.01$ by comparison (Wilcoxon 2-sample tests) with the asymptomatic group.
[b] Significance of $p < 0.05$ by comparison with the asymptomatic group.
RA, rheumatoid arthritis; SLE, systemic lupus erythematosus; OA, osteoarthritis. Human serum samples were provided by David E. Yocum, M.D., Arizona Arthritis Center, Tucson. "Blank" control plates did not receive antigen, but were blocked with the gelatin containing dilutant buffer.

epitopes from various groups of normal subjects (asymptomatic) and clinically ill individuals with RA, SLE, or osteoarthritis (OA). Osteoarthritis, which is not an autoimmune inflammatory disease, served as the control group for RA, as did the asymptomatic group. RA patients have been established to express relatively large quantities of autoantibodies, predominantly of the IgM class, that bind to human immunoglobulin determinants localized to the Fc fragment of the γ heavy chain (3,4). The majority of RA patients we studied displayed elevated levels of autoantibodies directed against TCR determinants, with the major reactivity directed towards the CDR1 peptide segment of our test Vβ sequence (9,11,35). It is interesting that the SLE and OA patients actually had significantly lower levels of IgM autoantibodies to TCR determinants than did the normal individuals. A comparison (not shown) of anti-TCR IgG autoantibodies showed slightly decreased levels in RA relative to the healthy and OA groups, but significantly elevated levels in the SLE group. Analysis of autoantibody binding to peptides duplicating the linear sequence of Vβ8.1, Vα1, and Vλ Mcg showed that the RA autoantibody profile was relatively simple, in that the major binding activity was in the IgM molecules and was restricted to the CDR1 peptide, the FR3 peptide, a joining segment peptide and the constant region loop. Little IgG autoantibody activity was detected. When present, the IgG activity was reactive with the same antigenic components. By contrast, sera from the SLE individuals had IgG autoantibodies reacting with a large group of different TCR β chain peptides. The IgM RA autoantibodies to the TCR epitopes were clearly distinct in specificity from the classical rheumatoid factors, which are directed against Fcγ.

4.2. Systemic Lupus Erythematosus

SLE patients contained IgG autoantibodies directed against numerous peptides of the TCR β chain, TCRα chain and CDR1 and FR3 peptides of the Mcg immunoglobulin λ light chain. One interesting observation was that SLE patients also had detectable autoantibodies against the CDR2 segment of the Vα construct. Such anti-Vα autoantibodies were not found in sera from normal women used as controls or in sera of pregnant women *(14)*. Overall, these studies suggest that the peptide-binding profiles of autoantibodies detected in various diseases are characteristic to individual diseases. We are presently testing the link between the antigenic specificity and the role of the autoantibodies in immunopathogenesis or immunoregulation, by developing monoclonal autoantibodies that replicate the activity of the patient antibodies and by study of their biological properties and gene usage.

5. ANALYSIS OF ANTI-TCR AUTOANTIBODIES IN RETROVIRUS INFECTIONS

5.1. Murine Retrovirally Induced Lymphoproliferative Disease (MAIDS)

Autoantibodies directed against immunoglobulin and TCR epitopes have been observed in autoimmune diseases, but the factors regulating the appearance of such antibodies are largely unknown. With respect to autoantibodies showing anti-immunoglobulin, rheumatoid factor type of activity, these have been shown to occur following infection as well as in rheumatoid arthritis. Such autoantibodies have been proposed to serve an immunoregulatory role both in normal physiological "immunization" and in infection *(1)*. Another class of RFs mediates pathological effects *(36)*. The infection of susceptible strains of mice, e.g., C57Bl/6, with the LP-BM5 retrovirus mixture induces a lymphoproliferative disease (MAIDS), beginning with lymphoid proliferation and expression of high levels of serum gamma-globulin, and followed by the generation of an acquired immunodeficiency disease *(37,38)*. B-cells are the major target of the LP-BM5 virus; B and T cells hyperproliferation, hypergammaglobulinemia, splenomegaly and lymphadenopathy result from the infection. Deghanpisheh et. al. *(18)* analyzed the production of IgG autoantibodies to TCR peptide epitopes following experimental infection with the LP-BM5 derivative of murine leukemia virus. Autoantibodies to particular Vβ CDR1 epitopes showed peak titers between 6-12 weeks following infection and generally diminished at the later time points. The infected animals did not show elevated levels of antibodies to the exogenous antigens, ovalbumin and bovine serum albumin, during this time period. Polyclonal autoantibody responses were evident, because specificities directed against murine Vβ1, Vβ8.1 and Vβ8.2, as well as against certain human peptide epitopes orthologous to murine Vβ11 were detected. Watson et al. *(18–20)* found that many of the immunological deficiencies resulting from the retroviral infection could be at least partially corrected by administration of certain TCR Vβ peptides shown to be highly autoantigenic in this infection/autoimmunity model. The infected mice tended to show an increase in the T_H2 type cytokine production and a decrease in the T_H1 type cytokine production cells. The cytokine shifts were significantly ameliorated by injection of human Vβ8.1 CDR1 peptide, but not by administration of a control peptide (the homologous sequence from the λ light chain Mcg). In addition, the B- and T-cell reactivities were substantially increased in the peptide-treated infected mice, and the animals regained the capacity to resist challenge with living cryptosporidium parasites. We generated monoclonal murine autoantibodies at the peak of the retrovirus-induced autoantibody production and analyzed the antibodies structurally and functionally. These results are consistent with a number of current studies showing that viral infection *(39)* and bacterial infection *(40)* can generate autoimmune reactivity.

5.2. Infection of Humans with HIV-1

Autoimmune reactivity is a frequent consequence of infection with human immunodeficiency virus *(41,42)*. Autoantibodies against a number of cell types and MHC antigen epitopes *(43)* and the Fab fragment of human IgG immunoglobulin following HIV infection have been documented *(5,6)*. Some workers observed an inverse relationship between the levels of the autoantibodies and the $CD4^+$ cells in circulation *(5)*. In our initial studies, Lake et al. *(16)* investigated the serological crossreactions of purified IgG from sera of HIV-infected individuals (HIVIG) by using nested sets of synthetic overlapping peptides duplicating the covalent structures of TCRs and immunoglobulin λ light chains. We concluded that two processes of autoantibody production occurred in HIV-infected subjects. In the first process, IgG autoantibodies to putative regulatory variable region CDR1 and FR3 epitopes were detected in HIVIG at levels approx 10-fold greater than in IVIG prepared from pooled sera of healthy humans. The second evident process is the involvement of antigen mimicry in anti-TCR autoimmunization. A conserved peptide sequence in the major neutralizing V3 loop determinant of HIV-1 gp120 and the FR4 segment of the TCR Vβ chain was identified. Affinity-purified antibodies to the synthetic V3 loop peptide were bound by a recombinant single chain TCR and by a synthetic TCR joining segment peptide containing the FR4 sequence. The two cross reactive peptide sequences are as follows:

Synth V3(IIIB):   R I H I Q R G P G - R A F Y T T K

Synth Jβ (1.2): A N Y G Y T F G S G T R L T V V

Conversely, affinity-purified autoantibodies to the TCR FR4 peptide from pooled IgG of HIV-1 infected individuals were bound by the V3 loop peptide and the single chain TCR. Inhibition studies indicated that the crossreactive immunizing antigen was the V3 loop of the viral glycoprotein. These results substantiated the conclusion that the anti-TCR autoantibody production was a consequence of retroviral infection, and localized the antigenic epitopes within the Vβ/Vα constructs. The finding that retrovirus-infected individuals reacted to a highly antigenic portion of the gp120 by forming antibodies crossreactive

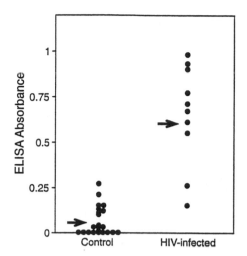

Fig. 3. Comparison of individual values for IgG autoantibody binding to the single chain TCR by 10 HIV+ patients and 22 healthy, uninfected individuals. Individual sera were assayed in triplicate by ELISA at a dilution of 1/200. "Blank" values of binding of each serum to pig gelatin were subtracted from each value. The means of the two populations (normals 0.06 ± 0.02: HIV+ 0.62 ± 0.09) differ significantly with $p < 0.01$. The means of the ELISA absorbances are indicated by arrows. (Taken from ref. *17*).

with TCR epitopes raises cautions regarding the choice of peptides for potential vaccination against HIV.

Subsequently, we performed longitudinal studies of anti-TCR autoantibodies in HIV-1 infected individuals, sera from uninfected individuals and sera from individuals infected with a nonviral agent, the fungus *Coccidioides immitis (17)*. We quantitated the levels of autoantibodies by titration using enzyme-linked-immunosorbent assay. The use of the intact TCR and its synthetic epitopes permitted the characterization of "autoantibody CDR recognition spectrotypes" in individual sera. The autoantibody levels against certain synthetic epitopes were substantially elevated in HIV-1 infected subjects relative to the reactivities in the control groups. Certain HIV sera showed relatively high level autoantibodies to a subset of the CDR1 peptide epitopes. Two patients who subsequently developed AIDS showed particularly high reactivity to human Vβ2.1, 8.1, 10.1, and 22.1 epitopes. The patients followed in this longitudinal study were generally healthy, although the autoantibody levels to the TCR epitopes and the recombinant single chain TCR (Fig. 3) were high at initial presentation and remained high during a two year course of follow-up. The results indicated that production of autoantibodies to TCR Vβ epitopes is a general consequence of HIV infection, with the response being individualized and showing some restriction in specificity for different subsets of Vβ CDR1 markers. Shifts in autoantibody subpopulations reactive with different TCR epitopes often occurred with time. Collaborative studies with Süsal's group (Marchalonis, J. J., Garza, A., Lake, D. F., Landsperger, W. J. ,and Susal, C., submitted) established that affinity-purified autoantibodies against immuno-globulin Fab determinants contain subpopulations of antibodies cross-reactive with TCR variable region markers. To establish the specificity and biological roles of such autoantibodies, it is necessary to generate monoclonal autoanti-bodies and assess them structurally and functionally.

6. MONOCLONAL AUTOANTIBODIES TO TCR VARIABLE DOMAIN EPITOPES

6.1. Generation and Specificity of Human Autoantibodies

Our studies with human sera and purified intravenous immunoglobulin preparations established that autoantibodies to TCRs can be both the IgM and IgG isotypes. We used several strategies to isolate naturally occurring mono-clonal antibodies with anti-TCR activity, i.e., human myeloma proteins *(24)*, and monoclonal immunoglobulin preparations with this activity derived by transformation of human B-cells with Epstein–Barr virus *(23)*, formation of murine hybridomas by fusion of spleen cells of 21-d old motheaten (mev) mice *(26)*, fusion of splenic B-cells of LP-BM5 retrovirally infected mice *(27)*, for-mation of heterohybridomas using peripheral blood B-cells of healthy humans or RA subjects, and formation of heterohybridomas using B-cells from syn-ovial tissue of RA patients *(25)*.

Two of 70 EBV- transformed human B-cell lines reacted with peptide-defined TCR epitopes. A $\kappa\mu$ autoantibody (IARC 307) that was studied in detail showed marked specificity for the CDR1 peptide of the human Vβ8.1 gene product *(23)*. The κ chain of this monoclonal autoantibody had a Vκ3 sequence related to the "a" group and used the Jκ2 segment. The heavy chain had a V$_H$3 sequence essentially identical to the germline sequence DP54 and incorporated the J$_H$6C minigene. The murine $\kappa\mu$ antibody (UN37-5) derived from mev mice used a gene from the V$_H$ J606 family. This V$_H$ gene is similar to a previously reported germline V$_H$ gene representing the unique J606 family V$_H$ gene used by mev-derived monoclonal antibodies directed against thymocyte and red blood cell antigens *(44)*. The V$_L$ gene sequence of the autoantibody to TCRs belongs to the Vκ4/5 gene family and showed 87% homology to the VKOX-1 germline gene *(45)*. Interestingly, the anti-TCR Vκ sequence showed greater than 95% identity at the amino acid level with Vκ chains from IgM hybridomas specific for DNA and the influenza virus hemagglutinin. This Vκ sequence has not been previously reported to be utilized in autoantibodies derived from viable motheaten mice *(44)*. Several monoclonal IgM autoantibodies were derived from the spleens of retrovirally infected C57/Bl6 mice *(27)* that were capable of binding recombinant single chain TCRs, intact T-cells bearing the appropri-ate TCRα/β and certain CDR1 peptides in the set of 24 human Vβ sequences. Two such antibody molecules were characterized in detail. The first antibody

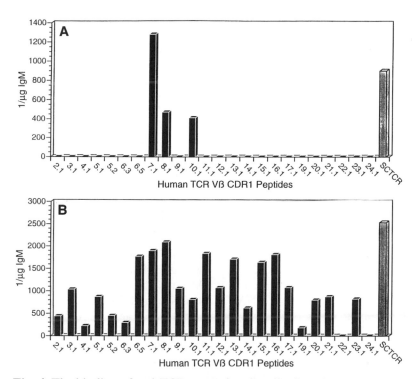

Fig. 4. The binding of anti-TCR monoclonal antibodies (**A**) ATM-1; (**B**) ATM 2 to the panel of synthetic human TCR Vβ CDR1 peptides and to a recombinant human single chain TCR *(30)*, as measured by ELISA. In these assays, serial two-fold dilutions of cell culture supernatants were carried out in duplicate. An absorbance of 0.250 at 405 nm was taken as the minimum value indicating positive binding. The concentration of antibody in the cell culture supernatants was determined using an antigen capture ELISA carried out simultaneously with the binding assay. The graphed data are the inverse of the amount of antibody that would give an absorbance of 0.250. The inverse of the amount of antibody is used to provide a datum point that correlates positively with increased binding. (Taken from ref. *27*).

showed specificity restricted to Vβ7.1, 8.1, and 10.1 gene segments, whereas the second antibody bound to the majority of CDR1 peptide homologs tested. This is illustrated in Fig. 4. These two IgM monoclonals utilized V_H genes exhibiting dissimilarities to one another in their FR and CDR amino acid sequences. One of these V_H genes (ATM-2) had greater homology to the full length V_H p.10.15.1 *(46)*, which is utilized by an IgG molecule capable of binding 4-hydroxy-3-nitrophenol-acetyl. The germline gene exhibiting the highest homology was the V130 germline V_H. With the exception of a two residue deletion in FR1, all of the residues in the second monoclonal anti-TCR appear to be in the germline configuration. The germline V_H gene with the greater homology to the other monoclonal antibody (ATM-1) is V23 (47) . This V_H gene specifies

```
                                    * * * *CDR1*  * *  * * * * * * *
IARC307       E I V̇ M T Q S P A T L S V S P G E R A T L S C R A S Q S V S S N L A - - - -
UN37-5        Q I V L T Q S P A I M S A S P G G K V T I S C S A S S S V S Y M Y - - - - -
N-anti-HIVᵃ   D I V M T Q S P D S L A V S L G E R A T I N C K S S Q S V L Y S S N N Y L A
P-anti-DNAᵇ               T Q S P S S L S A S V G D R V T I T C R A S Q S T G S F L N - - - -
Anti IgGᶜ     E I V L T Q S P G T L S L S P G E R A T L S C R A S Q S V S S S Y L A - - -

                                    * * CDR2  * *
IARC307       W Y Q Q K P G Q A P R L L I Y G A S I R A T G I P D R F S G S G S G T E F T
UN37-5        W Y Q Q K P G S S P K P W I Y R T S N L A S G V P A R F S G S G S G T S Y S
N-anti-HIVᵃ   W Y Q Q K P G K P P K L L I Y W A S T R E S G V P D R F S G S G S G T D F T
P-anti-DNAᵇ   W Y Q Q K P G K A P K L L I Y A A S S W Q N G V P S R F S G S G S G T D F T
Anti IgGᶜ     W Y Q Q K P G Q A P R L L I Y G A S S R A T G I P D R F S F S F S F T D F T

                                    * * CDR3* * * * * *
IARC307       L T I S S L Q S E D F A V Y Y C Q Q Y N N W P H - - - F G Q G T K L E I - K
UN37-5        L T I S S M E A E D A A T Y Y C Q Q Y H S Y P P T - F G A G T K L E L - K
N-anti-HIVᵃ   L T I S S L Q A E D V A V Y Y C Q Q Y Y S T P P L T F G G G T K V G I L R
P-anti-DNAᵇ   L T I S S L Q P E D F A T Y F C Q Q S Y S T P - L T F G G G T K V E I - K
Anti IgGᶜ     L T I S R L E P E D F A V Y Y C Q Q Y G S S P - L T F G G G T K V E I - K
```

Fig. 5. Comparative alignments of complete Vκ sequences of one human (IARC307) and one murine (UN37.5) monoclonal IgM autoantibody to Vβ CDR1 peptide epitopes and a naturally occurring IgM autoantibody to HIV (N-anti-HIV), a pathological autoantibody to DNA (P-anti-DNA) and the Vκ3 sequence of a monoclonal myeloma protein having rheumatoid factor activity. IARC307, *(23)*. UN37.5, *(26)*. N-anti-HIV, *(49)*. P-anti-DNA, *(50)*. Anti-IgG; Vκ3 myeloma protein GLO, WA idiotype, *(51)*.

the heavy chain of a monoclonal IgM autoantibody that binds spectrin, fluorescein, and interestingly, when used by another antibody, 4-hydroxyl-3-nitrophenol-acetyl. Overall, the IgM autoantibodies to TCR VβCDR1 segments do not show significant sequence relatedness to rheumatoid factors, a finding consistent with the evident differences in antigenic specificity.

Detailed comparisons of the complete Vκ/V$_H$ sequences of the anti-TCR autoantibodies with corresponding Vκ/V$_H$ sequences of natural antibodies and rheumatoid factors are illustrated in Figs. 5 and 6, respectively. Although the sample is too small to draw definitive conclusions, it is interesting that there is a high degree of identity in all three CDR segments of the Vκ segments. With respect to the CDR3 segment, the four human Vκs as well as the murine sequence begin with QQ and have a universally conserved P at position 7. The V$_H$ comparisons, however, show considerable sequence diversity in the CDR3 segments. The pathologic anti-DNA sequence in Fig. 6 represents the human V$_H$4 subgroup, whereas the remaining human sequences are of the V$_H$3 subgroup. It is most noteworthy that the pathologic anti-DNA CDR3 sequence *(50)* is considerably longer than CDR3 found in the other antibodies. Perhaps this is the structural correlate of the mono- versus poly-specificity of the antibodies. The murine ATM-1 CDR3 sequence is quite short. Interestingly, this molecule is extremely specific in its peptide recognition capacity, whereas the ATM-2 molecule is more promiscuous in its capacity to recognize the Vβ CDR1 synthetic peptide epitopes *(27)*. Nevertheless, both are capable of binding human

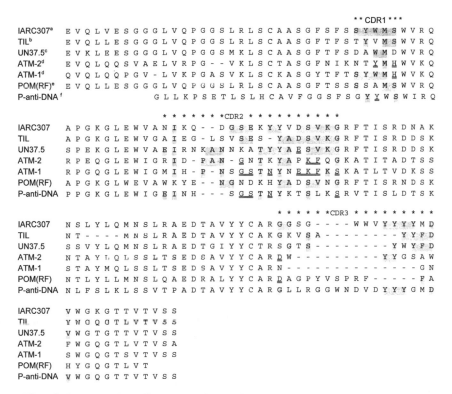

Fig. 6. Comparative alignment of complete V_H sequences of human and murine monoclonals autoantibodies to TCR Vβ epitopes. IARC307, TIL, UN37.5, ATM-2, ATM-1 with V_H of a rheumatoid factor and that of a pathological anti-DNA molecule. (**A**) *(23)*; (**B**) *(52)*; (**C**) *(26)*; (**D**) *(27)*; (**E**) *(53)*; (**F**) *(50)*.

monoclonal T-cells bearing the proper Vβ (Vβ8.1) and can synergize with microbial enterotoxins superantigens in activating murine T-cell subsets bearing the appropriate Vβ products. The five monoclonal autoantibodies to TCRs epitopes do not show particularly striking homologies with one another.

Although the transformed and hybridoma monoclonal antibodies studied to date are all of the IgM isotype, monoclonal IgG myeloma proteins that show specificity for TCR variable region epitopes *(24)* have also been identified. In a screen of more than 20 human IgG myeloma proteins for binding to a recombinant single chain TCR containing the complete Vβ 8.1 and Vα1 structures; the sets of synthetic peptide epitopes corresponding to a complete TCR β chain; a set of CDR1 epitopes corresponding to 24 human Vβ gene products; and intact monoclonal T-cells, two antibodies were found that displayed strong binding to the recombinant TCR. Five antibodies displayed binding to a synthetic peptide corresponding to the CDR1 segment of the YT35 Vβ8.1. On a mass basis, the binding activity was approx thousandfold greater than present in pooled polyclonal IVIG. The binding activity was confined to the $(Fab)_2$

fragment, and it was specifically inhibited by appropriate peptide determinants. Consistent with the previous results, the different TCR-binding IgG monoclonal antibodies showed distinct binding patterns when tested against the set of 24 synthetic Vβ sequences, ranging from highly specific to relatively promiscuous reactivity. At this point in time, it is clear that all autoantibodies directed against TCR peptide epitopes do not bind to intact recombinant TCR and intact T-cells. However, examples of both IgM and IgG autoantibodies have now been identified that bind to the intact TCRs as determined by immunofluorescence in flow cytometry studies *(11,15,27)*. Further, such autoantibodies are shown to functionally synergize with superantigens in the activation of T-cell subsets *(27)*. The molecules identified so far do not have unusually long or particularly distinct V_H CDR3 segments. We hypothesize that these autoantibodies can serve both immunoregulatory and pathogenic roles. The binding affinities and monogamy/promiscuity of TCR V region recognition can be anticipated to contribute to the functional role of the autoantibodies.

7. CONCLUSIONS AND DISCUSSION

Autoantibodies against TCRs arise under normal physiological conditions such as aging and pregnancy, in autoimmune diseases, in allografting and in viral infections. Less dramatic, but often significant increases in autoantibody titers have also been observed following fungal infections in humans *(17)* and in mice injected intraperitoneally with mineral oils *(48)*. In general, the levels of such autoantibodies are highest in autoimmune diseases and at certain time points following retroviral infections. We have found anti-TCR activity in IgM, IgG and IgA molecules e.g., the high level IgM activity in RA and the high level IgG activity in SLE and infection with HIV-1. Although patients show individual differences, certain common features of the activity profiles against Vβ CDR1 homologs (spectrotype analysis) were found in transplant patients, RA patients and HIV-1 infected individuals. Further study is required is to establish definitive correlation between the characteristic CDR-peptide binding spectrotypes and the individual diseases. Monoclonal anti-TCR autoantibodies have been generated in humans and mice that were not purposefully immunized with TCR antigens. Some of these monoclonal autoantibodies were bound by intact TCRs as well as by its peptide epitopes, and could modulate the in vitro cellular response to Vβ-specific antigens. We hypothesize that distinct subsets of autoantibodies to TCR-V-domain epitopes, particularly regulatory idiotopes defined by CDR1 and CDR4 sequences (the latter is a subsegment of the FR3), can be either immunoregulatory or pathogenic. An interesting feature of certain monoclonal anti-TCR autoantibodies that might bear significantly on the biological function is their apparent specificity for only a few of the CDR-1 peptide epitopes from the set of Vβ gene products tested. Other anti-TCR autoantibodies bind the majority of synthetic CDR1. Monoclonal TCRs are known to show promiscuous binding to different peptide epitopes presented by MHC molecules *(49)*. The finding that monoclonal antibodies can show broad spectrum recognition of homologous peptides presents interesting parallels. Functional consequences of the elaboration of anti-TCR autoantibodies probably follow from the recognition specificity and use of particular isotypes. We propose that continued functional studies of the monoclonal autoantibodies generated in infections and in autoimmune diseases will help resolve specific questions related to normal immunoregulation, as opposed to the generation and maintenance of autoimmune disease.

8. SUMMARY

Asymptomatic humans and mice have low constitutive levels of autoantibodies directed against autologous TCRs, particularly peptide-defined and conformational epitopes associated with the variable domains. Because of the highly orthologous relationships among many Vβ genes of humans and mice, it is possible to analyze the responses of both species using the same gene probes and autoantibodies. The quantitative levels (titers) and isotypes of autoantibodies vary with autoimmune disease, aging, allotransplantation, pregnancy, and microbial infections. In particular, retroviral infections of both species cause a pronounced increase in autoantibodies against defined TCR epitopes, which in HIV-infected humans, may represent responses to mimicry of self antigens and dysregulation of the autoimmune process. Monoclonal autoantibodies have been generated from both species, with some antibody molecules showing exquisite specificity for Vβ CDR1 synthetic epitopes and other antibodies reacting with a broad spectrum of epitopes ("Promiscuity in recognition"). These molecules can interact directly with TCR αβ-bearing T-cells and can modulate immunological processes such as cellular activation by microbial enterotoxin superantigens. We hypothesize that autoantibodies against TCR variable region epitopes can carry out both immunoregulatory functions and participate in the generation of autoimmune disease. The mechanisms underlying the specific differences in functional activity of different antibodies and at different disease stages remain to be determined.

ACKNOWLEDGMENTS

This work was supported in part by grant #9517 from Arizona Disease Control Research Commission, and a grant from Baxter Biotechnology, Hyland Division. The authors would like to thank Diana Humphreys for expert assistance in preparation of the manuscript.

REFERENCES

1. Carson, D. A., Chen, P. P., Fox, R. I., Kipps, T. J., Jirik, F., Goldfien, R. D., et al. (1987) Rheumatoid factor and immune networks. *Ann. Rev. Immunol.* **5,** 109–126.
2. Artandi, S. E., Calame, K. L., Morrison, S. L., and Bonagura, V. R. (1992) Monoclonal IgM rheumatoid factors bind to IgG at a discontinuous epitope comprized of amino acid loops from heavy-chain constant-region domain-2 and domain-3. *Proc. Natl. Acad. Sci. USA* **89,** 94–98.

3. Artandi, S. E., Calame, K. L., Morrison, S. L., and Bonagura, V. R. (1992) Monoclonal IgM rheumatoid factors bind to IgG at a discontinuous epitope comprized of amino acid loops from heavy-chain constant-region domain-2 and domain-3. *Proc. Natl. Acad. Sci. USA* **89,** 94–98.

4. Sasso, E. H., Barber, C. V., Nardella, F. A., Yount, W. J., and Mannik, M. (1988) Antigenic specificities of human monoclonal and polyclonal IgM rheumatoid factors. The Cγ2-Cγ3 interface region contains the major determinants. *J. Immunol.* **140,** 3098–3107.

5. Süsal, C., Daniel, V., Oberg, H. H. Terners, P., Hüth-Kühne, A., Zimmermann, R., et al. (1992) Striking inverse association of IgG anti-Fab antibodies and CD4 counts in patients with acquired immunodeficiency syndrome (AIDS)/AIDS-related complex. *Blood* **79,** 954–957.

6. Silvestria, D., Di Loreto, M., Romito, A., Grizzuti, M. A., and Dammacco, F. (1994) Distribution and antigenic analysis of circulating F(ab')2-reactive IgG in patients with HIV-1 infection. *Clin. Immunol. Immunopathol.* **73,** 229–234.

7. Kazim, A. L. and Atassi, M. Z. (1980) A novel and comprehensive synthetic approach for the elucidation of protein antigenic structures. *Biochem. J.* **191,** 261–265.

8. Marchalonis, J. J., Kaymaz, H., Dedeoglu, F., Schluter, S. F., Yocum, D. E., and Edmundson, A. B. (1992) Human autoantibodies reactive with synthetic auto-antigens from T-cell receptor β chain. *Proc. Natl. Acad. Sci. USA* **89,** 3325–3329.

9. Marchalonis, J. J., Kaymaz. H., Schluter, S. F., and Yocum, D. E. (1993) Human autoantibodies to a synthetic putative T-cell receptor β-chain regulatory idiotype: expression in autoimmunity and aging. *Exp. Clin. Immunogenet.* **10,** 1–15.

10. Marchalonis, J. J., Schluter, S. F., Wilson, L., Yocum, D. E., Boyer, J. R., and Kay, M. M. B. (1993) Natural human antibodies to synthetic peptide autoantigens: correlations with age and autoimmune disease. *Gerontology* **39,** 65–79.

11. Marchalonis, J. J., Schluter, S. F., Wang, E., Dehghanpisheh, K., Lake, D., Yocum, D. E., et al. (1994) Synthetic autoantigens of immunoglobulins and T-cell receptors: their recognition in aging, infection and autoimmunity. *Proc. Soc. Exp. Biol.* **207,** 129–147.

12. Lake, D. F., Bernstein, R. M. S., Hersh, E. M., Kaymaz, H., Schluter, S. F., and Marchalonis, J. J. (1994) Construction and serological characterization of a recombinant human single chain T-cell receptor (single chain TCR). *Biochem. Biophys. Res. Commun.* **201,** 1502–1509.

13. Lake, D. F., Landsperger, W. J., Bernstein, R. M. S., Schluter, S. F., and Marchalonis, J. J. (1995) Characterization of autoantibodies directed against T cell receptors. *Adv. Exp. Med. Bio.* **383,** 223–229.

14. Wang, E., Lake, D., Winfield, J. B., and Marchalonis, J. J. (1994) IgG autoantibodies to "switch peptide" determinants of Tcr α/β in human pregnancy. *Clin. Immunol. Immunopathol.* **73,** 224–228.

15. Marchalonis, J. J., Kaymaz, H., Schluter, S. F., Lake, D. F., Landsperger, W. J., and Sucui-Foca, N. (1997) Autoantibodies to Tcr β chains in human heart transplantation: epitope and spectrotype analyses and kinetics of response. *Exp. Clin. Immunogenet.* **13,** 181–191.

16. Lake, D. F., Schluter, S. F., Wang, E., Bernstein, R. M. S., Edmundson, A. B., and Marchalonis, J. J. (1994) Autoantibodies to the α/β T-cell receptors in human

immunodeficiency virus (HIV) infection: dysregulation and mimicry. *Proc. Natl. Acad. Sci. USA* **91**, 10,849–10,853.

17. Marchalonis, J. J., Ampel, N. M., Schluter, S. F., Garza, A., Lake, D. F., Galgiani, J. N., et al. (1997) Analysis of autoantibodies to T-cell receptors among HIV-infected individuals: epitope analysis and time course. *Clin. Immunol. Immunopathol.* **82**, 174–189.

18. Dehghanpisheh, K., Huang, D., Schluter, S. F., Watson, R. R., and Marchalonis, J. J. (1995) Production of IgG autoantibodies to T-cell receptors in mice infected with the retrovirus LP-BM5. *Intl. Immunol.* **7**, 31–36.

19. Watson, R. R., Dehghanpisheh, K., Huang. D. S., Wood, S., Ardestani, S. K., Laing, B., et al. (1995) T-cell receptor Vβ CDR1 peptide administration moderates immune dysfunction and cytokine dysregulation induced by murine retrovirus infection. *J. Immunol.* **155**, 2282–2291.

20. Liang, B., Marchalonis, J. J., Zhang, Z., and Watson, R. R. (1996) Effects of vaccination against different T-cell receptors on maintenance of immune function during murine retrovirus infection. *Cell. Immunol.* **172**, 126–134.

21. Liang, B., Ardestani, S., Marchalonis, J. J., and Watson, R. R. (1996) Effects of T cell receptor dose and term of application during murine retrovirus infection and maintenance of immune function. *Immunology* **87**, 198–204.

22. Liang, B., Marchalonis, J. J., and Watson, R. R. (1997) Prevention of immune dysfunction, vitamin E deficiency and loss of *Cryptosporidium* resistance during murine retrovirus infection by T cell receptor peptide immunization. *Nutr. Res.* **17**, 677–692.

23. Dedeoglu, F., Kaymaz, H., Klein, G., and Marchalonis, J. J. (1993) Light and heavy chains specifying a human IgM κ autoantibody to a T-cell receptor Vβ-antigen. *Immunol. Lett.* **38**, 223–227.

24. Marchalonis, J. J., Garza, A., Landsperger, W. J., Schluter, S. F., and Wang, A-C. (1997) Binding of human IgG myeloma proteins to autologous T-cell receptor determinants. *Crit. Rev. Immunol.*, in press.

25. Schluter S. F., Marchalonis, J. J., and Yocum, D. E. unpublished observations.

26. Dehghanpisheh, K., Bona, C. A., and Marchalonis, J. J. (1996) Peptide Epitope Binding Specificity and Vκ and V$_H$ gene usage in a monoclonal IgM natural autoantibody to T-cell receptor CDR1 from a viable motheaten mouse. *Immunol. Investigations* **25**, 241–252.

27. Dehghanpisheh, K. and Marchalonis, J. J. (1997) Retrovirally induced mouse anti-TCR monoclonals can synergize the in vitro proliferative T cell response to bacterial superantigens. *Scand. J. Immunol.* **45**, 645–654.

28. Marchalonis, J. J. and Byers, V. S. (1997) Use of synthetic T-cell receptor derived peptides in therapy for autoimmunity and retroviral infections. *The Chemist* **74**, 3–9.

29. Liang, B., Zhang, Z., Inserra, P., Jiang, S., Lee, J., Garza, A., et al. unpublished observations.

30. Loke, Y. W. and King, A. (1991) Recent developments in the human maternal-fetal immune interaction. *Curr. Opin. Immunol.* **3**, 762–766.

31. Duffy, B. F., Mathew, J. N., Flye, M. W., and Mohanakumar, T. (1993) Development of autoantibodies to T-cell clonotypic structures in a liver-kidney allograft recipient. *Transplant.* **56**, 212-216.

32. Liu, Z., Sun, Y. K., Xi, Y. P., Hong, B., Harris, P. E., Reed, E. F., et al. (1993) Limited usage of T-cell receptor Vβ genes by allopeptide-specific T cells. *J. Immunol.* **150,** 3180–3186.

33. Hand, S. L., Alter, M. D., and Finn, O. J. (1996) T cell receptor β-chain repertoires are nonrandomly selected in responses to HLA-DR1. *Transplant.* **61,** 1084–1094.

34. Husby, S., Oxelus, V. A., Teisner, B., Jensenius, J. C. D., and Svehag, S. E. (1985) Humoral immunity to dietary antigens in healthy adults. *Int. Arch. Allergy Appl. Immun.* **77,** 416–422.

35. Landsperger, W. J., Schluter, S. F., Garza, A., Yocum, D. E., and Marchalonis, J. J. (1997) Fine specificity analysis of autoantibodies to T-cell receptor CDR1 segments in rheumatoid arthritis. *Ann. NY Acad.* **815,** 459–461.

36. Stewart, J. J., Agostoa, H., Litwin, S., Welsh, J. D., Shlomchik, M., Weigert, M., et al. (1997) A solution to the rheumatoid factor paradox. Pathologic rheumatoid factors can be tolerized by competition with natural rheumatoid factors. *J. Immunol.* **159,** 1728–1738.

37. Jolicoeur, P. (1991) Murine acquired immunodeficiency syndrome (MAIDS): an animal model to study the AIDS pathogenesis. *FASEB J.* **5,** 2398–2402.

38. Mosier, D. E., Yetter, R. A., and Morse, H. C., III. (1985) Retroviral induction of acute lymphoprolyferative disease and profound immunosuppression in adult C57BL/6 mice. *J. Exp. Med.* **161,** 766.

39. Faxvaag, A., Moen, T., and Dalen, A. B. (1993) Polyclonal activation of B-lymphocytes and induction of autoimmunity in retrovirus infected NMRI mice. *Scand. J. Immunol.* **38,** 459–462.

40. Luo, G., Fan, J.-L., Seetharamaiah, G. S., Desai, R. K., Dallas, J. S. D., Wagle, N., et al. (1993) Immunization of mice with *Yersinia enterocolitica* leads to the induction of antithyrotropin receptor antibodies. *J. Immunol.* **151,** 922–928.

41. Shearer, G. M. (1983) Allogeneic leukocytes as a possible factor in induction of aids in homosexual men. *N. Engl. J. Med.* **308,** 223–224.

42. Silvestris, F., Williams, R. C., Jr., and Dammacco, F. (1995) Autoreactivity in HIV-1 infection: The role of molecular mimicry. *Clin. Immunol. Immunopathol.* **75,** 197–205.

43. Golding, H., Robey, F. A., Gates, F. T., Linder, W., Beining, P. R., Hoffman, T., et al. (1988) Identification of homologous regions in human immunodeficiency virus I gp41 and human MHC class II β1 domain. I. Monoclonal antibodies against the gp41-derived peptide and patients' sera react with native HLA Class II antigens, suggesting a role for autoimmunity in the pathogenesis of acquired immune deficiency syndrome. *J. Exp. Med.* **167,** 914.

44. Kasturi, K. N., Mayer, R., Bona, C. A., Scott, V. R., and Sidman, C. L. (1990) Germline V genes encode viable motheaten mouse antibodies against thymocytes and red blood cells. *J. Immunol.* **145,** 2304–2311.

45. Griffiths, G. M., Berek, C., Kaartinen, M., and Milstein, C. (1984) Somatic mutation and the maturation of immune response to 2-phenyl oxazolone. *Nature* **312,** 271-275.

46. Boersch-Supan, M. E., Agarwal, S., Wenti-Scharf, M. E., and Imanski-Kari, T. (1985) Heavy chain variable region. Multiple gene segments encode anti-4-(hydroxy-3-nitro-phenyl)acetyl idiotypic antibodies. *J. Exp. Med.* **161,** 1271–1292.

47. Bothwell, A. L., Paskind, M., Reth, M., Imanishi-Kari, T., Rajewsky, K., and Baltimore, D. (1981) Heavy chain variable region contribution to the Npb family of antibodies: somatic mutation evident in a γ 2a variable region. *Cell* **124,** 625–637.

48. Satoh and Marchalonis, unpublished observations.
49. Harindranth, N., Ikematsu, H., Notkins, A. L., and Casali, P. (1993) Structure of the V_H and V_L segments of polyreactive and monoreactive human natural antibodies to HIV-1 and *Escherchia coli* β-galactosidase. *Intern. Immunol.* **5,** 1523–1533.
50. Waisman, A., Schoenfeld, Y., Blank, M., Ruiz, P. J., and Mozes, E. (1995) The pathogenic human monoclonal anti-DNA that induces experimental systemic lupus erythematosus in mice is encoded by a V_H4 gene segment. *Intern. Immunol.* **7,** 689–696.
51. Capra, J. D. and Kehoe, J. M., (1975) Hypervariable regions, idiotypy and the antibody combining site. *Adv. Immunol.* **20,** 1–40.
52. Wang, A-C., Wang, I. T., and Fudenberg, H. H. (1977) Immunoglobulin structure and genetics. Identity between variable regions of a μ and γ2 chain. *J. Biol. Chem.* **252,** 7192–7199.
53. Kabat, E. A., Wu, T. T., Perry, H. M., Gottesman, K. S., and Foeller, C. (1991) *Sequences of proteins of immunological interest,* 5th ed. U.S. Dept. Health & Human Services. Public Health Service, National Inst. Health, Bethesda, MD, p. 326.

15
Autoantibody Catalysis

Sudhir Paul

1. INTRODUCTION

Why should the immunologist be interested in yet another new phenomenon, i.e., autoantibody catalysis, elucidation of the functional importance of which will undoubtedly require years of effort and millions of dollars? This chapter endeavors to answer this question by collating the evidence indicating the following:

1. Efficient catalytic antibodies exist.
2. Autoimmune disease is associated with the synthesis of antibodies specialized to recognize autoantigens.
3. The biological efficacy of catalytic antibodies is quantitatively greater and qualitatively different compared to their noncatalytic counterparts.
4. Various functional roles for catalytic antibodies in innate and adaptive immunity can be posited on theoretical grounds, which, if validated experimentally, will explain certain aspects of self-tolerance and the destructive responses in autoimmune diseases.

2. BINDING AND CATALYSIS AS EFFECTOR FUNCTIONS

Interactions that lead only to the binding of the reactants and those that go on to effect the chemical transformation of one or more reactant have very different biological outcomes. In the case of an interaction limited to binding, one of the reactants serves as the *receptor*, acting as a switch to transduce the binding event into a signal recognizable by other proteins. For instance, the binding of an antigen by an antibody expressed as a receptor on the B-cell surface can serve as the signal to drive the cells into clonal proliferation, and the binding of an antigen to a soluble antibody can promote the interaction of complement components with the F_c segment of the antibodies, leading, eventually to activation of the complement cascade. Molecular interactions resulting in chemical catalysis, on the other hand, serve roles that include but are not limited to the signaling transducing function. The two defining features of a catalyst are: 1) it must transform the substrate (i.e., the ligand, the antigen) chemically and 2) it must turn over, i.e., a single catalyst molecule must be capable of being reused for the chemical transformation of multiple substrate molecules.

Contemporary Immunology: Autoimmune Reactions
Edited by: S. Paul © Humana Press Inc., Totowa, NJ

Thus, the biological functions of a protein antigen can be anticipated to be irreversibly altered by a catalytic antibody. In the case of cleavage of peptide bonds in a protein antigen by a catalytic antibody, the function of the protein may be lost permanently, or a new function may be acquired upon its fragmentation. Cleavage of the HIV-1 protein gp120 at certain peptide bonds, for instance, inactivates the infective capability of HIV-1 *(1)*, and cleavage of the neuropeptide substance P at certain bonds can generate smaller peptides with a biological activity profile different from that of the parent peptide *(2)*. The turnover capability implies that on a molar basis, a catalytic antibody will be biologically more potent than a noncatalytic antibody that binds the antigen stoichiometrically. In the latter case, dissociation of the antigen from the antibody restores its biological activity, and only one antigen molecule can be neutralized per antigen binding site expressed by the antibody.

3. OVERVIEW OF CATALYTIC ANTIBODIES

Contrary to the traditional view that antibodies exist only to bind antigens, there has been a steady accumulation of evidence that antibodies can develop catalytic activities (Fig. 1). Biochemical and structural characterization of antibodies carried out by the author and other groups support the following hypothses: A germline encoded peptidase activity resides in the VL domain. The magnitude and quality of the peptidase activity encoded by the VL domain is susceptible to maturation by somatic means, i.e., mutation and pairing with VH domains. Preferential utilization of this germline activity and (or) dysfunctional somatic diversification mechanisms lead to increased synthesis of catalytic antibodies in autoimmune disease.

The *natural* origin of the antibodies discussed here distinguishes these molecules from designer catalytic antibodies elicited by immunization with transition state analogs (TSAs; *see* Subheading 7).

3.1. Autoantibody Catalysis

The first indication that antibodies can express peptidase activity came from data that vasoactive intestinal peptide (VIP) is cleaved by antibodies from asthma patients *(3,4)*, which has been reproduced independently by Suzuki et al. *(5)*. The phenomenon of autoantibody catalysis is not restricted to VIP. Autoantibodies in Hashimoto's thyroiditis were found catalyze the cleavage of thyroglobulin *(6)*. Further evidence for autoantibody catalysis has been provided by reports of the DNase action of antibodies from lupus patients *(7,8)* and of a protein kinase activity of antibodies isolated from human milk *(9)*. The bias towards catalytic antibody synthesis in autoimmune disease is supported by observations that mouse strains with a genetic predisposition to autoimmune disease produce esterase antibodies at higher levels compared to control mouse strains immunized with a transition state analog *(10)*.

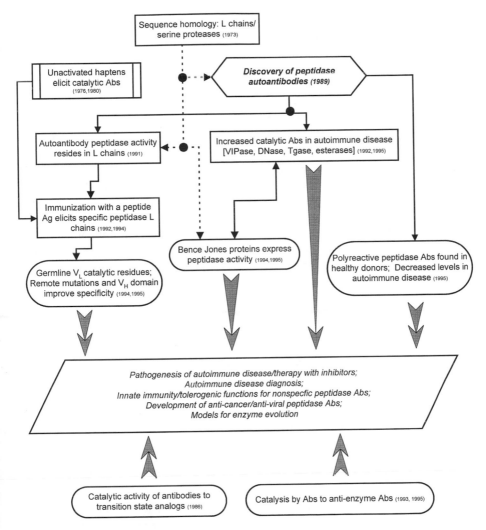

Fig. 1. History, current concepts, and implications of the field of catalytic antibodies with year of publication shown in parentheses. *See* text for references.

3.2. L Chain Catalysis

Erhan and Greller predicted immunoglobulins to possess peptidase activity based on sequence homology between the CDR1 of Bence Jones proteins (monoclonal L chains) and the region surrounding the active site Ser residue of serine proteases *(11)*. Fulfilment of this prediction came from our observations of the VIPase activity of L chains isolated from human autoantibodies *(12,13)*. Subsequently, Matsuura et al. *(14)* and we *(15)* showed the cleavage of synthetic protease substrates by a majority of monoclonal L chains isolated from multiple myeloma patients. Some of these L chains have been found to cleave physiologically relevant antigens like Arg-vasopressin *(16)*, VIP *(15)*, thyroglobulin (L. Lan and S. Paul, unpublished) and the HIV-1 protein gp120 *(17)*.

3.3. Peptidase L Chain Isolated by Immunization with VIP

Antibodies produced by immunization with phosphopyridoxyl tyrosine were shown in 1975 to accelerate Schiff's base formation between pyridoxal phosphate and tyrosine *(18)*. Then, three reports appeared showing that antibodies to the stable ground state structures of dinitrophenol and testosterone express esterase activities *(19–21)*. We found the L chain subunit of an antibody made by immunization with VIP to cleave VIP by a serine protease mechanism *(22–26)*. Mutagenesis studies suggested that the catalytic residues are encoded by a VL germline gene, and that somatic mutations are important in developing specificity for VIP *(25)*. Pairing the VL domain with the appropriate VH domain increased the specificity for VIP, indicating a second somatic mechanism responsible for specialization of the VIPase activity *(26)*. Other groups have recently identified additional catalytic antibodies (27,28) and L chains *(29)* by immunization with substrate analogs and analogs of a comparatively stable reaction intermediate (as opposed to TSAs).

3.4. Polyreactive Peptidase Antibodies in Unimmunized Individuals

The hypothesis that the peptidase activity is encoded by a germline gene(s) is supported by the presence of comparatively nonspecific antibodies capable of cleaving synthetic peptide substrates in all serum sample examined from healthy humans and unimmunized mice *(30)*. These antibodies are designated "polyreactive" because they can cleave very short peptides and are not specific for a particular antigen.

3.5. Catalytic Activity of Antibodies to Antienzyme Antibodies

Autoantibodies to enzymes found in autoimmune disease *(31)* could potentially stimulate the formation of anti-idiotypic antibodies that contain a replica of the enzyme active site. Recently, immunization with anticholinesterase and anti-DNaseI antibodies has been reported to elicit antibodies with cholinesterase and DNase activity, respectively *(32,33)*.

4. IMMUNOLOGICAL ORIGIN OF CATALYTIC ACTIVITY

4.1. Germline Origin

The peptidase activity of certain antibodies has been observed to derive from a catalytic site located in the L chain subunit *(12)*. The L chain of an antibody raised to vasoactive intestinal polypeptide (VIP) displays the ability to cleave this peptide. Molecular modeling of the VIPase L chain showed that its Ser27a, His 93, and Asp1 residues (Kabat numbering) can be precisely superimposed

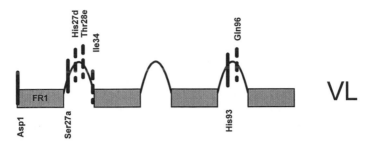

Fig. 2. Catalytic residues in anti-VIP light chain (clone c23.5) shown as solid vertical lines. The VL domain differs in its amino acid sequence from its germline counterpart in four positions (shown as broken lines). The three catalytic residues are germline encoded.

on the corresponding active site Ser, His, and Asp residues of a nonantibody serine protease, subtilisin *(24)*. Mutants containing an Ala residue instead of the wildtype Ser27a, His93, or Asp1 displayed loss of the peptidase activity, indicating that these residues constitute the catalytic site (Fig. 2) *(25,* Paul et al. unpublished observations). The VIPase VL domain contains four amino acid replacements compared to its germline VL (GenBank number Z72384) and Jk1 gene counterparts, of which three are located in CDR1 (His27d:Asp, Thr28e:Ser and Ile34:Asn; germline encoded residues shown second) and one at the junction of the VL and J segments (Gln96:Trp). Even though the three catalytic residues in the VIPase VL domain (Ser27a, His93, Asp1) are present in the germline VL gene, it could be argued that conformational changes induced by somatic mutations at remote sites are essential for the catalytic activity. To study this possibility, the germline configuration protein of the VIPase L chain was constructed by introducing the required four mutations as described previously *(25)*. The purified germline L chain expressed catalytic activity at about 3.5-fold lower level than the mature L chain, as detected by cleavage of the synthetic protease substrate Pro-Phe-Arg-MCA (S. Paul and G. Golobov, unpublished data). We concluded that the somatic mutations in the V domain are not obligatory for expression of the catalytic activity.

Replacement of the components of the catalytic triad by mutagenesis was without effect on the affinity of the L chain for VIP, as indicated by near equivalent K_m values of the wildtype and catalytically deficient mutants *(25)*. This observation can be understood from the transition state theory, which holds that catalyst binding to the unstable reaction intermediate between the reactant and the products, the transition state, reduces the activation energy and accelerates the reaction *(34)*. In the case of the L chain, the catalytic residues are important in binding the VIP transition state, but not the stable state of the peptide. These observations suggest that the catalytic subsite is physically and functionally distinct from the conventional antigen binding site.

Additional support for the central argument advanced above, i.e., a conserved, germline encoded site is responsible for the catalysis, can be adduced from observations of polyreactive catalytic antibodies *(30)*. These antibodies recognize small synthetic peptides with low affinity, cleave peptides with quite different sequences, and are present in unimmunized donors, suggesting an unspecialized nature. This behavior is reminiscent of polyreactive antigen binding by certain antibodies *(35)*, which are thought to be synthesized by CD5+ B-cells *(36)*, contain germline or minimally mutated V regions *(37)*, and can bind structurally different antigens with low affinity *(38)*.

4.2. Somatic Maturation

The germline origin of the catalytic subsite, while suggesting that the catalytic function is an expression of innate immunity, does not exclude a possible improvement in this function over the course of adaptive antibody responses. Polyclonal catalytic antibodies isolated from patients with autoimmune disease display high affinities for their autoantigens, i.e., VIP *(3,4)*, thyroglobulin *(6)* and DNA *(7,8)*, which is the classical sign that the antibodies have beeen subjected to somatic mutations and clonal selection. Further, two recombinant light chains with efficient VIP cleaving activities have been found to be extensively mutated in comparison to their germline VL gene counterparts *(13)*.

Pairing of the catalytic VL domain with the appropriate VH domain constitutes a second somatic process whereby the activity of the germline site can be modulated. This is suggested by observations of improved catalysis by linking the model VIPase VL domain with its natural VH domain partner but not an irrelevant VH domain *(26)*. Such improvements could potentially be mediated by allosteric effects that result in improved spatial positioning of the catalytic site for transition state binding, or by introduction of new chemical functionalities in the catalytic subsite that may participate directly in the mechanism of catalysis.

5. DYSFUNCTIONAL CATALYTIC FUNCTION IN AUTOIMMUNE DISEASE

5.1. VIP Cleaving Antibodies in Asthma

VIP binding autoantibodies were observed in a subpopulation of patients with asthma *(39)*. Some of these antibodies catalyzed the hydrolysis of VIP *(4,40)*. The activity was characterized as belonging to antibodies by several criteria, including electrophoretic purity of the IgG, binding of the activity by immobilized protein G (a bacterial IgG-binding protein that binds the F_c region), and by anti-human IgG; and, presence of the activity in Fab fragments. The VIP-hydrolyzing activity of IgG purified from 19 nonasthmatics and 33 asthmatic subjects was compared. Approximately 50% of IgG samples from asthmatic subjects displayed VIP-hydrolyzing activity $>$ mean $\pm$ 2 SD for IgG samples from the nonasthmatic controls ($P < 0.001$, Mann–Whitney U-test). The strong binding affinities (K_d, K_m) are typical of antibodies. Fragments of VIP produced by the antibodies were separated by reversed-phase HPLC and identified by N-terminal sequencing. Seven antibody-sensitive peptide bonds were identified *(4)*, of which six were clustered between residues 14–22. The epitope specificity of an antibody that cleaved a single bond in VIP [Gln(16)-Met(17)] was determined using synthetic fragments corresponding to linear, overlapping subsequences of VIP *(41)*. VIP[15–28], a large C-terminal subsequence, was deduced to be the antibody-reactive epitope because it was bound with high affinity. A shorter subsequence, VIP[22–28] was bound by the antibody with low affinity and inhibited the hydrolysis of VIP competitively. VIP[22–28], which is located four residues distant from the cleavage site, is evidently a subepitope that participates in antibody binding.

5.2. Thyroglobulin Cleaving Antibodies in Autoimmune Thyroiditis

Thyroglobulin (Tg), the precursor of thyroid hormones, is an established target of antibodies in autoimmune thyroid disease. Cleavage of ^{125}I-labeled Tg was studied by SDS-electrophoresis and autoradiography. Following treatment with Tg-specific autoantibodies isolated from a patient with Hashimoto's thyroiditis, disappearance of the 330 kDa Tg monomer and formation of a major 15 kDa product and minor 125 kDa, 60 kDa, and 25 kDa products were observed *(6)*. Control experiments showed the activity to belong to Tg-specific antibodies. The K_m for Tg was 39 nM, indicating high affinity Tg recognition. The Tg antibodies also cleaved Pro-Phe-Arg-MCA with low affinity (K_m ~430-fold greater than for Tg). Pro-Phe-Arg-MCA hydrolysis was inhibited competitively and potently by Tg (K_i 20 nM), suggesting that the same catalytic site is responsible for cleavage of both substrates.

5.3. Inverse Relationships Between Antigen-Specific and Polyreactive Peptidase Antibodies in Autoimmune Disease

We have previously reported that patients with rheumatoid arthritis display decreased polyreactive proteolytic activity, determined by measuring the cleavage of a peptide-MCA substrate *(30)*. To compare the levels of antigen-specific and polyreactive antibody activities in the same patients, cleavage of the peptide-MCA substrate and Tg by IgG from healthy subjects, lupus patients, and autoimmune thyroiditis patients was determined *(42)*. Decreased peptide-MCA hydrolysis was evident in the SLE and autoimmune thyroiditis patients ($P < 0.002$). Both types of patients showed increased hydrolysis of thyroglobulin compared to the control healthy subjects ($P < 0.001$). No cleavage of thyroglobulin by IgG purified from HIV-1 positive subjects or from mice hyperimmunized with an albumin-hapten conjugate was observed, indicating that the development of the catalytic activity is not a nonspecific event accompanying V-region maturation.

The observations summarized above suggest increased expression of *antigen-specific* and *efficient* peptidase activities in lupus, autoimmune thyroiditis, and asthma. In contrast, *unspecialized* peptidase activities are decreased in autoimmune disease compared to nondiseased controls. A possible explanation for this phenomenon is that genetic or cellular factors unique to autoimmune disease permit the increased recruitment of germline V-region genes encoding the unspecialized catalytic activity, followed by their specialization via the process of autoantigen-driven clonal selection of B-cells. The hypothesis that autoimmune disease is associated with biased usage of different V-genes is well-established in the literature *(43)*. Other genes relevant to antibody expression may also contribute to catalytic activity levels in autoimmune disease. The MRL/*lpr* mouse is known to be a good catalytic antibody producer *(10)*. In this mouse strain, a mutation of the *Fas* apoptosis gene is believed to permit proliferation of T- and B-cells and expression of lupus-like disease *(44)*.

6. FUNCTIONAL SIGNIFICANCE
OF AUTOANTIBODY CATALYSIS

As noted in Subheading 2., catalysts can be anticipated to exert a quantitatively greater and, in some cases, a qualitatively different biological effect compared to their reversibly binding counterparts. The main focus of researchers in this field until now, however, has been to validate and characterize the catalytic antibodies, and only recently has attention been devoted to study of the functions of the antibodies.

The case of catalytic antibodies to VIP is described here. Cleavage of any bond in VIP will lead to loss of its smooth muscle relaxant and antiinflammatory effects, because the entire sequence of VIP is necessary for its biological activity *(45)*. Recombinant VIP cleaving antibodies with catalytic proficiency comparable to a nonantibody protease, trypsin, have been isolated *(13)*. Based on the magnitude of the catalytic activities, it is a safe to predict that when present, the catalytic autoantibodies may regulate the concentrations of the substrate polypeptide. In multiple myeloma, the antibody and L chain products of the tumor cells accumulate in serum and urine to millimolar levels *(46; see also* Sinohara and Matsuura, this volume). Some L chains isolated from myeloma patients express the ability to cleave VIP, an activity that might cause the depletion of the peptide in these patients.

High affinity binding of neuronally released VIP by G-protein coupled receptors expressed on airway cells stimulates cyclic AMP synthesis and mediates, in part, the biological effects of of VIP *(47)*. Binding of VIP by receptors in guinea pig lung membranes was measured as described in our previous studies *(48)*, following incubation of the peptide with the wild type and His93:Arg mutant of a catalytic L chain (Fig. 3). The mutant and wildtype L chains bind VIP with equivalent affinity, but the mutant is 100-fold less active catalytically *(25)*. Near-complete inhibition of binding of VIP to the lung receptors by the wild type protein was evident, whereas the mutant effect was minimal. It may be concluded that the catalytic function confers an enhanced VIP neutralizing potency to the L chain.

Administration of a monoclonal antibody with VIP cleaving activity to experimental animals increased the number of inflammatory cells and the thromboxane

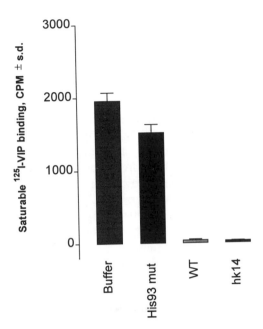

Fig. 3. Neutralization of VIP receptor binding by peptidase L chains. WT, wild type clone c23.5; His93 mut, catalytically deficient c23.5 mutant (His93:Arg); hk14, clone hk14 isolated from an asthma patient. ^{125}I-VIP (100 pM) was incubated (3 h) with assay buffer or the recombinant L chains (1 μM). Receptor binding of the ^{125}I-VIP in 10-fold diluted reaction mixtures was measured by incubation with guinea pig lung membranes (33 μg protein) as in ref. *48*. Saturable binding represents the binding to receptors displaceable by excess unlabeled VIP.

B2 levels in the airways, suggesting an inflammatory reaction *(49)*. These effects of the antibody are in line with the known actions of VIP. Release of VIP from nerve endings in the airway wall is believed to suppress inflammatory processes in the respiratory system, including release of inflammatory eicosanoid mediators *(50)*, interleukin production *(51)* and the injurious effects of reactive oxygen radicals *(52)*. A deficiency of VIP may be responsible for the airway inflammation in severe asthmatics *(53)*. Immunization of cats with VIP decreases the relaxation of airway smooth muscle in response to electrical stimulation *(54)*. VIPase antibodies are also found in lupus patients. This is interesting because of the generalized tendency toward inflammatory processes and the frequent occurrence of respiratory disorders in lupus *(55)*.

A case could also be made that antibody catalysis is beneficial under certain circumstances. According to Grabar *(56)*, efficient autoantigen clearance will reduce the exposure of the immune system to autoantigens, and thus suppress autoimmune reactions. The possibilities of pathological versus beneficial effects are not mutually exclusive, in that the antibody functions can vary depending on their properties and biological location. Observations of *increased* occurrence of autoantigen-specific catalytic antibodies in autoimmune disease accompanied by *decreased* occurrence of the polyreactive catalytic antibodies provide justification for the hypothesis that the former are harmful and the latter are beneficial. Tg, which fulfills its physiological function entirely within the thyroid, is found at very low levels in blood. Clearance of blood-borne thyroglobulin by catalytic antibodies can arguably reduce further autoimmune reactions against this protein. On the other hand, if thyroglobulin cleaving catalytic antibodies permeate the thyroid or are made by thyroidal lymphocyte *(57)*, destruction of the protein will lead to depletion of the thyroid hormones T3 and T4, which are formed from Tg by an orderly iodination and peptidase processing mechanism.

A possible role for catalytic antibodies in antigen presentation can be conceived, but has not been studied experimentally. It could be hypothesized that antigen digestion by antibodies produces epitopes that bind MHC antigens efficiently, thus permitting enhanced antigen presentation to T-cells and enhanced T-cell recruitment. Conversely, recruitment of autoantigen-specific T-cells will be reduced if the antibodies generate epitopes incapable of binding MHC molecules.

7. BIOTECHNOLOGICAL POTENTIAL OF AUTOANTIBODY CATALYSIS

Notwithstanding the likely pathogenic nature of autoantibody catalysis, this phenomenon can potentially be put to beneficial uses. The isolation of catalytic antibodies suitable for immunotherapy of tumors and microbial infections has been a long-standing goal. The autoimmune repertoire available in the lupus MRL/*lpr* mouse strain is an appropriate starting point in the search for such antibodies. Regardless of the reasons for the increased catalytic antibody synthesis, immunization with the desired tumor-specific or microbial antigen may yield catalytic antibodies suitable for clinical applications.

A search for the term *catalytic antibodies* in Medline will yield a plethora of reports dealing with designer antibodies raised by immunization with transition state analogs (TSAs). These reports can be traced back to Pauling *(58)* and Jencks *(59)*, who suggested that proteins become capable of catalysis when they acquire the capability to recognize the unstable reaction intermediate (or transition state) corresponding to the highest energy point in the reaction pathway from substrate to product. The current generation of phosphonate TSAs can be used to elicit antibodies capable of catalyzing comparatively undemanding reactions like ester bond cleavage, but because of various limitations in the structure of these TSAs, they do not elicit antibodies that cleave energetically demanding reactions such as peptide bond hydrolysis *(see* ref. *60* for discussion).

A fruitful intersection of the fields of autoantibody catalysis and designer antibody catalysis can be conceived, in that immunization of autoimmune mice with TSAs capable of recognizing the germline encoded, serine protease site in antibodies can be applied towards generation of efficient peptidase antibodies (if human antibodies are desired, the human antibody locus grafted in autoimmune mice can serve as the host).

8. CONCLUSIONS

The L chains of certain antibodies contain a serine protease-like catalytic site capable of cleaving peptide bonds. The catalytic site is encoded by a germline VL gene. The catalytic activity can potentially be improved by somatic sequence diversification and pairing of the light chain with the appropriate heavy chain. Autoimmune disease is associated with increased synthesis of antigen-specific antibodies, but the reasons for this phenomenon are not known. Only recently has attention turned to the functional role of the catalytic function. Preliminary studies confirm that the catalytic cleavage of peptide bonds is a more potent means to achieve antigen neutralization compared to reversible antigen binding. Administration of a monoclonal antibody to VIP in experimental animals induces an inflammatory response in the airways, suggesting that catalytic autoantibodies to this peptide found in airway disease and lupus are capable of causing airway dysfunction. The phenomenon of autoantibody catalysis can potentially be applied to isolate efficient catalysts directed against tumor or microbial antigens, by exposing the autoimmune repertoire to such antigens or their analogs capable of recruiting the germline VL gene encoding the catalytic site.

ACKNOWLEDGMENTS

This work was supported by the USPHS under grants HL44126 and AI31268. The author is grateful to his coworkers who have coauthored our papers cited here and to Bob Dannenbring for technical assistance.

REFERENCES

1. Pollard, S., Meier, W., Chow, P., Rosa, J., and Wiley, D. (1991) CD4-binding regions of human immunodeficiency virus envelope glycoprotein gp120 defined by proteolytic digestion. *Proc. Natl. Acad. Sci. USA* **88**, 11,320–11,324.
2. Martins, M. A., Shore, S. A., Gerard, N. P., Gerard, C., and Drazen, J. M. (1990) Peptidase modulation of the pulmonary effects of tachykinins in tracheal superfused guinea pig lungs. *J. Clin. Invest.* **85**, 170–176.
3. Paul, S., Volle, D. J., Beach, C. M., Johnson, D. R., Powell, M. J., and Massey, R. J. (1989) Catalytic hydrolysis of vasoactive intestinal peptide by human autoantibody. *Science* **244**, 1158–1162.
4. Paul, S., Sun, M., Mody, R., Eklund, S. H., Beach, C. M., Massey, R. J., et al. (1991) Cleavage of vasoactive intestinal peptide at multiple sites by autoantibodies. *J. Biol. Chem.* **256**, 16,128–16,134.
5. Suzuki, H., Imanishi, H., Nakai, T., and Konishi, Y. K. (1992) Human autoantibodies that catalyze the hydrolysis of vasoactive intestinal polypeptide. *Biochem. (Life Sci. Adv.)* **11**, 173–177.
6. Li, L., Kaveri, S., Tyutyulkova, S., Kazatchkine, M., and Paul, S. (1995) Catalytic activity of anti-thyroglobulin antibodies. *J. Immunol.* **154**, 3328–3332.
7. Shuster, A. M., Gololobov, G. V., Kvashuk, O. A., Bogomolova, A. E., Smirnov, I. V., and Gabibov, A. G. (1992) DNA hydrolyzing autoantibodies. *Science* **256**, 665–667.

8. Gololobov, G. V., Chernova, E. A., Schourov, D. V., Smirnov, I. V., Kudelina, I. A., and Gabibov, A. G. (1995) Cleavage of supercoiled plasmid DNA by autoantibody Fab fragment: Application of the flow linear dichroism technique. *Proc. Natl. Acad. Sci. USA* **92,** 254–257.

9. Kit, Y.-Y., Semenov, D. V., and Nevinsky, G. A. (1996) Phosphorylation of different human milk proteins by human catalytic secretory immunoglobulin A. *Biochem. Molec. Biol. Intl.* **39,** 521–527.

10. Tawfik, D., Chap, R., Green, B., Sela, M., and Eshhar, Z. (1995) Unexpectedly high occurrence of catalytic antibodies in MRL/lpr and SJL mice immunized with a transition state analog. Is there a linkage to autoimmunity? *Proc. Natl. Acad. Sci. USA* **92,** 2145–2149.

11. Erhan, S. and Greller, L. D. (1974) Do immunoglobulins have proteolytic activity? *Nature* **251,** 353–355.

12. Sun, M., Mody, B., Eklund, S. H., and Paul, S. (1991) VIP hydrolysis by antibody light chains. *J. Biol. Chem.* **266,** 15,571–15,574.

13. Tyutyulkova, S., Gao, Q.-S., Thompson, A., Rennard, A., and Paul, S. (1996) Effcient vasoactive intestinal polypeptide hydrolyzing antibody light chains selected from an asthma patient by phage display. *Biochem. Biophys. Acta* **1316,** 217–223.

14. Matsuura, K., Yamamoto, K., and Sinohara, H. (1994) Amidase activity of human Bence Jones proteins. *Biochem. Biophys. Res. Commun.* **204,** 57–62.

15. Paul, S., Li, L., Kalaga, R., Wilkins-Stevens, P., Stevens, F. J., and Solomon, A. (1995) Natural catalytic antibodies: Peptide hydrolyzing activities of Bence Jones proteins and V_L fragment. *J. Biol. Chem.* **270,** 15,257–15,261.

16. Matsuura, K. and Sinohara, H. (1996) Catalytic cleavage of vasopressin by human Bence Jones proteins at the arginylglycinamide bond. *Biol. Chem.* **377,** 587–589.

17. Kalaga, R., Huang, H., Stevens, F. J., Solomon, A., and Paul, S. (1995) gp120 hydrolysis by catalytic antibody light chain. *The 9th International Congress of Immunology,* San Francisco, CA, July 23–29, abstract #4893, 825.

18. Raso, V. and Stollar, B. D. The antibody-enzyme analogy. (1975) Comparison of enzymes and antibodies specific for phosphopyridoxyltyrosine. *Biochemistry* **14,** 591–599.

19. Kohen, F., Kim, J. B., Barnard, G., and Linder, H. R. (1979) A steroid immunoassay based on antibody-enhanced hydrolysis of a steroid umbelliferone conjugate. *FEBS Lett.* **100,** 137–140.

20. Kohen, F., Kim, J. B., Linder, H. R., Eshhar, Z., and Green, B. (1980) Monoclonal immunoglobulin G augments hydrolysis of an ester of the homologous hapten: An esterase-like activity of the antibody-containing site. *FEBS Lett.* **111,** 427–431.

21. Kohen, F., Kim, J.-B., Barnard, G., and Lindner, H. (1980) Antibody-enhanced hydrolysis of steroid esters. *Biochem. Biophys. Acta* **629,** 328–337.

22. Paul S., Sun, M., Mody, R., Tewary, H. K., Mehrotra, S., Gianferrara, T., et al. (1992) Peptidolytic by a neuropeptide. *J. Biol. Chem.* **267,** 13,142–13,145.

23. Sun, M., Gao, Q-S., Li, L., and Paul, S. (1994) Proteolytic activity of an antibody light chain. *J. Immunol.* **153,** 5121–5126.

24. Gao, Q.-S., Sun, M., Tyutyulkova, S., Webster, D., Rees, A., Tramontano, A., et al. (1994) Molecular cloning of a proteolytic antibody light chain. *J. Biol. Chem.* **269,** 32,389–32,393.

25. Gao, Q.-S., Sun, M., Rees, A., and Paul, S. (1995) Site-directed mutagenesis of proteolytic antibody light chain. *J. Mol. Biol.* **253**, 658–664.
26. Sun, M., Gao, Q.-S., Kirnarskiy, L., Rees, A., and Paul, S. (1997) Cleavage specificity of a proteolytic antibody light chain and effects of the heavy chain variable domain. *J. Mol. Biol.* **271**, 374–385.
27. Savitsky, A. P., Nelen, M. I., Yatsmirsky, A. K., Demcheva, M. V., Ponomarev, G. V., and Sinikov, I. V. (1994) Kinetics of oxidation of o-dianisidine by hydrogen peroxide in the presence of antibody complexes of iron(III) coproporphyrin. *Appl. Biochem. Biotechnol.* **47**, 317–327.
28. Gramatikova, S. and Christen, P. (1996) Pyridoxal 5'-phosphate-dependent catalytic antibody. *J. Biol. Chem.* **271**, 30,583–30,586.
29. Takagi, M., Kohda, K., Hamuro, T., Harada, A., Yamaguchi, H., Kamachi, M., et al. (1995) Thermostable peroxidase activity with a recombinant antibody L chain-porphyrin Fe(III) complex. *FEBS Lett.* **375**, 273–276.
30. Kalaga, R., Li, L., O'Dell, J., and Paul, S. (1995) Unexpected presence of polyreactive catalytic antibodies in IgG from unimmunized donors and decreased levels in rheumatoid arthritis. *J. Immunol.* **155**, 2695–2702.
31. Dolman, K. M., Van de Wiel, B. A., Kam, C.-M., Kerrigan, J. E., Hack, C. E., Von dem Borne, A. E. G. K., et al. (1993) Proteinase 3: Substrate specificity and possible pathogenetic effect of Wegener's granulomatosis autoantibodies (C-ANCA) by dysregulation of the enzyme. *Adv. Exp. Med. Biol.* **336**, 55–60.
32. Izadyar, L., Friboulet, A., Remy, M. H., Roseto, A., and Thomas, D. (1993) Monoclonal anti-idiotypic antibodies as functional internal images of enzymes active sites: Production of a catalytic antibody with a cholinesterase activity. *Proc. Natl. Acad. Sci. USA* **90**, 8876–8880.
33. Crespeau, H., Laouar, A., and Rochu, D. (1994) Un abzyme DNase polyclonal produit par la méthode de image interne anti-idiotypique. *C. R. Acad. Sci. Paris de la vie/Life Sciences* **317**, 819–823.
34. Schowen, R. L. *Transition States of Biochemical Processes* (Gandour, R. D. and Schowen, R. L., eds.), Plenum, New York, ch. 2, 1978.
35. Avrameas, S. (1991) Natural autoantibodies: from "horror autotoxicus" to "gnothi seauton". *Immunol. Today* **12**, 154–159.
36. Casali, P. and Notkins, A. L. (1989) CD5+ B lymphocytes, polyreactive antibodies and the human B-cell repertoire. *Immunol. Today* **10**, 364–368.
37. Harindranath, N., Ikematsu, H., Notkins, A. L., and Casali, P. (1993) Structure of the VH and VL segments of polyreactive and monoreactive human natural antibodies to HIV-1 and Escherichia coli beta-galactosidase. *Int. Immunol.* **5**, 523–1533.
38. Guilbert, B., Dighiero, G., and Avrameas, S. (1982) Naturally occurring antibodies against nine common antigens in human sera. I. Detection, isolation and characterization. *J. Immunol.* **128**, 2779–2787.
39. Paul, S., Said, S. I., Thompson, A. B., Volle, D. J., Agrawal, D. K., Foda, H., and de la Rocha, S. (1989) Characterization of autoantibodies to VIP in asthma. *J. Neuroimmunol.* **23**, 133–142.
40. Paul, S. (1994) Catalytic activity of anti-ground state antibodies, antibody subunits and human autoantibodies. *Appl. Biochem. Biotechnol.* **47**, 241–255.
41. Paul, S., Volle, D. J., Powell, M. J., and Massey, R. J. (1990) Site specificity of a catalytic vasoactive intestinal peptide antibody: An inhibitory VIP subsequence distant from the scissile peptide bond. *J. Biol. Chem.* **265**, 11,910–11,913.

42. Paul, S., Li, L., Kalaga, R., O'Dell, R. E., Dannenbring, Jr., R. E., Swindells, S., et al. (1997) Characterization of thyroglobulin-directed and polyreactive catalytic antibodies in autoimmune disease, *J. Immunol.* **159,** 1530–1536.
43. Schwartz, R. S. (1993) Autoimmunity and autoimmune diseases, in *Fundamental Immunology* (Paul, W. E., ed.), Raven, New York, 3rd edition, pp. 1033–1097.
44. Watanabe-Fukunaga, R., Brannan, C. I., Copeland, N. G., Jenkins, N. A., and Nagata, S., (1992) Lymphoproliferation disorder in mice explained by defects in *Fas* antigen that mediates apoptosis. *Nature* **356,** 314–317.
45. Couvineau, A., Rouyer, F. C., Fournier, A., St. Pierre, S., Pipkorn, R., and Laburthe, M. (1984) Structural requirements for VIP interaction with specific receptors in human and rat intestinal membranes: Effect of nine partial sequences. *Biochem. Biophys. Res. Commun.* **121,** 493–498.
46. Nelson, M., Brown, R. D., Gibson, J., and Joshua, D. E. (1992) Measurement of free kappa and lambda chains in serum and the significance of their ratio in patients with multiple myeloma. *Br. J. Haematol.* **81,** 223–230.
47. Paul, S. and Ebadi, M. (1993) Vasoactive intestinal peptide: its interactions with calmodulin and catalytic antibodies. *Neurochem. Int.* **23,** 197–214.
48. Paul, S., and Said S.I. (1987) Characterization of receptors for vasoactive intestinal peptide solubilized from the lung. *J. Biol. Chem.* **262,** 158–162.
49. Paul, S. (1997) Relevance of catalytic anti-VIP antibodies to the airway, in *Pro-Inflammatory and Anti-Inflammatory Peptides, Lung Biology in Health and Disease* (Sami Said, ed.), Marcel Dekker, New York, pp. 459–475.
50. Ciabattoni, G., Montuschi, P., Curro, D., Togna, G., and Preziosi, P. (1993) Effects of vasoactive intestinal peptide on antigen-induced bronchoconstriction and thromboxane release in guinea-pig lung. *Br. J. Pharmacol.* **109,** 243–250.
51. Sun, L. and Ganea, D. (1993) Vasoactive intestinal peptide inhibits interleukin (IL)-2 and IL-4 production through different molecular mechanisms in T cells activated via the T cell receptor/CD3 complex. *J. Neuroimmunol.* **48,** 59–70.
52. Said, S. I. (1991) VIP as a modulator of lung inflammation and airway constriction. *Am. Rev. Respir. Dis.* **143,** S22–S24.
53. Ollerenshaw, S., Jarvis, D., Woolcock, A., Sullivan, C., and Scheibner, T. (1989) Absence of immunoreactive vasoactive intestinal polypeptide in tissue from the lungs of patients with asthma. *N. Engl. J. Med.* **320,** 1244–1248.
54. Hakoda, H., Zhouqiu, X., Aizawa, H., Inoue, H., Hirata, M. and Ito, Y. (1991) Effects of immunization against VIP on neurotransmission in cat trachea. *Am. J. Physiol.* **261,** L341–L348.
55. Martin, L., Edworthy, S. M., Ryan, J. P., and Fritzler, M. J. (1992) Upper airway disease in systemic lupus erythematosus: A report of 4 cases and a review of the literature. *J. Rheum.* **19,** 1186–1190.
56. Grabar, P. (1983) Autoantibodies and the physiological role of immunoglobulins. *Immunol. Today* **4,** 337–340.
57. Kofler, R. and Wick, G. (1978) Immunofluorescent localization of thyroglobulin-autoantibody producing strains in various organs of obese strain (OS) chicken. *Z. Immunitatsforsch Immunobiol.* **154,** 88–93.
58. Pauling, L. (1946) Molecular architecture and biological reactions. *Chem. Eng. News* **24,** 1375–1377.
59. Jencks, W. P. (1975) Binding energy, specificity, and enzymatic catalysis: the circe effect. *Adv. Enzymol. Relat. Areas Mol. Biol.* **43,** 219–410.
60. Paul, S. (1996) Proteolytic antibodies. *Isr. J. Chem.* **36,** 207–214.

16

Is the Catalytic Activity of Bence Jones Proteins an Autoimmune Effector Mechanism in Multiple Myeloma?

Hyogo Sinohara and Kinji Matsuura

1. INTRODUCTION

On Friday, October 30, 1845, W. MacIntire, physician to the Metropolitan Convalescent Institution and to the Western General Dispensary, St. Marylebone, was called to see a patient who had been treated by T. Watson for several months (1,2). Since the patient had a history of edema, MacIntire examined the urine and noted the peculiar physical properties of the urinary protein (precipitation with heating at 40–60°C, disappearance with boiling, and reappearance with cooling). He wrote: "I was at first inclined to think that some mistake had occurred, but on repeated trials with other specimens, and closely watching their course, the results were always found to be the same" (2). Watson had evidently not examined the urine when the patient had been under his care, but was present when MacIntire performed urinalysis. In those days, it was customary for the specialist services to be provided by practicing physicians and surgeons. Urine specimens were sent to Henry Bence Jones, physician to St. George's Hospital and professor of forensic medicine of the Medical College associated with the Hospital. Jones was then 31 yr old, but had already established a reputation as a chemical pathologist. He confirmed the MacIntire results and examined the protein in some detail. The patient died six weeks later, and an autopsy was performed by Shaw, surgeon to the Middlesex Hospital, in the presence of Watson, Jones, Ridge, and MacIntire, none of whom thought that the peculiar urinary protein was related to the disease, mollities ossium, later called multiple myeloma (2). Jones included this peculiar protein in his Gulstonian Lectures on chemical pathology to Royal College of Physicians in London (3): "On the last day of October, a peculiar state of urine was discovered, through the carefulness of Dr. MacIntire." Jones further added: "it differs entirely from the oxides of protein. The quantity of carbon, oxygen, nitrogen, differ also remarkably from fibrin and albumen, but agree very nearly with tritoxide of protein." This lecture gave him credit for the discovery of Bence Jones protein. On the other hand, MacIntire's paper was concerned with clinical

Contemporary Immunology: Autoimmune Reactions
Edited by: S. Paul © Humana Press Inc., Totowa, NJ

features and postmortem examination, as well as the properties of the urinary protein *(2)*. At the end of the paper, MacIntire wrote: "I shall be content if I have succeeded in pointing out to future observers, gifted with the requisite qualifications for conducting researches of a higher order, certain definite and distinctive characters by which a peculiar and hitherto unrecorded pathological condition of the urine may be recognized and identified." One and a half centuries have passed, however, before MacIntire's modest wish is fulfilled, and the discovery of Bence Jones protein has become more than obscure history. Many investigators began to use the hyphenated name, i.e., Bence-Jones protein, leading to the misunderstanding that this protein had been discovered by Bence and Jones. In 1961, at the ninth Colloquium of Protides of the Biological Fluids at Brugge, Belgium, a medal which bore two figures in relief was distributed to all participants. According to the organizer *(4)*, "Bence and Jones are reproduced on our Colloquium medal this year." However, Bence and Jones were the middle and last names of the same person, but he occasionally spelled out his middle name possibly to avoid confusion with Dr. H(andbied) Jones working then at the same hospital *(5)*.

In 1962, Edelman and Gally *(6)* found that the light chain from a serum immunoglobulin G of myeloma was identical with the Bence Jones protein in the urine of the same patient. This was the first landmark in the research of Bence Jones protein. Since then, enormous progress has been made in our understanding of structure and function of immunoglobulins because of Bence Jones proteins, which are of monoclonal origin and readily available in large quantity. In 1974, Erhan and Greller *(7)* pointed out the statistically significant amino acid identity between antibody light chains and the active site region of serine proteinases. The significance of this paper was unnoticed for about 20 years until Paul et al. showed that immunoglobulin light chains were capable of hydrolyzing peptide and amide bonds *(8–11)*. Matsuura et al. *(12,13)* also made similar observations. In striking contrast to common assumption that catalysis by antibodies is a rare phenomenon, the majority of monoclonal light chains (Bence-Jones proteins) isolated from multiple myeloma patients have been found capable of hydrolyzing synthetic proteinase substrates *(11–13)*. These results raise the possibility that the catalytic activity of Bence Jones proteins may underlie the diverse clinical spectrum associated with multiple myeloma and other lymphoproliferative diseases *(14–16)*. There is at present virtually no direct evidence for this possibility. The purpose of this chapter is to call attention to this issue in the hope of stimulating studies of this "new class of autoimmune disease" as well as of satisfying the humble wish made by MacIntire some 150 years ago.

2. CATALYTIC ACTIVITIES OF BENCE JONES PROTEINS

Recently, numerous monoclonal antibodies (MAbs) that can catalyze more than 50 chemical reactions have been elicited *(17)*. Furthermore, Paul suggested that certain catalytic antibodies may evolve at relatively high frequency in the

Table 1
Cleavage of Various Chromogenic
Peptide Substrates by Bence Jones Proteins

Substrate[a]	Bence Jones proteins		
	HIR[b]	B6[c]	RHY[c]
Carbobenzoxy-Ile-Glu-Gly-Arg-pNa	+		
t-butyloxycarbonyl-Ile-Glu-Gly-Arg-MCA		+	+
Carbobenzoxy-Val-Gly-Arg-pNA	+		
t-butyloxycarbonyl-Glu-Arg-MCA		+	+
Pro-Phe-Arg-pNA	−		
Succinyl-Ala-Ala-Ala-pNA	−		
Ala-Ala-Ala-MCA		−	+
Leu-Leu-Val-Phe-MCA		−	−

[a] Abbreviation: pNA, *p*-nitroanilide; MCA, methylcoumarinamide.
[b] Data taken from ref. *12*.
[c] Data taken from ref. *11*.

normal immune response *(18)*. Virtually nothing is known, however, as to whether light chains from these catalytic antibodies are also capable of catalyzing the same reactions. The exception is the cleavage of certain amide and peptide bonds, which will be discussed below.

2.1. Amidolytic Activity

While studying urinary trypsin inhibitors, we made the serendipitous observation that five monoclonal Bence Jones proteins examined were all capable of hydrolyzing synthetic chromogenic substrates for trypsin (12). This was in agreement with the results of Paul et al. *(11)* who showed that 16 of 21 Bence Jones proteins examined were capable of hydrolyzing peptide-methylcoumarinamides, with substrate preference directed to basic amino acids, especially arginine (Table 1).

2.2. Peptidolytic Activity

The synthetic amide substrates used for the above assays are generally unstable, and undergo slow, spontaneous hydrolysis even at neutral pH. This is in marked contrast to peptide bonds, which are very stable and the hydrolysis of which requires exposure to harsh conditions such as boiling temperatures in strong mineral acid. As judged from their K_m or K_d values *(18–20)*, catalytic autoantibodies generally have high affinity to their antigens, which may be sufficient to hydrolyze the peptide bonds at rates that are physiologically significant. On the other hand, it seems likely that most interactions between Bence Jones proteins and their "pseudosubstrates" are generally of low affinity and comparatively nonspecific. In our studies, arginine vasopressin was hydrolyzed at the arginyl-glycinamide bond by four Bence Jones proteins examined *(13)*. The peptidolytic activity was saturable, it obeyed typical Michaelis–Menten kinetics with

Table 2
Kinetic Parameters for Peptidolysis by Monoclonal Bence Jones Proteins

Protein	Substrate	K_m (M)	k_{cat} (min^{-1})	k_{cat}/K_m (M^{-1}min^{-1})
HIR[a]	vasopressin	1.9×10^{-3}	1.1×10^{-2}	5.8
YUK[a]	vasopressin	0.7×10^{-3}	2.1×10^{-3}	3.1
LAYM[b]	VIP	1.4×10^{-3}	1.4×10^{-2}	1.0×10^5
rREC[b,c]	VIP	2.1×10^{-7}	1.0×10^{-3}	4.9×10^4

[a] Data taken from ref. *13*.
[b] Data taken from ref. *11*.
[c] Recombinant light chain fragment from ref. *13*.

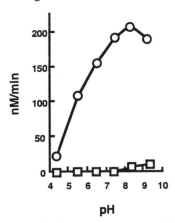

Fig. 1. Release of glycinamide from vasopressin by Bence Jones protein as a function of pH. Circles and squares indicate the presence and absence of Bence Jones protein, respectively, in the incubation mixture. Reprinted from *(13)* with permission.

K_m values in the low millimolar range (Table 2), and it was greatest at pH 8.2 (Fig. 1). Over the course of 24 h, there was a linear accumulation of glycinamide, the reaction product. The final concentration of glycinamide at termination of the reaction was much greater than that of the Bence Jones protein. This indicates that the Bence Jones protein is capable of substrate turnover, which is a defining feature of a true catalyst. Under the same conditions, desmopressin and oxytocin (Fig. 2) were not hydrolyzed at all. Paul et al. *(11)* showed that four of 21 Bence Jones proteins and 1 of 3 recombinant variable domains of light chain were capable of detectable cleavage of vasoactive intestinal peptide (VIP), and that the k_{cat}/K_m values for VIP hydrolysis were in the range of 10^4 M^{-1} min^{-1}, about four orders of magnitude greater than those of Bence Jones proteins for vasopressin (Table 2). The large differences in catalytic efficiency are owing mainly to the K_m values (0.14–0.21 µM for VIP versus 0.7–1.9 mM for vasopressin). The K_m value of a light chain subjected to denaturing solvent (guanidine hydrochloride) has been observed to be about

Cys-Tyr-Phe-Gln-Asn-Cys-Pro-Arg-GlyNH$_2$ arginine vasopressin

Cys$^+$-Tyr-Phe-Gln-Asn-Cys-Pro-Arg*-GlyNH$_2$ desmopressin

Cys-Tyr- Ile -Gln-Asn-Cys-Pro-Leu-GlyNH$_2$ oxytocin

Cys$^+$, deamino-cysteine; Arg*, D-arginine

Fig. 2. Amino acid sequences of arginine vasopressin, oxytocin, and desmopressin.

10-fold greater than that of the native light chain *(18)*. Thus, the catalytic efficiency also depends on the conformation of Bence Jones protein. Since the structure of the variable region is extremely diverse, individual Bence Jones proteins may differ enormously from each other in the K_m values, and hence in the level of catalytic activities and the scissile bond specificities. Paul et al. *(10,18)* showed that the light chain of a monoclonal antibody raised to VIP cleaved several peptide bonds (Gln-Met, Met-Ala, Ala-Val, Lys-Lys, and Lys-Tyr) which were clustered between residues 16 and 22 in VIP. The substrate specificity was somewhat different between the native light chain and the denatured/renatured light chain *(18)*. The results suggest that the molecular mechanisms underlying the proteolysis catalyzed by different Bence Jones proteins are complex and diverse. Pauling *(21)* pointed out the fundamental difference between enzymes and antibodies: the former selectively bind the transition state structures of chemical reactions while the latter bind the stable ground state structures. Based on this concept, numerous catalytic antibodies were prepared by immunization with haptens that mimic the transition states *(17)*. In addition, a MAb antibody raised against the ground state of VIP was able to cleave VIP *(10)*. Thus, it appears that the catalytic antibodies and their light chains synthesized by entirely natural mechanisms are capable of binding the transition state as well as the ground state of their antigens. Paul pointed out an essential feature of catalytic antibodies, i.e., a large turnover rate may be associated with reduced substrate specificity *(18)*. The same feature can be extrapolated to most Bence Jones proteins, which show a broad substrate specificity.

2.3. Nucleolytic Activity

It has been shown that autoantibodies present in sera of patients with systemic lupus erythematosus and their Fab fragments had the potential to hydrolyze DNA *(22)*. Some anti-DNA autoantibodies are known to traverse the cell and nuclear membranes to localize within the nuclei of cultured cells *(23)*. We found that one of four Bence Jones proteins unrelated to antinuclear antibodies had a DNA-hydrolyzing activity. This Bence Jones protein was taken up by cultured LLC-PK1 cells derived from renal proximal tubular epithelium and localized in the perinuclear region (unpublished data).

3. METABOLISM OF BENCE JONES PROTEINS

3.1. Biosynthesis of Light and Heavy Chains in Plasma Cells

The human genes encoding the κ and λ light chains of immunoglobulin are located on chromosomes 2 and 22, respectively, whereas the genes for all of the heavy chains reside on chromosome 14 *(24)*. Thus, the light and heavy chains are synthesized on separate ribosomes, and disulfide bonding of light and heavy chains occurs during or shortly after heavy chain synthesis, eventually forming an intact immunoglobulin molecule. The light chains are usually produced in excess over the heavy chains, and the level of the intracellular free light chain is assumed to play a regulatory role in the production and secretion of intact immunoglobulin *(25)*. This mechanism, designated isotype suppression, is lost in many patients with multiple myeloma at an early stage, resulting occasionally in massive production of Bence Jones protein.

3.2. Renal Handling of Bence Jones Proteins

Bence Jones proteins exist in plasma as monomers or dimers. There are roughly equal amounts of covalent and noncovalent dimers of κ chain, whereas the majority of λ chain dimers are covalently linked by disulfide bridge. Monomeric Bence Jones proteins are almost freely filtered through the glomerulus, whereas the clearance of dimers is about as half as great as that of monomers *(26)*. As the monomers are filtered through the glomerulus, a progressive dissociation of noncovalently linked dimers to monomers takes place in plasma, facilitating the urinary excretion of the light chains. One of the main functions of proximal renal tubules is the reabsorption and degradation of filtered proteins *(26,27)*. These proteins adhere to the brush border of tubular cells, possibly at specific receptor sites expressed by the cells, and are engulfed into pinocytotic vesicles. The vesicles are then pinched off and move into cytoplasm. The conventional view is that the vesicles fuse with lysosomes, which contain many proteolytic enzymes. When the enzymatic digestion is complete, free amino acids diffuse across the basement or basolateral membranes to the extracellular space. Some Bence Jones proteins remain intact within the cells and traverse the cytoplasm to reach the nucleus, although the exact mechanism of their uptake and transport as well as their final fate is not clear at present. Smaller oligopeptides are known to be hydrolyzed at the luminal surface of the brush border of proximal tubular cell *(27)*. This process is essentially the same as membrane digestion (also known as contact digestion) seen at the brush border of intestinal epithelial cells. It is likely, however, that the molecular size of Bence Jones proteins is too large to enter this catabolic pathway. Intact immunoglobulins are not filtered by glomerulus and hence their catabolism occurs by pathways different from that of Bence Jones proteins.

3.3. Reabsorptive Capacity of Renal Tubules

The reabsorptive capacity of the entire proximal tubule for proteins exceeds the amount of proteins filtered by the normal glomerulus. Polyclonal light chains are secreted into urine in the amounts of 5–50 mg per day in healthy subjects *(28)*. If the tubular function is not impaired, much greater loads of filtered proteins are reabsorbed. When the endocytotic receptors involved in reabsorption become saturated, the Bence Jones proteins in multiple myeloma patients pass to the distal tubules and into the urine (overflow proteinuria). Reabsorption of proteins beyond the convoluted proximal tubule is virtually absent. Patients with monoclonal gammopathies of undetermined significance secrete as much as 0.8 g light chains/d, while the patients with multiple myeloma excrete much larger amounts, up to 50 g light chains/d *(16,28–30)*. Impairments of the tubular function can also contribute towards increased excretion of Bence Jones proteins (tubular proteinuria).

3.4. Body Pool of Bence Jones Proteins

In the human body, water comprises approx 60% of the body weight and exists inside and outside the cell. The extracellular fluid comprises approx 60% of the total body water, and can be subdivided into three pools: vascular, interstitial, and transcellular fluids. The interstitial fluid is the solution surrounding the cells and accounts for approx 20% of the body water, whereas the transcellular pool includes the digestive juice, as well as cerebrospinal and synovial fluids. Proteins with relatively low molecular mass, such as Bence Jones proteins, are evenly distributed in vascular and interstitial fluids, irrespective of their body location. In steady state, the plasma concentration of Bence Jones protein approaches millimolar levels in some patients *(28–30)*. It can be concluded, therefore, that all cells facing the extracellular space are in persistent contact with millimolar levels of Bence Jones proteins.

4. DEPOSITION OF BENCE JONES PROTEIN IN VIVO

Bence Jones proteinuria is associated with a number of systemic diseases such as amyloidosis and light chain deposition disease (LCDD) as well as with a variety of renal disorders such as cast nephropathy *(14–16,31–35)*. These diseases result from the deposition of Bence Jones proteins in the form of amyloid, nonamyloid precipitates, and renal tubular casts. Gradual increases in these deposits ultimately lead to disorganization of tissue architecture, resulting in the impairment of renal and other organ functions. These changes were considered to account for much of the morbidity observed in patients with Bence Jones proteinuria. Since the Bence Jones proteins exist mainly in the body fluids and in the epithelial cells of the proximal renal tubules, the pathological changes take place most often in these two locations.

4.1. Systemic Deposits

Amyloidosis, which was named by Virchow in 1854, is now defined as a group of biochemically diverse conditions characterized by systemic tissue deposition of various fibrillar proteins, such as the Bence Jones proteins and transthyretin *(31–33)*. These fibrils consist of proteins that are structurally characterized by the antiparallel β-pleated sheet conformation, regardless of their chemical composition. The fibrils are deposited mainly outside the cell and are generally resistant to proteolytic digestion. The light chain-related amyloid, now termed AL, consists of partially digested light chains containing the variable region. The LCDD is characterized by polyvisceral extracellular deposition of an amorphous material which contains Bence Jones protein or its fragments, but does not have the intrinsic properties necessary to form β-pleated sheets *(34)*. Amyloidosis and LCDD are thought to proceed through two phases, with a lag between the individual phases *(33)*. The first phase involves partial proteolysis of Bence Jones protein, while the second phase is recognized by the deposition of the proteolytic fragments.

4.2. Local Deposits

Tamm–Horsfall glycoprotein is synthesized and secreted by cells of the thick ascending limb of the loop of Henle *(35)*. This glycoprotein has a high binding affinity for Bence Jones proteins, and with the two types of proteins coprecipitating to form proteinaceous casts, leads to the obstruction of distal tubules *(35)*. The resulting renal failure is called cast nephropathy or myeloma kidney.

5. PATHOGENESIS OF RENAL DYSFUNCTION

Among various symptoms associated with multiple myeloma, the renal dysfunction is the first clinical symptom in about 2/3 of cases and a major cause of their death *(14–16)*. The etiology of renal failure is multifactorial, but may be categorized into four mechanisms that are not mutually exclusive.

5.1. Mechanical or Cast Hypothesis

According to this hypothesis, the filtered Bence Jones protein does not damage the proximal tubule epithelium, but overloads the reabsorptive capacity of the proximal tubules. This leads to the increased delivery of the Bence Jones protein to the distal tubules, where it coprecipitates with Tamm–Horsfall glycoprotein. Mechanical obstruction of the distal nephron damages renal function. When rats were infused with Bence Jones proteins, tubular obstruction with impaired renal function was observed *(28)*, consistent with this hypothesis.

5.2. Alternative Mechanical Hypothesis

The above hypothesis was modified by Sanders *(31)* who showed that in experimental animals, Bence Jones proteins were endocytosed into proximal tubule cells, and some were precipitated within lysosomes. These cells were subsequently damaged, and debris from the disrupted cells filled the lumen of the tubules. It is proposed that as the epithelial cell function deteriorates progressively, the increased load of Bence Jones protein must be excreted by fewer number of nephrons, and the increased intratubular Bence Jones protein concentration favors its precipitation, resulting in cast formation. According to this hypothesis, the mechanical disruption of lysosomes is the initial event leading to the development of myeloma kidney.

5.3. Chemical or Nephrotoxicity Hypothesis

DeFronzo et al. *(36)* showed that the presence of renal insufficiency correlated best with tubular atrophy and degeneration, but not with the presence of obstructing intratubular casts. Cast formation, therefore, is the likely result, but not cause, of renal dysfunction. In animal experiments, similar results were obtained *(37)*. These investigators proposed that direct cytotoxic effects of Bence Jones proteins are the major mechanism of renal dysfunction. There are number of reports consistent with this hypothesis. Adult Fanconi syndrome (increased loss of glucose and amino acids) and defects in the ability to acidify and to concentrate the urine in the absence of renal casts were reported in at least 30 patients with Bence Jones proteinuria (reviewed in ref. *38*), and it was suggested that the prevalence of such defects would be even greater if all patients were to be tested for renal dysfunction (38). By using rat and rabbit kidney slices or membrane fractions, Bence Jones proteins were shown to block the transport of p-aminohippuric acid, ammonium, amino acids, and glucose, as well as to inhibit the activity of Na,K-ATPase (reviewed in ref. *38*).

5.4. Catalytic Hypothesis

The foregoing, taken together, suggest that the initial event in the pathogenesis for nephropathy is chemical rather than mechanical, although additional factors may contribute to variable levels of damage in the kidney. Virtually nothing is known, however, of the molecular mechanism underlying the chemical nephrotoxicity of Bence Jones protein. It is reasonable to propose that the catalytic acitvity of Bence Jones proteins may be responsible for the nephrotoxicity. The Bence Jones proteins may slowly hydrolyze either the extracellular membrane components such as cytokine receptors and ion channels, or upon internalization into cells, intracellular enzymes and nucleic acids. Cleavage of a single bond in these macromolecules would be sufficient to cause a loss or a decrease in their physiological function, ultimately leading to renal dysfunction.

6. PATHOGENESIS OF EXTRARENAL DISORDERS

Extrarenal disorders associated with Bence Jones proteinuria are mainly due to the aggregation of these proteins, the mechanism being mechanical rather than chemical. As discussed above, precipitation of Bence Jones protein is strongly facilitated by partial proteolysis, the enzymes responsible for which are thought to be released from neutrophils or macrophages. However, these cells begin to emigrate to the sites of amyloid or light chain deposition after, but not before, the formation of such deposits. Thus, the first phase is triggered by proteinases other than those released from inflammatory cells where we have occasionally observed the autocatalytic cleavage of Bence Jones protein. It is possible, therefore, that the first phase of amyloid or light chain deposition is triggered by an autocatalytic cleavage of Bence Jones proteins, although further work is needed to substantiate this possibility.

There are certain other extrarenal disorders associated with Bence Jones proteinuria. Coagulation abnormalities are found in many patients, and thought to be caused by the binding of the myeloma protein to fibrin during coagulation *(14)*. It is possible that a partial cleavage of clotting factors may underlie the coagulation abnormalities. Neurological symptoms, such as nonspecific higher cerebral dysfunction and peripheral sensorimotor neuropathies, occur in some patients *(14)*. Asthma has been associated with depletion of VIP in the airway *(39)*, which may be owing to the cleavage of VIP by catalytic autoantibodies *(18)*. By analogy, it is possible that partial hydrolysis of neuropeptides by Bence Jones protein may result in a variety of neurological manifestations in multiple myeloma patients.

7. CONCLUDING REMARKS

In this chapter, we proposed the possibility that the catalytic activity of Bence Jones proteins plays an important role for the pathogenesis of multiple myeloma. The question arises: Are polyclonal light chains present in healthy subjects capable of hydrolyzing some body constituents to any significant extent? Our answer is "probably not," since their concentrations in body fluids are very low, and since their k_{cat}/K_m values, which differ from protein to protein, may be, on average, much lower than of a pathogenic monoclonal Bence Jones protein. Furthermore, the intact antibody directed to the same antigen as the light chain may inhibit the catalytic activity by binding the ground state of the antigen and protecting it from contact with the light chain *(18)*. On the other hand, it is likely that the catalytic activity becomes significant in patients with multiple myeloma, in whom the concentrations of Bence Jones proteins reach up to millimolar levels. This situation is analogous to the one found in patients with diabetes mellitus. At the normal blood level, glucose does not damage body constituents, but when the concentration is several-fold elevated, slow glycation of a number of proteins can occur, ultimately leading to diverse symptoms seen in the diabetes patients. Therefore, it is possible, that the catalytic activity of the Bence Jones proteins, albeit weak, may underlie the diverse symptoms under conditions permitting massive production of these proteins. Note also that Bence Jones proteins contain hypervariable sequence regions, and certain clones of Bence Jones proteins might express high levels of catalytic activity.

Bence Jones proteins possess two independent globular domains, constant and variable regions that are linked by a short peptide segment. The constant region confers the common characteristics to all Bence Jones proteins, whereas the variable region is responsible for the diversity of chemical, physicochemical, and biological characteristics of the individual proteins. The catalytic activity as well as amyloidogenic and cast-forming potentials resides in the variable region *(18)*. This explains the great difference in the pathogenic potentials among Bence Jones proteins. Some Bence Jones proteins may be devoid of pathogenic potential. For example, patients with massive Bence Jones proteinuria, such as daily urinary excretion of 20–50 g for many years *(28)*, without developing systemic symptoms have been reported. Further work, such as the relationship between the catalytic activity of Bence Jones proteins and the severity of clinical symptoms, is needed to substantiate the catalytic hypothesis. It will not only lead to better understanding of the disease pathogenesis, but also to development of a new therapeutic approach for multiple myeloma.

ACKNOWLEDGMENTS

This research was supported in part by grants from the Japan Private School Promotion Foundation and the Environmental Science Research Institute of Kinki University.

REFERENCES

1. Clamp, J. R. (1967) Some aspects of the first recorded case of multiple myeloma. *Lancet* **2**, 1354–1356.
2. MacIntire, W. (1850) Case of mollities and fragilitas ossium, accompanied with urine strongly charged with animal matter. *Med. Chir. Trans.* **33**, 211–232.
3. Jones, B. H. (1847) Papers on chemical pathology; prefaced by the Gulstonian Lectures, read at the Royal College of Physicians, 1846. *Lancet* **2**, 88–92.
4. Peeters, H. (chairman) and 21 other participants (1961) Round table conference: New methods and recent results in protide chemistry. *Protides Biol. Fluids* **9**, 359–370.
5. Migita, S. (1965) The story of Bence Jones protein (in Japanese). *Kyudai Iho* **35**, 205–209.
6. Edelman, G. M. and Gally, J. A. (1962) The nature of Bence Jones proteins: chemical similarities to polypeptide chains of myeloma globulins and normal γ-globulins. *J. Exp. Med.* **116**, 207–227.
7. Erhan, S., and Greller, L. D. (1974) Do immunoglobulins have proteolytic activity? *Nature* **251**, 353–355.
8. Mei, S., Mody, R., Ekulund, S. H., and Paul, S. (1991) Vasoactive intestinal peptide hydrolysis by antibody light chains. *J. Biol. Chem.* **266**, 15,571–15,574.
9. Gao, Q.-S., Sun, M., Tyutyukova, S., Webster, D., Rees, A., Tranibtabim A., et al. (1994) Molecular cloning of a proteolytic antibody light chain. *J. Biol. Chem.* **269**, 32,389–32,393.
10. Sun, M., Gao, Q.-S., Li, L., and Paul, S. (1994) Proteolytic activity of an antibody light chain. *J. Immunol.* **153**, 5121–5126.
11. Paul, S., Li, L., Kalga, R., Wilkins-Stevens, P., Stevens, F. J., and Solomon, A. (1995) Natural catalytic antibodies: peptide-hydrolyzing activities of Bence Jones proteins and VL fragment. *J. Biol. Chem.* **270**, 15,257–15,262.

12. Matsuura, K., Yamamoto, K., and Sinohara, H. (1994) Amidase activity of human Bence Jones proteins. *Biochem. Biophys. Res. Commun.* **204,** 57–62.
13. Matsuura, K. and Sinohara, H. (1996) Catalytic cleavage of vasopressin by human Bence Jones proteins at the arginylglycinamide bond. *Biol. Chem.* **377,** 587–589.
14. Selby, P. and Gore, M. (1995) Myeloma and other plasma cell malignancies, in *Oxford Textbook of Oncology* (Peckham, M., Pinego, H., and Veronesi, U., eds.) vol. 1, pp. 1852–1878.
15. Buxbaum, J. (1992) Mechanisms of disease: Monoclonal immunoglobulin deposition. *Hematol. Oncol. Clin. N. Am.* **6,** 323–346.
16. Pascali, E. and Pezzoli, A. (1988) The clinical spectrum of pure Bence Jones proteinuria. *Cancer* **62,** 2408–2415.
17. Lerner, R. A., Benkovic, S. J., and Schultz, P. G. (1991) At the crossroads of chemistry and immunology: catalytic antibodies. *Science* **252,** 659–667.
18. Paul, S. (1996) Natural catalytic antibodies. *Mol. Biotechnol.* **5,** 197–207.
19. Li, L., Paul, S., Tyutyukova, S., Kazatchkine, M., and Kaveri, S. (1995) Catalytic activity of anti-thyroglobulin antibodies. *J. Immunol.* **154,** 3328–3332.
20. Paul, S., Volle, D. J., Beach, C. M., Johnson, D. R., Powell, M. J., and Massey, R. J. (1989) Catalytic hydrolysis of vasoactive intestinal peptide by human autoantibody. *Science* **244,** 1158–1162.
21. Pauling, L. (1946) Molecular architecture and biological reactions. *Chem. Eng. News* **24,** 1375–1377.
22. Shuster, A. M., Gololobov, G. V., Kvashuk, O. A., Bogomolova, A. E., Smirnov, I. V., and Gabibov, A.G. (1992) DNA hydrolyzing autoantibodies. *Science* **256,** 665–667.
23. Yanase, K., Smith, R. M., Cizman, B., Foster, M. H., Peachey, L. D., Jarett, L., et al. (1994) A subgroup of murine monoclonal antideoxyribonucleic acid antibodies traverse the cytoplasm and enter the nucleus in a time- and temperature-dependent manner. *Lab. Invest.* **71,** 52–60.
24. Levinson, S. S. and Keren, D. F. (1994) Free light chains of immunoglobulins: clinical laboratory analysis. *Clin. Chem.* **40,** 1869–1878.
25. Ioannidis, R. A., Joshua, D. E., Warburton, P. T., Francis, S. E., Brown, R. D., Gibson, J., et al. (1989) Multiple myeloma: evidence that light chains play an immunoregulatory role in B-cell regulation. *Hematol. Pathol.* **3,** 169–175.
26. Maack, T., Johnson, V., Kau, S. T., Figueiredo, J., and Sigulem, D. (1979) Renal filtration, transport, and metabolism of low-molecular-weight proteins: a review. *Kidney Int.* **16,** 251–270.
27. Carone, F. A., Peterson, D. R., Oparil, S., and Pullman, T. N. (1979) Renal tubular transport and catabolism of proteins and peptides. *Kidney Int.* **16,** 271–278.
28. Solomon, A., Weiss, D. H., and Kattine, A. A. (1991) Nephrotoxic potential of Bence Jones proteins. *N. Engl. J. Med.* **324,** 1845–1851.
29. Dammacco, F. and Waldenstrom, J. (1968) Serum and urine light chain levels in benign monoclonal gammopathies, multiple myeloma and Waldenstrom's macroglobulinemia. *Clin. Exp. Immunol.* **3,** 911–921.
30. Nelson, M., Brown, R. D., Gibson, J., and Joshua, D. E. (1992) Measurement of free kappa and lambda chains in serum and the significance of their ratio in patients with multiple myeloma. *Br. J. Haematol.* **81,** 223–230.
31. Sanders, P. W. (1994) Pathogenesis and treatment of myeloma kidney. *J. Lab. Clin. Med.* **124,** 484–488.

32. Kyle, R. A. and Gertz, M. A. (1995) Primary systemic amyloidosis: clinical and laboratory features in 474 cases. *Semin. Hematol.* **32,** 45–59.
33. Shirahama, T., Miura, K., Ju, S.-T., Kisilevsky, R., Gruys, E., and Cohen, A. S. (1990) Amyloid enhancing factor-loaded macrophages in amyloid fibril formation. *Lab. Invest.* **62,** 61–68.
34. Preud'homme, J.-L., Aucouturier, P., Touchard, G., Striker, L., Khamlichi, A. A., Rocca, A., et al. (1994) Monoclonal immunoglobulin deposition disease (Randall type). Relationship with structural abnormalities of immunoglobulin chains. *Kidney Int.* **46,** 965–972.
35. Huang, Z.-Q., Kirk, K. A., Connelly, K. G., and Sanders, P. W. (1993) Bence Jones proteins bind to a common peptide segment of Tamm-Horsfall glycoprotein to promote heterotypic aggregation. *J. Clin. Invest.* **92,** 2975–2983.
36. DeFronzo, R. A., Cooke, C. R., Wright, J. R., and Humphrey, R. L. (1978) Renal function in patients with multiple myeloma. *Medicine* **57,** 151–166.
37. Yokota, N., Yamamoto, Y., Kitamura, K., Kuroki, N., Hisanaga, S., Fujimoto, S., et al. (1991) Renal tubular lesions induced by human Bence Jones protein in the rat: N-acetyl-b-D-glucosaminidase as a sensitive marker. *J. Exp. Pathol.* **72,** 255–262.
38. Fang, L. S. T. (1985) Light-chain nephropathy. *Kidney Int.* **27,** 582–592.
39. Ollerenshaw, S., Jarvis, D., Woolcock, A., Sullivan, C., and Scheibner, T. (1989) Absence of immunoreactive vasoactive intestinal polypeptide in tissue from the lungs of patients with asthma. *N. Engl. J. Med.* **320,** 1244–1248.

17

Kidney Damage in Autoimmune Disease

Gerald C. Groggel

1. INTRODUCTION

In 1641, Daniel Sennet noted the association of scarlatina and dropsy *(1)*, but it was not until 40 years ago that Mellors first demonstrated in human kidney biopsies the deposition in the glomerulus of gamma globulins *(2)*. Since that time, there has been a tremendous amount of work, both experimental and clinical, demonstrating that the kidney is an important site of injury in auto-immune disease. In systemic lupus erythematous, the prototypic autoimmune disorder, the kidney is the organ most commonly affected. By kidney biopsy, at least mild abnormalities are seen in all patients with lupus.

2. IMMUNE REACTIONS IN KIDNEYS

This chapter will review immune injury in the kidney, concentrating on the glomerulus which is the primary site of damage in autoimmune disorders of the kidney. Immune injury in the kidney can involve either humoral or cellular immune responses to a variety of antigens, both endogenous and exogenous *(3)*. The humoral response involves antibodies, which are deposited in the kidney by two mechanisms: 1) the deposition of circulating immune complexes or 2) *in situ* binding of antibodies to antigens present within the kidney *(3)*. The antigens present within the kidney can either be structural elements of the kidney, such as components of the glomerular basement membrane, or anti-gens trapped or planted in the kidney. Antibodies can also interact with soluble antigens to form immune complexes in the circulation and those immune com-plexes which escape clearance by the mononuclear phagocytic system can accu-mulate within the kidney, particularly the glomerulus. These immune complexes can then undergo continuous rearrangement. Once an antibody is deposited in the kidney, a variety of other mediators will be activated. Recently, a new mech-anism whereby antibodies can activate immunologic responses within the kidney has been identified. Antibodies to constituents of neutrophil granules have been dentified as antineutrophil cytoplasmic antibodies (ANCA) *(4)*, which may induce immune injury by activating neutrophils. Certain autoimmune diseases such as Wegener's granuloma have active inflammatory changes within the glomerulus,

Contemporary Immunology: Autoimmune Reactions
Edited by: S. Paul © Humana Press Inc., Totowa, NJ

although glomerular antibody deposits are not detected. The presence of ANCA in the circulation often is associated with such diseases.

The second type of immune reaction in the kidney is the cell-mediated immune response, which involves activated T-cells, monocytes and macrophages *(3)*. Antigen specific T-cells can respond to their specific antigens in a delayed-type hypersensitivity reaction, accompanied by the release of various lympho-kines and a consequent recruitment of monocytes and macrophages. Sensitization to kidney antigens can also result in development of cytotoxic T-cells, which can directly damage kidney cells.

After initiation of the immune response, either cellular or humoral, a variety of mediators of inflammation are recruited *(5)*. The identity of the mediators of the immune injury varies, depending on the initial immune response as well as the location of the response in the kidney. The two major sites where immune responses can occur in the kidney are the glomerulus and the tubulointerstitium. The response of the kidney, and particularly the glomerulus, to the immuno-logical mediators is rather uniform, and includes 1) cellular proliferation and hypertrophy, 2) the synthesis and deposition of extracellular matrix within the glomerulus, which can lead to sclerosis and scarring, and 3) the expression of new antigens on the glomerular cells *(6)*. These responses often involve the synthesis and secretion of multiple growth factors. The major emphasis of this review will be on the mediators of the glomerular immune response.

3. MECHANISMS AND SITES OF IMMUNE DEPOSIT FORMATION

The humoral and cellular immune responses, as well as the mediators of inflammation, have been studied most extensively in experimental animal models of glomerular injury. Much of this chapter deals with the animal model studies, but there is accumulating evidence for similar immune responses in the patho-genesis of human renal disease as well.

Dixon proposed a classification of glomerulonephritis based on the evident pathogenetic mechanisms *(7)*. He proposed two basic forms of glomerulone-phritis: the one induced by circulating antibodies reacting with fixed structural antigens of the glomerular basement membrane (GBM) and producing linear IgG deposition in the glomeruli seen by immunofluorescence microscopy and the other induced by the deposition of circulating immune complexes in the glomerulus and producing granular immune deposits (Fig. 1). This classifica-tion has recently been expanded by the identification of an *in situ* mechanism for the development of immune deposits within the glomeruli *(8,9)*. Thus, granular immune deposits can result from trapping of circulating immune com-plexes, but they also can result from antigen or antibody binding to a glomeru-lar structure followed by immune complex formation *in situ* *(8)*. Although antibodies reacting with an intrinsic glomerular antigen can produce either linear or granular types of deposits (Fig. 1), immune injury may occur in the absence of

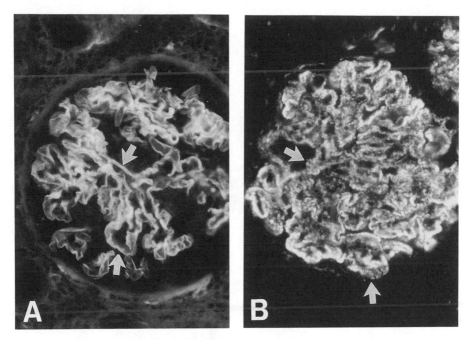

Fig. 1. Immunofluorescence micrographs comparing linear and granular stain-ing. A. Smooth linear deposits of anti-GBM antibody (arrows) are present along the glomerular basement membrane in a patient with anti-GBM glomeruloncphritis. B. Irregular granular deposits of IgG (arrows) are present along the glomerular capillary walls. (Fluorescein isothiocyanate conjugated anti-human IgG; original magnification × 832).

visible deposits. In this case, the injury is thought to be mediated by immune cells rather than by immunoglobulins.

An alternative classification of renal immunological disease relies on the histologic appearance and divides glomerular disorders into inflammatory and noninflammatory types *(5)*. In a third classification scheme, the glomerular injury can be classified according to the site of the immune deposits and the nature of the injury *(10)*. The deposits may lie within the subepithelial space, the subendothelial space, the GBM itself, or the mesangium (Fig. 2). The site of the immune deposit in the glomerulus is an important determinant of the consequent functional and histological lesions, and of the mediators involved in the immune injury.

4. MEDIATORS OF IMMUNE INJURY

Considerable recent research has been aimed at identifying the factors which mediate kidney damage in immunologic renal disease. The functional mani-festations of the injury include changes in glomerular filtration rate and proteinuria,

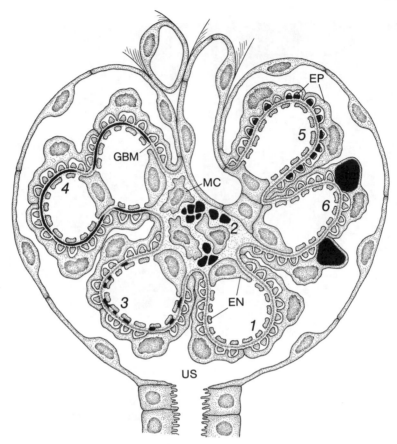

Fig. 2. Schematic representation of a single glomerulus illustrating the various sites of immune complex deposits. Loop 1 represents a normal glomerular capillary wall with endothelial cells (EN), glomerular basement membrane (GBM) and epithelial cells (EP). MC represents mesangial cells and US is the urinary space. Shown in 2 are immune complex deposits within the mesangial matrix as found in IgA nephropathy. Loop 3 demonstrates subendothelial immune deposits such as is found in membranoproliferative glomerulonephritis. Shown in loop 4 are the linear deposits along the GBM found in anti-GBM glomerulonephritis. In loop 5 are the diffuse subepithelial deposits of membranous nephropathy. Shown in loop 6 are the subepithelial humps found in post-streptococcal glomerulonephritis.

reflecting defects in glomerular permeability. The structural manifestations include GBM thickening, cellular proliferation, necrosis, thrombosis, crescent formation, and sclerosis.

A variety of mediators of immune glomerular injury have been identified *(5)*. The pathways by which the glomerular immune response leads to injury to capillary wall injury are shown in Fig. 3. These include: 1) cellular elements consisting of polymorphonuclear cells, mononuclear cells (including monocytes

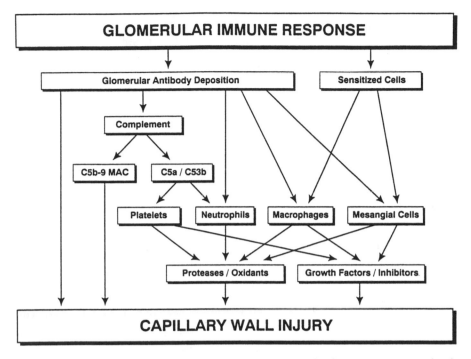

Fig. 3. Shown is a schematic by which the glomerular immune response leads to capillary wall injury through a variety of mediators (adapted from ref. 5).

and macrophages), lymphocytes, platelets, and also mesangial cells *(3)* and 2) soluble elements including antibody, complement (particularly the membrane attack complex), fibrinogen, prostanoids, leukotrienes, platelet activating factor, interleukins (IL), tumor necrosis factor (TNF), nitric oxide, endothelin, angiotensin II, and antineutrophil cytoplasmic antibodies.

The contribution of the individual mediators varies depending on the particular disease, and the stage and severity of the disease. The roles of these mediators have been most extensively studied in antibody-mediated experimental models of glomerular immune injury. It is hoped that a better understanding of the mediators will allow therapeutic interventions in various types of immune renal injuries, even without a complete elucidation of the underlying immune response.

4.1. Antibody

Antibody alone may produce injury without the participation of any other mediators. In nephrotoxic nephritis in the guinea pig, anti-GBM antibody produces proteinuria without the involvement of complement or cells *(11)*. In the isolated perfused rat kidney, anti-GBM antibody can produce changes in glomerular permeability without other mediators *(12)*. In passive Heymann nephritis, administration of the F(ab')$_2$ or F(ab') fragments of heterologous anti-Fx1A antibody produces proteinuria in the rat without fixing complement *(13)*. Monoclonal antibodies (MAbs) to the glomeruler epithelial cell (GEC) membrane or to the GEC slit diaphragm have been shown to cause proteinuria in the rat independent of other mediators *(14,15)*.

The mechanism(s) whereby antibody alone produces injury in these models is not known. Injury to the glomerular epithelial cells (GEC) could include detachment of the cells from the basement membrane, which could then lead to alterations in permeability. Alternatively, the GEC may be stimulated to produce substances that damage the glomerular capillary wall. GEC in culture have been shown to produce a neutral proteinase capable of digesting type IV collagen and the GBM *(16)*.

4.2. Complement

The usual mechanism whereby immune deposits and antibody are thought to initiate injury is through the activation of the complement system *(17,18)*. The complement system can be activated by either the classical pathway which is initiated by IgG or IgM, or by the alternative pathway which can be initiated by IgA or by nonimmunological agents like polysaccharides and bacteria *(19)*. Both pathways lead to the formation of a C3 convertase to form C3b *(19)*. This leads to the generation of a C5 convertase responsible for forming C5a and C5b. Generation of C5b from either pathway initiates self-assembly of C5b-9, which is the membrane attack complex.

The classical role for complement in immune injury is the generation of chemotactic factors, particularly C5a, which attract neutrophils to the site of immune deposits *(20)*. Neutrophils may also be attracted by immune adherence mechanisms involving C3b. The ability of neutrophils to produce injury is discussed in Subheading 4.3. The best examples of complement-neutrophil mediated glomerulonephritis are the heterologous and autologous phases of anti-GBM nephritis *(20)*. Depletion of complement in this model prevents neutrophil recruitment and injury *(20)*. Neutrophil depletion also prevents injury and repletion of neutrophils produces proteinuria *(21)*. Note that the neutrophils may be capable of mediating glomerulonephritis even in the absence of complement activation. Recent work has also shown that complement activation promotes the recruitment of platelets to the sites of immune deposits.

A role for complement in noninflammatory immunologic injury has been identified, which does not involve the recruitment of neutrophils, but rather, the formation of the membrane attack complex (C5b-9) (MAC) *(22)*. A role for the MAC was first shown in passive Heymann nephritis in the rat, a model of human membranous nephritis *(22)*. After administration of heterologous anti-Fx1A antibody to the animals, immune deposits form in the subepithelial space as a result of antibody binding to an antigen expressed on the GEC. The antibody activates complement and the MAC is formed. Depletion of complement with cobra venom factor in this model prevents injury without affecting the level of antibody deposition. In contrast, neutrophil-depletion does not ameliorate the injury. In rabbits unable to form the MAC because of a deficiency in the sixth component of complement, injury is prevented in a model of induced membranous nephropathy *(23)*. Similarly, in the isolated perfused kidney, no injury is evident following administration of antibody to Fx1A antigen if the perfusion is conducted with C6 or C8 deficient serum, but proteinuria develops immediately by perfusion with normal serum containing all of the complement components *(24)*. The participation of the MAC in glomerular disease is not confined to membranous nephropathy. Proteinuria is reduced and renal function is preserved in the heterologous phase of anti-GBM nephritis in rabbits deficient in C6 *(25)*. Deposits of the MAC have been detected at the sites of immune injury in experimental models of complement-dependent renal injury *(26)*.

The MAC formation is initiated by proteolytic cleavage of C5 to form C5b *(27)*. The C5b combines with C6 and C7, forming the C5b67 complex, which can bind to cell membranes or to S-protein (vitronectin) in the plasma. The C5b67 complex on the cell membranes binds C8 and multiple C9 molecules, and becomes capable of inserting into and disrupting the lipid bilayer, leading to lysis of the cell. If the S-protein binds the C5b67, the resultant complex can still bind C8 and C9, but it cannot insert into membranes.

The mechanism whereby the MAC produces injury in the kidney is not known fully. C5b-9 may activate cells such as the GEC in Heymann nephritis, which could lead to the release of inflammatory mediators. Antibody to GEC combined with sublytic concentrations of complement has been shown to induce noncytolytic injury in vitro *(28)*. The sublytic C5b-9 attack mechanism is associated with the following: increased intracellular calcium, activation of phospholipase C, increased IP2, IP3, diacylglycerol, and phosphatidic acid, and the release of PGF2 and thromboxane *(29)*. Further, exposure of glomerular mesangial cells in culture to sublytic amounts of C5b-9 leads to release of hydrogen peroxide and superoxide anion *(30)*. A second possible mechanism for the MAC-induced injury is the increased production of extracellular matrix components by GEC (such as type IV collagen production upon exposure to C5b-9) *(31)*. Last, but not least, activation and formation of MAC on the GEC surface may detach these cells, which can be anticipated to cause proteinuria.

Interestingly, a deficiency of C6 increases the severity of nephritis in rabbits administered sheep IgG followed by a subnephrotoxic dose of sheep anti-rabbit GBM *(32)*. On day five, after injection of the anti-GBM antibody, the C6-deficient rabbits had the same degree of proteinuria as the normocomplementemic control animals, greater loss of renal function, and more severe histologic damage. The C6-deficient animals also had displayed persistent immune deposits in the kidney as evident by measurement of sheep IgG in isolated glomeruli *(32)*. Thus, in this model, the complement deficient animals had more severe injury presumably because of a failure to clear the immune deposits. This suggests a role for the MAC in the solubilization and clearance of glomerular immune deposits. It is evident, therefore, that complement may play multiple roles in immune-mediated renal injury.

Another important function of complement is its role in the removal of immune complexes from the circulation via the complement receptor CR1, which is specific for C3b *(33,34)*. In primates, immune complexes are transported to the fixed macrophage system by erythrocytes, which express the CR1 receptors *(33,34)*. Immune complexes that activate complement contain bound C3b. The C3b binds its receptor CR1 on the surface of red blood cells and the cell-bound immune complexes are carried to the liver. The immune complexes are internalized by phagocytes and the erythrocytes are returned to the circulation *(34)*. The binding of the immune complexes to the erythrocytes prevents their deposition in organs such as the kidney. When complement is depleted in experimental animals, a large proportion of exogenously administered immune complexes are deposited in the kidney rather than being cleared by the liver *(32)*. Transport of immune complexes by erythrocytes thus has a protective function, ensuring their safe delivery to the mononuclear phagocyte system where they are eliminated. These findings may explain why patients with complement deficiencies have a higher incidence of immune complex-mediated diseases *(34)*.

4.3. Neutrophils

The site of antibody and immune complex deposition plays an important role in directing the infiltration of neutrophils *(10)*. In the subendothelial and mesangial areas, immune deposits are accessible to the neutrophils and the neutrophils can localize to these areas in response to a variety of mediators, including C5a, platelet activating factor and products of the lipoxygenase pathway. Neutrophils may adhere to tissue components containing immune deposits via their receptors for the F_c portion of the immunoglobulin molecule and for C3b. Leukocyte adhesion molecules expressed by kidney cells, including integrins, intracellular adhesions molecules, vascular cell adhesion molecules and selectins may promote neutrophil localization *(35)*. The neutrophils can then release various proteinases and oxidants to produce tissue injury. The subepithelial space is not accessible to neutrophils.

The importance of the polymorphonuclear leukocyte (PMN) has been established in several models of immune glomerular injury. Perhaps best documented is the participation of PMNs in nephrotoxic nephritis. Cochrane et al. showed a rapid influx of PMNs into rat glomeruli peaking at about two hours after injection of nephrotoxic serum (NTS) *(20)*. Rats depleted of PMNs had markedly lower levels of proteinuria following NTS administration, and the reduced proteinuria persisted throughout the first week of nephritis. Naisch et al. *(36)* extended these observations, documenting the participation of PMNs in the autologous phase of nephrotoxic nephritis. Rabbits depleted of PMNs by either nitrogen mustard or antipolymorphonuclear cell serum displayed a reduction in the autologous phase-induced proteinuria, fibrin deposition, and azotemia. A correlation between fibrin deposition and PMN accumulation was also noted by Hooke et al. *(37)* who used monoclonal antibodies to characterize the cellular infiltration in several forms of glomerular and interstitial disease.

PMNs, normally found in small numbers along with monocytes in the glomeruli, were increased in postinfectious glomerulonephritis and, to a lesser degree, in crescentic glomerulonephritis. In a model less commonly thought of as involving PMNs, in-situ immune complex glomerulonephritis, Cook et al. *(38)* documented an infiltration of PMNs within 30 min of immune complex formation. The neutrophil infiltration was superceded in the subsequent 24 h by an accumulation of macrophages.

It seems then that PMNs can be important effector cells, either because of their predominance in an infiltrating cell population or their early appearance in an infiltrate with an evolving constitution. The PMNs may potentially be functionally important in producing proteinuria, azotemia, or fibrin deposition. A surprising finding in a study by Cochrane *(20)* was that PMNs produced negligible glomerular destruction in the early phase of nephrotoxic nephritis. Ultrastructural analysis showed that the PMNs displaced endothelial cells away from the basement membrane. Even though endothelial cell apposition was restored after 12–24 h, the accompanying proteinuria persisted. The importance of PMNs in decreasing glomerular filtration was emphasized by Tucker et al. *(39)* in a rat model of nephritis induced by anti-GBM antibody. They showed that the glomerular ultrafiltration coefficient and the single nephron glomerular filtration rate did not decrease in rats depleted of PMNs prior to injection of anti-GBM antibody.

The central role of PMNs in producing mediators of tissue injury has drawn considerable attention from renal pathophysiologists. Specifically, PMNs are well known for their ability to produce oxygen free radicals (OFR) and tissue proteinases, substances that have gained increasing recognition as contributing to the pathogenesis of glomerular injury.

Study of the heterologous phase of nephrotoxic nephritis has offered the strongest evidence for the direct participation of reactive oxygen species in injury. Adachi et al. *(40)* administered nephrotoxic serum to rats followed by the daily administration of superoxide dismutase (SOD). The SOD treated rats displayed lower levels of proteinuria than control rats, as well as lesser mesangial thickening and lesser capillary obliteration. Rehan et al. *(41)* injected nephrotoxic serum directly into the renal artery of the rat, producing significant proteinuria, which was prevented by treatment with catalase. An inverse relationship between the dose of catalase and the proteinuria was evident. The calalase-treated animals showed lower degrees of endothelial cell injury and epithelial cell foot process fusion than the controls, but there was no improvement of the glomerular filtration rate. In a model of immune complex disease in which neutrophils were exposed to aggregated IgG, the cells were shown to elaborate superoxide anion *(42)*.

4.4. Proteases

Proteases are produced by inflammatory cells and mediate tissue damage. There are four major classes of proteases which are named for the chemical

Table 1
Classes of Proteases

Protease class	pH range	Location	Examples
Serine	7–9	Intra- and extracellular	Elastase, Cathepsin G, Plasmin
Cysteine	3–7	Intralysosomal	Cathepsin B and L
Aspartic	2–6	Intralysosomal	Cathepsin D
Metalloenzymes	5–9	Intra- and extracellular	Gelatinase, Type IV Collagenase

Adapted from ref. *43*.

species at their enzymatic active site, i.e., serine, cysteine and aspartic proteases, and metalloenzymes (Table 1) *(42)*. These enzymes differ in their cells of origin, their intralysosomal location, extracellular secretion pattern, and the pH at which they are optimally active (Table 1) *(43)*.

The evidence that proteases contribute to kidney disease is derived from four types of observations: 1) the capacity of various classes of proteases to digest different constituents of the kidney in vitro, 2) the presence of proteases at high levels in various models of glomerular disease in vivo, 3) the occurence of glomerular dysfunction following administration of proteases to experimental animals, and 4) the ability of protease inhibitors to ameliorate the histologic and functional indicators of induced kidney disease.

Because they are the predominant species within the azurophil granules of PMNs and are most active at neutral pH, the serine proteases (including, elastase, Cathepsin G, and plasmin) are considered to be of major importance in inflammatory reactions. Davies et al. *(44)* demonstrated substantial dissolution of collagen, measured as the release of hydroxyproline, upon incubation of GBM with either elastase or Cathepsin G. Serine protease inhibitors are effective in preventing neutrophil mediated detachment of endothelial cell monolayers from culture wells *(45)*. A metalloproteinase activated by a product of the myeloperoxidase-hydrogen peroxide-halide system is shown to mediate the degradation of GBM by neutrophils stimulated with PMA. Further, a neutral metalloproteinase capable of digesting GBM was also produced by glomerular mesangial cells in culture *(47)*. This proteinase specifically degraded both the soluble and insoluble forms of type IV collagen, a major component of the GBM. Baricos et al. *(48)* purified the lysosomal cysteine proteases, Cathepsin B and L, from human kidney and observed these enzymes to degrade the GBM at acid pH *(48)*. The presence of Cathepsin B in isolated glomeruli was evident in the absence of PMNs.

Johnson et al. *(49)* demonstrated that injection of the serine proteases, elastase and Cathepsin G into the renal arteries caused dose-dependent proteinuria. Invasion by white blood cells or proliferation of the resident glomerular cells was not seen. Despite the induction of significant proteinuria, no glomerular histologic changes were noted. Davin et al. *(50)* studied the role of neutral proteinases and metalloproteinases in two models of glomerular disease, accelerated nephrotoxic serum nephritis (NSN) and puromycin aminonucleoside nephrosis (PAN). In both models, urinary excretion of neutral proteinases was greatly increased and parallelled the excretion of type IV collagen and laminin. Whereas normal urine contained mainly serine proteinases, both serine and metalloproteinases were found in urine in infiltrating and noninfiltrating disease models. Schrijver et al. *(51)* studied the course of PMN-dependent, complement-independent NSN in Beije mice, in which the PMNs are deficient in both elastase and Cathepsin G. Administration of even the highest doses of the nephrotoxic serum in the Beije mice caused only a small increment in proteinuria, despite an influx of glomerular PMNs comparable to that in control mice receiving NSN. The proteinases must contribute substantially, therefore, in the proteinuria observed in this model. Despite the difference in proteinuria, the damage to endothelial cells in the Beije and control mice was comparable. The ameliorative effect of a specific cysteine proteinase inhibitor, trans-epoxy-succinyl-2-leucylamido- (4-guanidine) butane (E-64) has been studied in a complement- and neutrophil-independent model of anti-GBM antibody disease *(52)*. Administration of E-64 prior to and following anti-GBM antibody administration significantly reduced the degree of proteinuria. The specific activity of Cathepsin B and L in the glomeruli was found to be decreased.

Plasmin is a serine protease capable of degrading extracellular matrix as well as fibrin *(53)*. Plasmin is generated from plasminogen by two plasminogen activators, tissue-type plasminogen activator (t-PA) and urokinase-type plasminogen activator (u-PA) *(53)*. Several inhibitors of this system exist, the most important being plasminogen activator inhibitor 1 (PAI-1) *(53)*. PAI-1 can inhibit both t-PA an u-PA. PAI-1 is often found in extracellular matrix in association with vitronectin. Plasmin can degrade extracellular matrix directly and it is also able to activate metalloproteases *(54)*. All of the components of this system are produced within the glomerulus. Mesangial cells synthesize t-PA and PAI-1 and express the u-PA receptor on their cell surface *(55,56)*. PAI-1 is found in the mesangial matrix *(57)*. The GEC synthesizes primarily u-PA and PAI-1 and expresses both the u-PA receptor and a plasminogen/plasmin receptor *(58,59)*. The components of this system are upregulated by a number of cytokines, including tumor necrosis factor-α (TNF-α), transforming growth factor-β (TGF-β), and interleukin 1 (IL-1). Cultured mesangial cells from the kidney have been demonstrated to degrade extracellular matrix only in the presence of plasminogen *(60)*.

Distinct roles for the plasminogen/plasmin system have been identified in certain models of glomerular immune injury. In antithymoctye serum induced glomerulonephritis in the rat, the isolated glomeruli express decreased plasminogen activator activity, increased synthesis of PAI-1 and increased PAI-1 deposition in the matrix *(61)*. When an antibody to TGF-β was administered to these animals, there was a decrease in glomerular PAI-1 deposition. In an accelerated model of anti-GBM glomerulonephritis in the rat, increased expression of glomerular PAI mRNA and increased PAI-1 bioactivity with no change in expression of t-PA or u-PA mRNA are evident *(62)*. Increased expression of PAI-1 mRNA, which correlated with increased PAI-1 biologic activity, are evident in a rat model of anti-TBM antibody-associated tubulointerstitial nephritis. The net effect of the increased PAI-1 will be a decrease in plasmin formation, which could lead to an accumulation of the extracellular matrix.

4.5. Mononuclear Cells

Mononuclear cells, particularly monocytes and macrophages, are also important mediators of immune injury *(64)*. Monocytes and macrophages have been identified in the glomeruli in certain models of glomerulonephritis, particularly in proliferative glomerulonephritis *(64)*. Schreiner et al. *(65)* first showed depletion of monocytes to be a protective maneuver in accelerated anti-GBM nephritis. In models associated with crescent formation, macrophages are an important component of the crescents. Macrophage depletion prevents the glomerular fibrin deposition and markedly decreases the level of procoagulant activity *(66)*. The glomerular macrophage accumulation generally precedes glomerular fibrin deposition and coincides with increased glomerular procoagulant activity *(67)*. The macrophage is an important effector cell in immune injury because it synthesizes and releases a number of inflammatory mediators *(68)*. These include a procoagulant tissue-factor-like activity, reactive oxygen species, tumor necrosis factor, proteolytic enzymes, prostaglandins, polypeptide growth factors, and complement components. Further, macrophages can be activated by cytokines produced by sensitized lymphocytes. Accumulations of monocytes in the glomeruli correlate particularly strongly with fibrin deposition. Like other effector cells, monocytes and macrophages are capable of playing multiple roles in immune injury.

A role for lymphocytes, and especially T-lymphocytes, has been suspected in glomerular immune injury although the details are yet to be worked out. The infiltration of lymphocytes very early in the development of anti-GBM nephritis has been described *(69)*. Anti-GBM nephritis in the chicken can be mediated by T-lymphocytes *(70)* suggesting that cell mediated immunity alone, in the absence of antibody, can induce glomerulonephritis. T-lymphocytes produce several lymphokines which control the immune response, which could serve to stimulate macrophages and recruit other T- and B-cells.

4.6. Platelets

Platelets have long been known to be important in hemostasis. Recently, they have been shown to be effector cells in glomerular immune injury *(71)*. When activated, platelets release many inflammatory mediators including growth factors, proteases, vasoactive amines, thromboxane, cationic proteins and platelet activating factor *(71)*. Platelets are found within the glomeruli in many types of glomerulonephritis.

In subendothelial proliferative glomerulonephritis induced by concanavalin A, the phenomenon of very early accumulation of platelets was identified before the appearance of neutrophils. Complement depletion with cobra venom factor completely prevented the platelet infiltration and platelet-depletion reduced the albuminuria significantly *(72,73)*. Similarly, in mesangial proliferative glomerulonephritis induced by anti-Thy 1 antibody, platelet depletion reduced the degree of mesangial cell proliferation and improved the renal function *(74)*, and complement depletion with cobra venom factor markedly reduced the glomerular platelet accumulation *(75)*. In the latter model, both platelet depletion and complement depletion reduced the levels of glomerular platelet-derived growth factor (PDGF), PDGF mRNA, PDGF receptor, and PDGF receptor mRNA *(76)*. This suggests that the platelets can stimulate mesangial cells to release growth factors, which may act in an autocrine fashion to stimulate mesangial cell proliferation.

Platelets appear to mediate several roles in glomerular immune injury *(71)*. Their infiltration may lead to glomerular thrombosis by augmenting tissue factor release from monocytes and macrophages, or to glomerulosclerosis, by releasing growth factors such as PDGF and TGF-β. Platelets may also affect glomerular hemodynamics through the release of vasoactive substances, which can contract mesangial cells.

4.7. Mesangial Cells

The glomerular mesangium consists of an extracellular matrix and intrinsic smooth muscle-like contractile mesangial cells *(77,78)*. A second bone marrow-derived cell type is present in the mesangium, making up less than 5% of the cells. The mesangium is covered only by a fenestrated endothelium. There is no basement membrane, so that circulating macromolecules such as immune complexes can easily enter into the mesangium. The mesangium can regulate the glomerular filtration rate by controlling the surface area available for filtration through contraction and relaxation of the mesangial cells (79). Further, mesangial cells respond to various stimuli and produce a number of biologically active substances *(77)*.

Mesangial cell proliferation is a feature of many types of glomerular immune injury in humans *(80)*. These diseases include IgA nephropathy, Henoch Schonlein purpura, lupus nephritis, mesangial proliferative glomerulonephritis (such as found in steroid-resistant nephrotic syndrome), and membranoproliferative glomerulonephritis. The mesangial cells are proposed to play a pivotal role in many types of immune injury.

Mesangial cells respond to a variety of stimuli, including PDGF, epidermal growth factor (EGF), TGF, insulin-like growth factor 1 (ILGF-1), insulin, thrombin, IL-1, IL-6, TNF, fibronectin, endothelin, prostaglandins, angiotensin II, vasopressin, lipids, immune complexes, MAC of complement, heparan sulfate proteoglycan, and aggregated immunoglobulin *(78,80)*. The responses can range from proliferation, hypertrophy, contraction, migration, a changing matrix metabolism, and synthesis of inflammatory mediators. The mediators produced by the cells include neutral proteinases, plasminogen activators, plasminogen activator inhibitors, IL-1, platelet-activating factor, PDGF, ILGF-1, basic fibroblast growth factor, eicosanoids and oxygen radicals *(77,81)*. Mesangial cells are also responsible for the synthesis of many components of the extracellular matrix *(82)*.

Deregulated growth of mesangial cells may be important in glomerulosclerosis and progressive renal disease *(83)*. Recently, heparan sulfate, a component of the glomerular basement membrane and mesangial matrix, has been demonstrated to regulate mesangial cell growth *(84)*. When the glycosaminoglycan form of heparan sulfate is added to mesangial cells in culture, their growth is significantly inhibited *(84)*. The effect is reversible and unique to heparan sulfate, since chondroitin sulfate, another glycosaminoglycan found in the glomerulus, had no effect. The inhibitory action of heparan sulfate requires certain defined structural characteristics, particularly a low degree of sulfation (84). In both immune and nonimmune glomerular injury, the structure of glomerular heparan sulfate is altered *(85,86)*. Thus, changes in the structure of heparan sulfate produced in immunologic injury of the glomerulus may be important in the development of progressive renal disease. Heparan sulfate has also been shown to stimulate the synthesis of certain extracellular matrix components including laminin, fibronectin, and type V collagen *(82)*.

In mesangial proliferative glomerulonephritis induced by anti-Thy 1 antibody, increased production of PDGF and its receptor by mesangial cells is evident *(76)*. Administration of a neutralizing antibody to PDGF caused a significant decrease in mesangial cell proliferation. Increased gene expression of PDGF has been demonstrated in several proliferative glomerular immune lesions in humans *(87)*. In an immune complex glomerulonephritis model in the rat, the antithymocyte serum-induced glomerulonephritis, the mesangial cells synthesize and release a GBM degrading neutral proteinase *(88)*.

4.8. Antibodies to Cytoplasmic Neutrophil Antigens

Even antibodies to cytoplasmic antigens, which have traditionally been held to be beyond the purview of humoral immunity, can mediate immune injury in the kidney. This is a group of autoantibodies referred to as anti-neutrophil cytoplasmic antibodies (ANCA) *(89)* which react with the constituents of neutrophil azurophilic granules and monocyte lysosomes *(4)*. There are two types of ANCAs as defined by immunofluorescence staining patterns of ethanol fixed neutrophils exposed to ANCA. One is characterized by a cytoplasmic staining pattern and is directed to the granule constituent serine proteinase 3. The other manifests a perinuclear pattern of staining, and the antigen is usually myeloperoxidase. ANCAs have been found in the serum of patients with vasculitis either involving the kidney alone or other organs as well *(2)*.

ANCAs are able to induce neutrophils to undergo an oxidative burst, causing the release of reactive oxygen species *(90)*. Priming of the neutrophils with cytokines such as tumor necrosis factor enhances this effect, possibly by inducing expression of antigens reactive with ANCA on the cell surface. Antimyeloperoxidase autoantibodies have been demonstrated to stimulate neutrophils to damage endothelials cells in culture *(91)*.

5. PERSPECTIVES

This review has attempted to provide an overview of the mechanisms of injury in autoimmune disease in the kidney. The emphasis has been on the variety of mediators of glomerular immune injury. Multiple mediators are clearly involved in the development and course of glomerular immune injury, as depicted in Fig. 3. The multiplicity may be a consequence of the presence of redundant mediator systems in the immune system, presumably designed to provide more efficient protection from infections. In regard to therapy of autoimmune injury to the kidney, however, the plethora of mediators imposes serious obstacles. Inhibition of individual mediators will have a limited impact on the course of the immune injury. For instance, in rabbits deficient in the sixth component of complement and unable to form the MAC, the development of induced membranous nephropathy is delayed, but as other mediators are recruited, full development of the autoimmune injury occurs *(23)*. Clearly, it would be preferable to target the initiators of the autoimmune response once these are identified.

REFERENCES

1. Sennet, D. (1641) De febribus libri IV: Accessit ad calcem, ejusdem de dysenteria tractatus: E. movossoma. cie accessit fasciculus medicamentorum contra pestum Venetiis (Venice): F. Baba, 178–190.
2. Mellors, R. C. and Ortega, L. G. (1956) Analytical pathology: II New observations on the pathogenesis of glomerulonephritis, lipoid nephrosis, periarteritis nodosa and secondary amyloidosis in man. *Amer. J. Pathol.* **32,** 455–499.
3. Wilson, C. B. (1991) The renal response to immunologic injury, in *The Kidney* (Brenner, B. M. and Rector, F. C., eds.), 4th edn., Saunders, Philadelphia, PA, pp. 1062–1181.
4. Falk, R. J. and Jennette, J. C. (1991) Wegener's granulomatosis, systemic vasculitis and anti-neutrophil cytoplasmic autoantibodies. *Ann. Rev. Med.* **42,** 456–469.
5. Couser, W. G. (1990) Mediation of immune glomerular injury. *J. Amer. Soc. Neph.* **1,** 13–29.
6. Johnson, R. J. (1994) The glomerular response to injury: Progression or resolution? *Kidney Int.* **45,** 1769–1782.
7. Dixon, F. J. (1968) The pathogenesis of glomerulonephritis. *Amer. J. Med.* **44,** 493–498.
8. Couser, W. G. and Salant, D. J. (1980) Immune complex formation and glomerular injury. *Kidney Int.* **17,** 1–13.
9. Couser, W. G. (1985) Mechanisms of glomerular injury in immune-complex disease. *Kidney Int.* **28,** 569–583.
10. Salant, D. J., Adler, S., Darby, C., Capparell, N. J., Groggel, G. C., Feintzeig, I. D., et al. (1985) Influence of antigen distribution on the mediation of immunologic glomerular injury. *Kidney Int.* **27,** 938–950.
11. Couser, W. G., Stilmant, M. M., and Jermanovich, N. B. (1977) Complement-independent nephrotoxic nephritis in the guinea pig. *Kidney Int.* **11,** 170–180.
12. Couser, W. G., Darby, C., Salant, D. J. Adler, S., Stilmant, M. M., and Lowenstein, L. M. (1985) Anti-GBM antibody induced proteinuria in isolated perfused rat kidney. *Amer. J. Physiol.* **249,** F241–F250.

13. Salant, D. J., Madaio, M. P., Adler, S., Stilmant, M. M., and Couser, W. G. (1981) Altered glomerular permeability induced by F(ab')2 and Fab' antibodies to rat renal tubular epithelial antigen. *Kidney Int.* **21**, 36–43.
14. Mendrick, D. L. and Rennke, H. G. (1988) Induction of proteinuria in the rat by a monoclonal antibody against SGP-115/107. *Kidney Int.* **33**, 818–830.
15. Orikasa, M., Matsui, K., Oite, T., and Shimizu, F. (1988) Massive proteinuria induced in rats by a single intravenous injection of a monoclonal antibody. *J. Immunol.* **141**, 807–814.
16. Johnson, R., Yamabe, H., Chen, Y-P, Campbell, C., Gordon, K., Baker, P., et al. (1992) Glomerular epithelial cell secrete a glomerular basement membrane-degrading metalloproteinase. *J. Amer. Soc. Nephrol.* **2**, 1388–1397.
17. Couser, W. G., Baker, P. J., and Adler, S. (1985) Complement and the direct mediation of immune glomerular injury: a new perspective. *Kidney Int.* **28**, 879–890.
18. Cybulsky, A. V., Quigg, R. J., and Salant, D. J. (1988) Role of the complement membrane attack complex in glomerular injury, in *Immunopathology of Renal Disease* (Brenner, B. M. and Stein, J., eds.), Churchill, Livingstone, New York, pp. 57–86.
19. Schreiber, R. D. and Muller-Eberhard, H. J. (1979) Complement and renal disease, in *Immunologic Mechanisms of Renal Disease* (Brenner, B. M. and Stein, J., eds.), Churchill, Livingstone, New York, pp. 67–105.
20. Cochrane, C. G., Unanue, E. R., and Dixon, F. J. (1965) A role of polymorphonuclear leukocytes and complement in nephrotoxic nephritis. *J. Exp. Med.* **122**, 99–116.
21. Henson, P. M. (1972) Pathologic mechanisms in neutrophil-mediated injury. *Amer. J. Path.* **68**, 593–605.
22. Salant, D. J., Belok, S., Madaio, M. P., and Couser, W. G. (1980) A new role for complement in experimental membranous nephropathy in rats. *J. Clin. Invest.* **66**, 1339–1350.
23. Groggel, G. C., Adler, S., Rennke, H. G., Couser, W. G., and Salant, D. J. (1983) Role of the terminal complement pathway in experimental membranous nephropathy in the rabbit. *J. Clin. Invest.* **72**, 1948–1957.
24. Cybulsky, A. V., Rennke, H. G., Feintzeig, I. D., and Salant, D. J. (1986) Complement-induced glomerular epithelial cell injury. Role of the membrane attack complex in rat membranous nephropathy. *J. Clin. Invest.* **77**, 1096–1107.
25. Groggel, G. C., Salant, D. J., Darby, C., Renke, H. G., and Couser, W. G. (1985) Role of terminal complement pathway in the heterologous phase of antiglomerular basement membrane nephritis. *Kidney Int.* **27**, 643–651.
26. Falk, R. J., Dalmasso, A. P., Kim, Y., Tsai, C. H., Scheinman, J. I., Gerwurz, H., et al. (1983) Neoantigen of the polymerized ninth component of complement. Characterization of a monoclonal antibody and immunohistochemical localization in renal disease. *J. Clin. Invest.* **72**, 560–573.
27. Muller-Eberhard, H. J. (1988) Molecular organization and function of the complement system. *Ann. Rev. Biochem.* **57**, 321–347.
28. Quigg, R. J., Cybulsky, A.V., Jacobs, J. B., and Salant, D.J. (1988) Anti-Fx1A produces complement-dependent cytotoxicity of glomerular epithelial cells. *Kidney Int.* **34**, 43–52.
29. Cybulsky, A. V., Salant, D. J., Quigg, R. J., Badalamenti, J., and Bonventre, J. V. (1989) Complement C5b-9 complex activates phospholipases in glomerular epithelial cells. *Amer. J. Physiol.* **257**, F826–F836.

30. Adler, S., Baker, P. J., Johnson, R. J., Ochi, R. F., Pritzl, P., and Couser, W. G. (1986) Complement membrane attack complex stimulates production of reactive oxygen metabolites by cultured rat mesangial cells. *J. Clin. Invest.* **77,** 762–767.
31. Torbohm, I., Schonermark, M., Wingen, A. M., Berger, B., Rother, K., and Hansch, G. M. (1990) C5b-8 and C5b-9 modulate the collagen release of human glomerular epithelial cells. *Kidney Int.* **37,** 1098–1104.
32. Groggel, G. C. and Terreros, D. A. (1990) Role of the terminal complement pathway in accelerated autologous anti-glomerular basement membrane nephritis. *Amer. J. Pathol.* **136,** 533–540.
33. Hebert, L. A. and Cosio, F. G. (1987) The erythrocyte-immune complex-glomerulonephritis connection in man. *Kidney Int.* **31,** 877–885.
34. Schifferli, J. A., Ng, Y. C., and Peters, D. K. (1986) The role of complement and its receptor in the elimination of immune complexes. *N. Engl. J. Med.* **315,** 488–495.
35. Brady, H. R. (1994) Leukocyte adhesion molecules and kidney diseases. *Kidney Int.* **45,** 1285–1300.
36. Naisch, P. F., Thomson, N. M., Simpson, I. J., and Peters, D. K. (1975) The role of polymorphonuclear leukocytes in the autologous phase of nephrotoxic nephritis. *Clin. Exp. Immunol.* **22,** 102–111.
37. Hooke, D. H., Gee, D. C., and Atkins, R. C. (1987) Leucocyte analysis using monoclonal antibodies in human glomerulonephritis. *Kidney Int.* **31,** 964–972.
38. Cook, H. T., Smith, J., and Cattell, V. (1987) Isolation and characterization of inflammatory leukocytes from glomeruli in an in situ model of glomerulonephritis in the rat. *Amer. J. Pathol.* **126,** 126–136.
39. Tucker, B. J., Gushwa, L. C., and Wilson, C. B. (1985) Effect of leucocyte depletion on glomerular dynamics during active glomerular immune injury. *Kidney Int.* **28,** 28–35.
40. Adachi, T., Fukuta, M., Ito, Y., Hirano, K., Sugiura, M., and Sugiura, K. (1986) Effect of superoxides dismutase on glomerular nephritis. *Biochem Pharmacol.* **35,** 341–345.
41. Rehan, A., Johnson, K. J., Wiggins, R. C., Kunkel, R. G., and Ward, P. A. (1984) Evidences for the role of oxygen radicals in acute nephrotoxic nephritis. *Lab. Invest.* **51,** 96–403.
42. Johnson, R. B. and Lehmeyer, J. E. (1976) Elaboration of toxic oxygen by-products by neutrophils in a model of immune complex disease. *J. Clin. Invest.* **57,** 836–841.
43. Baricos, W. H. and Shah, S. V. (1991) Proteolytic enzymes as mediators of glomerular injury. *Kidney Int.* **40,** 161–173.
44. Davies, M., Barrett, A. J., Travis, J., Sanders, E., and Coles, G. A. (1978) The degradation of human glomerular basement membrane with purified lysosomal proteinases: evidence for the pathogenic role of the polymorphonuclear leukocyte in glomerulonephritis. *Clin. Sci. Mol. Med.* **54,** 233–240.
45. Harlan, J. M., Killen, P. D., Harker, L. A., and Striker, G. E. (1981) Neutrophil mediated endothelial injury in vitro mechanisms of cell detachment. *J. Clin. Invest.* **68,** 1394–1403.
46. Shah, S. V., Baricos, W. H., and Basci, A. (1987) Degradation of human glomerular basement membrane by stimulated neutrophils activation of a metalloproteinase by reactive oxygen metabolites. *J. Clin. Invest.* **79,** 25–31.
47. Lovett, D. H., Sterzel, B. R., Kashgarian, M., and Ryan, J. L. (1983) Neutral proteinase activity produced in vitro by cells of the glomerular mesangium. *Kidney Int.* **23,** 342–349.

48. Baricos, W. H., Cortez, S. L., Le, Q. C., Zhou, Y., Dicarlo, R. M., O'Connor, S. F., et al. (1990) Glomerular basement membrane degradation by endogenous cysteine proteinases in isolated rat glomeruli. *Kidney Int.* **38,** 395–401.

49. Johnson, R. J., Couser, W. G., Alpers, C. E., Vissers, M., Schulze, M., and Klebanoff, S. J. (1988) The human neutrophil serine proteinases elastase and cathepsin G can mediate glomerular injury in vivo. *J. Exp. Med.* **168,** 1169–1174.

50. Davin, J. C., Davies, M., Foidart, J. M., Foidart, J. B., Dechenne, C. A., and Mahieu, P. R. (1987) Urinary excretion of neutral proteinases in nephrotic rats with a glomerular disease. *Kidney Int.* **31,** 32–40.

51. Schrijver, G., Schwalkwijk, J., Robben, J. C. M., Assmann, K. J. M., and Koene, R. A. P. (1989) Antiglomerular basement membrane nephritis in Beije mice. *J. Exp. Med.* **169,** 1435–1448.

52. Baricos, W. H., O'Connor, S. E., Cortez, S. L., Wu, L.-T., and Shah, S. V. (1988) The cysteine proteinase inhibitor, E-64, reduces proteinuria in an experimental model of glomerulonephritis. *Biochem. Biophys. Res. Comm.* **155,** 1318–1323.

53. Vassalli, J. D., Sappino, A.-P., and Belin, D. (1991) The plasminogen activator/plasmin system. *J. Clin. Invest.* **88,** 1067–1072.

54. He, C. S., Wilhelm, S. M., Pentland, A. P., Marmer, B. L., Grant, G. A., Eisen, A. Z., et al. (1989) Tissue cooperation in a proteolytic cascade activating human interstitial collagenase. *Proc. Natl. Acad. Sci. USA* **86,** 2632–2636.

55. Lacave, R., Rondeau, E., Ochi, S., Delaure, F., Schleuning, W. D., and Sraer, J.-D. (1989) Characterization of a plasminogen activator and its inhibitor in human mesangial cells. *Kidney Int.* **35,** 806–811.

56. Nguyen, G., Li, X.-M., Peraldi, M.-N., Zacharias, U., Hagege, J., Rondeau, E., et al. (1994) Receptor binding and degradation of urokinase-type plasminogen activator by human mesangial cells. *Kidney Int.* **46,** 208–215.

57. Hagege, J., Peraldi, M. N., Rondeau, E., Adida, C., Delarue, F., Medcalf, R., et al. (1992) Plasminogen activator inhibitor-1 deposition in the extracellular matrix of cultured human mesangial cells. *Amer. J. Pathol.* **141,** 117–128.

58. Rondeau, E., Ochi, S., Lacave, R., He, C.-J., Medcalf, R., Delrue, F., et al. (1989) Urokinase synthesis and binding by glomerular epithelial cells in culture. *Kidney Int.* **36,** 593–600.

59. Becquemont, L., Nguyen, G., Peraldi, M.-N., He, C.-J., Sraer, J.-D., and Rondeau, E. (1994) Expression of plasminogen/plasmin receptors on human glomerular epithelial cells. *Amer. J. Physiol.* **267,** F303–F310.

60. Wong, A. P., Cortez, S. L., and Baricos, W. H. (1992) Role of plasmin and gelatinase in extracellular matrix degradation by cultured rat mesangial cells. *Amer. J. Physiol.* **263,** F1112–F1118.

61. Tomooka, S., Border, W. A., Marshall, B. C., and Noble, N. A. (1992) Glomerular matrix accumulation is linked to inhibition of the plasmin protease system. *Kidney Int.* **42,** 1462–1469.

62. Feng, L., Tang, W. W., Wilson, C. B., and Loskutoff, D. J. (1993) Dysfunction of glomerular fibrinolysis in experimental antiglomerular basement membrane antibody glomerulonephritis. *J. Amer. Soc. Nephrol.* **3,** 1753–1764.

63. Tange, W. W., Feng, L., Xia, Y., and Wilson, C. B. (1994) Extracellular matrix accumulation in immune-mediated tubulointerstitial injury. *Kidney Int.* **45,** 1077–1084.

64. Schreiner, G. F. (1991) The role of the macrophage in glomerular injury. *Semin. Nephrol.* **11,** 268–275.

65. Schreiner, G. F., Cotran, R. S., Pardo, U., and Uhane, E. R. (1978) A mononuclear cell component in experimental immunological glomerulonephritis. *J. Exp. Med.* **147**, 369–384.
66. Holdsworth, S. R. and Tipping, P. G. (1987) Macrophage-induced glomerular fibrin deposition in experimental glomerulonephritis in the rabbit. *J. Clin. Invest.* **76**, 1367–1374.
67. Tipping, P. G. and Holdsworth, S. R. (1986) The participation of macrophages, glomerular procoagulant activity, and Factor VIII in glomerular fibrin deposition. *Amer. J. Pathol.* **124**, 10–17.
68. Nathan, C. F. (1987) Secretory products of macrophages. *J. Clin. Invest.* **79**, 319–326.
69. Kreisberg, J. I., Wayne, D. B., and Karnovsky, M. D. (1979) Rapid and focal loss of negative charge associated with mononuclear cell infiltration early in nephrotoxic serum nephritis. *Kidney Int.* **16**, 290–300.
70. Bolton, W. K., Tucker, F. L., and Sturgill, C. (1984) New avian model of experimental glomerulonephritis consistent with mediation by cellular immunity. *J. Clin. Invest.* **73**, 1263–1276.
71. Johnson, R. J. (1991) Platelets in inflammatory glomerular injury. *Semin. Nephrol.* **11**, 276–284.
72. Johnson, R. J., Alpers, C. E., Pritzl, P., Schulze, M., Baker, P., Pruchno, C., et al. (1988) Platelets mediate neutrophil-dependent immune complex nephritis in the rat. *J. Clin. Invest.* **82**, 1225–1235.
73. Johnson, R. J., Alpers, C. E., Pruchno, C., Schulze, M., Baker, P. J., Pritzl, P., et al. (1989) Mechanisms and kinetics for platelet and neutrophil localization in immune complex nephritis. *Kidney Int.* **36**, 780–789.
74. Johnson, R. J., Garcia, R. I., Pritzl, P., and Alpers, C. E. (1990) Platelets mediate glomerular cell proliferation in immune complex nephritis induced by anti-mesangial cell antibodies in the rat. *Amer. J. Pathol.* **136**, 369–374.
75. Johnson, R. J., Pritzl, P., Iida, H., and Alpers, C. E. (1991) Platelet-complement interactions in mesangial proliferative nephritis in the rat. *Amer. J. Pathol.* **138**, 313–321.
76. Iida, H., Seifert, R., Alpers, C. E., Gronwald, R. G. K., Phillips, P. E., Pritzl, P. G., et al. (1991) Platelet-derived growth factor (PDGF) and PDGF receptor are induced in mesangial proliferative nephritis in the rat. *Proc. Natl. Acad. Sci. USA* **88**, 6560–6569.
77. Abboud, H. E. (1991) Resident glomerular cells in glomerular injury: mesangial cells. *Semin. Nephrol.* **11**, 304–310.
78. Mene, P., Simonson, M. S., and Dunn, M. J. (1989) Physiology of the mesangial cell. *Physiol. Rev.* **69**, 1347–1424.
79. Schlondorff, D. (1987) The glomerular mesangial cell: an expanding role for a specialized pericyte. *FASEB J.* **1**, 272–281.
80. Kreisberg, J. I., Venkatachalam, M., and Troyer, D. (1985) Contractile properties of cultured glomerular mesangial cells. *Amer. J. Physiol.* **249**, F457–F463.
81. Sterzel, R. B. and Lovett, D. H. (1988) Interactions of inflammatory and glomerular cells in the response to glomerular injury, in *Immunopathology of Renal Disease* (Wilson, C. B., Brenner B. M., and Stein, J. H., eds.), Churchill, Livingstone, New York, pp. 137–173.
82. Groggel, G. C. and Hughes, M. L. (1995) Heparan sulfate stimulates extracellular matrix component synthesis by mesangial cells. *Nephron.* **71**, 197–202.

83. Striker, L. J., Peten, E. P., Elliot, S. J., Doi, T., and Striker, G. E. (1991) Biology of disease: mesangial cell turnover: effect of heparin and peptide growth factors. *Lab. Invest.* **64,** 446–456.

84. Groggel, G. C., Marinedes, G. M., Hovingh, P., Hammond, E., and Linker, A. (1990) Inhibition of rat mesangial cell growth by heparan sulfate. *Amer. J. Physiol.* **258,** F259–F265.

85. Groggel, G. C., Hovingh, P., Border, W. A., and Linker, A. (1987) Changes in glomerular heparan sulfate in puromycin aminonucleoside nephrosis. *Amer. J. Path.* **128,** 521–527.

86. Groggel, G. C., Stevenson, J., Hovingh, P., Linker, A., and Border, W. A. (1988) Changes in heparan sulfate correlate with increased glomerular permeability. *Kidney Int.* **33,** 517–523.

87. Gesualdo, L., Pinzani, M., Floriano, J. J., Hassan, M. O., Nagy, N. U., Schena, F. P., et al. (1991) Platelet-derived growth factor expression in mesangial proliferative glomerulonephritis. *Lab. Invest.* **65,** 160–167.

88. Lovett, D. H., Johnson, R. J., Marti, H. P., Martin, J., Davies, M., and Couser, W. G. (1992) Structural characterization of the mesangial cell type IV collagenase and enhanced expression in a model of mmune complex-mediated glomerulonephritis. *Amer. J. Pathol.* **141,** 85–98.

89. Falk, R. J. and Jennette, J. C. (1988) Anti-neutrophil cytoplasmic autoantibodies with specificity for myeloperoxidase in patients with systemic vasculitis and idiopathic necrotizing and crescentic glomerulonephritis. *N. Engl. J. Med.* **318,** 1651–1657.

90. Falk, R. J., Terrell, R. S., Charles, L. A., and Jennette, J. C. (1990) Anti-neutrophil cytoplasmic autoantibodies induce neutrophils to degranulate and produce oxygen radicals in vitro. *Proc. Natl. Acad. Sci. USA* **87,** 4115–4119.

91. Ewert, B., Jennette, J. C., and Falk, R. (1992) Anti-myeloperoxidase antibodies stimulate neutrophils to damage human endothelial cells. *Kidney Int.* **41,** 375–383.

18

DNA as Immunogen for the Induction of Immune and Autoimmune Antibody in Mice

Tony N. Marion

1. INTRODUCTION

Mice from strains genetically predisposed to the development of systemic auto-immune diseases have been an invaluable experimental resource for research efforts to understand the basis for the human autoimmune disease systemic lupus erythematosus (SLE) *(1)*. There are clear differences in the clinical presentation of lupus in mice compared to the human patients *(2)*. Nevertheless, much useful information has been gained by studies in mice, particularly those from the MRL *lpr/lpr*, NZB, NZW, and (NZB × NZW)F_1 strains. Studies in these mouse strains have been particularly informative in helping us to understand the basis for the autoimmune antibody responses to DNA. Lupus in humans as defined by the American Rheumatism Association is a much more heterogeneous disease than that in the lupus-prone mouse strains *(3,4)*. The presence of serum antibody to nuclear antigens, in particular to DNA, is only one of the diagnostic criteria In this regard, mouse lupus may only be representative of the form of human lupus that is associated with autoantibodies to nuclear antigens, of which the most important for lupus nephritis are antibodies to DNA. The objective of this chapter is to review results derived from studies of anti-DNA antibodies in mice. For the most part, the review will concentrate on results obtained with (NZB × NZW)F_1 mice. Although the underlying genetic bases for the autoimmune phenotype may be different in other autoimmune mouse strains, such as the MRL *lpr/lpr*, BXSB, and motheaten mice *(1)*, the characteristics of the autoimmune DNA antibody responses are similar.

The most significant point is that autoimmunity to DNA in (NZB × NZW)F_1 mice appears to be both initiated and sustained as an antigen-induced immune response to DNA *(5)*. DNA, most likely in the form of DNA-protein complexes, is the probable immunogen responsible for inducing the autoimmune DNA antibodies. The results supporting this conclusion are presented in Subheading 2. The immunogenicity of DNA-peptide and DNA-protein complexes, and the potential of such complexes to induce DNA antibodies in mice not genetically predisposed to autoimmunity is the subject of the second section.

Contemporary Immunology: Autoimmune Reactions
Edited by: S. Paul © Humana Press Inc., Totowa, NJ

Subheading 3. deals with the way in which environmental antigens may influence or participate in the generation of autoimmune DNA antibody, and Subheading 4. describes how DNA driven selection affects the specificity and function of autoimmune anti-DNA antibodies. The last section provides a discussion of the results from experimental lupus in mice relevant to understanding the anti-DNA antibody specificity to the pathogenesis of human lupus. For the sake of brevity, this chapter does not include an exhaustive review of the literature and the author has tried as much as possible to include critical references. For those whose work may not have been referenced, it no way reflects a qualitative assessment of importance.

2. ANTIGEN DRIVEN SELECTION IN THE AUTOIMMUNE RESPONSE TO DNA IN MICE

The clinical association of anti-nuclear antibodies, particularly anti-DNA with SLE, has been known and studied for more than forty years (6–8). The specificity of the antibodies for native DNA was held to be the most remarkable characteristic and was the focus of much of the early research (9). Throughout this chapter, the terms native DNA and dsDNA (double stranded DNA) will refer to the duplex, B-form, mammalian DNA. The early work of several groups, Stollar et al. in particular, demonstrated clearly that antibody to denatured DNA, i.e., single stranded DNA(ssDNA) could be readily induced by immunization of rabbits or mice with ssDNA in a noncovalent complex with methylated bovine serum albumin (mBSA) (10). Antibodies have also been induced by immunization with dsDNA in conformations other than B-form (11), particularly the Z-form DNA (12), and by immunization with chemically modified DNA (13). Repeated attempts to induce antibody with specificity for dsDNA, however, were generally unsuccessful (14). This led to the prevailing opinion at the time that autoimmunity to DNA in both murine and human lupus could not be attributed to a specific immune response to DNA. Rather, autoimmune anti-DNA antibody was thought to be the byproduct of a generalized B-cell hyperactivity, either as an intrinsic B-cell defect or through the general loss of functional regulation of B-cell responses to self antigens, including DNA (15).

2.1. Monoclonal Anti-DNA Antibodies

The advent of monoclonal antibody (MAb) technology provided a critical and useful tool for the analysis of anti-DNA autoantibodies particularly in mice (16). Numerous laboratories were able to generate B-cell hybridomas producing monoclonal antibodies with specificity for DNA. Hybridomas producing monoclonal ssDNA-binding antibodies were obtained from fusions of splenic B-cells from various strains of mice, both those genetically predisposed to autoimmunity and those with no genetic autoimmune tendencies. The resultant antibodies from the latter types of strains were almost always of the IgM class, and were classified as natural autoantibodies (17). With respect to the DNA specificity, such antibodies bind to ssDNA but not dsDNA. Fusions of splenic B-cells from mice genetically prone to autoimmune disease, such as (NZB × NZW)F₁ *(18–20)* and MRL *lpr/lpr (21)*, on the other hand, almost always yield hybridomas producing dsDNA-specific monoclonal antibodies of the IgG class, depending on the age and stage of autoimmune disease in the donor mice. We obtained hybridomas from fusions of the lipopolysaccharide-stimulated B-cells of non-autoimmune-prone mice that produced monoclonal dsDNA-binding antibodies. The antibodies, however, were of the IgM class and bound dsDNA with very low avidity (M. Krishnan and T. Marion, submitted). These observations establish an important characteristic of autoimmune anti-DNA antibodies first deduced from the analyses of serum anti-DNA antibody in (NZB × NZW)F₁ mice. Anti-DNA autoantibodies from autoimmune mice and humans, unlike the so called natural DNA autoantibodies found in all mice, belong to the IgG class and they bind dsDNA with relatively high avidity *(22–25)*.

By analyzing a relatively large number of DNA-specific hybridomas derived from individual mice and compiling the results from such analyses from several mice, we and others have been able to develop an understanding of the autoimmune response to DNA *(5,20,21,25–34)*. Studies in both MRL and (NZB×NZW)F₁ mice have indicated that the autoimmune antibody response to DNA has all of the characteristics of a normal, secondary antibody response. Autoimmune antibodies to DNA initially are IgM but later switch to IgG. The sequence of the light and heavy chain variable regions from autoimmune monoclonal anti-DNA antibodies contains structural characteristics consistent with an antigen-selected, oligoclonal derivation. This is true both for the early-appearing IgM anti-DNA as well as the later-appearing IgG anti-DNA *(16,35,36)*. Further, the patterns of somatic mutations displayed by monoclonal anti-DNA from autoimmune mice are consistent with the antigen-driven, oligoclonal B-cell selection process. The antibody response to DNA undergoes specificity and affinity maturation as the response matures from the primary IgM form to the secondary IgG form. As discussed below, the antigen likely to be responsible for initiating and sustaining the autoimmune response is DNA, most likely in the form of DNA-protein complexes.

2.2. Preferential V_H and V_L Gene Expression Among Anti-DNA

An important structural characteristic of antibodies to haptens such as phosphorylcholine, nitrophenol, arsonate, and dinitrophenol is the remarkably limited number of light and heavy chain variable region genes (V_L and V_H) that encode the *VL* and *VH* protein domains, respectively, of these antibodies *(37)*. This *V* region restriction has been fundamentally important for studies aimed at understanding how antibody *V* region diversity is applied to generate antigen specific antibodies. In contrast, *V* gene expression among DNA autoantibodies is not restricted *(5,16)*. In fact, V_H and V_L gene usage among DNA autoantibodies is remarkably heterogeneous. In mice, the estimated numbers of germline V region genes that can encode V regions for DNA antibodies are 50 for

V_H and 36 for V_L *(16)*. Our statistical estimates of V_L/V_H gene usage in anti-DNA antibodies are based upon study of 257 monoclonal DNA antibodies for which we have obtained the complete *VH* and *VL* nucleotide sequences. Among all of the monoclonal DNA antibodies we analyzed, one or more germline V_H genes from each of the V_H7183, V_HQ52, V_HS107, V_H36-60, V_HJ606, V_H10, V_H12, and V_HJ558 families was found. One or more V_L genes from each of the V_κ1, V_κ2, V_κ4/5, V_κ8, V_κ9A, V_κ10, V_κ12, V_κ19, V_κ20, V_κ21, V_κ23, V_κRF V_λ1, and V_λ2 families were observed to encode the *VL*. Within the heterogeneous gene sets used for the generation of the anti-DNA antibodies, certain V_H and V_κ genes are found to encode the *VH* and *VL* far more often than would be predicted from chance alone. This is apparent from both the preferential and the recurrent expression of particular *V* genes among anti-DNA MAbs derived from individual mice as well as mice from different autoimmune-prone strains *(5,34–36)*. Among the anti-DNA MAbs for which we determined the *V* region structures, several V_H genes from the V_H558 family were expressed preferentially, most notably the V_H gene for antibody BWDNA7 *(5,38)*, followed by the V_H7183 genes for 163.1 and 111.55 *(5)*. With respect to the light chain, the V_κ1A gene for antibody MRLDNA4 *(5,38)* and the V_κ8A gene for DNA5 *(5)* were expressed preferentially. The preferential V_H and V_L gene expression was evident in IgM hybridomas obtained from mice early in the autoimmune response to DNA, as well as IgG hybridomas obtained later in the response *(5)*. These results imply that B cells expressing anti-DNA specificity derived from particular V_H and V_L genes are selectively expanded in both the early and late stages of the anti-DNA response. The structural correlate of this conclusion is that the preferentially expressed V genes have the greatest potential to develop into dsDNA-specific *VH* and *VL* domains. Within the individual autoimmune mice, most of the anti-DNA hybridomas, particularly those obtained late in the autoimmune response after the IgM to IgG switch had occurred, appeared to be derived from a relatively small number of B-cell precursors.

2.3. Specificity and Affinity Maturation of Autoimmune Anti-DNA

The maturation of specificity for DNA became apparent from our analyses of hybridomas obtained from partial splenectomies *(5)*. Partial splenectomies were performed on autoimmune mice when their serum IgM anti-DNA titer was 1000 or more, and prior to the appearance of IgG anti-DNA antibodies in the serum. Hybridomas were generated from each individual spleen fragment. The mice were allowed to recover, and when the serum IgG anti-DNA titers in the same mice reached 1000 or more, the remaining spleen halves were used to generate hybridomas. The results indicated that the autoimmune antibody response progresses from one with specificity primarily for ssDNA to one with specificity for dsDNA. The majority of hybridomas obtained from fusions in the early stages of antibody production were IgM producers, and they appeared to be clonally heterogeneous. The monoclonal antibodies from these hybridomas bound ssDNA but not dsDNA. In contrast, the hybridomas obtained from the remaining spleen halves synthesized IgG antibodies and appeared to be of oligoclonal origin. Most of the MAbs obtained from the later fusions bound both ssDNA and dsDNA. In a limited number of mice, hybridomas derived from the later fusion set were clonally related to the hybridomas obtained in the first fusion (early set). In one example, the IgM hybridomas obtained in the first fusion were specific for ssDNA only; the clonally related IgG hybridoma obtained in the second fusion was specific for both ssDNA and dsDNA. The acquisition of dsDNA binding capability was correlated to a mutation in the VH expressed by the IgG hybridoma.

Affinity maturation of antibody responses is dependent on two major processes. One is the selective clonal expansion of B-cells specific for the relevant immunogen *(39–43)*. The other is somatic hypermutation of antibody *V* regions *(44–47)*. B cells expressing immunoglobulin receptors with the highest affinity for the relevant immunogen are selectively stimulated to expand clonally. As a result, particular V_H and V_L genes are selected by the immunogen to dominate the antigen specific antibody response. As clones of B-cells expand, the V_H and V_L genes expressed by the cells acquire random somatic mutations at the rate of approx one per cell division *(48)*. If a mutation improves the specificity of a particular B-cell for the relevant immunogen, the cell has a greater selective advantage for continued antigen-driven clonal expansion *(40)*. The antigen-specific B-cells tend to selectively accumulate mutations in the complementarity determining regions (CDR), even though somatic *V* region hypermutation is a random process *(49,50)*. Replacement mutations in CDR are more likely to influence and potentially improve the antibody specificity. Framework (FR) mutations are less likely to improve the specificity and are more likely to detrimentally affect antibody function. This is immediately apparent when one examines the pattern of *V* region mutations in antigen-specific, IgG hybridomas derived from B-cells. The ratio of replacement to silent mutations (R/S) is generally higher in the CDRs than is expected based on chance, and the ratio is usually lower than expected in the framework regions (FR) *(21)*. The differences become progressively more apparent among hybridomas obtained following secondary and tertiary immunizations with the antigen.

The pattern of V region somatic mutations observed in the DNA-specific, IgG hybridomas from autoimmune mice is consistent with an antigen selected derivation *(36)*. The R/S ratio for CDR mutations is generally higher than expected by chance. The R/S ratio for FR mutations is lower than expected by chance with one exception. The exception occurs at amino acid position 76 in FR3. The R/S ratio at this position is similar to that for the CDRs. Many replacement mutations in CDRs and FR position 76 generate arginines or asparagines. Because of their ability to hydrogen bond with paired bases and with the deoxyribose phosphate backbone of DNA (51), the arginine and asparagine mutations may increase the DNA binding potential of the antibody *V* regions.

In summary, the DNA autoantibodies have all of the structural characteristics expected for antibodies produced in response to a specific immunogen. These include the IgG class, an oligoclonal origin, an antigen-driven variable region selection process, and the presence of V region somatic mutations that favor antigen binding. The maturation of the antibody specificity from the predominant ssDNA to predominant dsDNA indicates that DNA, or more likely DNA-protein complexes, must provide the immunogenic stimulus.

3. VARIABLE REGION STRUCTURES IMPORTANT FOR ANTI-DNA SPECIFICITY

One of the characteristic features common to most anti-DNA antibodies but uncommon among antibodies with other specificities is the presence of one or more arginines in the third complementarity-determining region (CDR3) of *VH* *(5,25,28,30,31,52)*. The *VH*-CDR3 is encoded by one or more D genes, the 5' end of a J_H gene, and nontemplate encoded nucleotides, the N and P sequences, which are added randomly to the V_H-D_H and D_H-J_H junctions. Generally, the structure of *VH*-CDR3 in antibodies with specificities to antigens other than DNA is dominated by tyrosines and serines. The coding sequence(s) for arginine in *VH*-CDR3 is generated somatically either by N sequence addition, recombination of a D gene into reading frame (RF) 3 rather than RF1 *(53)*, or somatic mutation during antigen-induced B-cell clonal expansion *(28,30,31)*.

3.1. VH-CDR3 Arginines and DNA Specificity

A remarkably strong correlation exists between the specificity for dsDNA and the presence of the arginines in *VH*-CDR3 in antibodies that utilize gene families V_H7183, V_HQ52, and V_HS107, but not the V_H 558 family *(52)*. Among MAbs without arginine in *VH*-CDR3, only those with V_H encoded by V_H558 family V genes were able to bind dsDNA. MAbs without arginines in *VH*-CDR3 and *VH* encoded by V_H7183, V_HQ52, and V_HS107 family genes bound only to ssDNA. Among MAbs with at least one arginine in VH-CDR3, there was a strong correlation between the specificity for dsDNA and the position of the arginine(s). This is illustrated in Fig. 1. The arginines in the anti-ssDNA antibodies were found more frequently at positions 95–98 in the amino terminal end of *VH*-CDR3. Arginines in the anti-dsDNA antibodies were found more frequently at amino acid positions 98–100a in the middle of *VH*-CDR3. Statistical comparison of the ssDNA versus dsDNA-binding MAbs indicated that arginine expression in amino acid position 100 of *VH*-CDR3 was most strongly correlated with the dsDNA specificity.

These results are remarkably consistent with computer models *(5,54–57)* and X-ray crystallographic data for dsDNA-binding MAbs *(57)*. The molecular models indicate that the *VH*-CDR3 loop forms an important contact region with dsDNA. The average length of *VH*-CDR3 in dsDNA-binding MAbs is 11 amino acids. Amino acid position 100 is located at the apex of a *VH*-CDR3 loop of 11

95	96	97	98	99	100	100a	100b	c-102	
3	2	2	1	0	2	1	0	1	low
19	16	10	11	7	9	5	3	3	ssDNA
11	16	2	22	20	37	23	7	10	dsDNA
63	56	34	28	33	30	14	8	11	None

Fig. 1. Frequency of arginines at different amino acid positions in VH-CDR3 among DNA-binding and non DNA-binding MAbs. The MAbs were grouped according to DNA specificity as determined by a competitive inhibition ELISA: low, MAbs that were competitively inhibited from binding to solid phase CT-DNA by > 2 μg/mL DNA; ssDNA, MAbs that were competitively inhibited from binding to solid phase CT-DNA by < 2 μg/mL ssDNA but not dsDNA; dsDNA, MAbs that were competitively inhibited from binding to solid phase CT-DNA by < 2 μg/mL dsDNA. The VH-CDR3 structures for the non DNA-binding MAbs were obtained from the Kabat D region database maintained by the National Center for Biotechnology Information. The total number of MAbs in each group was: low, 29; ssDNA, 112; dsDNA, 112, and none, 945. Amino acid positions in VH-CDR3 are as defined by Kabat et al. (107). J_H1 and J_H4 encode amino acids 100h to 102; J_H2 and J_H3, amino acids 100j to 102. Amino acids 95 to 100g are encoded by D genes or N and P nucleotides.

amino acids. Arginine at position 100 would be capable of forming hydrogen bonds with either the G-C base pair through the major groove or with the phosphate oxygen in the deoxyribose phosphate backbone of DNA. A computer-generated model demonstrating how arginine in the center of the VH-CDR3 loop may participate in forming the antibody combining site for dsDNA is presented in Fig. 2. The structural analyses illustrate the importance of VH-CDR3 structure in determining the DNA specificity. They also indicate that V_H genes from the V_H558 family may have an inherent potential to encode antibodies with a dsDNA-binding activity, without the requirement for arginines in VH-CDR3. This may explain in part why the V_H domain encoded by V_H558 family V genes is present so frequently in murine anti-DNA antibodies.

3.2. VL Structure and DNA Specificity

The importance of VL structures in DNA specificity can be inferred not only from the model presented in Fig. 2 but also in the preferential expression of particular V_κ genes and somatically derived structures in anti-DNA antibodies. As

A

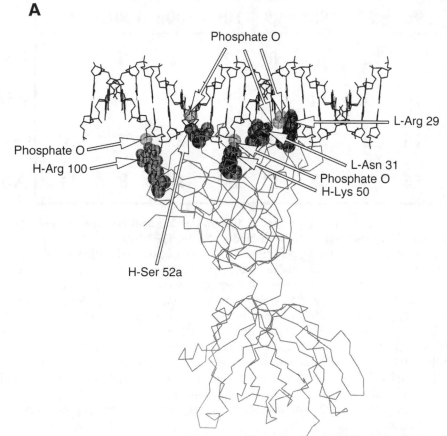

Fig. 2. A hypothetical computer-generated model of anti-DNA antibody binding to duplex, B-form DNA. A model of the 163.1 Mab *Fab* is presented as a stick figure of the α-carbon amino acid chain without *R* groups. The model is based on the crystallographic coordinates for the monoclonal antibody HyHEL5 *(108)*. The DNA model is that for 16 base pairs of poly(dA-dT)-poly(dA-dT), B form, double helical DNA (supplied with the software). Those amino acids in positions that would allow hydrogen bonding with the indicated phosphate oxygens on the DNA backbone are represented as dotted Van der Waals spheres of the *R* groups. (**A**) View perpendicular to the linear axis of the DNA. Facing the model, H-Arg 100, L-Arg 29, and L-Asn 31 are on the front side of the double helix and H-Lys 50 and H-Ser 52a are on the back side.

noted above, V_κ genes from the $V_\kappa 1$ and $V_\kappa 8$ families are expressed preferentially in anti-DNA MAbs *(35,36)*. A recurrent, somatically derived VL structure in anti-DNA MAbs, particularly in the MAbs that bind to dsDNA and contain the $J_\kappa 1$ gene, is the presence of arginine at position 96 *(5)*. The codon for this recurrent arginine was most likely generated by junctional diversification during *V-J* recombination. The first codon in the germline $J_\kappa 1$ gene is TGG, encoding

B

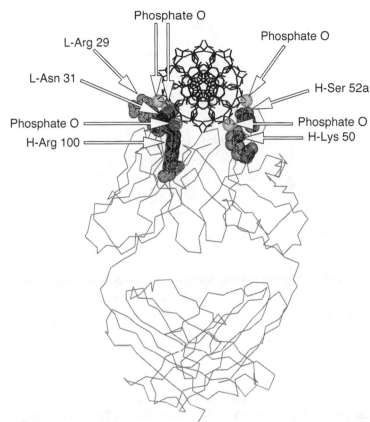

Phosphate O

Phosphate O

L-Arg 29

L-Asn 31

H-Ser 52a

Phosphate O

H-Arg 100

Phosphate O

H-Lys 50

Fig. 2. (Continued) (**B**) View down the linear axis of the DNA obtained by rotating the right side of the model (as seen in A) 90° out of the plane of the page.

tryptophan. The arginine codon (CGG) may be generated by exonucleolytic removal of the T and joining of the resulting $J_{\kappa}1$ to a C present at the 3' end of most germline V_{κ} genes. The effects of V_L gene usage on the specificity of anti-DNA MAbs has been demonstrated elegantly by Ibrahim et al. *(58)*. These investigators used mice transgenic for the γ2b heavy chain constant region and 3H9 VH *(21)*. The original 3H9 MAb contains a $V_{\kappa}4$ derived V_L and binds dsDNA. The DNA and phospholipid binding specificity of various MAbs encoded by the 3H9-γ2b transgene and *VL* domains from different V_{κ} families was observed to vary depending upon the particular *VL* *(58)*.

4. IMMUNOGENICITY OF DNA-PEPTIDE AND DNA-PROTEIN COMPLEXES

The *V* region structure analyses of anti-DNA MAbs from autoimmune mice indicated that the antibodies are produced in response to antigen-specific stimu-

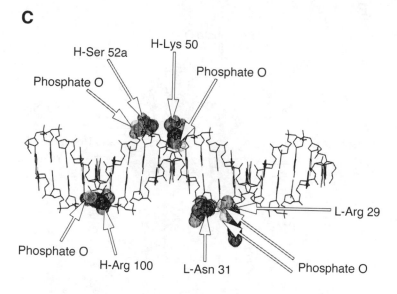

Fig. 2. (Continued) **(C)** View from the top of the combining site with the α-carbon chain removed to improve visualization of the orientation of the indicated amino acids relative to the DNA. The model was generated with the SYBYL software package (Tripos Associates, Inc., St. Louis, MO) running on a Sun 4-260 and displayed on an Evans and Sutherland PS390 graphics display terminal. Reprinted with permission from ref. *(35)*.

lation by DNA or DNA containing complexes. In other words, within the appropriate immunological context, DNA, even dsDNA, can be immunogenic. This conclusion is somewhat contrary to the results from numerous attempts to induce duplex, B-form DNA-specific antibody by experimental immunization *(14,59,60)*. Although some types of DNA have been reported to be capable of polyclonal B-cell stimulation *(61)*, DNA alone is not immunogenic. The secondary response characteristics of the mouse antibodies to DNA suggested that the DNA-specific B-cells require T-cell help either directly or indirectly. Antibody to ssDNA, Z-form DNA, and chemically modified DNA can be readily induced by immunization with the appropriate DNA as a complex with mBSA (methylated bovine serum albumin) *(10,13,59,60,62)*. As discussed in the following section, complexes formed between mBSA and either bacterial or viral DNA will induce the IgG class of anti-DNA antibody; however, in neither case does the induced antibody bind to mammalian dsDNA. Complexes of mammalian B-form duplex DNA and mBSA have not been reported to induce antibody to dsDNA. The general conclusion from these studies was that the dsDNA is not immunogenic even in a complex with an immunogenic protein *(14)*. Adding to this conundrum was the conflicting hypothesis that autoimmunity to DNA must be initiated as a byproduct of nonselective, polyclonal B-cell hyperactivity in autoimmune mice, particularly (NZB × NZW)F$_1$ *(35)*. In an attempt to resolve this conundrum, we reasoned that the appropriate immunological context necessary for the dsDNA to be immunogenic involves the recruitment of T-cell help stimulated by a protein or peptide bound to the dsDNA. Since mBSA has not worked effectively in stimulating the synthesis of antibody to dsDNA, we attempted to induce the antibody using DNA-peptide complexes generated with a strongly immunogenic DNA-binding peptide. As described below, this attempt was successful.

4.1. Induction of Anti-dsDNA by Immunization with DNA-Peptide Complexes

The dsDNA-binding Fus1 peptide was used to generate immunogenic complexes with mammalian dsDNA-Fus1. It is a synthetic peptide derived from the sequence of a ubiquitin carboxy-extension protein (CEP) from *Trypanasoma cruzi* *(63)*. Fus1 is 27 amino acids in length and has the structural features of a single zinc-finger DNA-binding motif. The CEP protein is highly conserved among all eukaryotes and in yeast is thought to be important in ribosome biogenesis *(64)*. Fus1 and CEP bind avidly and noncovalently to DNA to form complexes that vary in size and solubility depending upon the relative amounts of DNA and peptide *(16,65)*. We have no indication that Fus1 or CEP binding to DNA is dependent on the nucleotide sequence of the latter molecule. Complexes generated at a ratio of approximately 1 Fus1 molecule per 50 base pairs of DNA have been most successful for inducing dsDNA-binding anti-DNA.

After three to four immunizations, mice from strains generally not considered to be prone to autoimmune disease, such as BALB/c, C3H, and NZW, all produced IgG antibody to dsDNA, i.e., the mammalian, duplex, B-form DNA *(65)*. In aged autoimmune-disease prone mice, e.g., NZW mice six months or older, interpretation of the immunization experiments has sometimes been difficult because of the tendency of these animals to spontaneously produce the anti-DNA antibody. The subclass of the induced anti-DNA was predominantly IgG$_{2a}$, similar to the spontaneously produced anti-DNA antibody in autoimmune mice. The IgG subclass of Fus1-binding antibody in the same mice was either IgG$_1$ or IgG$_{2a}$, with the IgG$_1$ predominating. In mice immunized with Fus1 alone, the predominant subclass of anti-DNA antibody was IgG$_1$. Similar to the spontaneously appearing anti-DNA in autoimmune mice, the specificity of the DNA-Fus1 induced antibody was initially predominantly for ssDNA, with the dsDNA specificity being acquired over time and following tertiary and quaternary immunizations. Many of the mice that developed dsDNA-specific antibody following DNA-Fus1 immunization also developed proteinuria and had glomerular IgG deposits, both indicators of lupus-like glomerulonephritis. The IgG antibody eluted from the kidneys of these mice was bound by DNA. Mice immunized only with Fus1 and producing only Fus1-specific antibody did not develop any signs of glomerulonephritis or glomerular IgG deposition. Monoclonal antibodies generated from DNA-Fus1 immunized mice have *H* and *L* chain *V* region structures that are very similar if not identical to those of autoimmune anti-DNA antibodies *(66)*. The specificities of the MAbs for ssDNA and dsDNA have likewise been very similar to those of autoimmune anti-DNA antibodies. The specificity and other characteristics of the anti-DNA induced by DNA-Fus1 and other mammalian DNA-protein complexes are quite different from those of anti-DNA antibodies induced by DNA from viruses or bacteria as discussed below.

These results provided convincing evidence that dsDNA can be immunogenic when provided as a complex with an appropriate peptide carrier for stimulating T-cell help. They also demonstrated that mice not prone to autoimmune disease have the potential to produce anti-DNA antibodies with the same characteristics as autoimmune anti-DNA. Similar results have been reported recently from experiments in which mice were immunized with DNA complexed to other DNA-binding proteins, particularly DNaseI *(67)*. Datta et al. have accumulated substantial results demonstrating that nucleosome-specific T-cells in both mice *(68)* and humans *(69)* with lupus may provide the necessary T-cell help to promote anti-DNA antibody production by splenic B-cells. More important, such T-cells capable of providing B-cell help have been isolated as cell lines and hybridomas from mice and humans with SLE. The specificity for some if not all of such T-cells is for histone-derived peptides *(70)*. Histones, thus, are attractive candidates as stimulants of the T-cell help necessary to sustain autoimmune anti-DNA antibody production.

5. ANTI-DNA INDUCED WITH BACTERIAL DNA

As discussed in the previous section, the mammalian B-form of dsDNA can induce anti-DNA antibody when combined with an appropriate T_H cell stimulating carrier such as Fus1. Bacterial DNA even when complexed with a carrier such as mBSA will also induce anti-DNA with an IgG isotype *(71)*. Mice not prone to autoimmune disease produce anti-DNA antibody that binds to the bacterial B-form dsDNA when immunized with DNA from *Escherichia coli* complexed to mBSA. Unlike the anti-DNA antibodies induced with mammalian DNA, however, the antibodies induced by bacterial DNA do not bind mammalian DNA. Autoimmune anti-DNA antibodies bind native DNA from all species tested; however, the avidity of binding varies depending upon the species from which the DNA was isolated *(72,73,* and D. Desai and T. Marion, submitted). This implies the presence of structural differences in DNA derived from different species that can be distinguished by the anti-DNA antibodies. The results from bacterial DNA immunizations suggest that structures associated with bacterial DNA but not mammalian DNA may be immunogenic *(74)*. Anti-DNA that binds bacterial but not mammalian DNA may qualify as an example of the so-called natural autoantibodies. Perhaps the occurrence of such antibodies is induced by bacteria commonly encountered in the environment. Open to question is whether an immune response to bacterial DNA has any role in autoimmunity to DNA or in autoimmune disease. There is little indication that autoimmunity to DNA in mice and humans is dependent upon bacterial infection or symbiotic colonization.

Bacterial DNA in addition to being immunogenic can stimulate lymphocytes, including T-cells, B-cells, and NK-cells, through mechanisms that would appear to be independent of clonotypic immunoglobulin or T-cell receptors. The nonclonotypic, polyclonal stimulation of T- and B-cells appears to be dependent upon the presence of unmethylated CpG dinucleotides with two 5' flanking purines and two 3' flanking pyrimidines *(61)*. This sequence motif is far more prevalent in bacterial than mammalian DNA. Bacterial DNA and synthetic CpG dinucleotide-containing DNA are reported to stimulate the production of polyclonal IgM, interleukins 6 (IL-6), interleukin-12 (IL-12), and γ-interferon (IFNγ). The mechanism by which the CpG dinucleotide-containing DNA induces these effects is presently unknown. It is also unclear how such biological activities may be related to the specific immune responses and autoimmune responses to DNA.

6. ANTI-DNA INDUCED BY VIRUSES

There was considerable support in the seventies for the idea that autoimmunity to DNA, particularly in NZB and (NZB × NZW)F_1 mice, could be caused by endogenous retroviruses *(75)*. This idea lost favor when it was shown that autoimmunity to DNA was genetically independent of the inheritance of endogenous retroviruses *(76)*. In later studies, Rekvig et al. were able to induce anti-DNA and antihistone antibody by inoculation of either rabbits or mice with live BK virus or infectious circular viral DNA *(77)*. BK is a horizontally transmitted polyoma virus in humans *(78)*. Virtually all humans are infected with this virus very early in life, after which the virus remains latent. The anti-DNA antibodies induced by BK inoculation were of the IgG class, they were bound by mammalian duplex DNA, and they expressed *V* region structures similar to those of autoimmune anti-DNA antibodies *(79–81)*. Neither the inactivated virus nor linear viral DNA were able to induce the synthesis of anti-DNA antibodies. BK DNA-mBSA complexes induced anti-DNA that bound to native BK DNA but not native mammalian DNA *(80,82)*. Even though BK cannot establish productive infections in mice, cells infected with the BK virus nevertheless synthesize viral proteins, most notably the BK large T-antigen. This protein binds both viral and host cell DNA *(83)*. Rekvig and colleagues hypothesized that the large T-antigen bound to mouse chromatin in infected cells represents an immunogenic DNA complex. Chromatin-viral protein complex can be seen as the natural analog of the DNA-Fus1 complex, with the large T-antigen providing the necessary carrier function for stimulating helper T-cells. Vaccination of mice with plasmid DNA in which the constitutive expression of cloned cDNA for large T-antigen is driven by an appropriate promoter elicits antibodies to DNA, histones and the large T-antigen. Mice vaccinated with a similar plasmid containing the gene for a mutant, non-DNA-binding form of large T-antigen produced antibody to large T-antigen but not to DNA or to histones. Recent results from studies in SLE patients have revealed a remarkably strong correlation between the anti-DNA antibody production and BK virus reactivation *(85)*. Further studies are needed to study a possible cause and effect relationship between BK reactivation and the induction of anti-DNA production in SLE patients. It will be interesting to know whether and how an autoimmune response to DNA dependent on T-cell help induced by a viral protein is related to the autoimmune anti-DNA response dependent upon the histone-specific or the nucleosome-specific T-cell help.

7. DIFFERENCES BETWEEN THE INDUCED IMMUNE AND AUTOIMMUNE RESPONSE TO DNA

The results summarized in the preceding sections support the hypothesis that autoimmunity to DNA is both initiated and sustained as an antigen-specific, clonally selected immune response to DNA-protein complexes. The results also indicate that normal, nonautoimmune prone mouse strains inherit and can express the immunological potential to produce antibody specific for native mammalian DNA (including autologous DNA). Unlike the anti-DNA response in mice genetically predisposed to autoimmunity, the anti-DNA response in non-susceptible, normal mice immunized with DNA-Fus1 or other DNA immunogens is not sustained unless further immunizations are carried out *(16,65)*. Once the antibody response to DNA is initiated in autoimmune mice, the response is sustained until the death of the mice. The anti-DNA antibodies induced by DNA-Fus1 immunization, on the other hand, wax and wane with each cycle of immunization, just like the antibody responses to conventional, nonself-immunogens. This has also been true for the anti-DNA antibodies induced by viral and bacterial DNA. Whether the difference in immune responsiveness to DNA between normal and autoimmune mice is due to differences in B-cell tolerance to DNA, T-cell tolerance to DNA-bound proteins, or the availability of immunogenic DNA-protein complexes is not clear. The existence of histone-specific T-cells capable of promoting anti-DNA antibody production by B-cells in autoimmune mice may be critical for sustained production of anti-DNA antibodies.

7.1. Tolerance vs Immunity to DNA

There are important differences between the induced and autoimmune responses to duplex, B-form DNA and those to conventional foreign antigens, within which class can be included Z-DNA, chemically modified DNA, and even ssDNA. As elaborated by Stollar in a recent workshop review *(86)*, hapten-protein conjugates including Z-DNA-mBSA induce milligram per milliliter concentrations of specific serum antibody in mice (serum antibody titers equal to 10^5 and higher). Serum titers of induced antibody to duplex, B-form DNA in mice rarely exceed a few thousand. Even in autoimmune disease-prone mice, the serum concentrations of the antibody do not exceed 100 µg/mL. Although we have been able to consistently induce IgG type of anti-DNA antibody in the sera of nonautoimmune prone mice by immunization with DNA-Fus1 and DNA-CEP complexes, we are unable to consistently generate hybridomas producing IgG anti-DNA MAbs (D. Desai, M. Krishnan, and T. Marion, unpublished). The anti-DNA hybridomas generated from the mice immunized with DNA-

Fus1 generally secrete IgM, even though the serum of the splenocyte donors contained IgG with DNA binding titers of 2000 or more. In comparison, autoimmune (NZB × NZW)F$_1$ mice with serum anti-DNA titers of 2000 or more have consistently yielded at least a dozen or more DNA-specific IgG-producing hybridomas per fusion. The reason for the low success rate in obtaining IgG anti-DNA hybridomas in the nonautoimmune prone mice is not known. The problem does not seem to be the localization of immune B-cells to lymph nodes instead of the spleen or the timing of the fusion of splenocytes following the booster immunization (unpublished). An interesting possibility is that efficient peripheral tolerance mechanisms in mice not prone to autoimmune disease limit the clonal expansion of DNA-specific B-cells. We have observed no differences, however, in the responses of autoimmune (NZB × NZW)F$_1$ mice and nonautoimmune prone mice to a model antigen, DNP-OVA (dinitrophenyl hapten conjugated to ovalbumin). The kinetics and duration of the serum antibody response to DNP in the autoimmune mice, BALB/c mice and C57Bl/6 mice were similar (M. Krishnan and T. Marion, unpublished). There was no difference in the affinity of anti-DNP antibodies produced in the different mouse strains, and there was no indication that DNP-OVA immunization in any way influenced the anti-DNA response in (NZB × NZW)F$_1$. It appears, therefore, that the sustained antibody production to DNA in (NZB × NZW)F$_1$ mice is not due to a general failure to down-regulate the immune response. These results do not preclude selective deficiencies in either peripheral or central tolerance as contributing to the development of autoimmunity to DNA. In fact, recent results from several laboratories indicate that the development of tolerance to DNA may be less efficient in the autoimmune disease prone mice *(87–89)*.

8. BINDING OF ANTI-DNA ANTIBODIES TO KIDNEY

The clinical course of SLE has long been known to be associated with specificity of serum antibodies to dsDNA *(90,91)*. Antibodies eluted from diseased kidneys from mice *(92,93)* and humans *(94,95)* with lupus display the ability to bind dsDNA. Generally, the dsDNA-directed antibodies will bind to the glomerular basement membrane, but ssDNA specific antibodies will not. The specificity and affinity maturation of the autoimmune anti-DNA response results in progressively increasing specificity for dsDNA *(5)*. This progressive increase in specificity for dsDNA is accompanied by a progressive increase in the pathogenic potential of the antibodies due to glomerular deposition (M. Krishnan, R. Holder, and T. Marion, submitted).

Until recently, deposition of anti-DNA in the glomeruli was perceived to occur by binding of immune complexes formed either in circulation or *in situ* along the glomerular basement membrane. In both processes, the anti-DNA antibodies are thought to bind mononucleosomes or polynucleosomes. Basic proteins present in the nucleosomes are thought to promote binding to acidic glomerular membrane structures. The anti-DNA binding can be reproduced experimentally by provision of the individual components of the anti-DNA-

Table 1
Monoclonal Anti-DNA Binding to Basement Membrane

	Direct binding[a] (μg/mL MAb)			Competitive binding[b] (μg/mL competitor)	
Number MAbs	DNA	Chromatin	Basement membrane	ssDNA	dsDNA
ssDNA- 16	0.06	2.22	N.B.	0.25	N.I.
specific 2	4.64	0.06	N.B.	0.24	>10
2	0.26	1.73	5.53	1.58	N.I.
dsDNA- 20	2.01	0.02	1.90	0.87	1.98
specific 2	0.07	0.42	1.84	N.I.	4.15
7	1.52	0.07	N.B.	0.47	3.95

[a] Forty-nine MAbs were assayed for binding to DNA, chromatin, and synthetic basement membrane in a solid phase ELISA. The mean concentration of the MAbs in each designated group required to generate 50% of maximum binding in the assay is indicated. "N.B." means no binding by any of the MAbs in the respective group.

[b] Likewise for each MAb group, the mean concentration of ssDNA or dsDNA competitor required to generate 50% inhibition in a competitive ELISA is indicated. "N.I." means no inhibition by any of the MAbs in the respective group.

nucleosome complexes to the glomerular basement membrane both in vitro and in vivo *(96–101)*. Based on these studies, there is no doubt that the anti-DNA antibodies can bind to nucleosomes deposited along glomerular basement membrane. What is not as clear is whether the glomerular basement membrane in normal subjects or in patients with autoimmune disease has sufficient DNA bound as nucleosomes to permit anti-DNA binding in vivo.

Results from several laboratories including our own suggest that direct glomerular binding of anti-DNA antibodies may be important in disease pathogenesis *(102–105,* M. Krishnan, R. Holder, and T. Marion, submitted). Anti-DNA antibodies specific for ssDNA, do not bind the glomerular basement membrane either in vitro or in vivo in our experiments, even though most anti-ssDNA MAbs bind chromatin with high avidity. On the other hand, the majority of MAbs capable of binding dsDNA with moderate to high avidity also bind chromatin and the basement membrane in vitro and in vivo (Table 1). Some dsDNA-binding MAbs do not bind the glomerular basement membrane even though they bind to both dsDNA and chromatin with avidities equal to or better than those of the MAbs that do bind to basement membrane. When two anti-DNA hybridomas were grown simultaneously in the same mouse, the monoclonal anti-DNA known to bind the basement membrane in vitro was deposited in the kidneys. The second antibody, which did not bind to basement membrane in vitro, was not deposited in kidneys. Both antibodies had similar avidities for chromatin and dsDNA. Both were present in nearly identical concentrations in the sera and ascites fluid obtained from the mice. The two MAbs could be distinguished because they were of different IgG subtypes. The IgG subtype did not influence the ability of anti-DNA to bind to the basement membrane either in vitro or in vivo. These results suggest that binding to DNA or chromatin is not required for anti-DNA deposition in kidneys. Obviously, the results do not preclude immune complex formation either in the circulation or *in situ* as a mechanism for glomerular anti-DNA deposition.

9. WHAT STUDIES OF LUPUS MICE TEACH US ABOUT HUMAN LUPUS

The studies of murine autoimmunity to DNA in (NZB × NZW)F$_1$ may be informative in two important aspects in regard to the therapy of lupus. The mouse studies suggest that the autoimmune anti-DNA antibodies are generated in response to specific stimulation by DNA-protein complexes, rather than as a byproduct of generalized immune dysfunction. Immune therapies designed to inhibit selectively the autoimmune anti-DNA response may be better than current, nonselective immunosuppressive therapies to remedy the pathogenesis induced by anti-DNA antibodies.

The mouse studies may also provide important insight about how anti-DNA antibodies participate in the pathogenesis of human lupus. Although serum anti-DNA, particularly anti-dsDNA, is a diagnostic criterion for lupus, the correlation between disease activity and the anti-DNA titer is not always apparent *(106)*. Patients may present with extremely high serum anti-dsDNA but with little or no indication of disease activity measured as glomerulonephritis or other chronic inflammation. In such patients, very high serum anti-dsDNA levels may be maintained for extended periods in the absence of clear disease activity. On the other hand, patients may present with a history of low serum anti-dsDNA activity but with devastating glomerulonephritis. One could account for such results if the anti-DNA B-cells clonally selected and expanded in the first type of patient produced anti-DNA with high avidity to dsDNA, but little to no avidity for binding to glomerular basement membrane. Likewise, results observed in the second type of patient could be explained if the DNA-specific B-cells initially selected and expanded produced anti-DNA with a strong propensity for glomerular binding. Although present research results are insufficient to provide a clear understanding about how the specificity and structure of anti-DNA antibodies determines their pathogenetic potential, they do indicate that such an understanding should be forthcoming. Finally, recent developments in the research tools available to study the basis for tolerance and immune responsiveness to DNA enormously enhance the potential to understand fully how and why autoimmunity to DNA develops.

ACKNOWLEDGMENTS

The author wishes to acknowledge D. Desai for careful review and criticism of the manuscript. This work was supported by the NIH under Grants NIAID (AI26833) and NIAMS (AR42519).

REFERENCES

1. Theofilopoulos, A. N. and Dixon, F. J. (1985) Murine models of systemic lupus erythematosus. *Adv. Immunol.* **37,** 269–389.
2. Andrews, B. S., Eisenberg, R. A., Theofilopoulos, A. N., Izui, S., Wilson, C. B., McConahey, P. J., et al. 1978) Spontaneous murine lupus-like syndromes. Clinical and immunopathological manifestations in several strains. *J. Exp. Med.* **148,** 1198–1215.
3. Tan, E. M., Cohen, A. S., Fries, J. F., Masi, A. T., McShane, D. J., Rothfield, N. F., et al. (1982) The 1982 revised criteria for the classification of systemic lupus erythematosus. *Arthritis Rheum.* **25,** 1271–1277.
4. Liang, M. H., Socher, S. A., Larson, M. G., and Schur, P. H. (1989) Reliability and validity of six systems for the clinical assessment of disease activity in systemic lupus erythematosus. *Arthritis Rheum.* **32,** 1107–1118.
5. Tillman, D. M., Jou, N.-T., and Marion, T. N. (1992) Both IgM and IgG anti-DNA antibody are the products of clonally selective B cell stimulation in (NZB × NZW)F$_1$ mice. *J. Exp. Med.* **176,** 361–380.
6. Miescher, P. and Fauconnet, M. (1954) L'absorption du facteur "L.E." par des noyaux cellulaires isoles. *Experientia* **10,** 252–253.
7. Ceppellini, R., Polli, E., and Celada, F. (1957) A DNA-reacting factor in serum of a patient with Lupus Erythematosus Diffusus. *Proc. Soc. Exp. Bio. Med.* **96,** 572–574.
8. Robbins, W. C., Holman, H. R., Deicher, H., and Kunkel, H. G. (1957) Complement fixation with cell nuclei and DNA in Lupus Erythematosus. *Proc. Soc. Exp. Bio. Med.* **96,** 575–579.
9. Tan, E. M. (1982) Autoantibodies to nuclear antigens (ANA): their immunobiology and medicine. *Adv. Immunol.* **33,** 167–243.
10. Stollar, B. D., Fuchs, S., and Mozes, E. (1973) Immune response of mice to nucleic acids: strain dependent differences in magnitude and class of antibody production. *J. Immunol.* **111,** 121–129.
11. Stollar, B. D. (1970) Double-helical polynucleotides: immunochemical recognition of differing conformations. *Science* **169,** 609–611.
12. Lafer, E. M., Möller, A., Nordheim, A., Stollar, B. D., and Rich, A. (1983) Antibodies specific for left-handed Z-DNA. *Proc. Natl. Acad. Sci. USA* **78,** 3546–3550.
13. Lee, J. S., Woodsworth, M. L., and Latimer, J. P. (1984) Monoclonal antibodies specific for poly(dG). poly(dC) and poly(dG).poly(dm5C). *Biochemistry* **23,** 3277–3281.
14. Stollar, B. D. (1986) Antibodies to DNA. *CRC Critical Rev. Biochem.* **20,** 1–36.
15. Klinman, D. M. and Steinberg, A. D. (1987) Systemic autoimmune disease arises from polyclonal B cell activation. *J. Exp. Med.* **165,** 1755–1760.
16. Marion, T. N., Krishnan, M. R., Desai, D. D., Jou, N.-T., and Tillman, D. M. (1997) Monoclonal anti-DNA antibodies: structure, specificity, and biology, in *Anti-DNA Antibodies: Induction and Role in Autoimmunity* (Marion, T. N., ed.). Methods: A Companion to Methods in Enzymology (Abelson, J. N., Adolph, K. W., Cohn, P. M., Langone, J. J., and Simon, M. I., eds.), Academic, NY, pp. 3–11.
17. Ternynck, T. and Avrameas, S. (1986) Murine natural monoclonal autoantibodies: a study of their polyspecificities and their affinities. *Immunol. Rev.* **94,** 99–112.

18. Andrzejewski, C., Rauch, J., Lafer, E., Stollar, D., and Schwartz, R. (1980) Antigen-binding diversity and idiotypic cross-reactions among hybridoma autoantibodies to DNA. *J. Immunol.* 226–231. **126,**

19. Marion, T. N. and Briles, D. E. (1981) Analysis of autoimmune anti-DNA antibody responses using somatic cell hybridization, in *Monoclonal Antibodies and T Cell Hybridomas* (Hammerling, G. J., Hammerling, U., and Kearney, J. F., eds.), Elsevier-North Holland, Amsterdam, pp. 251–258.

20. Eilat, D., Hochberg, M., Pumphrey, J., and Rudikoff, S. (1984) Monoclonal antibodies to DNA and RNA from NZB/NZW F1 mice: antigenic specificities and NH2 terminal amino acid sequences. *J. Immunol.* **133,** 489–494.

21. Shlomchik, M. J., Aucoin, A. H., Pisetsky, D. S., and Weigert, M. G. (1987) The structure and function of anti-DNA autoantibodies derived from a single autoimmune mouse. *Proc. Natl. Acad. Sci. USA* **84,** 9150–9154.

22. Steward, M. W. and Hay, F. C. (1976) Changes in immunoglobulin class and subclass on anti-DNA antibodies with increasing age in NZB/W F1 hybrid mice. *Clin. Exp. Immunol.* **26,** 363–370.

23. Steinberg, A. D., Klassen, L. W., Raveche, E. S., Gerber, N. L., Reinertsen, J. L., Krakauer, R. S., et al. (1978) Study of multiple factors in the pathogenesis of autoimmunity in New Zealand mice. *Arthritis Rheum.* **21,** s190–S201.

24. Papoian, R., Pillarisetty, R., and Talal, N. (1977) Immunological regulation of spontaneous antibodies to DNA and RNA. II. Sequential switch from IgM to IgG in NZB/NZW F1 mice. *Immunology* **32,** 75–79.

25. Marion, T. N., Bothwell, A. L. M., Briles, D. E., and Janeway, C. A. (1989) IgG anti-DNA autoantibodies within an individual autoimmune mouse are the products of clonal selection. *J. Immunol.* **142,** 4269–4274.

26. Marion, T. N., Lawton, I., Kearney, J. F., and Briles, D. E. (1982) Anti-DNA autoantibodies in (NZB × NZW)F1 mice are clonally heterogeneous, but the majority share a common idiotype. *J. Immunol.* **128,** 668–674.

27. Trepicchio, W., Jr. and Barrett, K. J. (1987) Eleven MRL-*lpr/lpr* anti-DNA autoantibodies are encoded by genes from four V_H gene families: a potentially biased usage of V_H genes. *J. Immunol.* **138,** 2323–2331.

28. Eilat, D., Webster, D. M., and Rees, A. R. (1988) V region sequences of anti-DNA and anti-RNA autoantibodies from (NZB × NZW)F$_1$ mice. *J. Immunol.* **141,** 1745–1753.

29. Eilat, D., Hochberg, M., Tron, F., Jacob, L., and Bach, J.-F. (1989) The V_H gene sequences of anti-DNA antibodies in two different strains of lupus-prone mice are highly related. *Eur. J. Immunol.* **19,** 1241–1246.

30. Marion, T. N., Tillman, D. M., and Jou, N.-T. (1990) Interclonal and intraclonal diversity among anti-DNA antibodies from an (NZB × NZW)F1 mouse. *J. Immunol.* **145,** 2322–2332.

31. Shlomchik, M., Mascelli, M., Shan, H., Radic, M. Z., Pisetsky, D., Marshak-Rothstein, A., and Weigert, M. (1990) Anti-DNA antibodies from autoimmune mice arise by clonal expansion and somatic mutation. *J. Exp. Med.* **171,** 265–297.

32. Eilat, D. (1990) The role of germline gene expression and somatic mutation the generation of auto antibodies to DNA. *Mol. Immunol.* **27,** 203–210.

33. Behar, S. M., Lustgarten, D. L., Corbet, S., and Scharff, M. D. (1990) Characterization of somatically mutated S107 VH11-encoded anti-DNA autoantibodies derived from autoimmune (NZB × NZW)F1 mice. *J. Exp. Med.* **173,** 731–741.

34. Eilat, D. and Fischel, R. (1991) Recurrent utilization of genetic elements in V regions of antinucleic acid antibodies from autoimmune mice. *J. Immunol.* **147,** 361–368.

35. Marion, T. N., Tillman, D. M., Jou, N.-T., and Hill, R. H. (1992) Selection of immunoglobulin variable regions in autoimmunity to DNA. *Immunol. Rev.* **128,** 123–149.

36. Radic, M. Z. and Weigert, M. (1994) Genetic and structural evidence for antigen selection of anti-DNA antibodies. *Ann. Rev. Immunol.* **12,** 487–520.

37. Davie, J. M., Seiden, M. V., Greenspan, N. S., Lutz, C. T., Bartholow, T. L., and Clevinger, B. L. (1986) Structural correlates of idiotopes, in *Ann. Rev. Immunol.* (Paul, W. E., ed.). Annual Reviews, Palo Alto, CA pp. 147–165.

38. Kofler, R., Strohal, R., Balderas, R. S., Johnson, M. E., Noonan, D. J., Duchosal, M. A., et al. (1988) Immunoglobulin k light chain variable region gene complex organization and immunoglobulin genes encoding anti-DNA autoantibodies in lupus mice. *J. Clin. Invest.* **82,** 852–860.

39. McKean, D., Huppi, K., Bell, M., Staudt, L., Gearhard, W., and Weigert, M. (1984) Generation of antibody diversity in the immune response of BALB/c mice to influenza virus hemagglutinin. *Proc. Natl. Acad. Sci. USA* **81,** 3180–3184.

40. Manser, T., Huang, S.-Y., and Gefter, M. L. (1984) Influence of clonal selection on the expression of immunoglobulin variable regions. *Science* **226,** 1283–1288.

41. Clarke, S. H., Huppi, K., Ruezinsky, D., Staudt, L., Gearhard, W., and Weigert, M. (1985) Inter- and intra-clonal diversity in the antibody response to influenza hemagglutinin. *J. Exp. Med.* **161,** 687–704.

42. Berek, C., Griffiths, G. M., and Milstein, C. (1985) Molecular events during maturation of the immune response to oxazolone. *Nature* **316,** 412–418.

43. Blier, P. R. and Bothwell, A. (1987) A limited number of B cell lineages generates the heterogeneity of a secondary immune response. *J. Immunol.* **139,** 3996–4006.

44. Crews, S., Griffin, J., Huang, H., Calame, K., and Hood, L. (1981) A single VH gene segment encodes the immune response to phosphorylcholine: somatic mutation is correlated with the class of the antibody. *Cell* **25,** 59–66.

45. Griffiths, G. M., Berek, C., Kaartinen, M., and Milstein, C. (1984) Somatic mutation and the maturation of immune response to 2-phenyl oxazolone. *Nature* **312,** 272–275.

46. Wysocki, L., Manser, T., and Gefter, M. (1986) Somatic evolution of variable region structures during an immune response. *Proc. Natl. Acad. Sci. USA* **83,** 1847–1851.

47. Hartmann, A. B. and Rudikoff, S. (1984) V(H) genes encoding the immune response to beta-(1,6)-galactan: somatic mutation in IgM molecules. *EMBO J.* **3,** 3023.

48. Siekevitz, M., Kocks, C., Rajewsky, K., and Dildro, R. (1987) Analysis of somatic mutation and class switching in naive and memory B cells generating adoptive primary and secondary responses. *Cell* **48,** 757–770.

49. Gorski, J., Rollini, P., and Mach, B. (1983) Somatic mutations of immunoglobulin variable genes are restricted to the rearranged V gene. *Science* **220,** 1179–1181.

50. Heinrich, G., Traunecker, A., and Tonegawa, S. (1984) Somatic mutation reates diversity in the major group of mouse immunoglobulin kappa-light chains. *J. Exp. Med.* **159,** 417– 35.

51. Pabo, C. O. and Sauer, R. T. (1984) Protein-DNA recognition. *Ann. Rev. Biochem.* **53,** 293–321.

52. Krishnan, M. K., Jou, N.-T., and Marion, T. N. (1996) Correlation between the amino acid position of arginine in VH-CDR3 and specificity for native DNA among autoimmune antibodies. *J. Immunol.* **157,** 2430–2439.

53. Kaartinen, M. and Mäkelä, O. (1985) Reading of D genes in variable frames as a source of antibody diversity. *Immunol. Today* **6,** 324–326.

54. Cygler, M., Boodhoo, A., Lee, J. S., and Anderson, W. F. (1987) Crystallization and structure determination of an autoimmune anti-poly (dT) immunoglobulin Fab fragment at 3.0 A resolution. *J. Biol. Chem.* **262,** 643–648.

55. Radic, M. Z., Mackle, J., Erikson, J., Mol, C., Anderson, W. F., and Weigert, M. (1993) Residues that mediate DNA binding of autoimmune antibodies. *J. Immunol.* **150,** 4966–4977.

56. Barry, M. M., Mol, C. D., Anderson, W. F., and Lee, J. S. (1994) Sequencing and modeling of anti-DNA immunoglobulin Fv domains. Comparison with crystal structures. *J. Biol. Chem.* **269,** 3623–3632.

57. Mol, C. D., Muir, A. K., Lee, J. S., and Anderson, W. F. (1994) Structure of an immunoglobulin Fab fragment specific for poly(dG). poly(dC). *J. Biol. Chem.* **269,** 3605–3614.

58. Ibrahim, S. M., Weigert, M., Basu, C., Erikson, J., and Radic, M. Z. (1995) Light chain contribution to specificity in anti-DNA antibodies. *J Immunol.* **155,** 3223–3233.

59. Fournie, G. J., Lambert, P., Bankhurst, A., and Miescher, P. (1976) Features of the immune response to DNA in mice. *Clin. Exp. Immunol.* **26,** 52–56.

60. Madaio, M. P., Hodder, S., Schwartz, R. S., and Stollar, B. D. (1984) Responsiveness of autoimmune and normal mice to nucleic acid antigens. *J. Immunol.* **132,** 872–876.

61. Krieg, A. M., Yi, A. K., Matson, S., Waldschmidt, T. J., Bishop, G. A., Teasdale, R., et al. (1995) CpG motifs in bacteria DNA trigger direct B-cell activation. *Nature* **374,** 546–549.

62. Brigido, M. M. and Stollar, B. D. (1991) Two induced anti-Z-DNA monoclonal antibodies use VH gene segments related to those of anti-DNA autoantibodies. *J. Immunol.* **146,** 2005–2009.

63. Swindle, J. T., Ajioka, J., Eisen, H., Sanwal, B., Jacquemot, C., Browder, Z., et al. (1988) The genomic organization and transcription of the ubiquitin genes of Trypanosoma cruzi. *EMBO J.* **7,** 1121–1127.

64. Finley, D., Bartel, B., and Varshavsky, A. (1989) The tails of ubiquitin precursors are ribosomal proteins whose fusion to ubiquitin facilitates ribosome biogenesis. *Nature* **338,** 394–401.

65. Desai, D. D., Krishnan, M. R., Swindle, J. T., and Marion, T. N. (1993) Antigen-specific induction of antibodies against native mammalian DNA in nonautoimmune mice. *J. Immunol.* **151,** 1614–1626.

66. Krishnan, M. K. and Marion, T. N. (1993) Structural similarity of antibody variable- regions from immune and autoimmune anti-DNA antibodies. *J. Immunol.* **150,** 4948–4957.

67. Marchini, B., Puccetti, A., Dolcher, M. P., Madaio, M. P., and Migliorini, P. (1995) Induction of anti-DNA antibodies in nonautoimmune mice by immunization with a DNA-DNAase I complex. *Clin. Exp. Rheumatol.* **13,** 7–10.

68. Mohan, C., Adams, S., Stanik, V., and Datta, S. K. (1993) Nucleosome: a major immunogen for pathogenic autoantibody-inducing T cells of lupus. *J. Exp. Med.* **177,** 1367–1381.
69. Desai-Mehta, A., Mao, C., Rajagopalan, S., Robinson, T., and Datta, S. K. (1995) Structure and specificity of T cell receptors expressed by potentially pathogenic anti-DNA autoantibody-inducing T cells in human lupus. *J. Clin. Invest.* **95,** 531–541.
70. Kaliyaperumal, A., Mohan, C., Wu, W., and Datta, S. K. (1996) Nucleosomal peptide epitopes for nephritis-inducing T helper cells of murine lupus. *J. Exp. Med.* **183,** 2459–69.
71. Gilkeson, G. S., Grudier, J. P., Karounos, D. G., and Pisetsky, D. S. (1989) Induction of anti-double stranded DNA antibodies in normal mice by immunization with bacterial DNA. *J. Immunol.* **142,** 1482–1486.
72. Stollar, B. D., Levine, L., and Marmur, J. (1962) Antibodies to denatured deoxyribonucleic acid in lupus erythematosus serum. II. Characterization of antibodies in several sera. *Biochim. Biophys. Acta* **61,** 7.
73. Desai, D. and Marion, T. (1994) Differences in the reactivity of autoimmune anti-DNA antibodies to DNA from different species. *J. Cell. Biochem.* **18D,** 315.
74. Pisetsky, D. S. (1997) Specificity and immunochemical properties of antibodies to bacterial DNA, in *Anti-DNA Antibodies: Induction and Role in Autoimmunity* (Marion, T. N., ed.). Methods: A Companion to Methods in Enzymology (Abelson, J. N., Adolph, K. W., Cohn, P. M., Langone, J. J., and Simon, M. I., eds.), Academic, NY, pp. 55–61.
75. Lambert, P. H. and Dixon, F. J. (1970) Genesis of antinuclear antibody in NZB/NZW mice. *Clin. Exp. Immunol.* **6,** 829–839.
76. Datta, S. K. and Schwartz, R. S. (1976) Genetics of expression of xenotropic virus and autoimmunity in NZB mice. *Nature* **263,** 412–415.
77. Flaegstad, T., Fredriksen, K., Dahl, B., Traavik, T., and Rekvig, O. P. (1988) Inoculation with BK virus may break immunological tolerance to histone and DNA antigens. *Proc. Natl. Acad. Sci. USA* **85,** 8171–8175.
78. Mäntijärvi, R. A., Meurman, O. H., Vihma, L., and Berglund, B. (1973) A human papovavirus (BK), biological properties and seroepidemiology. *Ann. Clin. Res.* **5,** 283–287.
79. Fredriksen, K., Traavik, T., and Rekvig, O. P. (1990) Anti-DNA antibodies induced by BK virus inoculations. *Scand. J. Immunol.* **32,** 197–203.
80. Rekvig, O. P., Fredriksen, K., Brannsether, B., Moens, U., Sundsfjord, A., and Traavik, T. (1992) Antibodies to eukaryotic, including autologous, native DNA are produced during BK virus infection, but not after immunization with non-infectious DNA. *Scand. J. Immunol.* **36,** 487–495.
81. Rekvig, O. P., Fredriksen, K., Hokland, K., Moens, U., Traavik, T., Krishnan, M. R., et al. (1995) Molecular analyses of anti-DNA antibodies induced by polyomavirus BK in BALB/c mice [*Erratum* appears in *Scand. J. Immunol.* (1995) Aug. **42:**286]. *Scand. J. Immunol.* **41,** 593–602.
82. Fredriksen, K., Brannsether, B., Traavik, T., and Rekvig, O. P. (1991) Antibodies to viral and mammalian native DNA in response to BK virus inoculation and subsequent immunization with calf thymus DNA. *Scand. J. Immunol.* **34,** 109–119.
83. Bondeson, K., Ronn, O., and Magnusson, G. (1995) Preferred DNA-binding-sites of polyomavirus large T-antigen. *Eur. J. Biochem.* **227,** 359–366.

84. Moens, U., Seternes, O.-M., Hey, A. W., Silsand, Y., Traavik, T., Johansen, B., et al. (1995) In vivo expression of a single viral DNA-binding protein generates systemic lupus erythematosus-related autoimmunity to double-stranded DNA and histones. *Proc. Natl. Acad. Sci. USA* **92,** 12,393–12,397.

85. Rekvig, O. P., Moens, U., Sundsfjord, A., Bredholt, G., Osei, A., Haaheim, H., et al. (1997) Experimental expression in mice and spontaneous expression in human SLE of polyomavrius T-antigen: a molecular basis for induction of antibodies to DNA and eukaryotic transcription factors. *J. Clin. Invest.* **99,** 2045–2054.

86. Kalden, J. and Marion, T. N. Environmental and other stimuli for DNA antibody production. *Lupus,* in press.

87. Roark, J. H., Kuntz, C. L., Nguyen, K.-A., Mandik, L., Cattermole, M., and Erikson, J. (1995) B cell selection and allelic exclusion of an anti-DNA Ig transgene in MRL-lpr/lpr mice. *J. Immunol.* **154,** 4444–4455.

88. Roark, J. H., Kuntz, C. L., Nguyen, K. A., Caton, A. J., and Erikson, J. (1995) Breakdown of B cell tolerance in a mouse model of systemic lupus erythematosus. *J. Exp. Med.* **181,** 1157–1167.

89. Spatz, L., Iliev, A., Saenko, V., Jones, L., Irigoyen, M., Manheimer-Lory, A., et al. (1997) Studies on the structure, regulation, and pathogenic potential of anti-dsDNA antibodies, in *Anti-DNA Antibodies: Induction and Role in Autoimmunity* (Marion, T. N., ed.). Methods: A Companion to Methods in Enzymology (Abelson, J. N., Adolph, K. W., Cohn, P. M., Langone, J. J., and Simon, M. I., eds.), Academic, NY, pp. 70–78.

90. Koffler, D., Carr, R., Agnello, V., Thoburn, R., and Kunkel, H. G. (1971) Antibodies to polynucleotides in human sera: antigenic specificity and relation to disease. *J. Exp. Med.* **134,** 294–312.

91. Koffler, D. (1974) Immunopathogenesis of systemic lupus erythematosus. *Annu. Rev. Med.* **25,** 149–173.

92. Lambert, P. H. and Dixon, F. J. (1968) Pathogenesis of the glomeulonephritis of NZB/W mice. *J. Exp. Med.* **127,** 507–523.

93. Ebling, F. and Hahn, B. H. (1980) Restricted subpopulations of DNA antibodies in kidneys of mice with systemic lupus. Comparison of antibodies in serum and renal eluates. *Arthritis Rheum.* **23,** 392–403.

94. Koffler, D., Schur, P. H., and Kunkel, H. G. (1967) Immunological studies concerning the nephritis of systemic lupus erythematosus. *J. Exp. Med.* **126,** 607–624.

95. Andres, G. A., Erlanger, B. F., Hsu, K. C., and Seegal, B. C. (1970) Localization of fluorescein-labeled anti-nucleoside antibodies in glomeruli of patients with active systemic lupus erythematosus nephritis. *J. Clin. Invest.* **49,** 2106–2118.

96. Schmiedeke, T. M., Stockl, F. W., Weber, R., Sugisaki, Y., Batsford, S. R., and Vogt, A. (1989) Histones have high affinity for the glomerular basement membrane. Relevance for immune complex formation in lupus nephritis. *J. Exp. Med.* **169,** 1879–1894.

97. Termaat, R. M., Assman, K. M., Dijkman, H. M., Smeenk, R. T., and Berden, J. M. (1991) Nephritogenic anti-DNA monoclonal antibodies bind to the glomerulus via two distinct mechanisms. *J. Am. Soc. Nephritis* **2,** 565–571.

98. Kramers, C., Hylkema, M. N., van Bruggen, M. C., van de Lagemaat, R., Dijkman, H. B., Assmann, K. J., et al. (1994) Anti-nucleosome antibodies complexed to nucleosomal antigens show anti-DNA reactivity and bind to rat glomerular basement membrane in vivo. *J. Clin. Invest.* **94,** 568–577.

99. Morioka, T., Woitas, R., Fujigaki, Y., Batsford, S. R., and Vogt, A. (1994) Histone mediates glomerular deposition of small size DNA anti-DNA complex. *Kidney Int.* **45,** 991–997.
100. Morioka, T., Fujigaki, Y., Batsford, S. R., Woitas, R., Oite, T., Shimizu, F., et al. (1996) Anti-DNA antibody derived from a systemic lupus erythematosus (SLE) patient forms histone-DNA-anti-DNA complexes that bind to rat glomeruli in vivo. *Clin. Exp. Immunol.* **104,** 92–96.
101. Di Valerio, R., Bernstein, K. A., Varghese, E., and Lefkowith, J. B. (1995) Murine lupus glomerulotropic monoclonal antibodies exhibit differing specificities but bind via a common mechanism. *J. Immunol.* **155,** 2258–2268.
102. Sabbaga, J., Line, S. R. P., Potocnjak, P., and Madaio, M. P. (1989) A murine nephritogenic monoclonal anti-DNA autoantibody binds directly to mouse laminin, the major non-collagenous protein component of the glomerular basement membrane. *Eur. J. Immunol.* **19,** 137–143.
103. Madaio, M. P., Carlson, J., Cataldo, J., Ucci, A., Migliorini, P., and Pankewycz, O. (1987) Murine monoclonal anti-DNA antibodies bind directly to glomerular antigens and form immune deposits. *J. Immunol.* **138,** 2883–2889.
104. Madaio, M. P., Schattner, A., Shattner, M., and Schwartz, R. S. (1986) Lupus serum and normal human serum contain anti-DNA antibodies with the same idiotype marker. *J. Immunol.* **137,** 2535–2540.
105. Raz, E., Brezis, M., Rosenmann, E., and Eilat, D. (1989) Anti-DNA antibodies bind directly to renal antigens and induce kidney dysfunction in the isolated perfused rat kidney. *J. Immunol.* **142,** 3076–3082.
106. Gladman, D. D., Urowitz, M. B., and Keystone, E. C. (1979) Serologically active clinically quiescent systemic lupus erythematosus: a discordance between clinical and serological features. *Am. J. Med.* **66,** 210–215.
107. Kabat, E. A., Wu, T. T., Perry, H. M., Gottesman, K. S., and Foeller, C. (1991) Sequences of proteins of immunological interest. U. S. Gov. Print. Office, Bethesda, MD.
108. Sheriff, S., Silverton, E. W., Padlan, E. A., Cohen, G. H., Smith-Gill, S. J., Finzel, B. C., et al. (1987) Three-dimensional structure of an antibody-antigen complex. *Proc. Natl. Acad. Sci. USA* **84,** 8075–8079.

19

Cellular Entry and Nuclear Localization of Anti-DNA Antibodies

Kumiko Yanase and Michael P. Madaio

1. INTRODUCTION

The production of elevated quantities of autoantibodies is characteristic of individuals with systemic lupus erythematosus (SLE) and other autoimmune diseases *(1,2)*. In lupus, the autoantibodies react with a wide variety of ubiquitous intracellular, membrane-associated and circulating autoantigens, whereas in other autoimmune disorders the autoantibodies typically are more organ-specific *(3)*. Anti-DNA antibodies are the prototypic lupus autoantibodies. Their levels often fluctuate with disease activity; they can be demonstrated within immune deposits in the kidneys and other organs; and their deposition in various tissues (along with other autoantibodies) initiates an inflammatory response that frequently leads to organ failure despite intensive immunosuppressive therapy *(1,2)*. Nevertheless, the features that distinguish pathogenic from nonpathogenic autoantibodies have been the subject of considerable debate.

2. HETEROGENEITY OF ANTIBODY BINDING TO KIDNEY CONSTITUENTS

We and others have evaluated the capacity of murine monoclonal autoantibodies derived from lupus-prone mice, to induce disease upon transfer to normal mice (reviewed in ref. *4*). A few concepts emerged from the results. As expected, not all monoclonal autoantibodies are pathogenic. Of particular relevance to the variable disease patterns commonly found in patients with lupus nephritis, individual murine autoantibodies produced different disease phenotypes *(5–9)*. For example, individual monoclonal (MAbs) anti-DNA antibodies produced either basement membrane, subendothelial, mesangial, intraluminal or intranuclear deposits, and each of these profiles were associated with distinct light microscopic and clinical features *(5,6)*. The disease phenotypes appear to be influenced by both the location and nature of the target antigen engaged by the pathogenic antibody within the glomerulus, along with the capacity of the deposited immunoglobulin to recruit inflammatory mediators *(4,5)*. Others

Contemporary Immunology: Autoimmune Reactions
Edited by: S. Paul © Humana Press Inc., Totowa, NJ

have found that some autoantibodies form immune deposits by local complex formation with circulating autoantigens within the glomerular capillary wall. In this case, the autoantigen binds to various glomerular constituents, and the site of the antigen deposition influences both the site of immunoglobulin deposition and the disease phenotype. The most carefully studied example of this phenomenon involves the binding of nucleosomes to glomeruli, followed by binding of the nucleosomes to anti-DNA, antihistone and antinucleosome antibodies *(10)*. The differences in antibody interactions with kidney constituents contribute to the phenotypic diversity among individuals with lupus nephritis.

3. INTERNALIZATION OF ANTIBODIES

During our investigations, an intriguing subset of pathogenic anti-DNA antibodies was identified: anti-DNA antibodies that enter cells and localize within nuclei, in vivo *(6)*. Following implantation of murine anti-DNA antibody producing hybridomas (derived from different lupus prone strains) in normal mice, immunoglobulins were detected within the nuclei of cells in several organs. In the kidney, immunoglobulins were observed within glomerular, tubular, and vascular cells. This phenomenon was associated with glomerular hypercellularity, mesangial fiber bundles, epithelial foot process fusion, and proteinuria. Nuclear localization was present after injection of $F(ab)'_2$ fragments of these anti-DNA antibodies, indicating that localization occurred through the antigen binding region of the molecule and was F_cR-independent. The hypercellularity and proteinuria were not associated with complement deposition, cellular infiltration or platelets, suggesting that the morphologic and functional abnormalities were mediated by a direct effect of intranuclear antibodies within glomerular cells.

The capacity of immunoglobulins to penetrate cells and induce functional perturbations has been debated for more than 20 yr, since Alarcon-Segovia et al. initially described the phenomenon *(11–23)*. Intranuclear immunoglobulin deposits have been found in the skin, kidneys and other organs of 5–30% of lupus patients *(17,19–26)*. Some have argued that the immunoglobulins moved into the cell as an artifact of tissue fixation, whereas others have suggested that the effects of intracellular immunoglobulins are inconsequential, because they are often detected in noninflammatory tissues *(18,27)*. Furthermore, since intracellular transit of large proteins was poorly understood, it was uncertain how large extracellular proteins like immunoglobulins can transit across the cell membrane, through the cytoplasm, and into the nucleus. Tissue culture studies of polyclonal lupus serum with living cells have led to conflicting interpretations.

Initial studies using monoclonal lupus autoantibodies also produced somewhat controversial interpretations, although recent evidence (including results from our laboratory), indicates that internalized monoclonal autoantibodies behave like their polyclonal counterparts *(13)*. The phenomenon of internalization of autoantibodies is now supported by multiple laboratories as described below. Nevertheless, some have continued to hold that the cytoplasmic and/or nuclear localization of monoclonal immunoglobulins occurs because of the fixation process. In one recent study, antinucleosomal antibodies that had been deposited in vivo in a "nuclear pattern" as well as extracellularly were found to be internalized in tissue culture experiments into the cytoplasm of cultured cells, but the antibodies did not enter the nucleus *(27)*. From these results, the conclusion was made that anti-DNA/nucleosome antibodies can enter cells but cannot enter nuclei. On careful examination of the results, however, it turns out that the in vivo deposition of these autoantibodies was perinuclear (not intranuclear). It is not surprising, therefore, that these antibodies failed to enter the nuclei of cultured cells. On the other hand, the results clearly demonstrated that autoantibodies can be internalized into cells, and that the internalized immunoglobulins are transported within the cells to bind their target ligand.

With the identification of monoclonal antibodies with intracellular localizing and penetrating properties (such as ours), most of the recent debate has focused on the functional perturbations induced by the internalized autoantibodies, rather than the validity of the observation *(13,15,16,28–31)*. In this regard, the findings that the internalized human lupus autoantibodies with well characterized specificities (i.e., anti-SmRNP antibody activity) modify specific functions in living cells support the notion that these immunoglobulins enter cells, migrate to, and interact with, their intracellular target antigens *(16)*.

Recent reports from other laboratories support the occurrence of antibody internalization. Reichlin et al. recently found that internalized monoclonal anti-RNP antibodies persisted in the cytoplasm, mainly in mitochondria *(13)*. By contrast, Zack and Weisbart and Golan, Gharavi, and Elkon, demonstrated that anti-DNA antibodies enter cells, traverse the cytoplasm, and localize within the nucleus *(13,29,32)*. These results, obtained using MAbs, validate previous findings on polyclonal antiserum, and indicate that the ultimate location of the internalized antibodies is related to their antigen binding properties.

4. MECHANISM OF INTERNALIZATION

Ultrastructural and molecular analyses of the movement of large proteins between cellular compartments provide insights to the behavior of antibodies. It is now recognized that relatively large proteins can cross both the cell and nuclear membranes to deliver specific signals that influence transcription and translation, catalyze various reactions, and alter the transport of small molecules *(33–59)*. Furthermore, monoclonal immunoglobulins (and *Fv* fragments) produced in cells with specific localization sequences (as opposed to secretory or transmembrane sequences) migrate to their target antigen within the cell. These "intrabodies" have been used to target specific proteins and modulate their function within living cells *(60)*. Taken together, the results indicate that once internalized, the destination of the intracellular antibodies is determined by their autoantigen binding properties, and that the functional perturbation induced by the antibodies is related to the function of the target antigen within the cell.

To examine the mechanisms responsible for the cellular penetration and nuclear localization, a subset of monoclonal anti-DNA antibodies derived from MRL-*lpr/lpr* mice in our laboratory was studied. Using cultured living cell lines, multiple experimental approaches were employed, including immunofluorescence, confocal, and immunoelectron microscopy, and quantitative analysis of cellular and nuclear uptake of radiolabeled antibodies *(61)*. In the latter group of experiments, the requirements for nuclear localization were evaluated in nuclei isolated from cells cultured with radiolabeled antibodies under varying experimental conditions. Nuclear localization was observed only with the subset of anti-DNA antibodies that localized within the nuclei in vivo, i.e., were found in the nucleus in tissue sections. The anti-DNA antibodies that did not produce intranuclear deposits in vivo also did not do so in cultured cells. Furthermore, nuclear localization was dependent on the antigen binding region *(Fab)* of the antibodies. The specificity of these events was shown by the observation that both the cellular and the nuclear uptake of radiolabeled antibodies were significantly inhibited by unlabeled nuclear-localizing antibodies, but not by unlabeled anti-DNA antibodies that did not enter cells. Both the cellular localization and nuclear localization of the immunoglobulins were temperature dependent, consistent with an energy-dependent, specific process.

To more precisely examine these events, ultrastructural analyses of cells after incubation with tagged antibodies were performed. Following coculture of gold-labeled antibodies with cells, the cells were examined by electron microscopy. After progressive intervals, immunoglobulins were observed at the cell surface, within the cytoplasm, clustered at the nuclear pore and within the nucleus *(61)*. Of particular interest, a fraction of the internalized immunoglobulins was found to recycle and reappear on the cell surface. Similar time-dependent migration of the antibodies through the cell and into the nucleus was also observed by confocal microscopy.

Nucleotide sequence analysis of the immunoglobulins was also revealing. The results indicated the presence of nuclear localization-like motifs in CDR3 of the heavy chains *(62)*. Although an identical consensus sequence in the different nuclear localization antibodies was not evident, the antibodies shared a tertiary conformation not present in the nonnuclear localizing anti-DNA antibodies. All of the nuclear-localizing antibodies (3/3) contained multiple positively charged amino acids in their CDR regions, resembling the nuclear localization signals that direct protein import into the nucleus *(39,46,63,64)*. Furthermore, molecular modeling of the nuclear-localizing antibodies revealed a shared conformational motif in the heavy chain CDR3 region resembling the nuclear localization sequence. These results suggest that the CDR3 motif participates in nuclear import of the antibodies. The nuclear entry of antibodies is an energy requiring process. Following coculture of nuclear-localizing antibodies with digitonin-permeabilized cells, immunoglobulins were present at the nuclear membrane but not in the nucleus. However, when ATP was added, the antibodies were observed in the nucleus (Yanase and Madaio; unpublished observations).

The results of these experiments demonstrate that this subset of monoclonal anti-DNA antibodies traverse *both* the cell and nuclear membranes to localize within the nuclei of cultured cells. Furthermore, they indicate that nuclear localization of immunoglobulins is regulated in a manner analogous to that of other large cytoplasmic proteins that cross membranes and enter the nucleus *(57,65–67).* More recent results indicate that cellular entry is initiated by the binding of the nuclear-localizing anti-DNA antibodies to myosin 1, a 110-kD cell surface receptor *(68).* Particularly relevant to the internalization of anti-DNA antibodies is the finding that cell surface myosin 1 is expressed on the surfaces of many cell types (reviewed in ref. *69),* and it has been recently shown to modulate endocytosis in yeast *(70).* The role of this protein in internalization of the nuclear-localizing anti-DNA antibodies is under further investigation. Figure 1 illustrates the postulated transport pathways of anti-DNA antibodies.

5. FUNCTIONAL EFFECTS

The identification of myosin 1 as the candidate cell surface receptor modulating cellular entry of anti-DNA antibodies provides both a potential link to the functional perturbations produced by these antibodies in vivo (i.e., glomerular hypercellularity) and insight into the behavior of these antibodies within the cytoplasm en route to the nucleus. In this regard, we recently observed that all three nuclear-localizing anti-DNA antibodies cross-react with DNaseI and interfered with activity of the enzyme in vivo *(71).* Recent evidence from other laboratories suggests that myosin 1 forms a complex with calmodulin and DNaseI within the cytoplasm *(72).* Thus, internalization of anti-DNA antibodies by myosin 1 places them in proximity to DNaseI, and imparts to the antibodies the potential to interfere with the activity of the enzyme *within the cell.*

It is particularly relevant that DNaseI has been linked to apoptosis, although the primary role of this enzyme is still under debate *(73–77).* In some cell lines, this endonuclease appears critical for apoptosis, whereas in others its activity has been delinked from this process. Note that in studies of cell death, the nature of the apoptotic stimulus and the experimental conditions often confounds comparative analysis of different experimental systems, often leading to different conclusions. In our own studies, we tested the hypothesis that the interaction of the nuclear-localizing antibodies with DNaseI in the cytoplasm modulates apoptotic activity. We observed that preincubation of HL60 cells with the nuclear-localizing anti-DNA antibodies prior to challenge with an apoptotic stimulus inhibited the appearance of morphologic and biochemical markers of apoptosis *(78).* The intranuclear antibodies may only delay the inevitable, i.e., the occurrence of apoptosis, but regardless of the length of the delay, the observations indicate that the antibodies play a functional role during disease.

Previous debate over the pathogenic role of the anti-DNA antibodies can be reconciled by the observation of antibody-mediated inhibition of apoptosis. Since intranuclear immunoglobulins have been found within nuclei in both non-inflamed and inflamed tissues, it has been suggested that they are without pathologic

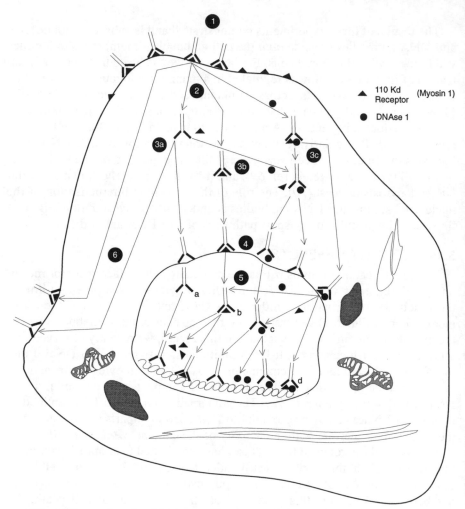

Fig. 1. Events involved in internalization, cellular transit and nuclear localization of anti-DNA antibodies: 1. Cell surface binding to myosin 1. 2. Energy-dependent internalization. 3. Intracytoplasmic transit (postulated): i) as unbound IgG, ii) as myosin 1-IgG complex, and iii) shuffling from myosin 1 to DNaseI and inactivation of DNaseI. 4. Binding of antibody to nuclear pore as either free antibody or part of myosin 1/DNaseI complex. 5. Transport of antibody (+/- complex) through nuclear pore complex into the nucleus, either as free antibody (a) or part of myosin 1 (b), and/or a DNaseI (c) complex, where it can bind to DNA (d); and 6. A fraction of internalized antibody is recycled back to the cell surface.

relevance. In the normal physiologic state, in which apoptosis occurs less frequently, intranuclear antibodies would not be expected to have a perceptible effect. During inflammation, however, the apoptotic activity is increased, and in some cases the increased activity may be relevant to the recovery of the kidney to a more healthy state *(79)*. Interference with the process of apoptosis by antibodies in the diseased state, therefore, could have dire effects. These observations are especially provocative in light of the glomerular hypercellularity observed in vivo in lupus. Taken together, the results implicate a novel pathogenic role for lupus autoantibodies. Further, these studies have provided unique tools to assess the functional role of DNaseI in apoptosis in future experiments.

Like the nuclear-localizing antibodies, the investigation of intracytoplasmic antibodies can also provide information relevant to the disease process. Intracytoplasmic immunoglobulins introduced into cells by artificial means behave like other intracytoplasmic proteins (reviewed in ref. *80*). Their movement and ultimate location within the cell is dependent on specific localization sequences contained within the antigen binding region. Recently, some investigators have taken advantage of this phenomenon by transfecting cells with antibody cDNA containing the localization sequences at their 5' end *(60)*. The 5' sequence that normally signals either surface membrane insertion or secretion is replaced by signal peptide sequences that facilitate the movement of immunoglobulins to specific sites within the cell. Once at the designated site, the immunoglobulins interact with their target antigen and either disrupt or facilitate specific cellular functions. These "intrabodies" have obvious potential use for evaluating and altering the function of specific target antigens within the cells. This approach is being used effectively in a variety of cell culture systems, although its utility in whole animals awaits better delivery and more specific expression techniques. In the context of the lupus antibodies, the emerging body of work lends further support to the notion that antibodies can move through cells, interact with specific molecules, and modulate their function.

Based on the consideration presented here, we hypothesize that the nuclear-localizing anti-DNA antibodies contain sequences that bind specific sites on myosin, which facilitates the internalization of the antibodies into the cell. Once internalized, further antibody transit is determined by both the trafficking sequences unique to these antibodies (i.e., nuclear localization sequences) and the antigen binding specificity of the antibodies (e.g., DNaseI). If the ligand is required for cell function, complexation of the ligand to an autoantibody within the cell may be predicted to alter the cellular properties.

ACKNOWLEDGMENTS

This work was supported by a George M. O'Brien Kidney and Urological Research Center Grant (DK45191), individual PHS Awards:DK 33694, AI 27915 to MPM and the DCI RED FUND. The authors thank Demetrios Vlahakos, Mary Foster, Robert Smith, Leonard Jarett, and Antonio Puccetti for their contributions to the work summarized in this review.

REFERENCES

1. Hahn, B. H. (1980) Systemic lupus erythematosus, in *Clinical Immunology* (Parker, C. W., eds.), W. B. Saunders, Philadelphia, PA, pp. 583-631.

2. Glassock, R. J., Cohen, A. H., Adler, S. G., and Ward, H. J. (1991) Secondary glomerular diseases, in *The Kidney* (Brenner, B. M. and Rector, F. C., eds.), W.B. Saunders, Philadelphia, PA, pp. 1280-1368.
3. Schwartz, R. S. and Stollar, B. D. (1985) Origins of anti-DNA autoantibodies. *J. Clin. Invest.* **75,** 321–327.
4. Foster, M. H., Cizman, B., and Madaio, M. P. (1994) Nephritogenic autoantibodies in systemic lupus erythematosus: Immunochemical properties, mechanisms of immune deposition and genetic origins. *Lab. Invest.* **69,** 494–507.
5. Vlahakos, D. V., Foster, M. H., Adams, S., Katz, M., Ucci, A. A., Barrett, K. J., et al. (1992) Monoclonal anti-DNA antibodies deroved from lupus-prone mice form immune deposits at distinct glomerular locations and induce different structural and functional abnormalities in vivo. *Kidney Int.* **41,** 1690–1700.
6. Vlahakos, D. V., Foster, M. H., Ucci, A. A., Barrett, K. J., Datta, S. K., and Madaio, M. P. (1992) Murine monoclonal anti-DNA antibodies penetrate cells, bind to nuclei, and induce glomerular proliferation and proteinuria in vivo. *J. Am. Soc. Neph.* **2,** 1345–1354.
7. Termaat, R. M., Brinkman, K., Gompel, F. V., Heuvel, L. P. W., Veerkamp, J., Smeenk, R. J. T., et al. (1990) Cross-reactivity of monoclonal anti-DNA antibodies with heparan sulfate is mediated via bound DNA/histone complexes. *J. Autoimmun.* **3,** 531–545.
8. Reininger, L., Berney, T., Shibata, T., Spertini, F., Merino, R., and Izui, S. (1990) Cryoglobulinemia induced by a murine IgG3 rheumatoid factor: skin vasculitis and glomerulonephritis arise from distinct pathogenic mechanisms. *Proc. Natl. Acad. Sci. USA* **87,** 10,038–10,042.
9. Gavalchin, J. and Datta, S. K. (1987) The NZBxSWR model of lupus nephritis. II. Autoantibodies deposited in renal lesions show a distinctive and restricted idiotypic diversity. *J. Immunol.* **138,** 138–148.
10. Termaat, R., Assmann, K. J. M., Dijkman, H. B. P. M., Gompel, F. V., Smeenk, R. J. T., and Berden, J. H. M. (1992) Anti-DNA antibodies can bind to the glomerulus via two distinct mechanisms. *Kidney Int.* **42,** 1363–1371.
11. Coons, A. H., Leduc, E. H., and Kaplan, M. H. (1951) Localization of antigen in tissue cells. VI. The fate of injecting foreign proteins into the mouse. *J. Exp. Med.* **93,** 173.
12. Rosenkranz, H. S., Erlanger, B. F., Tanenbaum, S. W., and Beiser, S. M. (1964) Purine- and pyrimidine-specific antibodies: effect on the fertilized sea urchin egg. *Science* **145,** 282–284.
13. Reichlin, M. (1995) Cell injury mediated by autoantibodies to intracellular antigens. *Clin. Immunol. Immunopath.* **76,** 215–219.
14. Alarcon-Segovia, D., Rutz-Arguelles, A., and Fishbein, E. (1978) Antibody to nuclear ribonucleoprotein penetrates live human mononuclear cells through Fc receptors. *Nature* **271,** 67–69.
15. Alarcon-Segovia, D., Ruiz-Arguelles, A., and Llorente, L. (1979) Antibody penetration into living cells. II. Antiribonucleoprotein IgG penetrates into T lymphocytes causing their deletion and the abrogation of suppressor function. *J. Immunol.* **122,** 1855–1862.
16. Alarcon-Segovia, D. and Lorente, L. (1983) Antibody penetration into living cells IV. Different effects of anti-native DNA and anti-ribonucleoprotein IgG on the cell cycle of activated T cells. *Clin. Exp. Immunol.* **52,** 365–371.

17. Andersen, I., Anderson, P., Elling, P., and Graudal., H. (1983) Epidermal nuclear immunoglobulin deposits in some connective tissue diseases: correlations with ENA antibodies. *Ann. Rheum. Dis.* **42,** 163–167.
18. Baart de la Faille-Kuyper, E. H. (1974) In vivo nuclear localization of immunoglobulins in clinically normal skin in systemic and procainamide induced lupus erythematosus. *Neth. J. Med.* **17,** 58.
19. Chen, Z., Dobson, R., Ainsworth, S., Silver, R., and Maricq, H. (1985) Epidermal nuclear immunofluorescence: serological correlations supporting an in vivo reaction. *Br. J. Dermatol.* **112,** 15–22.
20. Gilliam, J. N. and Prystowsky, S. D. (1977) Mixed connective tissue disease syndrome. *Arch. Dermatol.* **113,** 583–587.
21. Gilliam, J. N. (1975) The significance of cutaneous immunoglobulin deposits in lupus erythematosus and NZBxNZW/F1 hybrid mice. *J. Invest. Dermatol.* **65,** 154–161.
22. Izuno, G. T. (1978) Observations on the in vivo reaction of antinuclear antibodies with epidermal cells. *Br. J. Dermatol.* **98,** 391–398.
23. McCoy, R. C. (1972) Nuclear localization of immunoglobulins in renal biopsies of patients with lupus nephritis. *Am. J. Pathol.* **68,** 469–478.
24. Tan, M. and Kunkel, H. G. (1966) Immunofluorescent study of the skin lesions in systemic lupus erythematosus. *Arthritis Rheum.* **9,** 37–46.
25. Iwatsuki, K., Tagami, H., Imaizumi, S., Ginoza, M., and Yamada, M. (1982) The speckled epidermal nuclear immunofluorescence of mixed connective tissue disease seems to develop a an in vitro phenomenon. *Br. J. Dermatol.* **107,** 653–657.
26. Wells, J. V., Webb, J., Van Deventer, M., Fry, B., Pollard, K. M., Raftos, J., et al. (1979) In vivo anti-nuclear antibodies in epithelial biopsies in SLE and other connective tissue diseases. *Clin. Exp. Immunol.* **38,** 424–435.
27. Kramers, K., van Bruggen, M. C. J., Rijke-Schilder, T. P. M., Dijkman, H. B. P. M., Hylkema, M. N., Croes, H. J. E., et al. (1996) In vivo ANA is a fixation artifact: Nucleosome-complexed antinucleosome autoantibodies bind to cell surface and are internalized. *J. Am. Soc. Neph.* **7,** 946–954.
28. Alarcon-Segovia, D., Llorente, L., and Ruiz-Arguelles, A. (1982) Antibody penetration into living cells. III Effect of anti-ribonucleoprotein IgG on the cell cycle of human peripheral blood mononuclear cells. *Clin. Immunol. Immunopath.* **23,** 22–33.
29. Golan, T. D., Gharavi, A. E., and Elkon, K. B. (1993) Penetration of autoantibodies into living cells. *J. Invest. Derm.* **22,** 316–322.
30. Lee, L. A., Gaither, K. K., Coulter, S. S., Notis, D. A., and Harley, J. B. (1990) Patterns of cutaneous immunoglobulin deposition in subacue cutaneous lupus erythematosus is reproduced by infusing purified anti-Ro (SSA) autoantibodies into human skin grafted mice. *J. Clin. Invest.* **83,** 1556–1562.
31. Okudaira, K., Yoshizawa, H., and Williams, R. (1987) Mononuclear murine anti-DNA antibodies interacts with living mononuclear cells. *Arthritis Rheum.* **30,** 669–678.
32. Zack, D. and Weisbart, R. (1998) Cell and nuclear penetration by autoantibodies, this volume.
33. Dingwall, C. and Laskey, R. A. (1986) Protein import into the cell nucleus. *Annu. Rev. Cell. Biol.* **2,** 365–388.

34. Biocca, S., Neuberger, M. S., and Cattaneo, A. (1990) Expression and targeting of intracellular antibodies in mammalian cells. *EMBO J.* **9,** 101–108.
35. Blobel, G. (1980) Intracellular protein topogenesis. *Proc. Natl. Acad. Sci. USA* **77,** 1496–1500.
36. Dang, C. V. and Lee, W. M. F. (1989) Nuclear and nucleolar targeting sequences of c-*erb*-A, c-*myb*, N-*myc*, p53, HSP70, and HIV tat proteins. *J. Biol. Chem.* **264,** 18,019–18,023.
37. Einck, L. and Bustin, M. (1984) Functional histone antibody fragments traverse the nuclear envelope. *J. Cell. Biol.* **98,** 205–213.
38. Goidl, J. A. (1979) Insulin binding to isolated liver nuclei from obese and lean mice. *Biochemistry* **18,** 3674–3679.
39. Goldfarb, D. S., Gariepy, J., Schoolnik, G., and Kornberg, R. D. (1986) Synthetic peptides as nuclear localization signals. *Nature* **322,** 641–644.
40. Goldfine, I. D. (1981) Interaction of insulin, polypeptide hormones, and growth factors with intracellular membranes. *Biochem. Biophys. Acta* **650,** 53–67.
41. Goldstein, J. L., Brown, M., Anderson, R. G., Russell, D. W., and Schneider, W. (1985) Receptor-mediated endocytosis: Concepts emerging from the LDL receptor system. *Annu. Rev. Cell Biol.* **1,** 1–39.
42. Grenfell, S., Smithers, N., Miller, K., and Solari, R. (1989) Receptor-mediated endocytosis and nuclear transport of human interleukin 1α. *Biochem. J.* **264,** 813–822.
43. Gruenberg, J. and Howell, K. E. (1989) Membrane traffic in endocytosis: insights from cell-free assays. *Annu. Rev. Cell Biol.* **5,** 453–481.
44. Hunt, T. (1989) Cytoplasmic anchoring proteins and the control of nuclear localization. *Cell* **59,** 949–951.
45. Knutson, V. P. (1991) Cellular trafficking and processing of the insulin receptor. *FASEB J.* **5,** 2130–2138.
46. Lanford, R. E., Kanda, P., and Kennedy, R. C. (1986) Induction of nuclear transport with a synthetic peptide homologous to the SV40 T antigen transport signal. *Cell* **46,** 575–582.
47. Lee, B. A., Maher, D. W., Hannink, M., and Donoghue, D. J. (1987) Identification of a signal for nuclear targeting in platelet-derived-growth-factor-related molecules. *Mol. Cell Biol.* **7,** 3527–3537.
48. Lippincott-Schwartz, J., Yuan, L. C., Bonifacino, J. C., and Klawsner, R. D. (1989) Rapid redistribution of golgi proteins into the ER in cells treated with brefeldin A: evidence for membrane cycling from golgi to ER. *Cell* **56,** 80.
49. Moreland, R. B., Nam, H. G., Hereford, L. M., and Fried, H. M. (1985) Identification of a nuclear localization signal of a yeast ribosomal protein. *Proc. Natl. Acad. Sci. USA* **82,** 6561–6565.
50. Moreland, R. B., Langevin, G. L., Singer, R. H., Garcea, R. L., and Hereford, L. M. (1987) Amino acid sequences that determine the nuclear localization of yeast histone 2B. *Mol. Cell Biol.* **7,** 4048–4057.
51. Morgan, D. O. and Roth, R. (1988) Analysis of intracellular protein function by antibody injection. *Immunol. Today* **9,** 84–86.
52. Nehrbass, U. and Blobel, G. (1996) Role of the nuclear transport factor p10 in nuclear import. *Science* **272,** 120–122.
53. Newmeyer, D. D. and Forbes, D. J. (1988) Nuclear import can be separated into distinct steps in vitro: Nuclear pore binding and translocation. *Cell* **52,** 641–653.

54. Podlecki, D. A., Smith, R. M., Kao, M., Tsai, P., Huecksteadt, T., Brandenburg, D., et al. (1987) Nuclear translocation of the insulin receptor: a possible mediator of insulin's long term effects. *J. Biol. Chem.* **262,** 3362–3368.
55. Richardson, W. D., Roberts, B. L., and Smith, A. E. (1986) Nuclear location signals in polyoma virus large-T. *Cell* **44,** 77–85.
56. Richardson, W. D., Mills, A. D., Dilworth, S. M., Laskey, R. A., and Dingwall, C. (1988) Nuclear protein migration involves two steps: Rapid binding at the nuclear envelope followed by slower translocation through nuclear pores. *Cell* **52,** 655–664.
57. Silver, P. A. (1991) How proteins enter the nucleus. *Cell* **64,** 489–497.
58. Smith, R. M. and Jarett, L. (1987) Ultrastructural evidence for the accumulation of insulin in nuclei of intact 3T3-L1 adipocytes by an insulin-receptor mediated process. *Proc. Natl. Acad. Sci. USA* **84,** 459–463.
59. Thompson, K. A., Peralta Soler, A., Smith, R. M., and Jarett, L. (1989) Intranuclear localization of insulin in rat hepatoma cells: Insulin/matrix association. *Eur. J. Cell Biol.* **50,** 442–446.
60. Mhashilkar, A., Bagley, J., Chen, S., Zilvay, A., Helland, D., and Marasco, W. (1995) Inhibition of HIV-1 TAT-mediated LTR transactivation and HIV-1 infection by anti-TAT single-chain intrabodies. *EMBO J.* **14,** 1542–1551.
61. Yanase, K., Smith, R. M., Cizman, B., Foster, M. H., Peachey, L. D., Jarett, L., et al. (1994) A subgroup of murine monoclonal anti-DNA antibodies traverse the cytoplasm and enter the nucleus in a time and temperature dependent manner. *Lab. Invest.* **71,** 52–60.
62. Foster, M. H., Thompson, K., and Madaio, M. P. (1992) Heterogeneity in primary structure among nuclear localizing anti-DNA antibodies. *J. Am. Soc. Neph.* **3,** 588.
63. Valle, G., Jones, F. A., and Coleman, A. (1982) Anti-ovalbumin monoclonal antibodies interact with their antigen in internal membranes of Xenopus oocytes. *Nature* **300,** 71–74.
64. Boulikas, T. (1993) Nuclear localization signals (NLS). *Crit. Rev. Eukaryot. Gene Expr.* **3,** 193–227.
65. Hurt, E. C. (1996) Importins/karyopherins meet nucleoporins. *Cell* **84,** 509–515.
66. Rexach, M. and Blobel, G. (1995) Protein import into nuclei: Association and dissociation reactions involving transport substrate, transport factors and nucleoporins. *Cell* **83,** 683–692.
67. Silver, P. and Goodson, H. (1989) Nuclear protein transport. *Critic. Rev. Biochem. Mol. Biol.* **24,** 419–435.
68. Yanase, K., Smith, R., Puccetti, A., Jarett, L., and Madaio, M. (1997) Receptor-mediated cellular entry of nuclear localizing anti-DNA antibodies via myosin 1. *J. Clin. Invest.* **100,** 25–31.
69. Mooskeker, M. S. and Cheney, R. E. (1995) Unconventional myosins. *Annu. Rev. Cell. Dev. Biol.* **11,** 633–675.
70. Geli, M. I. and Riezman, H. (1996) Role of type 1 myosins in receptor-mediated endocytosis in yeast. *Science* **272,** 533–535.
71. Puccetti, A., Madaio, M. P., Bellese, G., and Migliorini, P. (1995) Anti-DNA antibodies bind to DNaseI. *J. Exp. Med.* **181,** 1797–1804.
72. Milligan, R. I. (1996) Protein-protein inteactions in the rigor actomyosin complex. *Proc. Natl. Acad. Sci. USA* **93,** 21–26.
73. Oberhammer, F., Wilson, J. W., Dive, C., Morris, I. D., Hickman, J. A., Wakeling, A. E., et al. (1993) Apoptotic death in epithelial cells: cleavage of DNA to 300

and/or 500 kb fragments prior to or in the absence of internucleosommal fragmentation. *EMBO J.* **12,** 3679–3684.

74. Cohen, G. M., Sun, X.-M., Snowden, R. T., Dinsdale, D., and Skilleter, D. N. (1992) Key morphologic features of apoptosis may occur in the absence of internucleosomal DNA fragmentation. *Biochem. J.* **286,** 331–334.

75. Peithsch, M., Polzar, B., Stephan, H., Crompton, T., MacDonald, H.-R., Mannherz, H. G., et al. (1993) Characterization of endogenous deoxyribonuclease involved in nuclear DNA degradation during apoptosis. *EMBO J.* **12,** 371–377.

76. Kroemer, G., Petit, P., Zamzami, N., Vayssiere, J.-L., and Mignotte, B. (1995) The biochemistry of programmed cell death. *FASEB* **9,** 1277–1287.

77. Steller, H. (1995) Mechanisms and genes of cellular suicide. *Science* **267,** 1445–1449.

78. Madaio, M., Fabbi, M., Tiso, M., Daga, A., and Puccetti, A. (1996) Spontaneously produced anti-DNA/DNase I autoantibodies modulate nuclear apoptosis in living cells. *Eur. J. Immunol.* **26,** 3035–3041.

79. Baker, A. J., Mooney, A., Hughes, J., Lombardi, D., Johnson, R., and Savill, J. (1994) Mesangial cell apoptosis—The major mechanism for resolution of glomerular hypercellularity in experimental mesangial proliferative nephritis. *J. Clin. Invest.* **94,** 2105–2116.

80. Biocca, S. and Cattaneo, A. (1995) Intracellular immunization: antibody targeting to subcellular compartments. *Trends Cell Biol.* **5,** 248–252.

20

Cell and Nuclear Penetration by Autoantibodies

Debra Jeske Zack and Richard H. Weisbart

1. INTRODUCTION

The idea that some antibodies possess the ability to penetrate both the cell and nuclear membranes of a living cell is still considered to be a controversial, if not heretical, notion. However, there is a considerable body of literature to support the idea that penetration of cells by certain antibodies can and does occur. The first reports observing the presence of immunoglobulin in the nuclei of cells were published over 30 yr ago. In these studies, skin (1) and renal (2) biopsy specimens from patients with systemic lupus erythematosus (SLE) were examined for the presence or absence of immunoglobulin by immunofluorescence staining with anti-IgG antisera. SLE is an autoimmune disease characterized by the production of a wide variety of autoantibodies. Within each tissue type, several different patterns of immunoglobulin deposition were seen. One recurrent pattern was the finding of nuclear deposits of immunoglobulin in either a homogenous or a speckled distribution. Implicit in this observation is the notion that the antibody deposition had occurred in vivo prior to the collection of the specimen, and by extension, that the deposits might somehow be involved in the pathogenesis of the skin findings. Only some individuals with the disease demonstrated the presence of penetrating antibodies and there was some suggestion that the penetrating antibodies showed tissue specificity (1).

Thus, the concept of in vivo ANA (antinuclear antibody) reactivity was born. Over the next decade, deposits of nuclear immunoglobulin were described in lesional and nonlesional skin (3–7), kidney (2,8–10), pneumocytes and pleural cells (11), and even vaginal epithelium (4) from patients with autoimmune disease. Contemporaneously, the association of the in vivo ANA with a variety of autoantibodies, including those to RNP (ribonucleoprotein), Sm (Smith antigen), Ro/SSA (Sjogren's syndrome A antigen), La/SSB (Sjogren's syndrome B antigen), and dsDNA (double stranded DNA), was elucidated (reviewed in refs. 12,13). Although several investigators maintained that the entire phenomenon resulted from fixation artifacts occurring during tissue processing (14,15), others presented strong arguments for in vivo deposition (reviewed most thoroughly in ref. 4). Many of these arguments were based on clinical studies as follows.

Contemporary Immunology: Autoimmune Reactions
Edited by: S. Paul © Humana Press Inc., Totowa, NJ

1. A patient found to have penetrating antibodies would continue to exhibit the in vivo phenomenon in the skin, for example, on repeated biopsies despite fluctuation in serum autoantibodies.
2. Different patients with similar titer and specificity of autoantibody would often show biopsy results that differed from one another.
3. Patients with high titer serum autoantibody capable of binding the nuclei of fixed cells did not necessarily exhibit nuclear deposition of antibody when biopsy material was examined.
4. Intracellular antibody deposition was present in some, but not all, tissues from an individual, even if all tissues were harvested on the same day.

Although these arguments are enumerated here chiefly to dispel the notion that circulating serum autoantibodies are the reason for nuclear staining of tissue biopsies, they can also be seen to contain the seeds of the ideas that only a subset of certain autoantibodies might possess the ability to penetrate living cells, and that the cellular targets of these antibodies might differ.

The next major advance was the demonstration by Alarcon-Segovia, Ruiz-Arguelles, and Fishbein *(16)* of anti-RNP IgG which could penetrate the nuclei of live mononuclear cells in vitro. Two other reports, published contemporaneously, also used anti-RNP sera to demonstrate penetration of the antibodies into the epidermal nuclei of freshly harvested skin sections *(5)* and into the nuclei of live isolated keratinocytes *(17)*. For the first time, antibody preparations could be tested directly for their ability to penetrate cells. This chapter will review the characterization of these and other published examples of antibodies with the ability to penetrate cells and nuclei. In particular, mechanisms of entry across cell and nuclear membranes and the functional outcomes of penetration will be discussed.

2. INTERACTION OF AUTOANTIBODIES WITH EXTRACELLULAR MATRIX AND CELL SURFACE MOLECULES

In order to thoroughly review the literature on penetrating antibodies, it is necessary to first discuss another related paradigm shift which has occurred concurrently. SLE, with its myriad of circulating autoantibodies, has historically been considered to be the prototype for "immune complex disease," particularly of the kidney. Anti-double stranded DNA (dsDNA) antibodies are found specifically in SLE and their levels correlate strongly with lupus nephritis. It was originally believed that circulating immune complexes consisting of anti-dsDNA antibodies and DNA deposited nonspecifically in the kidney, leading to damage by complement activation *(18,19)*. Several difficulties with this concept forced its reexamination. For example, if exogenous immune complexes were injected to simulate the circulating immune complexes of SLE, they were cleared by the liver and not deposited in the kidney at all *(20,21)*. More specific mechanisms of antibody deposition in the kidney have since been elucidated. These mechanisms basically fall into two groups; interaction with various extracellular matrix components of basement membrane and interaction directly with cell surface molecules.

Extracellular matrix components such as heparan sulfate and laminin have been proposed to interact directly with anti-DNA antibodies primarily on the basis of the anionic charge of the former molecules and the cationic nature of anti-DNA antibodies. If DNA were present, the anti-DNA/DNA complex would not be likely to deposit since the DNA and the extracellular matrix are both negatively charged (22) and would be expected to repel each other. Therefore, one would expect to find either the direct interaction of anti-DNA with the matrix component or the presence of positively charged intermediary molecules allowing the two negatively charged molecules to interact. In fact, both situations have been described. In one case, laminin was shown to be directly reactive with pathogenic lupus autoantibodies, with three 20-mer peptides of laminin defining the major reactive sites (23–25). In the second case, heparan sulfate serves as a major ligand for the deposition of positively charged histones (26), and the histones mediate the binding of DNA/anti-DNA complexes, leading to the formation of a multiple layer sandwich of immune complex *in situ* in the kidney (27).

Similar to the extracellular matrix binding, anti-DNA antibodies have been shown to bind to cell surface components either indirectly or directly. Antibodies can bind indirectly through DNA or nucleosomes to DNA/nucleosome receptors on the cell surface (28–30). In some cases, the antibodies are subsequently internalized into vesicles in the cytoplasm (29). In SLE, there is also evidence for direct binding to nucleosome receptors (31,32). Other investigators have shown direct binding to individual protein or glycoprotein antigens located on glomerular cell membranes (33–38), kidney tubules (39), and endothelia (34). The identity of these antigens is still under investigation. These latter targets are the most intriguing, as they represent potential organ-specific cell surface receptor candidates which might mediate internalization of autoantibodies across the cell membrane.

Anti-DNA antibody reactivity has also been described with novel antigens, the roles of which as matrix or cell membrane determinants have not yet been clearly defined. For example, a molecule designated HP8 was isolated from a cDNA expression library using an anti-DNA antibody as the probe (40). The same molecule has been isolated by another group and designated HEVIN (41). A 22-mer peptide derived from this molecule is reactive with a monoclonal (MAb) anti-DNA antibody and with some polyclonal lupus sera (40). This molecule shares homology with the SPARC group of extracellular matrix proteins, and is expressed by a variety of cells including high endothelial venules. Neither the function nor the accessibility of HP8 to antibodies is known at the present time.

While the preceding discussion reviews anti-dsDNA antibodies and their antigenic targets, it is important to note that many other autoantibodies under scrutiny in this chapter are directed against classical protein antigens found in

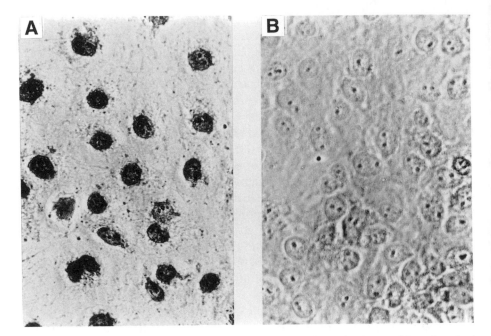

Fig. 1. Penetration of cells by MAb 3E10 Fab evident by immunhistochemical localization. (**A**) COS-7 cells were cotransfected with plasmids containing MAb 3E10 light chain cDNA and MAb 3E10 VH through CH1 cDNA. The heavy chain *V* region used for this experiment contains a mutation at position 31 as described in ref. *52*. Secreted *Fab* fragments penetrate the neighboring COS-7 cells and are evident as dark deposits in the nuclei. (**B**) Sham transfected COS-7 cells. Reprinted with permission from ref. *52*.

intracellular and intranuclear compartments. Like DNA, these protein antigens are usually sequestered away from detection by the humoral immune system. As in the case of the anti-DNA antibodies, the ability of anti-protein antibodies to recognize and penetrate particular cell types may involve more accessible, unknown targets in addition to their originally described antigenic specificities.

3. ANTIBODY ENTRY ACROSS THE CELL MEMBRANE

A wide variety of autoantibodies of differing specificities have been shown to penetrate the cell membrane. One can easily envision that the binding of an antibody to a surface receptor could lead to internalization via receptor mediated endocytosis and subsequent destruction within lysosomes. As illustrated in Fig. 1, however, autoantibody entry into cells often leads to pathways that allow the antibody to reach unexpected locations within the cell, such as the nucleus. Some examples of penetrating antibodies are summarized in Table 1. These include autoantibodies of different specificities such as RNP *(16,17, 42–44)*, dsDNA *(45–53)*, and the neuronal antigen Hu *(54)*. Penetrating antibodies with specificity for the Ro/SSA antigen *(55)*, ribosomal P protein *(56)*,

Table 1
Examples of Nuclear Penetrating Autoantibodies

Autoantibody	Source	Target cell	Entry mechanism	Time	Amount	Effect	Ref.
Polyclonal anti-RNP	Human	PBMC[a]	F_c receptor	1h	4.2 mg/mL	ND[b]	16
Polyclonal anti-RNP	Human	T-cells with $Fc\gamma R$	F_c receptor	2–4 d	4.2 mg/mL	Cell deletion	42
Polyclonal anti-dsDNA	Human	PBMC, T	F_c receptor, temp[c]	1 d	4.2 mg/mL	Cell deletion	45
Polyclonal anti-RNP	Human	Lymphocytes	Combined F_c and *Fab*	1 d	1 mg/mL	ND	44
Polyclonal anti-RNP	Human	Fresh keratinocytes	Not F; Con A inhibits	1 h	1/1000 dil	Viable	17
Polyclonal anti-dsDNA	Human	Epithelial cell lines	Not F_c; not C[d]; temp; cytochalasin blocks	30 min	1/50- dil	Viable	46
MAb anti-DNA (4B5)	Murine	PBMC, thymocytes	DNA or DNA-like; temp	15 h	100 μg/mL	Viable	47
MAb anti-dsDNA (BWds1) and Polyclonal anti-dsDNA	Murine Human	Fibroblasts, pig kidney cell line	Not F; Not DNA; antibodies crossreact with A and D snRNP	1–2 d	100 μg/mL	?C killing; cell dysfunction; mesangial proliferation	48 49
MAb anti-dsDNA (H7, H9, H72)	Murine	Mesangial, renal tubule, hepatoma, fibroblast; glomerulus in vivo	Not F_c; temp	1–5 h	ND	Inhibition of apoptosis	50 51
MAb anti-dsDNA (3E10)	Murine	Kidney cell line, fibroblast; renal tubule in vivo	Not F_c: monovalent; ?DNA or DNA-like not HP8[e]	1 h	10 μg/mL; 30–60 ng/mL for mutant	Viable	52
MAb anti-dsDNA (B3, 35.21)	Human	In vivo (SCID) glomerulus, skin, liver, spleen	Not DNA alone	3–7 wk	ND	Proteinuria	53
Polyclonal anti-Hu	Human	Hu expressing lines	?	4–24 h	100 μg/mL	Viable	54

[a] PBMN, peripheral blood mononuclear cells; [b] ND, not done; [c] Temp, temperature dependent; [d] C, complement; [e] HP8, HP8 is a protein isolated using 3E10 MAb.

and other autoantigens have also been described. Usually, only a subset of the antibodies with a given specificity are able to penetrate cells, and even within this subset, variability in the profile of tissues in which penetration occurs is encountered.

A variety of mechanisms for antibody entry can be conceived. The early studies by Alarcon-Segovia's group strongly implicated the F_c receptor *(16,42,45)*. Internalization of whole antibody was blocked with γ-globulin and $F(ab')_2$ fragments did not penetrate the cells. Studies by Ma et al. suggested that a combination of F_c and *Fab* determinants contributed to internalization *(43,44)*. Recent investigations have failed to implicate the F_c receptor, but the target cells studied have been different from those used originally in studies pointing to F_c receptor-mediated internalization. DNA has been proposed to promote internalization *(47)*, perhaps by binding of DNA/anti-DNA complexes to the nucleosome receptor *(28)*. However, it is difficult to implicate DNA/nucleosome receptors as a universal mechanism for autoantibody entry (particularly anti-DNA), primarily because many high affinity anti-DNA antibodies are unable to penetrate cells *(48,49,53)*.

Organ specific cell surface proteins which might serve as receptors and mediate antibody uptake have been sought. Several studies have shown that monoclonal anti-DNA antibodies have very specific patterns of deposition and internalization in different tissues, suggesting the existence of such cell surface receptor proteins. For example, some anti-DNA antibodies bind glomeruli in vivo, but do not penetrate the cells *(53)*, while others can penetrate multiple tissues such as skin, liver, and kidney *(53)*, and still others can penetrate only a few cell types, such as mesangial cells *(51)* or renal tubule cells *(52)*. Potential antibody receptors have been identified by immunoprecipitation studies using antibodies reactive with a specific tissue type. For example, Raz et al. identified proteins with mass 102, 80, 52, 35, and 31 kDa that are expressed in different combinations on various cell types *(33)*. D'Andrea and colleagues identified a 108-kDa protein on mesangial cells and a 47-kDa molecule on endothelia reactive with selected anti-DNA antibodies *(34)*. Two proteins of 88 and 68 kDa were immunoprecipitated from keratinocytes by Golan and coworkers using internalizable antibodies *(46)*. The functional role of these proteins must still be determined. In Heymann nephritis, a mouse model for autoimmune membranous glomerulonephritis, a complex of gp330 and a 44-kDa protein are present on proximal tubules. Antibodies to these proteins crossreact with glomerular antigens, leading to glomerular membrane binding and immune complex deposits *(57)*.

In addition, antigens previously thought of as being cytoplasmic proteins have sometimes been isolated from the cell surface. For example, Sun *(58)* and Koren *(59)* and their colleagues have identified the 38-kDa human acidic ribosomal phosphoprotein (ribosomal P protein) as being expressed on the surface of various cells, including mesangial, neuroblastoma, hepatoma, and fibroblast cells. The former group also suggested that cell surface expression of the ribosomal P protein may be dependent on the cellular activation state or the stage at which cells are located in the cell cycle. Elkon's group postulated that antibody penetration might be limited by the extent of cellular differentiation and the activation state of the cell *(46)*. Several stimuli have been shown to induce the expression of sequestered antigens such as Ro/SSA, La/SSB, RNP, Sm, and Ku on the cell surface. The increased antigen expression on the cell surface could then be postulated to result in increased penetration of cells by antibodies specific for these antigens. The most well-described stimuli are ultraviolet (UV) light *(60–62)* and apoptosis *(63)*. The idea that UV light could influence expression of autoantigens is intriguing, particularly in the context of the photosensitive pathology found in SLE.

Finally, the individual characteristics of the autoantibody itself play a role in cellular penetration. In one example using the same cell target, two monoclonal anti-dsDNA antibodies were bound to the cell surface after an 8-h incubation period, but only one antibody went on to penetrate the cells and their nuclei after 24 h *(48,49)*. The patterns of antibody interaction appear to depend, therefore, on several variables: the particular surface antigen recognized by the antibody, unidentified but unique characteristics of the antibody itself, and, perhaps, the state of activation of the target cell. It is possible, therefore, that multiple internalization pathways exist, and different antibodies utilize different pathways to penetrate the cells.

4. ANTIBODY ENTRY ACROSS THE NUCLEAR MEMBRANE

Once an antibody has traversed the cell membrane, it must still be transported through the cytoplasm and then achieve translocation across the nuclear membrane. Antibodies are too large to gain entry through the nuclear pores. Therefore, in order to gain entry into the nucleus, an antibody must either bind a transport molecule or must contain an internal transport signal. There is evidence that antibodies directed to transport proteins such as hsp70 will traverse the nuclear membrane after microinjection into the cytoplasm, whereas others without such reactivity will not *(64)*. Because autoantibodies have been shown to bind many diverse cytoplasmic and nuclear proteins, their potential reactivity with transport molecules remains a distinct possibility.

Alternatively, there are at least three different types of signals that, when present, may allow translocation of proteins into the nucleus: nuclear localization signals, glycosylation, and phosphorylation. Nuclear localization signals (NLS) are short stretches in the primary amino acid sequence that are rich in basic residues and that mediate translocation to the nucleus (reviewed in ref. *65*). Many anti-dsDNA antibodies contain a large number of basic amino acids (especially arginines) in their antigen combining sites *(66,67)*. Madaio's group has postulated that the uptake of certain anti-dsDNA antibodies into the nucleus is mediated by these runs of basic amino acids acting essentially as an NLS *(68)*. This is certainly quite feasible, as addition of an NLS structure has been shown to direct nuclear entry of non-antibody molecules *(69)*. Many other anti-dsDNA antibodies are not so heavily endowed with basic residues and may use

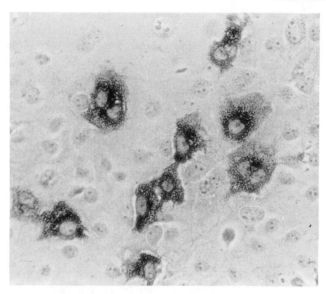

Fig. 2. Immunohistochemical localization of MAb 3E10 ($V_H 31$ mutant) devoid of signal peptide sequences. COS-7 cells were cotransfected with plasmids containing cDNA encoding MAb 3E10 VH mutant heavy chain and the light chain devoid of signal peptide sequences. MAb 3E10 is localized in the cytoplasm, evident as a dark deposit, but not in the nucleus. Reprinted with permission from ref. *52.*

signals other than NLS for nuclear entry. The following experiment examined one of these arginine poor antibodies *(52)* for the presence of an NLS. Synthesis of antibody molecules lacking signal peptides was obtained in the cytoplasm by transfection of cells with immunoglobulin heavy and light chain cDNA clones devoid of the leader sequences. If an NLS is present in the antibody primary structure, transport of the antibody into the nucleus *(70)* can be anticipated. The result is shown in Fig. 2. The antibody remains in the cytoplasm of the cell, suggesting the absence of an NLS sequence. In its physiological structure, this antibody is capable of nuclear entry. The absence of the leader peptide sequence in the recombinant version of the antibody could account for its failure to enter the nucleus. For instance, the leaderless antibody may not be trafficked appropriately to undergo posttranslational modifications necessary for nuclear translocation (*see* next paragraph). Alternatively, it is possible that the antibody must be secreted and interact with an appropriate cell surface molecule in order to be directed into the pathway leading to nuclear localization *(52).*

Two posttranslational modifications of proteins, i.e., glycosylation and phosphorylation have been shown to promote their nuclear localization. Glycosylation of molecules which are not normally transported into the nucleus has been shown to confer the ability to enter the nucleus *(71).* In some cases, the glycosylated proteins enter the nucleus by complexing with and being transported by lectin shuttles *(71,72).* Phosphorylation of proteins is another general mechanism cells use to tag molecules for nuclear entry. Protein kinase cascades activated during signal transduction are known to result in the phosphorylation and nuclear entry of many transcriptional factors. Specific phosphorylation of exogenous proteins such as viral proteins is known to target them for nuclear entry *(73,74)*. The importance of such posttranslational signals in the transport of nuclear penetrating antibodies is not known.

5. FUNCTIONAL CONSEQUENCES OF ANTIBODY PENETRATION

There are few well-defined functional consequences of antibody penetration into cells and nuclei *(see* Table 1). Non-penetrating antibodies bound to the cell surface mediate complement dependent cytotoxicity more potently than antibodies that bind the surface and then go on to penetrate cells *(48,49)*. DNA receptor dysfunction has been observed as a result of interaction with anti-DNA, antihistone, and antireceptor antibodies *(31)*, but it is not clear whether the effects are cell-surface related, whether the antibodies penetrated the cells and whether protein synthesis might have been affected by the antibodies. Penetration of cells by antibodies can influence protein synthesis processes. Reichlin and coworkers have identified anti-ribosomal P autoantibodies that penetrated live human hepatoblastoma cells and caused altered transmembrane calcium flux, decreased apolipoprotein B synthesis and increased intracellular accumulation of fat *(56)*.

The penetration of antibodies can also influence the cellular metabolism at the DNA and RNA level. The penetration of anti-RNP and anti-DNA antibodies into T-cells can arrest cell cycle progression, leading to protracted cell death *(75)*. Interestingly, the anti-DNA and anti-RNP antibodies caused cell cycle arrest at different stages in the cell cycle. Penetration of anti-RNP antibody into a subset of T-cells expressing the $F_c\gamma R$ resulted in the elimination of this subset, accompanied by loss of suppressor function and dysregulation of the immune response *(75)*.

The in vivo administration of anti-DNA antibodies induces cellular proliferation and foot process fusion in glomeruli and leads to proteinuria *(48–51)*. Dissecting the influence of immune deposition from that of cellular penetration, however, is somewhat difficult in the in vivo experiments. An intriguing mechanism that may be responsible for some cases of mesangial proliferation has been recently elucidated. In this case, the anti-DNA antibodies that penetrated mesangial cells were shown to cross-react with the active site of the enzyme DNase I *(76)*, an enzyme postulated to mediate DNA fragmentation during apoptosis. The antibodies blocked the enzymatic activity of DNase I both in vitro and in the nuclei of living cells. The antibody-containing cells were resistant to apoptotic stimuli *(77)*. Thus, the anti-DNA antibodies in this study presumably entered the cells via binding to a cell surface ligand, penetrated into the nuclei, and interacted with a second cross-reactive molecule, DNase I, resulting in the prevention of apoptosis and proliferation of the cells.

Other more subtle changes in cell function due to penetration of autoantibodies are possible. For example, although autoimmune disease is usually associated with inflammatory changes in tissues, often there appears to be organ dysfunction even in the absence of overt inflammation. Central nervous system disease in SLE frequently presents with this kind of bland histopathology. Another potential example of the effects of penetrating antibodies can be found in the association of paraneoplastic subacute sensory neuropathy and encephalomyelitis with anti-Hu antibodies. Anti-Hu antibodies do not cause either complement mediated lysis nor do they increase antibody-dependent cell-mediated cytotoxicity, but their presence appears to be intimately associated with the development of the disease *(54)*. The mechanism remains unidentified.

Finally, some penetrating autoantibodies may not have a significant effect on either cell viability or function. Further studies of this group of autoantibodies may allow their use as delivery vehicles into cells and nuclei.

6. CONCLUSIONS AND FUTURE DIRECTIONS

Penetration of cells and nuclei by autoantibodies can occur in vivo and in vitro with potential physiologic or pathologic consequences. Autoantibodies appear to use several different target molecules and entry pathways, as evidenced by the variety in the observed patterns of target cell penetration. Antibody penetration appears to be dependent upon the characteristics of the individual antibody, the location and nature of the target antigen, and possibly, the state of activation of the target cell. Heterogeneity in the response to antibody penetration is seen and some antibodies induce cell death upon penetration; other antibodies inappropriately prolong the life of the cells by blocking apoptosis. Antibody penetration can also block the synthesis of specific proteins. Thus, autoantibody penetration might initiate previously unappreciated pathogenic mechanisms operative in autoimmune disease. Conversely, some antibodies may penetrate cells to subserve physiological purposes.

Elucidation of the pathways for cellular penetration by antibodies may lead to the design of new delivery systems for therapeutic agents. Some internalized antibodies exert little or no pathological effect on the target cells. In these cases, the internalization signals could potentially be harnessed as tools to achieve delivery of therapeutic agents into the nuclei of specific cells.

REFERENCES

1. Tan, E. M. and Kunkel, H. G. (1966) An immunofluorescent study of the skin lesions in systemic lupus erythematosus. *Arthritis Rheum.* **9,** 37–46.
2. Freedman, P. and Markowitz, A. S. (1962) Gamma globulin and complement in the diseased kidney. *J. Clin. Invest.* **41,** 328–334.
3. Shu, S., Provost, T., Croxdale, M. B., Reichlin, M., and Beutner, E. H. (1977) Nuclear deposits of immunoglobulins in skin of patients with systemic lupus erythematosus. *Clin. Exp. Immunol.* **27,** 238–244.

4. Wells, J. V., Webb, J., Van Deventer, M., Fry, B., Pollard, K. M., Raftos, J., et al. (1979) In vivo anti-nuclear antibodies in epithelial biopsies in SLE and other connective tissue diseases. *Clin. Exp. Immunol.* **38**, 424–435.

5. Izuno, G. T. (1978) Observations on the in vivo reaction of antinuclear antibodies with epidermal cells. *Br. J. Dermatol.* **98**, 391–398.

6. Prystowsky, S. D. and Tuffanelli, D. L. (1978) Speckled (particulate) epidermal nuclear IgG deposition in normal skin. *Arch. Dermatol.* **114**, 705–710.

7. Baart de la Faille-Kuyper, E. H. (1974) In vivo nuclear localization of immunoglobulins in clinically normal skin in systemic and procainamide-induced lupus erythematosus. *Neth. J. Med.* **17**, 58–65.

8. Paroretto, F. and Koffler, D. (1965) Immunofluorescent localization of immunoglobulins, complement, and fibrinogen in human diseases: I. Systemic lupus erythematosus. *J. Clin. Invest.* **44**, 1657–1664.

9. Hench, P. K., Tan, E. M., and Wilson, C. B. (1969) In vivo fixation of gammaglobulin in renal cell nuclei of patients with systemic lupus erythematosus (SLE). *Arthritis Rheum.* **12**, 668.

10. McCoy, R. C. (1972) Nuclear localization of immunoglobulins in renal biopsies of patients with lupus nephritis. *Am. J. Pathol.* **68**, 469–478.

11. Pertschuk, L. P., Moccia, L. F., and Rosen, Y. (1977) Acute pulmonary complications in systemic lupus erythematosus: immunofluoresence and light microscopic study. *Am. J. Pathol.* **68**, 553–557.

12. Williams, W. V., Barjenbrach, P., Adelstein, E., Sharp, G. C., and Walker, S. E. (1986) The clinical significance of the in vivo antinuclear antibody phenomenon. *Arch. Pathol. Lab Med.* **110**, 798–802.

13. Velthuis, P. J., Kater, L., van der Tweel, I., Gmelig Meyling, F., Derksen, R. H. W. M., Hene, R. J., et al. (1990) In vivo antinuclear antibody of the skin: diagnostic significance and association with selective antinuclear antibodies. *Ann. Rheum. Dis.* **49**, 163–167.

14. Prystowsky, S. D., Gilliam, J. N., and Tuffanelli, D. L. (1978) Epidermal nucleolar IgG deposition in clinically normal skin (Clinical and serologic features of eight patients). *Arch. Dermatol.* **114**, 536–538.

15. Iwatsuki, K., Tagami, H., Imaizumi, S., Ginoza, M., and Yamada, M. (1982) The speckled epidermal nuclear immunofluoresence of mixed connective tissue disease seems to develop as an in vitro phenomenon. *Br. J. Dermatol.* **107**, 653–657.

16. Alarcon-Segovia, D., Rutz-Arguelles, A., and Fishbein, E. (1978) Antibody to ribonucleoprotein penetrates live human mononuclear cells through Fc receptors. *Nature* **271**, 67–69.

17. Galoppin, L. and Saurat, J. H. (1981) In vitro study of the binding of antiribonucleoprotein antibodies to the nucleus of isolated living keratinocytes. *J. Invest. Dermatol.* **76**, 264–267.

18. Koffler, D., Schur, P. H., and Kunkel, H. G. (1967) Immunological studies concerning the nephritis of systemic lupus erythematosus. *J. Exp. Med.* **126**, 607–624.

19. Lambert, P. H. and Dixon, F. J. (1968) Pathogenesis of the glomerulonephritis of NZB/W mice. *J. Exp. Med.* **127**, 507–522.

20. Emlen, W. and Mannik, M. (1982) Clearance of circulating DNA anti-DNA immune complexes in mice. *J. Exp. Med.* **155**, 1210–1215.

21. Emlen, W. and Burdick, G. (1988) Clearance and organ localization of small DNA anti-DNA immune complexes in mice. *J. Immunol.* **140**, 1816–1822.

22. Fournie, G. J. (1988) Circulating DNA and lupus nephritis. *Kidney Int.* **33,** 487–497.
23. Naparstek, Y. and Madaio, M. P. (1997) Are DNA antibodies actually pathogenic? *Lupus* **6,** 307–309.
24. Ben-Yehuda, A., Rasooly, L., Bar-Tana, R., Breuer, G., Tadmor, B., Ulmansky, R., et al. (1995) The urine of SLE patients contains antibodies that bind to the laminin component of the extracellular matrix. *J. Autoimmun.* **8,** 279– 291.
25. Foster, M. H., Sabbaga, J., Line, S. R. P., Thompson, K. S., Barrett, K. J., and Madaio, M. P. (1993) Molecular analysis of spontaneous nephrotropic anti-laminin antibodies in an autoimmune MRL-ipr mouse. *J. Immunol.* **151,** 814–824.
26. Schmiedeke, T. M. J., Stockl, F. W., Weber, R., Sugisaki, Y., Batsford, S. R., and Vogt, A. (1989) Histones have high affinity for the glomerular basement membrane. *J. Exp. Med.* **169,** 1879–1894.
27. Termaat, R. M., Brinkman, K., van Gompel, F., van de Heuvel, L. P. W. J., Veerkamp, J., Smeenk, R. J. T., et al. (1990) Cross-reactivity of monoclonal anti-DNA antibodies with heparan sulfate is mediated via bound DNA/histone complexes. *J. Autoimmun.* **3,** 531–545.
28. Bennett, R. M., Gabor, G. T., and Meritt, M. M. (1985) DNA binding to human leukocytes. Evidence for a receptor-mediated association, internalization, and degradation of DNA. *J. Clin. Invest.* **76,** 2182–2190.
29. Koutouzov, S., Cabrespines, A., Amoura, Z., Chabre, H., Lotton, C., and Bach, J. F. (1996) Binding of nucleosomes to a cell surface receptor: redistribution and endocytosis in the presence of lupus antibodies. *Eur. J. Immunol.* **26,** 472–486.
30. Jacob, L. and Viard, J. P. (1992) Anti-DNA antibodies and their relationships with anti-histone and anti-nucleosome specificities. *Eur. J. Med. 1,* 425–431.
31. Bennett, R. M., Kotzin, B. L., and Merritt, M. J. (1987) DNA receptor dysfunction in systemic lupus erythematosus and kindred disorders. Induction by anti-DNA antibodies, antihistone antibodies, and antireceptor antibodies. *J. Exp. Med.* **166,** 850–863.
32. Bennett, R. M., Cornell, K. A., Merritt, M. J., Bakke, A. C., Hsu, P. H., and Hefeneider, S. H. (1991) Autoimmunity to a 28-30 kD cell membrane DNA binding protein: occurrence in selected sera from patients with SLE and mixed connective tissue disease (MCTD). *Clin. Exp. Immunol.* **86,** 374–379.
33. Raz, E., Ben-Bassat, H., Davidi, T., Shlomai, Z., and Eilat, D. (1993) Crossreactions of anti-DNA autoantibodies with cell surface proteins. *Eur. J. Immunol.* **23,** 383–390.
34. D'Andrea, D. M., Coupaye-Gerard,B., Kleyman, T. R., Foster, M. H., and Madaio, M. P. (1996) Lupus autoantibodies interact directly with distinct glomerular and vascular cell surface antigens. *Kidney Int.* **49,** 1214–1221.
35. Sun, K.-H., Liu, W.-T., Tang, S.-J., Tsai, C.-Y., Hsieh, S.-C., Wu, T.-H., et al. (1996) The expression of acidic ribosomal phosphoproteins on the surface membrane of different tissues in autoimmune and normal mice which are the target molecules for anti-double-stranded DNA antibodies. *Immunology* **87,** 362–371.
36. Raz, E., Brezis, M., Rosenmann, E., and Eilat, D. (1989) Anti-DNA antibodies bind directly to renal antigens and induce kidney dysfunction in the isolated perfused rat kidney. *J. Immunol.* **142,** 3076–3082.
37. Madaio, M. P., Carlson, J., Cataldo, J., Ucci, A., Migliorini, P., and Pankewycz, O. (1987) Murine monoclonal anti-DNA antibodies bind directly to glomerular antigens and form immune deposits. *J. Immunol.* **138,** 2883–2889.

38. Jacob, L., Lety, M.-A., Louvard, D., and Bach, J.-F. (1985) Binding of a monoclonal anti-DNA autoantibody to identical protein(s) present at the surface of several human cell types involved in lupus pathogenesis. *J. Clin. Invest.* **75,** 315–317.

39. Van Leer, E. H. G., Bruijn, J. A., Prins, F. A., Hoedemaeker, P. H. J., and De Heer, E. (1993) Redistribution of glomerular dipeptidyl peptidase type IV in experimental lupus nephritis. *Lab. Invest.* **68,** 550–556.

40. Zack, D. J., Yamamoto, K., Wong, A. L., Stempniak, M., French, C., and Weisbart, R. H. (1995) DNA mimics a self protein that may be a target for some anti-DNA antibodies in systemic lupus erythematosus. *J. Immunol.* **154,** 1987–1994.

41. Girard, J.-P. and Springer, T. A. (1994) Cloning from purified high endothelial venule cells of hevin, a close relative of the antiadhesive extracellular matrix protein SPARC. *Immunity* **2,** 113–123.

42. Alarcon-Segovia, D., Ruiz-Arguelles, A., and Llorente, L. (1979) Antibody penetration into living cells: II. Anti-ribonucleoprotein IgG penetrates into T gamma lymphocytes causing their deletion and the abrogation of suppressor function. *J. Immunol.* **122,** 1855–1862.

43. Ma, J., Chapman, G. V., Chen, S. L., Melick, G., Penny, R., and Breit, S. N. (1991) Antibody penetration of viable human cells. I. Increased penetration of human lymphocytes by anti-RNP IgG. *Clin. Exp. Immunol.* **84,** 83–91.

44. Ma, J., King, N., Chen, S. L., Penny, R., and Breit, S. N. (1993) Antibody penetration of viable human cells. II. Anti-RNP antibodies binding to RNP antigen expressed on cell surface, which may mediate the antibody internalization. *Clin. Exp. Immunol.* **93,** 396–404.

45. Alarcon-Segovia, D., Llorente, L., Fishbein, E., and Diaz-Jouanen, E. (1982) Abnormalities in the content of nucleic acids of peripheral blood mononuclear cells from patients with systemic lupus erythematosus: relationship to DNA antibodies. *Arthritis Rheum.* **23,** 304–317.

46. Golan, T. D., Gharavi, A. E., and Elkon, K. B. (1993) Penetration of autoantibodies into living epithelial cells. *J. Invest. Dermatol.* **100,** 316–322.

47. Okudaira, K., Yoshizawa, H., and Williams, R. C. (1987) Monoclonal anti-DNA antibody interacts with living mononuclear cells. *Arthritis Rheum.* **30,** 669–678.

48. Reichlin, M., Hahn, B., and Koren, E. (1995) Characterization of anti-dsDNA antibodies: Cross-reaction with SnRNP polypeptides and cell-binding abilities. *The Immunologist* **3,** 84–88.

49. Koren, E., Koscec, M., Wolfson-Reichlin, M., Ebling, F. M., Tsao, B., Hahn, B. H., and Reichlin, M. (1995) Murine and human antibodies to native DNA that cross-react with the A and D SnRNP polypeptides cause direct injury of cultured kidney cells. *J. Immunol.* **154,** 4857–4864.

50. Vlahakos, D., Foster, M. H., Ucci, A. A., Barrett, K. J., Datta, S. K., and Madaio, M. P. (1992) Murine monoclonal anti-DNA antibodies penetrate cells, bind to nuclei, and induce glomerular proliferation and proteinuria in vivo. *J. Am. Soc. Nephrol.* **2,** 1345–1354.

51. Yanase, K., Smith, R. M., Cizman, B., Foster, M. H., Peachey, L. D., Jarett, L., et al. (1994) A subgroup of murine monoclonal anti-deoxyribonucleic acid antibodies traverse the cytoplasms and enter the nucleus in a time- and temperature-dependent manner. *Lab. Invest.* **71,** 52–60.

52. Zack, D. J., Stempniak, M., Wong, A. L., Taylor, C., and Weisbart, R. H. (1996) Mechanisms of cellular penetration and nuclear localization of an anti-double strand DNA autoantibody. *J. Immunol.* **157,** 2082–2088.
53. Ehrenstein, M. R., Katz, D. R., Griffiths, M. H., Papadaki, L., Winkler, T. H., Kalden, J. R., et al. (1995) Human IgG anti-DNA antibodies deposit in kidneys and induce proteinuria in SCID mice. *Kidney Int.* **48,** 705–711.
54. Hormigo, A. and Lieberman, F. (1994) Nuclear localization of anti-Hu antibody is not associated with in vitro cytotoxicity. *J. Neuroimmunol.* **55,** 205–212.
55. Lee, L. A., Weston, W. L., Krueger, G. G., Emam, M., Reichlin, M., Stevens, J. O., et al. (1986) An animal model of antibody binding in cutaneous lupus. *Arthritis Rheum.* **29,** 782–788.
56. Koscec, M., Koren, E., Wolfson-Reichlin, M., Fugate, R. D., Trieu, E., Targoff, I. N., and Reichlin, M. (1997) Autoantibodies to ribosomal P proteins penetrate into live hepatocytes and cause cellular dysfunction in culture. *J. Immunol.* **159,** 2033–2041.
57. Orlando, R. A., Kerjaschki, D., Kurihara, H., Biemesderfer, D., and Farquhar, M. G. (1992) gp330 associates with a 44-kDa protein in the rat kidney to form the Heymann nephritis antigenic complex. *Proc. Natl. Acad. Sci. USA* **89,** 6698–6702.
58. Sun, K.-H., Liu, W.-T., Tsai, C.-Y., Tang, S.-J., Han, S.-H., and Yu, C.-L. (1995) Anti-dsDNA antibodies cross-react with ribosomal P proteins expressed on the surface of glomerular mesangial cells to exert a cytostatic effect. *Immunology* **85,** 262–269.
59. Koren, E., Reichlin, M. W., Koscec, M., Fugate, R. D., and Reichlin, M. (1992) Autoantibodies to the ribosomal P proteins react with a plasma membrane-related target on human cells. *J. Clin. Invest.* **89,** 1236–1241.
60. Furukawa, F., Kashihara-Sawami, M., Lyons, M. B., and Norris, D. A. (1990) Binding of antibodies to the extractable nuclear antigens SS-A/Ro and SS-B/La is induced on the surface of human keratinocytes by ultraviolet light: Implications for pathogenesis of photosensitive cutaneous lupus. *J. Invest. Dermatol.* **94,** 77– 85.
61. Lefeber, W. P., Norris, D. A., Ryan, S. R., Huff, J. C., Lee, L. A., Kubo, M., et al. (1984) Ultraviolet light induces the binding of antibodies to selected nuclear antigens on cultured human keratinocytes. *J. Clin. Invest.* **74,** 1545–1551.
62. Golan, T. D., Elkon, K. B., Gharavi, A. E., and Krueger, J. G. (1992) Enhanced membrane binding of autoantibodies to cultured keratinocytes of systemic lupus erythematosus patients after ultraviolet B/ultraviolet A irradiation. *J. Clin. Invest.* **90,** 1067–1076.
63. Casciola-Rosen, L. A., Anhalt, G., and Rosen, A. (1994) Autoantigen targets in systemic lupus erythematosus are clustered in two populations of surface structures on apoptotic keratinocytes. *J. Exp. Med.* **179,** 1317–1330.
64. Moreau, N., Laine, M.-C., Billoud, B., and Angelier, N. (1994) Transcription of amphibian lampbrush chromosomes is disturbed by microinjection of HSP70 monoclonal antibodies. *Exp. Cell Res.* **211,** 108–114.
65. Silver, P. A. (1991) How proteins enter the nucleus. *Cell* **64,** 489–497.
66. Radic, M. Z., Mackle, J., Erikson, J., Mol, C., Anderson, W. F., and Weigert, M. (1993) Residues that mediate DNA binding of autoimmune antibodies. *J. Immunol.* **150,** 4966–4977.
67. Krishnan, M. R., Jou, N. T., and Marion, T. N. (1996) Correlation between the amino acid position of arginine in VH-CDR3 and specificity for native DNA among autoimmune antibodies. *J. Immunol.* **157,** 2430–2439.

68. Foster, M. H., Kieber-Emmons, T., Ohliger, M., and Madaio, M. P. (1994) Molecular and structural analysis of nuclear localizing anti-DNA lupus antibodies. *Immunol. Res.* **13,** 186–206.
69. Goldfarb, D. S., Gariepy, J., Schoolnik, G., and Kornberg, R. D. (1986) Synthetic peptides as nuclear localization signals. *Nature* **322,** 641–644.
70. Biocca, S., Neuberger, M. S., and Cattaneo, A. (1990) Expression and targeting of intracellular antibodies in mammalian cells. *EMBO.* **9,** 101–108.
71. Duverger, E., Carpenter, V., Roche, A.-C., and Monsigny, M. (1993) Sugar-dependent nuclear import of glycoconjugates from the cytosol. *Exp. Cell Res.* **207,** 197–201.
72. Wang, J. L., Laing, J. G., and Anderson, R. L. (1991) Lectins in the cell nucleus. *Glycobiology* **1,** 243–252.
73. Veronese, F. D., Copeland, T. D., Oroszlan, S., Gallo, R. C., and Sarngadharan, M. (1988) Biochemical and immunological analysis of human immunodeficiency virus gag gene products p17 and p24. *J. Virol.* **62,** 795–801.
74. Mervis, R. J., Ahman, N., Lillehoj, E. P., Raum, M. G., Salazar, F. H. R., Chan, H. W., et al. (1988) The gag gene products of human immunodeficiency virus type 1: alignment within the gag open reading frame, identification of posttranslational modifications and evidence for alterative gag precursors. *J. Virol.* **62,** 3993–4002.
75. Alarcon-Segovia, D. and Llorente, L. (1983) Antibody penetration into living cells: IV. Different effects of anti-native DNA and anti-ribonucleoprotein IgG on the cell cycle of activated T gamma cells. *Clin. Exp. Immunol.* **52,** 365–371.
76. Puccetti, A., Madaio, M. P., Bellese, G., and Migliorini, P. (1995) Anti-DNA antibodies bind to DNase I. *J. Exp. Med.* **181,** 1797–1804.
77. Madaio, M. P., Fabbi, M., Tiso, M., Daga, A., and Puccetti, A. (1996) Spontaneously produced anti-DNA/DNase I autoantibodies modulate nuclear apoptosis in living cells. *Eur. J. Immunol.* **26,** 3035–3041.

21

Alcohol, Anesthetics, and Analgesics in Autoimmune Reactivity

Geoffrey M. Thiele, Dean J. Tuma, and Lynell W. Klassen

1. INTRODUCTION

Alcohol, anesthetics, and analgesics in general are relatively safe and well tolerated. However, one of the most common side effects of these agents is the development of severe liver injury and death owing to liver failure. Hepatotoxicity is most likely owing to the fact that these agents are generally metabolized in the liver. The liver injury can involve direct cell toxicity (necrosis), cholestasis (cessation of bile flow), or steatosis (fatty liver). Recent attention has focused on the hepatocyte as a direct target for hepatotoxic agents because it makes up such a substantial portion of the liver and is the most active in the biotranformation of drugs to toxic metabolites. However, injury to the liver can also involve nonparenchymal cells such as Kupffer cells, endothelial cells, stellated cells, and other cells lining the hepatic sinusoids and bile ducts. The timing from administration of the agent to the onset of liver injury is variable, and it appears that only a small fraction of individuals receiving therapy are affected. In addition, the lesions often are not reproducible in experimental animals, leaving the mechanism(s) of immune-related injury caused by reactive metabolite(s) poorly understood. One important area of study concerns the identity of tissue proteins serving as targets of the reactive metabolites. A number of approaches have been developed for the sensitive detection, identification, and characterization of the protein targets, which have been utilized to characterize the autoantibody responses and the identification of proteins serving as auto-antigens in autoimmune hepatitis associated with alcohol, anesthetics and anti-inflammatory agents.

2. ALCOHOL

Alcohol abuse remains a major health risk and costs the United States more than $116 billion per year. It is a major cause of mortality, of which approx 19% of the deaths can be attributed to cirrhosis of the liver (1–3). However, the underlying mechanisms of alcohol-induced liver disease (ALD) remains unclear.

Contemporary Immunology: Autoimmune Reactions
Edited by: S. Paul © Humana Press Inc., Totowa, NJ

Most of the attention in the past has been directed at investigating the roles of altered nutrition, direct toxic action of alcohol or its metabolites *(3,4)*, hypermetabolic states of the liver *(5,6)*, lipid peroxidation *(7,8)*, or genetic factors *(9–13)* as causative events in the development of liver injury.

In recent years, increasing interest has centered around the possible role of immune mechanisms in the pathogenesis and perpetuation of ALD. Many of the clinical features of ALD suggest that immune effector mechanisms may contribute to liver tissue damage *(14)*. Interestingly, only 10–20% of alcoholics develop ALD, suggesting that host factor(s) may be involved in the susceptibility to the toxic effects of alcohol *(15)*. It is well known that liver injury can persist for some time after the withdrawal of alcohol, and that a number of patients who stop drinking and experience complete histological recovery from ALD rapidly redevelop alcoholic hepatitis on resumption of alcohol ingestion. The rapid disease recurrence suggests an anamnestic type of response reminiscent of adaptive immune reactions. Immune abnormalities such as hypergammaglobulinemia, circulating autoantibodies, and the presence of CD4$^+$ lymphoid cells in areas of hepatocyte degeneration have been described in ALD. In addition, a subgroup of patients with alcoholic hepatitis appears to respond favorably to corticosteroid therapy, indirectly suggesting that immune mechanisms may be involved *(16,17)*. Finally, the fact that hepatic fibrosis and cirrhosis tend to recur rapidly in a transplanted liver following the resumption of alcohol ingestion, suggests toxic reactions that could be immune mediated *(18)*.

Multiple effects of alcohol on cellular and humoral immune activity have been described. Alcohol appears to modulate the existing immune responses to foreign antigens and self-antigens. In addition, in vitro studies show that alcohol alters the levels of cytokines known to be directly involved in cytolysis, fibrosis, and cellular regeneration. Alcohol and its metabolites also may induce the formation of new antigenic structures on native-proteins (neoantigens) that can initiate immune responses in various experimental situations. The hypothesis that immune mechanisms are involved in recurrent alcoholic hepatitis, while not proven, is backed by substantial clinical and experimental evidence.

Several studies have indicated that the susceptibility to alcohol-induced liver injury may be associated with the human leukocyte antigen (HLA) B locus. British Caucasian patients showed an increased incidence of HLA-B8 in patients with alcohol-induced cirrhosis, and a normal incidence in patients with alcohol-induced steatosis *(10,19)*. In other studies, alcohol-induced cirrhosis was associated with B13 in Chilean patients *(20)*, and with BW40 in Scandinavian patients *(11,21)*. There is now considerable evidence that females are more susceptible to alcohol-induced liver injury than males *(22–26)*, which may be of interest because of the greater prevalence of autoimmune diseases in females.

Impaired immunity to foreign antigens is often cited as the cause of increased bacterial and viral infections in alcoholic individuals and may also be an important co-factor in provoking autoimmune responses *(10,12)*. On the other hand, immune "hyperfunction" to modified self-antigens has been proposed as a possible mechanism in the development and/or progression of alcoholic liver injury. An area of intense investigation is the possible structural modification of self-antigen(s) that could initiate the induction of a liver specific autoimmune disease, as discussed in Section 2.1.

2.1. Adducts Associated with ALD

Alcohol and its metabolites induce new antigenic structures on native proteins (neoantigens) that can initiate immune responses in experimental situations. Sorrell and Leevy first described the role that alcohol metabolites might play in inducing abnormal anti-liver immune responses in patients with ALD (27). Additional reports have since suggested that patients with alcohol-associated liver disease mount unique antigen-driven immune responses that target the liver. Leevy et al. *(28)* and Zetterman et al. *(29)* documented a cell-mediated immune response to alcoholic hyalin in patients with alcoholic hepatitis. Johnson and Williams *(30)* showed that T-lymphocytes of patients with ALD undergo blast transformation upon exposure to liver homogenates. Other studies have shown that lymphocytes from alcoholics can kill autologous hepatocytes in vitro *(31,32)*. Furthermore, hyalin obtained from patients with ALD induces cytokine secretion when mixed with autologous immune cells *(33)*. These studies have provided the impetus for the current efforts to identify the antigen(s) that might trigger the altered immune responses leading to recognition of the alcohol-exposed hepatocyte as nonself.

2.1.1. Acetaldehyde Adducts

The possibility that the covalent binding of acetaldehyde to proteins may contribute to liver injury was originally postulated by Sorrell and Tuma *(34)*. While acetaldehyde binding in vivo can directly alter both protein and cellular function, it is also clear that acetaldehyde adducts elicit unique and antigen-driven humoral and cellular immune responses *(35–47)*. Chronic alcohol ingestion causes both the production of acetaldehyde-protein adducts in liver tissue *(38–40,43,46,47)*, and the development of anti-acetaldehyde adduct antibodies in both human and animal models *(35,40–42,48)*. These findings have led to the hypothesis that acetaldehyde protein adducts are recognized as neoantigenic epitopes present in liver tissue *(33,34,36)*. It has been suggested that the resultant antibodies and cytotoxic T-cells can induce and/or potentiate liver damage in the setting of chronic alcohol exposure.

Several studies have used comparatively high concentrations of acetaldehyde for protein derivitization in the presence of reducing agents. This results predominantly in the formation of N-ethyllysine residues on proteins *(49)*. Although N-ethyllysine residues are immunogenic, recent work using monoclonal antibodies (MAbs) suggests that these reduced residues are not formed when acetaldehyde-protein adducts are prepared under physiological conditions. Further, the reduced adducts are not detected in the liver of alcohol-fed rats *(50,51)*. The biological significance of immune responses to the reduced protein adducts, thus, is ambiguous.

A recent report by Yokoyama et al. provides further evidence that immune recognition of acetaldehyde protein adducts may play a role in alcoholic liver injury *(45)*. In an experimental model of chronic oral alcohol exposure to guinea pigs, the combination of alcohol feeding and repeated immunizations with non-reduced acetaldehyde foreign protein adducts resulted in hepatic fibrosis in the periportal and perivenular areas. Serum antibodies to acetaldehyde adducts were detected in all animals immunized with acetaldehyde modified foreign proteins, regardless of the exposure to alcohol. However, significant fibrosis was only observed in immunized animals which had also ingested alcohol. It was suggested that chronic consumption of alcohol facilitated the formation of metabolically derived acetaldehyde adducts, and that immune responses directed against the adducts initiated an inflammatory response, leading eventually to hepatic fibrosis.

Although it is clear that acetaldehyde-protein adducts can form in vivo after alcohol consumption and that the adducts can induce specific immune responses, many important questions must be answered before the causal role of the adducts in ALD can be established *(38)*. It remains to be shown that immunological factors are directly responsible for liver necrosis, inflammation, or fibrosis. A major problem in establishing the causal role of immunological factors has been the non-availability of animal models in which spontaneous alcohol ingestion leads to immune-mediated hepatocyte dysfunction.

2.1.2. Malondialdehyde-Acetaldehyde Adducts

Several studies have suggested that chronic ethanol consumption induces hepatic lipid peroxidation, which in turn generates another reactive aldehyde, malondialdehyde (MDA) *(8,52,53)*. MDA-protein adducts have been detected in the liver following administration of agents that promote lipid peroxidation, such as carbon tetrachloride, iron overload, and chronic ethanol feeding *(54–56)*. Since the concentrations of acetaldehyde and MDA in the liver can reach similar levels over the course of ethanol metabolism *(53,57)*, it is not surprising that both acetaldehyde and MDA adducts have been detected in the liver of ethanol-fed animals *(56)*. This is particularly significant because MDA and mono-functional aldehydes (alkanals) have been shown to mutually enhance each other's reactivity towards primary amines, resulting in the formation of a distinct profile of conjugated products *(58)*. Tuma et al. *(59)* have studied the synergistic effect of acetaldehyde and MDA in forming protein adducts. MDA stimulated acetaldehyde binding to proteins can be monitored by the formation of highly fluorescent product(s). The hybrid adducts of MDA and acetaldehyde, designated MAA adducts, were detected in livers from ethanol-fed rats but not in pair-fed controls using affinity-purified polyclonal antibodies in a competitive ELISA. Recently, Thiele et al. have shown that the MAA adducts can induce antibody responses to the adduct and its carrier in the absence of adjuvant *(60)*. This is significant in that the concentrations of acetaldehyde and malondialdehyde used to generate the immunogen approached physiological levels that have been reported following ethanol ingestion.

2.1.3. Hydroxyethyl Radicals

Hydroxyethyl radicals can be generated during ethanol oxidation by liver microsomes *(61–65)*. The radicals can bind the microsomal proteins covalently *(66,67)*. Cytochrome P4502E1 (CYP2E1) catalyzes the formation of hydroxyethyl radicals, and modulation of CYP2E1 expression greatly influences the generation of hydroxyethyl radicals both in vitro and in vivo *(68,69)*. It has recently been reported that both chronically ethanol-fed rats and patients who abuse alcohol develop antibodies that bind the protein adducts of hydroxyethyl radicals *(70)*. These antibodies do not crossreact with acetaldehyde-modified proteins and appear to preferentially recognize microsomal proteins complexed with hydroxyethyl radicals *(70)*. One of the microsomal proteins recognized by the antibodies to hydroxyethyl adducts is CYP2E1, as determined by immunoblotting and immunoprecipitation experiments *(70)*. Cytochrome P450 isoenzymes, including CYP2E1, are expressed on rat and human hepatocyte plasma membranes, thus rendering the cells vulnerable to the antibodies *(71–73)*. Recently, Clot et al. *(74)* observed that human antibodies recognizing the hydroxyethyl radical-CYP2E1 adducts can bind to the surface of isolated hepatocytes exposed to alcohol. Further, the cells were lysed by an antibody dependent cell mediated cytoxicity process in the presence of the anti-adduct antibodies and normal human peripheral blood mononuclear cells. The cytochrome P450 adducts may, therefore, possess an important role in liver cell injury leading to ALD.

2.1.4. 4-HNE and Malondialdehyde

Low density lipoprotein (LDL) oxidation is a complex process initiated by a free-radical lipid-peroxidation mechanism *(75)*. The in vitro experiments show that LDL oxidation can be facilitated by endothelial cells *(76)*, smooth-muscle cells (77), monocytes and macrophages *(78)*, as well as bivalent transition-metal ions such as copper or iron *(79)*. Recent studies have shown that ALD is associated with increased lipid peroxidation, as indicated by the presence of increased hepatocellular lipid peroxidation products, MDA and 4-hydroxynonenal (HNE) *(53,80)*.

The process of lipid peroxidation not only results in the perturbation of cellular membrane lipids, but also is associated with the production of aldehyde products such as MDA and 4-HNE. These aldehydes can be toxic to cells *(81)*. If the enzymatic mechanisms for detoxification of the aldehydes are saturated, these metabolites can accumulate to toxic levels and potentiate ethanol-induced hepatocellular injury. 4-HNE-protein adducts have been found to localize in the areas of hepatic injury in rat experimental models of ALD (55). Further, acetaldehyde *(82,83)* as well as products of lipid peroxidation *(84,85)* can directly stimulate collagen production and collagen gene expression in cell cultures of fibroblasts and stellate cells, suggesting an involvement of these metabolites in fibrosis.

2.2. Autoantibodies

A number of nonorgan-specific and organ-specific autoantibodies have been reported in patients with ALD. It is unknown whether these autoantibodies cause or are the result of liver dysfunction.

2.2.1. Nonorgan Specific Autoantibodies

Autoantibodies at low titer are a common feature of ALD. No increase in the prevalence of antinuclear (ANF) and smooth muscle (SMA) autoantibodies were found in ALD *(10,19)*, but 12–25% of patients with cirrhosis are positive for these antibodies *(86–88)*.

2.2.2. Organ Specific Antibodies

Mallory body antigens were detected in the serum of patients with early alcoholic hepatitis using complement fixation and immune adherence methods. In more advanced hepatitis, Mallory body antibodies have been found *(29,89)*. These findings could not be confirmed by Kehl et al. *(90)*, who used a more sensitive solid phase radioimmunoassay method. The insolubility of Mallory bodies has limited the ability to investigate specific humoral or cellular immune responses to these unique epitopes.

LSP is a high molecular weight lipoprotein associated with the plasma membrane of hepatocytes and may also be present in other organs, such as the kidney *(91,92)*. Antibodies to LSP are detected in nearly all patients with untreated chronic active hepatitis, the antibody levels are correlated with the disease activity, and they are also correlated with the presence of piece-meal necrosis *(93)*.

Some antibodies react with a liver membrane antigen (LMA) that is distinct from LSP and is not species specific *(93)*. Using immunofluorescence methods, IgG and IgA antibodies to LMAs have been demonstrated in about 10% of ALD patients with fatty liver, in 24% with alcoholic hepatitis, in 30% with active cirrhosis, and in 62% with inactive cirrhosis *(94)*. Wiedmann et al. found IgA anti-LMAs in 57% of patients with alcoholic hepatitis, but no IgG antibodies with this specificity *(95)*.

2.3. Immune Complexes

Circulating IgA- and IgG-containing immune complexes have been reported in ALD, but attempts to isolate the antigen in these complexes have generally not been successful *(96–99)*. There is one report that Mallory body antigens were detected in IgA and IgG complexes isolated from eluates of the liver from alcoholic hepatitis and active cirrhosis patients *(100)*. It is uncertain whether the Ig deposits are immune complexes or antibody aggregates. Additionally, it is unknown whether the deposits can activate complement or other inflammatory responses.

2.4. Cytokines and Alcohol Liver Disease

ALD is associated with fever, malaise, anorexia, and leukocytosis *(101,102)*. Increased production of cytokines occurs in several models of alcohol-related liver injury. Rats fed ethanol chronically are more susceptible to endotoxin-mediated liver injury *(103,104)*. Ethanol-fed rats exposed to lipopolysaccharide display increased levels of TNF-α (105). These and related experiments *(106,107)* have prompted the suggestion that high serum concentrations of TNF-α are associated with liver injury. The Kupffer and endothelial cells are thought to be responsible for the increased synthesis of TNF-α *(107,108)*.

Other cytokines may also play important roles in the development and/or progression of ALD. Recent reports suggest that the IL-8 levels are increased in patients with alcoholic hepatitis and in alcohol-dependent patients without liver injury *(109)*. The hepatic levels of IL-8 appear to correlate with neutrophil infiltration *(110)*. Measurements of serum IL-1 using the thymocyte proliferation assay have shown increased levels of this cytokine in patients with alcoholic hepatitis *(111,112)*. Monocytes from patients with ALD secrete greater amounts of IL-1 in response to LPS than do monocytes from controls *(113)*. The serum concentrations of interleukin-6 (IL-6), the cytokine responsible for much of the hepatic acute phase response, are increased in patients with ALD *(114)*. In patients with alcoholic hepatitis, the plasma IL-6 concentrations are correlated with the biochemical and clinical features of the disease *(115,116)*, while a decrease in IL-6 levels correlates with clinical improvement. The pathogenic mechanisms leading to increased production of cytokines in ALD are not completely understood. Recent reports have suggested that the stimuli for production of cytokines by macrophages and other types of cells in the liver include endotoxin, prostanoids, glutathione, and various types of adducts of ethanol metabolites *(117–119)*.

In summary, the cytokine production is strongly correlated with ALD, suggesting that cytokines play an important role in alcohol-induced injury to the liver. The precise stimulus for the release of the cytokines remains to be determined. It is not clear whether the cytokine abnormalities are part of a nonspecific inflammatory response, or whether they are the result of antigen-specific immune responses.

3. ANESTHETICS

3.1. Halothane

Halothane hepatotoxicity may be manifested clinically as one of two distinct syndromes: 1) a rare, but often, fatal acute hepatitis and 2) a far more common, usually mild, form of hepatitis that occurs in up to 25% of patients *(120–125)*. An increasing body of evidence has suggested that the idiosyncratic hepatitis caused by halothane inhalation may be owing to immune reactions directed against liver proteins that are structurally altered by halothane *(122,126–128)*. The involvement of immunological factors is supported by the increased frequency of hepatotoxicity in patients who have had prior exposure to halothane, and the occurrence of systemic features such as fever and eosinophilia *(122,129–133)*.

Since halothane is not chemically reactive under physiological conditions, it appeared that a reactive metabolite of halothane was most likely responsible for the induction of serum antibodies capable of recognizing liver microsomal proteins following halothane exposure. The metabolite trifluoroacetyl chloride [CF_3COCl] is formed via the oxidative metabolism of halothane by cytochrome P-450 system *(134)*. An early study found two of six patients with halothane-associated liver cell necrosis express serum antibodies that bound trifluoro-acetylated rabbit serum albumin (TFA-RSA) *(135)*. An antibody was raised against the TFA hapten by immunizing rabbits with TFA-RSA, which was synthesized by the reaction of RSA with S-ethyl-trifluorothioacetate *(133)*. This reagent mainly reacts with lysine residues of proteins, which were assumed to be the sites of adduct formation of CF_3COCl with tissue proteins. Immunoblotting studies with microsomes from rats (136) and humans *(127)* treated with halothane revealed that the proteins recognized by the serum antibodies from patients also reacted with the anti-TFA antibodies. When the TFA hapten was removed from the liver microsomes, the antibodies from patients failed to recognize the micro-somal proteins *(136)*, showing that the TFA moiety was required for antibody binding. However, the patients' antibodies did not appear to be directed solely against the TFA hapten. The antigenic epitopes appeared to consist of the TFA hapten and undefined structures of the proteins, as suggested by findings of frequent differences in the patterns of protein recognition by patient antibodies and by incomplete inhibition of the antibody binding to TFA-microsomal pro-teins by the hapten derivative N^e-TFA-L-lysine. In contrast, the hapten deriva-tive abolished the binding of the rabbit anti-TFA antibodies to the TFA-liver microsomal proteins *(136,137)*. The hypothesis that the CF_3COCl metabolite of halothane preferentially forms stable covalent bonds with lysine residues of microsomal proteins has recently been confirmed by ^{19}F nuclear magnetic resonance studies *(138)*.

The purification and characterization of several TFA-labeled proteins from rat liver microsomes has been accomplished using the anti-TFA antibodies. A 59-kDa target protein was purified by affinity chromatography on an anti-TFA column and has been identified as a carboxylesterase *(133)*. TFA also binds a number of other proteins including:

1. A 100-kDa protein identified as Erp99 identical to a 94-kDa glucose-regulated protein, endoplasmin *(139)*,
2. A 76-kDa protein fraction that was resolved into two different proteins, an 80-kDa protein identical to Erp72 *(140)*, and an 82-kDa protein corre-sponding to a 78-kDa glucose-regulated protein, also known as Bip *(141)*,
3. A 57-kDa target protein identical to protein disulfide isomerase *(142)*,
4. A 54-kDa protein corresponding to an unidentified form of cytochrome P–450 *(134)*,
5. A 63-kDa protein corresponding to calreticulin *(143)*,
6. A 58-kDa protein *(144,145)*, which may be a member of the PDI family *(146)* and is most likely a cellular protease *(147)* or a carnitine medium/long-chain acyltransferase *(148)*.

The anti-TFA antibodies have been used to study several additional issues. In immunohistochemistry studies, the antibodies were employed to show that the perivenous region of the liver lobule was the major site of trifluoroacetylation of liver proteins and that surface macromolecules of hepatocytes were labeled by the trifluoroacetyl chloride metabolite of halothane *(133)*. Western blotting and immunohistochemical studies have revealed that small levels of TFA-proteins are formed in extrahepatic tissues, including the testes *(134)*, kidney *(149,150)*, heart *(151)*, lung *(150)*, and respiratory and olfactory epithelium of nasal tissue *(150)*. In the liver, low levels of TFA adducts have been found in Kupffer cells *(152)*. The anti-TFA antibodies also bind the target proteins of reactive metabolites derived from other halogenated hydrocarbons that form TFA adducts or adducts with structural similarity to the TFA adducts. The antibodies cross-react with CHF_2CS adducts formed by the reaction of tissue proteins with the difluorothionoacetylating metabolite CHF_2CSF derived from the nephrotoxic agent S-(1,1,2,2-tetrafluoroethyl)-L-cysteine (TFEC). When rats were treated with TFEC, immunohistochemical analysis revealed that CHF_2CS adducts in the kidney were localized to the damaged areas of the proximal tubules *(153)*.

3.2. Methoxyflurane

This agent causes a form of hepatic injury very similar to that associated with halothane. There is evidence for "cross reactivity," in that some patients with a history of exposure to methoxyflurane develop a reaction to halothane and vice-versa *(121,154,155)*. Methoxyflurane and halothane are known to cause hepatitis in individuals who have abused ("sniffed") these agents *(156–158)*.

3.3. Enflurane

Enflurane has been reported to cause liver injury *(155,159–161)*. The syndrome is clinically similar to halothane hepatitis and is associated with centrilobular necrosis. Prior exposure to either enflurane or halothane is a predisposing factor, and it shortens the latent period between exposure and clinical onset of illness *(160)*.

3.4. Isoflurane

This agent has the lowest association with liver injury, presumably because it is metabolized to a far lesser extent than halothane *(155,162,163)*. However, despite the rarity of severe acute isoflurane hepatitis, published case reports seem sufficiently suggestive of a causal relationship between isoflurane and liver damage *(164–166)*.

3.5. Desflurane, Sevoflurane

These newer agents appear to be relatively safe, but recent studies have suggested that similar liver responses can be observed as for halothane and isoflurane.

In summary, inhaled anesthetics undergo oxidative metabolism catalyzed by hepatic cytochrome P450 2E1. Exposure to halothane, enflurane, isoflurane, and desflurane produces TFA-labeled proteins. Furthermore, the extent of labeling with TFA parallels the degrees to which the individual anesthetics are metabolized. Serum antibodies from patients with halothane hepatitis react with acylated liver proteins from rats exposed to halothane. These findings support the view that the degree of metabolism of the fluorinated inhaled anesthetics influences their toxic potential, and suggests that minimally metabolized molecules are the safer anesthetic choices.

4. ANALGESICS

4.1. Acetaminophen

Acetaminophen has enjoyed a long history as a relatively safe and well-tolerated analgesic agent. However, it became evident in 1966 that the drug causes severe liver injury and death owing to liver injury when taken in very large doses. Similar to halothane hepatitis, the evidence indicates that acetaminophen hepatotoxicity is mediated by the formation of a toxic intermediate during the biotransformation of the parent compound *(167–169)*. The reactive metabolite that causes the hepatotoxicity produced by an acetaminophen overdose is *N*-acetyl-p-benzoquinone imine (NAPQI). This metabolite is formed by the oxidation of acetaminophen by cytochromes P-450 *(170,171)* and appears to bind covalently to cysteine residues of proteins *(167,172)*. Antibodies that bind NAPQI bound covalently to tissue proteins have been produced *(173,174)*, and have been used to detect adducts of NAPQI in tissues by immunohistochemical *(175,176)*, ELISA *(177)*, and immunoblotting methods *(176,178,179)*. The immunoblotting studies have revealed several protein targets of NAPQI. In the mouse liver, the major targets are a 44-kDa microsomal protein and a 55–58-kDa cytosolic protein *(176,178,179)*. The 55–58 kDa protein target has been purified and identified as a selenium binding protein *(180,181)*.

4.2. Sulfasalazine

This compound is split into its component sulfapyridine and 5-aminosalicylate moieties in the colon. The sulfapyridine is mostly absorbed and is believed to be responsible for hepatotoxic reactions. Liver injury has been reported in young patients treated with sulfasalazine for inflammatory bowel disease and rheumatoid arthritis. Typically, a florid hypersensitivity reaction with accompanying rash, lymphadenopathy, leukocytosis, eosinophilia, hypocomplementemia and circulating immune complexes begins within three weeks of starting the drug *(182,183)*. Fulminant hepatic failure occurs in spite of discontinuation of the drug. Resolution of the syndrome has been aided in anecdotal cases by high-dose intravenous corticosteroids *(182)*. The clinical picture of sulfasalazine hepatotoxicity is typical of sulfa drug hypersensitivity. The newer agents containing only 5-aminosalicylate and its derivatives are expected to produce far fewer adverse effects. Nonetheless, the 5-aminosalicylate moiety is not entirely exonerated, as evidenced by the rare occurrence of a hypersensitivity hepatitis to mesalazine after a previous episode of sulfasalazine-induced hepatitis *(184)*.

5. ANTI-INFLAMMATORY DRUGS

Induction of hepatitis by nonsteroidal anti-inflammatory drugs (NSAIDs) has received considerable attention in recent years *(185–187)*. A number of risk factors have been identified for the development of liver damage by NSAIDs, including: advanced age, renal insufficiency, multiple drug use, use of high NSAID doses, and concomitant alcohol use *(188)*. Of the currently available NSAIDs in the United States, diclofenac, sulindac, and phenylbutazone appear to carry the greatest risk of hepatotoxicity. Piroxicam, ibuprofen, naproxen, and fenoprofen carry an intermediate risk *(186)*. While there are suggestions of an autoimmune involvement for the development of hepatotoxicity induced by all of these NSAIDS, the strongest data comes from studies performed with diclofenac.

5.1. Diclofenac

One of the most widely prescribed NSAIDs is diclofenac. Although this drug is relatively safe, several cases of severe and even fatal hepatotoxicity have been reported to occur *(189–196)*. Some studies suggest a role for hypersensitivity in the toxicity *(190,194,196)*, while others favor a metabolic mechanism *(189,191–193)*. To investigate the possible role of diclofenac-protein conjugates in the hepatotoxicity produced by diclofenac, antisera have been developed to detect such conjugates in liver tissue.

The development of the antisera was based on the possible role of acyl-glucuronide metabolites of NSAIDs in mediating some of the toxicities *(197–199)*. The formation of acyl-glucuronides of NSAIDs is catalyzed by microsomal UDP-glucuronosyltransferase (UDPGT; EC 2.4.2.17). The acyl-glucuronide metabolites can covalently bind to tissue proteins by transacylation *(197–199)*. In the antibody studies, diclofenac was able to inhibit, at least in part, the reaction of the antisera with the diclofenac carrier conjugate. Therefore, the antibodies appear to bind glucuronide adducts as well as other possible covalent adducts of diclofenac. Using these antibodies, four major protein adducts of 50, 70, 110, and 140-kDa have been detected in liver homogenates from mice treated with diclofenac *(200)*. A 110-kDa adduct was found in the plasma membrane fraction of liver cells *(201)*, and its existence was corroborated by the immunohistochemical evidence of diclofenac adduct accumulation in canalicular plasma membranes in the perivenous region of the liver lobule *(201)*. Further study of the role of the adducts in diclofenac hepatotoxicity is ongoing.

6. POSSIBLE PATHWAYS OF AUTOIMMUNE REACTIONS

Following exposure to toxic agents, hepatocytes can produce the adducts described in Subheadings 2., 3., 4., and 5. These adducts may contribute to the functional impairment of hepatocytes and may eventually result in cellular

332

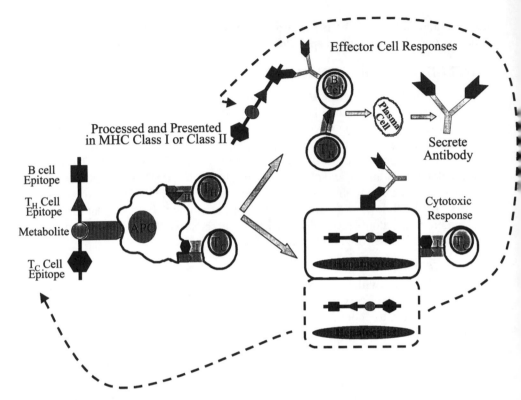

Fig. 1. Hypothetical mechanism of immunization by proteins modified by bioreactive metabolites. The covalent binding of reactive metabolites to hepatic proteins may lead, after the death of hepatocytes, to the release of modified proteins. In most instances, these modified proteins are removed by the cells of the secondary lymphoid tissues (lymph nodes, spleen, and so on), inciting antibody and T-cell responses to the selfprotein (carrier), the adduct (hapten), or the hapten-carrier. LECs, Kupffer cells, Ito cells, and hepatocytes may be activated to increase their expression of cytokines (IL-1, IL-6, IL-8, and TNF-α) and adhesion molecules (ICAM-1, P-selectin, L-selectin, Class I, or Class II). This results in the binding of macrophages, neutrophils, Th-cells and Tc-cells to LECs to extravasate into the area and increase the inflammatory response. Additionally, Tc-cells would bind to Class I on hepatocytes expressing the carrier or hapten-carrier; resulting in the further destruction of even more hepatocytes. The release of these materials will exacerbate the immune response resulting in autoimmune disease.

destruction (*see* Fig. 1). During the turnover of hepatocytes, proteins from the dying hepatocytes may be phagocytosed by antigen-presenting cells, such as macrophages, sinusoidal endothelial cells or B-lymphocytes. Inside these cells, the protein is degraded into small peptides, some of which are then presented on the cell surface by MHC Class II molecules. These materials can also escape the liver and move to the secondary lymphoid tissues. Here, they could be bound, internalized, degraded, and processed for presentation by MHC Class II molecules, resulting in sensitization of T-helper cells, T-cytotoxic cells, and B-cells to the drug metabolites and the self-proteins to which the metabolites are conjugated.

Upon further drug exposure, cellular activation with a concomitant upregulation of adhesion molecules, secretion of inflammatory cytokines, and antigen presentation in the context of MHC Class II may occur. The released cytokines (TNF-α, IL-1, IL-8, and so on) can be anticipated to promote infiltration of neutrophils, macrophages and T-cells. Binding of the cells to adhesion molecules on the activated LECs can be anticipated to allow for diapedisis into the liver. Additional tissue dysfunction can be predicted if the adducted proteins are presented by the MHC Class I pathway, enabling killing by sensitized cytotoxic T-cells.

The need for appropriate MHC Class I or Class II molecules to present the adducts of self-protein to T-cells might impose some selectivity to the consequences of alcohol, anesthetic, and analgesic exposure, although genetic predispositions toward disease have not been adequately described. While all individuals have the ability to respond with TNF-α, IL-1, or IL-8, there must be some specific initiator of the pathology, or everyone who was exposed to these agents would develop hepatitis.

7. CONCLUSIONS

Although the exact pathophysiology of hepatotoxicity in response to alcohol, anesthetics, and analgesics remains unsolved, there is substantial evidence that altered immune reactivity occurs as a consequence of exposure to these agents in both humans and animal models. The association of hepatotoxicity with circulating autoantibodies, antibodies to unique hepatic proteins, and cytotoxic lymphocytes that recognize autologous hepatocytes, strongly suggests that alterations in immune regulation occur, resulting in a break in tolerance to hepatic constituents.

The mechanism of immune responses generated by alcohol, anesthetics, and analgesics appears to involve their reactive metabolites. While these agents and their metabolites are too small to act as immunogens themselves, the metabolites react with membrane constituents of hepatocytes, and the resultant adducts can serve as neoantigens in causing the break in self-tolerance.

8. FUTURE DIRECTIONS

As a result of the advent of the immunochemical approach for identifying the targets of toxic reactive metabolites, many more protein targets of toxic reactive metabolites are likely to be identified. The functional consequences of protein adduct formation must still be resolved. If the target proteins possess important cellular functions, perhaps their reaction with the metabolites directly alters the functions. Alternatively, the immunogeneity of the protein adducts might be the cause of the subsequent pathological events. Note that not all reactions between the protein targets and reactive metabolites need be toxic. The proteins may also serve as scavengers to protect cells from toxic reactive metabolites.

ACKNOWLEDGMENT

The authors thank Crystal C. Miller for her expertise in the preparation of this manuscript.

REFERENCES

1. Harwood, H. J., Napcitano, D. M., and Kristiansen, P. L. (1984) Economic costs for society of alcohol and drug abuse and mental illness. Report submitted to the Alcohol, Drug, Abuse, and Mental Health Administration. Research Triangle Institute, Rockville, MD.
2. Board of Trustees Report (1986) Alcohol. Advertising, counter advertising, and depiction in the public media. *JAMA* **256,** 1485–1488.
3. Anonymous (1984) *Alcoholism and Related Problems: Issues for the American Public.* Prentice-Hall, Englewood Cliffs, NJ.
4. Bondy, S. C. (1992) Ethanol toxicity and oxidative stress. *Toxicol. Lett.* **63,** 231–241.
5. Israel, Y. and Orrego, H. (1984) Hypermetabolic state and hypoxic liver damage. *Recent Dev. Alcohol* **2,** 119–133.
6. French, S. W., Benson, N. C., and Sun, P. S. (1984) Centrilobular liver necrosis induced by hypoxia in chronic ethanol-fed rats. *Hepatology* **4,** 912–917.
7. DiLuzio, N. R. and Hartman, A. D. (1967) Role of lipid peroxidation in the pathogenesis of ethanol-induced fatty liver. *Fed. Proc.* **26,** 1436.
8. Dianzani, M. U. (1985) Lipid peroxidation in ethanol poisoning: a critical reconsideration. *Alcohol Alcohol* **20,** 161–173.
9. Robertson, D. M., Morse, R. M., Moore, S.B., O'Fallon, W. M., and Hurt, R. D. (1984) A study of HLA antigens in alcoholism. *Mayo Clin. Proc.* **59,** 243–246.
10. Bailey, R. J., Krasner, N., Eddleston, A. L., Williams, R., Tee, D. E., Doniach, D., et al. (1976) Histocompatibility antigens, autoantibodies, and immunoglobulins in alcoholic liver disease. *Br. Med. J.* **2,** 727–729.
11. Bell, H. and Nordhagen, R. (1978) Association between HLA-BW40 and alcoholic liver disease with cirrhosis. *Br. Med. J.* **1,** 822.
12. MacSween, R. N. (1985) Alcohol and liver injury: genetic and immunologic factors. *Acta Med. Scand. Suppl.* **703,** 57–65.
13. Jenkins, W. J. and Thomas, H. C. (1981) Genetic factors in determining susceptibility to alcohol dependence and development of alcohol-induced liver disease. *Clin. Gastroenterol.* **10,** 307–314.
14. Zetterman, R. K. and Sorrell, M. F. (1981) Immunologic aspects of alcoholic liver disease. *Gastroenterology* **81,** 616–624.
15. Baillie, M. (1971) Alcohol and the liver. *Gut* **12,** 222–229.
16. Carithers, R.L., Jr., Herlong, H. F., Diehl, A.M., Shaw, E. W., Combes, B., Fallon, H. J., et al. (1989) Methylprednisolone therapy in patients with severe alcoholic hepatitis. A randomized multicenter trial. *Ann. Intern. Med.* **110,** 685–690.
17. Ramond, M. J., Poynard, T., Rueff, B., Mathurin, P., Theodore, C., Chaput, J. C., et al. (1992) A randomized trial of prednisolone in patients with severe alcoholic hepatitis. *N. Engl. J. Med.* **326,** 507–512.
18. Baddour, N., Demetris, A. J., Shah, G., Tringali, R., and Van Thiel, D. H. (1992) The prevalence, rate of onset and spectrum of histologic liver disease in alcohol abusing liver allograft recipients. *Gastroenterology* **102,** A777(Abstract).

19. Morgan, M. Y., Ross, M. G., Ng, C. M., Adams, D. M., Thomas, H. C., and Sherlock, S. (1980) HLA-B8, immunoglobulins, and antibody responses in alcohol-related liver disease. *J. Clin. Pathol.* **33,** 488–492.
20. Melendez, M., Vargas-Tank, L., Fuentes, C., Armas-Merino, R., Castillo, D., Wolff, C., et al. (1979) Distribution of HLA histocompatibility antigens, ABO blood groups and Rh antigens in alcoholic liver disease. *Gut* **20,** 288–290.
21. Bell, H. and Nordhagen, R. (1980) HLA antigens in alcoholics, with special reference to alcoholic cirrhosis. *Scand. J. Gastroenterol.* **15,** 453–456.
22. Wilkinson, P., Santamaria, J. N., and Rankin, J. G. (1969) Epidemiology of alcoholic cirrhosis. *Australas. Ann. Med.* **18,** 222–226.
23. Krasner, N., Davis. M., Portmann, B., and Williams, R. (1977) Changing pattern of alcoholic liver disease in Great Britain: relation to sex and signs of autoimmunity. *Br. Med. J.* **1,** 1497–1500.
24. Morgan, M. Y. and Sherlock, S. (1977) Sex-related differences among 100 patients with alcoholic liver disease. *Br. Med. J.* **1,** 939–941.
25. Pequignot, G., Chabert, C., Eydoux, H., and Courcoul, M. A. (1974) Augmentation du risque de cirrhos en fonction de la rotion d'alcool. *Revue de l'Alcoolisme* **20,** 191–202.
26. Saunders, J. B., Wodak, A. D., Haines, A., Powell-Jackson, P. R., Portmann, B., Davis, M., et al. (1982) Accelerated development of alcoholic cirrhosis in patients with HLA-B8. *Lancet* **1,** 1381–1384.
27. Sorrell, M. F. and Leevy, C. M. (1972) Lymphocyte transformation and alcoholic liver injury. *Gastroenterology* **63,** 1020–1025.
28. Leevy, C. M., Zetterman, R., and Smith, F. (1975) Newer approaches to treatment of liver disease in the alcoholic. *Ann. NY Acad. Sci.* **252,** 135–144.
29. Zetterman, R. K., Luisada-Opper, A., and Leevy, C. M. (1976) Alcoholic hepatitis. Cell-mediated immunological response to alcoholic hyalin. *Gastroenterology* **70,** 382–384.
30. Johnson, R. D. and Williams, R. (1986) Immune responses in alcoholic liver disease. *Alcohol Clin. Exp. Res.* **10,** 471–486.
31. Izumi, N., Hasumura, Y., and Takeuchi, J. (1983) Lymphocyte cytotoxicity for autologous human hepatocytes in alcoholic liver disease. *Clin. Exp. Immunol.* **54,** 219–224.
32. Poralla, T., Hutteroth, T. H., and Meyer zum Buschenfelde, K. H. (1984) Cellular cytotoxicity against autologous hepatocytes in alcoholic liver disease. *Liver* **4,** 117–121.
33. Zetterman, R. K. (1986) Alcoholic liver disease. *Curr. Hepatol.* **6,** 93.
34. Sorrell, M. F. and Tuma, D. J. (1985) Hypothesis: alcoholic liver injury and the covalent binding of acetaldehyde. *Alcohol Clin. Exp. Res.* **9,** 306–309.
35. Israel, Y., Orrego, H., and Niemela, O. (1988) Immune responses to alcohol metabolites: pathogenic and diagnostic implications. *Semin. Liver Dis.* **8,** 81–90.
36. Tuma, D. J. and Klassen, L. W. (1992) Immune responses to acetaldehyde-protein adducts: role in alcoholic liver disease. *Gastroenterology* **103,** 1969–1973.
37. Crossley, I. R., Neuberger, J., Davis, M., Williams, R., and Eddleston, A. L. (1986) Ethanol metabolism in the generation of new antigenic determinants on liver cells. *Gut* **27,** 186–189.
38. Lin, R. C., Smith, R. S., and Lumeng, L. (1987) Detection of an ethylated liver protein in rats fed and ethanol-containing liquid diet. *Gastroenterology* **93,** 1751 (Abstract).

39. Niemela, O., Parkkila, S., Yla-Herttuala, S., Villanueva, J., Ruebner, B., and Halsted, C.H. (1995) Sequential acetaldehyde production, lipid peroxidation, and fibrogenesis in micropig model of alcohol-induced liver disease. *Hepatology* **22,** 1208–1214.

40. Hoerner, M., Behrens, U. J., Worner, T., and Lieber, C. S. (1986) Humora immune response to acetaldehyde adducts in alcoholic patients. *Res. Commun. Chem. Pathol. Pharmacol.* **54,** 3–12.

41. Worrall, S., de Jersey, J., Shanley, B. C., and Wilce, P. A. (1989) Ethanol induces the production of antibodies to acetaldehyde-modified epitopes in rats. *Alcohol Alcohol* **24,** 217–223.

42. Lin, R. C., Lumeng, L., Shahidi, S., Kelly, T., and Pound, D. C. (1990) Protein-acetaldehyde adducts in serum of alcoholic patients. *Alcohol. Clin. Exp. Res.* **14,** 438–443.

43. Niemela, O., Juvonen, T., and Parkkila, S. (1991) Immunohistochemical demonstration of acetaldehyde-modified epitopes in human liver after alcohol consumption. *J. Clin. Invest.* **87,** 1367–1374.

44. Terabayashi, H. and Kolber, M. A. (1990) The generation of cytotoxic T lymphocytes against acetaldehyde-modified syngeneic cells. *Alcohol Clin. Exp. Res.* **14,** 893–899.

45. Yokoyama, H., Nagata, S., Moriya, S., Kato, S., Ito, T., Kamegaya, K., et al. (1995) Hepatic fibrosis produced in guinea pigs by chronic ethanol administration and immunization with acetaldehyde adducts. *Hepatology* **21,** 1438–1442.

46. Worrall, S., de Jersey, J., and Wilce, P. A. (1992) Liver damage in ethanol-fed rats injected with acetaldehyde modified proteins. *Alcohol Clin. Exp. Res.* **16,** 623 (Abstract).

47. Israel, Y., Hurwitz, E., Niemela, O., and Arnon, R. (1986) Monoclonal and polyclonal antibodies against acetaldehyde-containing epitopes in acetaldehyde-protein adducts. *Proc. Natl. Acad. Sci. USA* **83,** 7923–7927.

48. Worrall, S., de Jersey, J., Shanley, B. C., and Wilce, P. A. (1990) Antibodies against acetaldehyde-modified epitopes: presence in alcoholic, non-alcoholic liver disease and control subjects. *Alcohol Alcohol.* **25,** 509–517.

49. Tuma, D. J., Newman, M. R., Donohue, T. M., Jr., and Sorrell, M. F. (1987) Covalent binding of acetaldehyde to proteins: participation of lysine residues. *Alcohol Clin. Exp. Res.* **11,** 579–584.

50. Klassen, L. W., Tuma, D. J., Sorrell, M. F., McDonald, T. L., DeVasure, J. M., and Thiele, G. M. (1994) Detection of reduced acetaldehyde protein adducts using a unique monoclonal antibody. *Alcohol Clin. Exp. Res.* **18,** 164–171.

51. Thiele, G. M., Wegter, K. M., Sorrell, M. F., Tuma, D. J., McDonald, T. L., and Klassen, L. W. (1994) Specificity of N-ethyl lysine of a monoclonal antibody to acetaldehyde-modified proteins prepared under reducing conditions. *Biochem. Pharmacol.* **48,** 183–189.

52. Cederbaum, A. I. (1989) Role of lipid peroxidation and oxidative stress in alcohol toxicity. *Free Radic. Biol. Med.* **7,** 537–539.

53. Kamimura, S., Gaal, K., Britton, R. S., Bacon, B. R., Triadafilopoulos, G., and Tsukamoto, H. (1992) Increased 4-hydroxynonenal levels in experimental alcoholic liver disease: association of lipid peroxidation with liver fibrogenesis. *Hepatology* **16,** 448–453.

54. Benedetti, A. and Comporti, M. (1987) Formation reactions and toxicity of aldehydes produced in the course of lipid peroxidation in cellular membranes. *Bioelectrochem. Bioenerg.* **18,** 187–202.

55. Houglum, K., Filip, M., Witztum, J. L., and Chojkier, M. (1990) Malondialdehyde and 4-hydroxynonenal protein adducts in plasma and liver of rats with iron overload. *J. Clin. Invest.* **86,** 1991–1998.
56. Niemela, O., Parkkila, S., Yla-Herttuala, S., Halsted, C., Witztum, J. L., Lanca, A., and Israel, Y. (1994) Covalent protein adducts in the liver as a result of ethanol metabolism and lipid peroxidation. *Lab. Invest.* **70,** 537–546.
57. Eriksson, C. J., Atkinson, N., Petersen, D. R., and Deitrich, R. A. (1984) Blood and liver acetaldehyde concentrations during ethanol oxidation in C57 and DBA mice. *Biochem. Pharmacol.* **33,** 2213–2216.
58. Ohya, T. (1993) Formation of a new 1,1,1 adduct in the reaction of malondialdehyde, hexylamine and alkanal under neutral conditions. *Biol. Pharm. Bull.* **16,** 137–141.
59. Tuma, D. J., Thiele, G. M., Xu, D. S., Klassen, L. W., and Sorrel, M. F. (1995) Acetaldehyde and malondialdehyde react together to generate distinct protein adducts in the liver during chronic ethanol administration. *Hepatology* **22,** 226A (Abstract).
60. Thiele, G. M., Tuma, D. J., Willis, M. S., Miller, J. A., McDonald, T. L., Sorrel, M. F., et al. (1997) Soluble proteins modified with the alcohol metabolites acetaldehyde and malondialdehyde are immunogenic in mice in the absence of adjuvant. *Alcoholism: Clin. Exp. Res.* (Submitted).
61. Albano, E., Tomasi, A., Goria-Gatti, L., and Dianzani, M. U. (1988) Spin trapping of free radical species produced during the microsomal metabolism of ethanol. *Chem. Biol. Interact.* **65,** 223–234.
62. Albano, E., Tomasi, A., and Ingelman-Sundberg, M. (1994) Spin trapping of alcohol-derived radicals in microsomes and reconstituted systems by electron spin resonance. *Meth. Enzymol.* **233,** 117–127.
63. Knecht, K. T., Bradford, B. U., Mason, R. P., and Thurman, R. G. (1990) In vivo formation of a free radical metabolite of ethanol. *Mol. Pharmacol.* **38,** 26–30.
64. Moore, D. R., Reinke, L. A., and McCay, P. B. (1995) Metabolism of ethanol to 1-hydroxyethyl radicals in vivo: detection with intravenous administration of alpha-(4-pyridyl-1-oxide)-N-t- butylnitrone. *Mol. Pharmacol.* **47,** 1224–1230.
65. Rao, D. N., Yang, M. X., Lasker, J. M., and Cederbaum, A. I. (1996) 1-Hydroxyethyl radical formation during NADPH- and NADH-dependent oxidation of ethanol by human liver microsomes. *Mol. Pharmacol.* **49,** 814–821.
66. Albano, E., Parola, M., Comoglio, A., and Dianzani, M. U. (1993) Evidence for the covalent binding of hydroxyethyl radicals to rat liver microsomal proteins. *Alcohol Alcohol* **28,** 453–459.
67. Moncada, C., Torres, V., Varghese, G., Albano, E., and Israel, Y. (1994) Ethanol-derived immunoreactive species formed by free radical mechanisms. *Mol. Pharmacol.* **46,** 786–791.
68. Albano, E., Tomasi, A., Persson, J. O., Terelius, Y., Goria-Gatti, L., Ingelman-Sundberg, M., et al. (1991) Role of ethanol-inducible cytochrome P450 (P450IIE1) in catalysing the free radical activation of aliphatic alcohols. *Biochem. Pharmacol.* **41,** 1895–1902.
69. Albano, E., Clot, P., Morimoto, M., Tomasi, A., Ingelman-Sundberg, M., and French, S. W. (1996) Role of cytochrome P4502E1-dependent formation of hydroxyethyl free radical in the development of liver damage in rats intragastrically fed with ethanol. *Hepatology* **23,** 155–163.

70. Clot, P., Bellomo, G., Tabone, M., Arico, S., and Albano, E. (1995) etection of antibodies against proteins modified by hydroxyethyl free radicals in patients with alcoholic cirrhosis. *Gastroenterology* **108**, 201–207.
71. Loeper, J., Descatoire, V., Maurice, M., Beaune, P., Feldmann, G., Larrey, D., et al. (1990) Presence of functional cytochrome P-450 on isolated rat hepatocyte plasma membrane. *Hepatology* **11**, 850–858.
72. Wu, D. and Cederbaum, A. I. (1992) Presence of functionally active cytochrome P-450IIE1 in the plasma membrane of rat hepatocytes. *Hepatology* **15**, 515–524.
73. Loeper, J., Descatoire, V., Maurice, M., Beaune, P., Belghiti, J., Houssin, D et al. (1993) Cytochromes P-450 in human hepatocyte plasma membrane: recognition by several autoantibodies. *Gastroenterology* **104**, 203–216.
74. Clot, P., Parola, M., Bellomo, G., Dianzani, M. U., Carini, R., Tabone, M., et al. (1995) Role of plasma membrane hydroxyethyl radical adducts in causing antibody-dependent cytotoxicity in hepatocytes exposed to alcohol. *Hepatology* **22**, 227A(Abstract).
75. Jurgens, G., Hoff, H. F., Chisolm G. M., III, and Esterbauer, H. (1987) Modification of human serum low density lipoprotein by oxidation—characterization and pathophysiological implications. *Chem. Phys. Lipids* **45**, 315–336.
76. Henriksen, T., Mahoney, E. M., and Steinberg, D. (1981) Enhanced macrophage degradation of low density lipoprotein previously incubated with cultured endothelial cells: recognition by receptors for acetylated low density lipoproteins. *Proc. Natl. Acad. Sci. USA* **78**, 6499–6503.
77. Henriksen, T., Mahoney, E. M., and Steinberg, D. (1983) Enhanced macrophage degradation of biologically modified low density lipoprotein. *Arteriosclerosis* **3**, 149–159.
78. Cathcart, M. K., Morel, D. W., and Chisolm, G. M., 3rd. (1985) Monocytes and neutrophils oxidize low density lipoprotein making it cytotoxic. *J. Leukoc. Biol.* **38**, 341–350.
79. Heinecke, J. W., Rosen, H., and Chait, A. (1984) Iron and copper promote modification of low density lipoprotein by human arterial smooth muscle cells in culture. *J. Clin. Invest.* **74**, 1890–1894.
80. Tsukamoto, H., Horne, W., Kamimura, S., Niemela, O., Parkkila, S., Yla-Herttuala, S., et al. (1995) Experimental liver cirrhosis induced by alcohol and iron. *J. Clin. Invest.* **96**, 620–630.
81. Esterbauer, H., Schaur, R. J., and Zollner, H. (1991) Chemistry and iochemistry of 4-hydroxynonenal, malonaldehyde and related aldehydes. *Free Radic. Biol. Med.* **11**, 81–128.
82. Casini, A., Cunningham, M., Rojkind, M., and Lieber, C. S. (1991) Acetaldehyde increases procollagen type I and fibronectin gene transcription in cultured rat fat-storing cells through a protein synthesis-dependent mechanism. *Hepatology* **13**, 758–765.
83. Pares, A., Potter, J. J., Rennie, L., and Mezey, E. (1994) Acetaldehyde activates the promoter of the mouse alpha 2(I) collagen gene. *Hepatology* **19**, 498–503.
84. Tsukamoto, H., Kim, C. W., and Luo, Z. Z. (1993) Role of lipid peroxidation in vivo and in vitro models of liver fibrogenesis. *Gastroenterology* **104**, A1012 (Abstract).
85. Parola, M., Pinzani, M., Casini, A., Albano, E., Poli, G., Gentilini, A., et al. (1993) Stimulation of lipid peroxidation or 4-hydroxynonenal treatment increases pro-

collagen alpha 1 (I) gene expression in human liver fat-storing cells. *Biochem. Biophys. Res. Commun.* **194**, 1044–1050.

86. Gluud, C., Tage-Jensen, U., Bahnsen, M., Dietrichson, O., and Svejgaard, A. (1981) Autoantibodies, histocompatibility antigens and testosterone in males with alcoholic liver cirrhosis. *Clin. Exp. Immunol.* **44**, 31–37.

87. Laskin, C. A., Vidins, E., Blendis, L. M., and Soloninka, C. A. (1990) Autoantibodies in alcoholic liver disease. *Am. J. Med.* **89**, 129–133.

88. Cunningham, A. L., Mackay, I. R., Frazer, I. H., Brown, C., Pedersen, J. S., Toh, B. H., et al. (1985) Antibody to G-actin in different categories of alcoholic liver disease: quantification by an ELISA and significance for alcoholic cirrhosis. *Clin. Immunol. Immunopathol.* **34**, 158–164.

89. Kanagasundaram, N., Kakumu, S., Chen, T., and Leevy, C. M. (1977) Alcoholic hyalin antigen (AHAg) and antibody (AHAb) in alcoholic hepatitis. *Gastroenterology* **73**, 1368–1373.

90. Kehl, A., Schober, A., Junge, U., and Winckler, K. (1981) Solid-phase radioimmunoassay for detection of alcoholic hyalin antigen (AHAg) and antibody (anti-AH). *Clin. Exp. Immunol.* **43**, 215–221.

91. Behrens, U. J. and Paronetto, F. (1979) Studies on "liver-specific" antigens. I. Evaluation of the liver specificity of "LSP" and "LP-2". *Gastroenterology* **77**, 1045–1052.

92. McFarlane, I. G., Wojcicka, B. M., and Williams, R. (1980) Antigens of the human liver. *Clin. Exp. Immunol.* **40**, 1–7.

93. Manns, M., Meyer zum Buschenfelde, K. H., and Hess, G. (1980) Autoantibodies against liver-specific membrane lipoprotein in acute and chronic liver diseases: studies on organ-, species-, and disease- specificity. *Gut* **21**, 955–961.

94. Burt, A. D., Anthony, R. S., Hislop, W. S., Bouchier, I. A., and MacSween, R. N. (1982) Liver membrane antibodies in alcoholic liver disease: 1. prevalence and immunoglobulin class. *Gut* **23**, 221–225.

95. Wiedmann, K. H., Bartholemew, T. C., Brown, D. J., and Thomas, H. C. (1984) Liver membrane antibodies detected by immunoradiometric assay in acute and chronic virus-induced and autoimmune liver disease. *Hepatology* **4**, 199–204.

96. Sancho, J., Egido, J., Sanchez-Crespo, M., and Blasco, R. (1982) Detection of monomeric and polymeric IgA containing immune complexes in serum and kidney from patients with alcoholic liver disease. *Clin. Exp. Immunol.* **97**, 327–335.

97. Penner, E., Albini, B., and Milgrom, F. (1978) Detection of circulating immune complexes in alcoholic liver disease. *Clin. Exp. Immunol.* **34**, 28–31.

98. Thomas, H. C., De Villiers, D., Potter, B., Hodgson, H., Jain, S., Jewell, D. P., et al. (1978) Immune complexes in acute and chronic liver disease. *Clin. Exp. Immunol.* **31**, 150–157.

99. Abrass, C. K., Border, W. A., and Hepner, G. (1980) Non-specificity of circulating immune complexes in patients with acute and chronic liver disease. *Clin. Exp. Immunol.* **40**, 292–298.

100. Kakumu, S., Arakawa, Y., Goji, H., Kashio, T., and Yata, K. (1979) Occurrence and significance of antibody to liver-specific membrane lipoprotein by double-antibody immunoprecipitation method in sera of patients with acute and chronic liver diseases. *Gastroenterology* **76**, 665–672.

101. Mezey, E. (1982) Alcoholic liver disease. *Prog. Liver Dis.* **7**, 555–572.

102. French, S. W. and Burbige, E. J. (1979) Alcoholic hepatitis: clinical, morphologic, pathogenic, and therapeutic aspects. *Prog. Liver Dis.* **6**, 557–579.

103. Bhagwandeen, B. S., Apte, M., Manwarring, L., and Dickeson, J. (1987) Endotoxin induced hepatic necrosis in rats on an alcohol diet. *J. Pathol.* **152,** 47–53.
104. Arai, M., Nakano, S., Okuno, F., Hirano, Y., Sujita, K., Kobayashi, T., et al. (1989) Endotoxin-induced hypercoagulability: a possible aggravating factor of alcoholic liver disease. *Hepatology* **9,** 846–851.
105. Honchel, R., Ray, M. B., Marsano, L., Cohen, D., Lee, E., Shedlofsky, S., et al. (1992) Tumor necrosis factor in alcohol enhanced endotoxin liver injury. *Alcohol Clin. Exp. Res.* **16,** 665–669.
106. Hansen, J., Cherwitz, D. L., and Allen, J. I. (1994) The role of tumor necrosis factor-alpha in acute endotoxin-induced hepatotoxicity in ethanol-fed rats. *Hepatology* **20,** 461–474.
107. Hoffmann, R., Grewe, M., Estler, H. C., Schulze-Specking, A., and Decker, K. (1994) Regulation of tumor necrosis factor-alpha-mRNA synthesis and distribution of tumor necrosis factor-alpha-mRNA synthesizing cells in rat liver during experimental endotoxemia. *J. Hepatol.* **20,** 122–128.
108. Thiele, G. M., Klassen, L. W., Miller, J. A., Hill, G. E., and Tuma, D. J. (1997) Binding of aldehyde-modified proteins to liver endothelial cells changes the adhesion molecule and TNF-alpha Expression. *J. Allergy Clin. Immunol.* **99(1),** 5195.
109. Hill, D. B., Marsano, L. S., and McClain, C. J. (1993) Increased plasma interleukin-8 concentrations in alcoholic hepatitis. *Hepatology* **18,** 576–580.
110. Sheron, N., Bird, G., Koskinas, J., Portmann, B., Ceska, M., Lindley, I., et al. (1993) Circulating and tissue levels of the neutrophil chemotaxin interleukin-8 are elevated in severe acute alcoholic hepatitis, and tissue levels correlate with neutrophil infiltration. *Hepatology* **18,** 41–46.
111. Khoruts, A., Stahnke, L., McClain, C. J., Logan, G., and Allen, J. I. (1991) Circulating tumor necrosis factor, interleukin-1 and interleukin-6 concentrations in chronic alcoholic patients. *Hepatology* **13,** 267–276.
112. McClain, C. J., Cohen, D. A., Dinarello, C. A., Cannon, J. G., Shedlofsky, S. I., and Kaplan, A. M. (1986) Serum interleukin-1 (IL-1) activity in alcoholic hepatitis. *Life Sci.* **39,** 1479–1485.
113. Deviere, J., Content, J., Denys, C., Vandenbussche, P., Schandene, L., Wybran, J., et al. (1990) Excessive in vitro bacterial lipopolysaccharide-induced production of monokines in cirrhosis. *Hepatology* **11,** 628–634.
114. Kishimoto, T. (1989) The biology of interleukin-6. *Blood* **74,** 1–10.
115. Deviere, J., Content, J., Denys, C., Vandenbussche, P., Schandene, L., Wybran, J., et al. (1989) High interleukin-6 serum levels and increased production by leucocytes in alcoholic liver cirrhosis. Correlation with IgA serum levels and lymphokines production. *Clin. Exp. Immunol.* **77,** 221–225.
116. Hill, D. B., Marsano, L., Cohen, D., Allen, J., Shedlofsky, S., and McClain, C. J. (1992) Increased plasma interleukin-6 concentrations in alcoholic hepatitis. *J. Lab. Clin. Med.* **119,** 547–552.
117. McClain, C., Hill, D., Schmidt, J., and Diehl, A. M. (1993) Cytokines and alcoholic liver disease. *Semin. Liver Dis.* **13,** 170–182.
118. Ulich, T. R., Guo, K., and del Castillo, J. (1989) Endotoxin-induced cytokine gene expression in vivo. I. Expression of tumor necrosis factor mRNA in visceral organs under physiologic conditions and during endotoxemia. *Am. J. Pathol.* **134,** 11–14.

119. Peristeris, P., Clark, B. D., Gatti, S., Faggioni, R., Mantovani, A., Mengozzi, M., et al. (1992) N-acetylcysteine and glutathione as inhibitors of tumor necrosis factor production. *Cell Immunol.* **140**, 390–399.
120. Pohl, L. R. and Gillette, J. R. (1982) A perspective on halothane-induced hepatotoxicity [letter]. *Anesth. Analg.* **61**, 809–811.
121. Neuberger, J. and Williams, R. (1984) Halothane anaesthesia and liver damage. *Br. Med. J. (Clin. Res. Ed.)* **289**, 1136–1139.
122. Neuberger, J. and Kenna, J. G. (1987) Halothane hepatitis: a model of immune mediated drug hepatotoxicity. *Clin. Sci.* **72**, 263–270.
123. Neuberger, J. M. (1990) Halothane and hepatitis. Incidence, predisposing factors and exposure guidelines. *Drug Saf.* **5**, 28–38.
124. Ray, D. C. and Drummond, G. B. (1991) Halothane hepatitis. *Br. J. Anaesth.* **67**, 84–99.
125. Elliott, R. H. and Strunin, L. (1993) Hepatotoxicity of volatile anaesthetics. *Br. J. Anaesth.* **70**, 339–348.
126. Satoh, H., Davies, H. W., Takemura, T., Gillette, J. R., Maeda, K., and Pohl, L. R. (1987) An immunochemical approach to investigating the mechanism of halothane-induced hepatotoxicity. *Prog. Drug Metab.* **10**, 187–206.
127. Pohl, L. R., Kenna, J. G., Satoh, H., Christ, D., and Martin, J. L. (1989) Neoantigens associated with halothane hepatitis. *Drug. Metab. Rev.* **20**, 203–217.
128. Kenna, J. G. (1991) The molecular basis of halothane-induced hepatitis. *Biochem. Soc. Trans.* **19**, 191–195.
129. Paronetto, F. and Popper, H. (1970) Lymphocyte stimulation induced by halothane in patients with hepatitis following exposure to halothane. *N. Engl. J. Med.* **283**, 277–280.
130. Williams, B. D., White, N., Amlot, P. L., Slaney, J., and Toseland, P. A. (1977) Circulating immune complexes after repeated halothane anaesthesia. *Br. Med. J.* **2**, 159–162.
131. Price, C. D., Gibbs, A. R., and Williams, W. J. (1977) Halothane macrophage migration inhibition factor test in halothane-associated hepatitis. *J. Clin. Pathol.* **30**, 312–316.
132. Vergani, D., Tsantoulas, D., Eddleston, A. L., Davis, M., and Williams, R. (1978) Sensitisation to halothane-altered liver components in severe hepatic necrosis after halothane anaesthesia. *Lancet* **2**, 801–803.
133. Satoh, H., Fukuda, Y., Anderson, D. K., Ferrans, V. J., Gillette, J. R., and Pohl, L. R. (1985) Immunological studies on the mechanism of halothane-induced hepatotoxicity: immunohistochemical evidence of trifluoroacetylated hepatocytes. *J. Pharmacol. Exp. Ther.* **233**, 857–862.
134. Kenna, J. G., Martin, J. L., Satoh, H., and Pohl, L. R. (1990) Factors affecting the expression of trifluoroacetylated liver microsomal protein neoantigens in rats treated with halothane. *Drug Metab. Dispos.* **18**, 788–793.
135. Satoh, H., Gillette, J. R., Takemura, T., Ferrans, V. J., Jelenich, S. E., Kenna, J. G., et al. (1986) Investigation of the immunological basis of halothane-induced hepatotoxicity. *Adv. Exp. Med. Biol.* **197**, 657–673.
136. Kenna, J. G., Satoh, H., Christ, D. D., and Pohl, L. R. (1988) Metabolic basis for a drug hypersensitivity: antibodies in sera from patients with halothane hepatitis recognize liver neoantigens that contain the trifluoroacetyl group derived from halothane. *J. Pharmacol. Exp. Ther.* **245**, 1103–1109.

137. Satoh, H., Martin, B. M., Schulick, A. H., Christ, D. D., Kenna, J. G., and Pohl, L. R. (1989) Human anti-endoplasmic reticulum antibodies in sera of patients with halothane-induced hepatitis are directed against a trifluoroacetylated carboxylesterase. *Proc. Natl. Acad. Sci. USA* **86,** 322–326.
138. Harris, J. W., Pohl, L. R., Martin, J. L., and Anders, M. W. (1991) Tissue acylation by the chlorofluorocarbon substitute 2,2-dichloro- 1,1,1-trifluoroethane. *Proc. Natl. Acad. Sci. USA* **88,** 1407–1410.
139. Thomassen, D., Martin, B. M., Martin, J. L., Pumford, N. R., and Pohl, L. R. (1990) The role of a stress protein in the development of a drug-induced allergic response. *Eur. J. Pharmacol.* **183,** 1138–1139.
140. Pumford, N. R., Martin, B. M., Thomassen, D., Burris, J. A., Kenna, J. G., Martin, J. L., et al. (1993) Serum antibodies from halothane hepatitis patients react with the rat endoplasmic reticulum protein ERp72. *Chem. Res. Toxicol.* **6,** 609–615.
141. Davila, J. C., Martin, B. M., and Pohl, L. R. (1992) Patients with halothane hepatitis have serum antibodies directed against glucose-regulated stress protein GRP78/BiP. *Toxicologist* **12,** 255.
142. Martin, J. L., Kenna, J. G., Martin, B. M., Thomassen, D., Reed, G. F., and Pohl, L. R. (1993) Halothane hepatitis patients have serum antibodies that react with protein disulfide isomerase. *Hepatology* **18,** 858–863.
143. Butler, L. E., Thomassen, D., Martin, J. L., Martin, B. M., Kenna, J. G., and Pohl, L. R. (1992) The calcium-binding protein calreticulin is covalently modified in rat liver by a reactive metabolite of the inhalation anesthetic halothane. *Chem. Res. Toxicol.* **5,** 406–410.
144. Martin, J. L., Pumford, N. R., LaRosa, A. C., Martin, B. M., Gonzaga, H. M., Beaven, M. A., et al. (1991) A metabolite of halothane covalently binds to an endoplasmic reticulum protein that is highly homologous to phosphatidylinositol-specific phospholipase C-alpha but has no activity. *Biochem. Biophys. Res. Commun.* **178,** 679–685.
145. Martin, J. L., Reed, G. F., and Pohl, L. R. (1993) Association of anti-58 kDa endoplasmic reticulum antibodies with halothane hepatitis. *Biochem. Pharmacol.* **46,** 1247–1250.
146. Srivastava, S. P., Chen, N. Q., Liu, Y. X., and Holtzman, J. L. (1991) Purification and characterization of a new isozyme of thiol: protein- disulfide oxidoreductase from rat hepatic microsomes. Relationship of this isozyme to cytosolic phosphatidylinositol-specific phospholipase C form 1A. *J. Biol. Chem.* **266,** 20,337–20,344.
147. Urade, R., Nasu, M., Moriyama, T., Wada, K., and Kito, M. (1992) Protein degradation by the phosphoinositide-specific phospholipase C- alpha family from rat liver endoplasmic reticulum. *J. Biol. Chem.* **267,** 15,152–15,159.
148. Murthy, M. S. and Pande, S. V. (1993) Carnitine medium/long chain acyltransferase of microsomes seems to be the previously cloned approximately 54 kDa protein of unknown function. *Mol. Cell. Biochem.* **122,** 133–138.
149. Huwyler, J., Aeschlimann, D., Christen, U., and Gut, J. (1992) The kidney as a novel target tissue for protein adduct formation associated with metabolism of halothane and the candidate chlorofluorocarbon replacement 2,2-dichloro-1,1,1-trifluoroethane. *Eur. J. Biochem.* **207,** 229–238.
150. Heijink, E., De Matteis, F., Gibbs, A. H., Davies, A., and White, I. N. (1993) Metabolic activation of halothane to neoantigens in C57Bl/10 mice: immunochemical studies. *Eur. J. Pharmacol.* **248,** 15–25.

151. Huwyler, J. and Gut, J. (1992) Exposure to the chlorofluorocarbon substitute 2,2-dichloro-1,1,1-trifluoroethane and the anesthetic agent halothane is associated with transient protein adduct formation in the heart. *Biochem. Biophys. Res. Commun.* **184,** 1344-1349.
152. Christen, U., Burgin, M., and Gut, J. (1991) Halothane metabolism: Kupffer cells carry and partially process trifluoroacetylated protein adducts. *Biochem. Biophys. Res. Commun.* **175,** 256–262.
153. Hayden, P. J., Ichimura, T., McCann, D. J., Pohl, L. R., and Stevens, J. L. (1991) Detection of cysteine conjugate metabolite adduct formation with specific mitochondrial proteins using antibodies raised against halothane metabolite adducts. *J. Biol. Chem.* **266,** 18,415–18,418.
154. Joshi, P. H. and Conn, H. O. (1974) The syndrome of methoxyflurane-associated hepatitis. *Ann. Intern. Med.* **80,** 395–401.
155. Njoku, D., Laster, M. J., Gong, D. H., Eger, E. I., II, Reed, G. F., and Martin, J. L. (1997) Biotransformation of halothane, enflurane, isoflurane, and desflurane to trifluoroacetylated liver proteins: association between protein acylation and hepatic injury. *Anesth. Analg.* **84,** 173–178.
156. Spencer, J. D., Raasch, F. O., and Trefny, F. A. (1976) Halothane abuse in hospital personnel. *JAMA* **235,** 1034–1035.
157. Min, K. W., Cain, G. D., Sabel, J. S., and Gyorkey, F. (1977) Methoxyflurane hepatitis. *South. Med. J.* **70,** 1363–1364.
158. Kaplan, H. G., Bakken, J., Quadracci, L., and Schubach, W. (1979) Hepatitis caused by halothane sniffing. *Ann. Intern. Med.* **90,** 797,798.
159. Kline, M. M. (1980) Enflurane-associated hepatitis. *Gastroenterology* **79,** 126–127.
160. Lewis, J. H., Zimmerman, H. J., Ishak, K. G., and Mullick, F. G. (1983) Enflurane hepatotoxicity. A clinicopathologic study of 24 cases. *Ann. Intern. Med.* **98,** 984–992.
161. White, L. B., DeTarnowsky, G. O., Mir, J. A., and Layden, T. J. (1981) Hepatotoxicity following enflurane anesthesia. *Dig. Dis. Sci.* **26,** 466–469.
162. Anonymous (1985) Isoflurane [editorial]. *Lancet* **2,** 537,538.
163. Zimmerman, H. (1991) Even isoflurane [editorial]. *Hepatology* **13,** 1251–1253.
164. Stoelting, R. K., Blitt, C. D., Cohen, P. J., and Merin, R. G. (1987) Hepatic dysfunction after isoflurane anesthesia. *Anesth. Analg.* **66,** 147–153.
165. Carrigan, T. W. and Straughen, W. J. (1987) A report of hepatic necrosis and death following isoflurane anesthesia. *Anesthesiology* **67,** 581–583.
166. Brunt, E. M., White, H., Marsh, J. W., Holtmann, B., and Peters, M. G. (1991) Fulminant hepatic failure after repeated exposure to isoflurane anesthesia: a case report. *Hepatology* **13,** 1017–1021.
167. Nelson, S. D. (1990) Molecular mechanisms of the hepatotoxicity caused by acetaminophen. *Semin. Liver Dis.* **10,** 267–278.
168. Clemens, D. L., Halgard, C. M., Miles, R. R., Sorrell, M. F., and Tuma, D. J. (1995) Establishment of a recombinant hepatic cell line stably expressing alcohol dehydrogenase. *Arch. Biochem. Biophys.* **321,** 311–318.
169. Tuma, D. J. and Sorrell, M. F. (1987) Functional consequences of acetaldehyde binding to proteins. *Alcohol Alcohol* **Suppl 1,** 61–66.
170. Thummel, K. E., Lee, C. A., Kunze, K. L., Nelson, S. D., and Slattery, J. T. (1993) Oxidation of acetaminophen to N-acetyl-p-aminobenzoquinone imine by human CYP3A4. *Biochem. Pharmacol.* **45,** 1563–1569.

171. Patten, C. J., Thomas, P. E., Guy, R. L., Lee, M., Gonzalez, F. J., Guengerich, F. P., et al. (1993) Cytochrome P450 enzymes involved in acetaminophen activation by rat and human liver microsomes and their kinetics. *Chem. Res. Toxicol.* **6**, 511–518.
172. Hoffmann, K. J., Streeter, A. J., Axworthy, D. B., and Baillie, T. A. (1985) Identification of the major covalent adduct formed in vitro and in vivo between acetaminophen and mouse liver proteins. *Mol. Pharmacol.* **27**, 566–573.
173. Roberts, D. W., Pumford, N. R., Potter, D. W., Benson, R. W., and Hinson, J. A. (1987) A sensitive immunochemical assay for acetaminophen-protein adducts. *J. Pharmacol. Exp. Ther.* **241**, 527–533.
174. Bartolone, J. B., Birge, R. B., Sparks, K., Cohen, S. D., and Khairallah, E. A. (1988) Immunochemical analysis of acetaminophen covalent binding to proteins. Partial characterization of the major acetaminophen-binding liver proteins. *Biochem. Pharmacol.* **37**, 4763–4774.
175. Roberts, D. W., Bucci, T. J., Benson, R. W., Warbritton, A. R., McRae, T. A., Pumford, N. R., et al. (1991) Immunohistochemical localization and quantification of the 3-(cystein-S-yl)-acetaminophen protein adduct in acetaminophen hepatotoxicity. *Am. J. Pathol.* **138**, 359–371.
176. Birge, R. B., Bartolone, J. B., Hart, S. G., Nishanian, E. V., Tyson, C. A., Khairallah, E. A., et al. (1990) Acetaminophen hepatotoxicity: correspondence of selective protein arylation in human and mouse liver in vitro, in culture, and in vivo. *Toxicol. Appl. Pharmacol.* **105**, 472–482.
177. Pumford, N. R., Roberts, D. W., Benson, R. W., and Hinson, J. A. (1990) Immunochemical quantitation of 3-(cystein-S-yl)acetaminophen protein adducts in subcellular liver fractions following a hepatotoxic dose of acetaminophen. *Biochem. Pharmacol.* **40**, 573–579.
178. Pumford, N. R., Hinson, J. A., Benson, R. W., and Roberts, D. W. (1990) Immunoblot analysis of protein containing 3-(cystein-S-yl)acetaminophen adducts in serum and subcellular liver fractions from acetaminophen- treated mice. *Toxicol. Appl. Pharmacol.* **104**, 521–532.
179. Birge, R. B., Bulera, S. J., Bartolone, J. B., Ginsberg, G. L., Cohen, S. D., and Khairallah, E. A. (1991) The arylation of microsomal membrane proteins by acetaminophen is associated with the release of a 44 kDa acetaminophen-binding mouse liver protein complex into the cytosol. *Toxicol. Appl. Pharmacol.* **109**, 443–454.
180. Pumford, N. R., Martin, B. M., and Hinson, J. A. (1992) A metabolite of acetaminophen covalently binds to the 56 kDa selenium binding protein. *Biochem. Biophys. Res. Commun.* **182**, 1348–1355.
181. Bartolone, J. B., Birge, R. B., Bulera, S. J., Bruno, M. K., Nishanian, E. V., Cohen, S. D., et al. (1992) Purification, antibody production, and partial amino acid sequence of the 58-kDa acetaminophen-binding liver proteins. *Toxicol. Appl. Pharmacol.* **113**, 19–29.
182. Boyer, D. L., Li, B. U., Fyda, J. N., and Friedman, R. A. (1989) Sulfasalazine-induced hepatotoxicity in children with inflammatory bowel disease. *J. Pediatr. Gastroenterol. Nutr.* **8**, 528–532.
183. Caspi, D., Fuchs, D., and Yaron, M. (1992) Sulphasalazine induced hepatitis in juvenile rheumatoid arthritis. *Ann. Rheum. Dis.* **51**, 275–276.
184. Hautekeete, M. L., Bourgeois, N., Potvin, P., Duville, L., Reynaert, H., Devis, G., et al. (1992) Hypersensitivity with hepatotoxicity to mesalazine after hypersensitivity to sulfasalazine. *Gastroenterology* **103**, 1925–1927.

185. Zimmerman, H. J. (1990) Update of hepatotoxicity due to classes of drugs in common clinical use: non-steroidal drugs, anti-inflammatory drugs, antibiotics, antihypertensives, and cardiac and psychotropic agents. *Semin. Liver Dis.* **10,** 322–338.

186. Tolman, K. G. (1990) Hepatotoxicity of antirheumatic drugs. *J. Rheumatol. Suppl.* **22,** 6–11.

187. Rabinovitz, M. and Van Thiel, D. H. (1992) Hepatotoxicity of nonsteroidal antiinflammatory drugs. *Am. J. Gastroenterol.* **87,** 1696–1704.

188. Bush, T. M., Shlotzhauer, T. L., and Imai, K. (1991) Nonsteroidal anti-inflammatory drugs. Proposed guidelines for monitoring toxicity. *West. J. Med.* **155,** 39–42.

189. Dunk, A. A., Walt, R. P., Jenkins, W. J., and Sherlock, S. S. (1982) Diclofenac hepatitis. *Br. Med. J. (Clin. Res. Ed.)* **284,** 1605–1606.

190. Schapira, D., Bassan, L., Nahir, A. M., and Scharf, Y. (1986) Diclofenac-induced hepatotoxicity. *Postgrad. Med. J.* **62,** 63–65.

191. Helfgott, S. M., Sandberg-Cook, J., Zakim, D., and Nestler, J. (1990) Diclofenac-associated hepatotoxicity. *JAMA* **264,** 2660–2662.

192. Iveson, T. J., Ryley, N. G., Kelly, P. M., Trowell, J. M., McGee, J. O., and Chapman, R. W. (1990) Diclofenac associated hepatitis. *J. Hepatol.* **10,** 85–89.

193. Purcell, P., Henry, D., and Melville, G. (1991) Diclofenac hepatitis. *Gut* **32,** 1381–1385.

194. Sallie, R. W., McKenzie, T., Reed, W. D., Quinlan, M. F., and Shilkin, K. B. (1991) Diclofenac hepatitis. *Aust. N. Z. J. Med.* **21,** 251–255.

195. Ouellette, G. S., Slitzky, B. E., Gates, J. A., Lagarde, S., and West, A. B. (1991) Reversible hepatitis associated with diclofenac. *J. Clin. Gastroenterol.* **13,** 205–210.

196. Breen, E. G., McNicholl, J., Cosgrove, E., McCabe, J., and Stevens, F. M. (1986) Fatal hepatitis associated with diclofenac. *Gut* **27,** 1390–1393.

197. Faed, E. M. (1984) Properties of acyl glucuronides: implications for studies of the pharmacokinetics and metabolism of acidic drugs. *Drug Metab. Rev.* **15,** 1213–1249.

198. Olson, J. A., Moon, R. C., Anders, M. W., Fenselau, C., and Shane, B. (1992) Enhancement of biological activity by conjugation reactions. *J. Nutr.* **122,** 615–624.

199. Spahn-Langguth, H. and Benet, L. Z. (1992) Acyl glucuronides revisited: is the glucuronidation process a toxification as well as a detoxification mechanism? *Drug Metab. Rev.* **24,** 5–47.

200. Pumford, N. R., Myers, T. G., Davila, J. C., Highet, R. J., and Pohl, L. R. (1993) Immunochemical detection of liver protein adducts of the nonsteroidal antiinflammatory drug diclofenac. *Chem. Res. Toxicol.* **6,** 147–150.

201. Myers, T. G., Pumford, N. R., Davila, J. C., and Pohl, L. R. (1992) Covalent binding of diclofenac to plasma membrane proteins of the bile canaliculi in the mouse. *Toxicologist* **12,** 253.

22

Paraneoplastic Autoimmune Reactions

Connie L. Sivinski, Richard M. Tempero, Michelle L. VanLith, and Michael A. Hollingsworth

1. INTRODUCTION

The purpose of this chapter is to describe inflammatory and autoimmune reactions that are secondary to the development of cancer. In some cases, it is believed that inflammatory and autoimmune reactions result from interactions between substances and cells of the immune responses that are directed against tumor cells but cross react with normal tissues.

Immune reactions that destroy tumors (tumor immunity) are desirable autoimmune reactions. The full extent of tumor immunity exhibited by normal individuals is not fully understood. Malignant tumors result when inherited or acquired mutations in a number of oncogenes, tumor suppressor genes, or other cell products cause dysfunction in the regulation of the growth properties of a cell, so that it begins to grow in an uncontrolled manner or in an inappropriate location. Somatic mutations can result in proteins with sequences distinct from "normal" self-antigens. The mutated protein can then be recognized as being foreign by the immune system, and cells expressing the mutated proteins can be rejected by immunological mechanisms similar to those mediating elimination of virally infected cells. These mutated proteins are ideal tumor-specific antigens (TSAs) to which therapy can be directed. The ability of the immune system to identify these antigens as foreign is determined by several parameters, including: the expression of the altered protein at the tumor cell surface either as an unprocessed antigen or as a processed peptide in association with MHC Class I or Class II molecules; the existence in the T-cell and B-cell repertoire of appropriate specificities capable of recognizing the mutated protein as an immunogenic stimulus; the anatomical location of the tumor and its physical accessibility to immunological effector cells. Although difficult to document, it is likely that immune responses to such tumor antigens occur regularly in most patients with cancer, and that these responses protect most healthy individuals from tumors during the course of their lives. The best evidence in support of this theory is the finding that individuals with conditions that cause immunosuppression from birth are more prone to the development of malignant

Contemporary Immunology: Autoimmune Reactions
Edited by: S. Paul © Humana Press Inc., Totowa, NJ

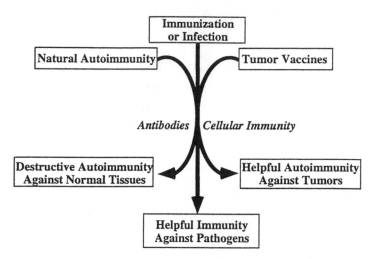

Fig. 1. The cost of immunological defense.

tumors than nonimmunosuppressed individuals. Moreover, animal studies have shown that the immune responses to certain mutated antigens expressed by tumors can confer protection against malignant tumor growth.

Another class of antigens expressed by tumors are tumor-associated antigens (TAAs). TAAs are proteins that are expressed on normal cell types, and they are expressed in an altered form or manner by tumors. Immune responses to these antigens may result in rejection of the tumor, and, simultaneously, some measure of autoimmunity due to the development of antibody or cellular responses to crossreactive antigens expressed on tumors and their normal cellular counterparts (Fig.1). Immunological tolerance to such antigens can be seen as permitting rapid tumor growth, while ameliorating destructive autoimmune responses.

Many tumors produce cytokines and other molecules that are capable of modifying immune responses to tumors (and presumably normal tissues). Thus, we will consider the possibility that aberrant expression of such compounds by malignant tumors can alter immunological homeostasis in the immune system. This may result in suppression of the normal immune responses, and thus influence an organism's ability to mount an effective immune response. One consequence would be an increase in the development of infections in some cancer patients. Alternatively, effects on the normal mechanisms that regulate tolerance to self-proteins may result in autoimmune or inflammatory disorders.

2. AUTOIMMUNE-RELATED PARANEOPLASTIC SYNDROMES IN HUMANS

Paraneoplastic syndromes develop as a result of factors produced by the tumor that act at sites distal to the primary tumor site and its metastases, and may be the first signs of sickness the patient experiences. Frequently, a paraneoplastic syndrome parallels the course of the malignant disease and disappears when the tumor is removed or destroyed. Approximately 7–15% of cancer patients are affected by these syndromes. A smaller percentage of these cancer patients experience paraneoplastic syndromes that have an autoimmune etiology, and may include the production of autoantibodies. In some cases, plasma exchange or treatment with immunosuppressants can alleviate symptoms experienced by these patients. Several mechanisms have been suggested to account for autoimmunity evident in these syndromes: expression of antigens normally restricted to immunologically privileged sites by the tumor, such as central nervous system antigens; secretion of soluble factors by the tumor, which enter the circulation and modify normal self-antigens in such a way as to make them immunogenic to the host *(1)*; production of antibodies directed against the idiotype of antitumor antibodies, which are cross-reactive with normal self-proteins *(2)*; impairment of suppressor T-cell function by factors produced by the tumor, resulting in induction of self-reactive B-cells *(3)*; and production of autoantibodies by the malignant cells themselves, as has been suggested for a number B-cell malignancies *(4,5)*. Table 1 provides a summary of a number of paraneoplastic syndromes with which the presence of autoantibodies has been associated.

Neurological paraneoplastic syndromes, such as paraneoplastic encephalomyelitis or myasthenia gravis, can affect either the central nervous system (CNS) or the peripheral nervous system (PNS) and are associated with specific tumors that are often of neuroectodermal origin *(6)*. Autoantibodies have been identified in the sera of patients with these syndromes; certain antigens reactive with these antibodies have been defined. These include neuronal antigens expressed by tumors outside the central nervous system, in particular, by small cell lung cancers (Table 1). This tumor type is probably of neuroectodermal origin and hence may express cross-reacting neuronal antigens.

Anemia and hemolysis owing to red blood cell (RBC)-specific autoantibodies are the primary clinical features associated with autoimmune hemolytic anemia and cold agglutinin disease (Table 1). These paraneoplastic hematological syndromes are commonly associated with lymphoid malignancies and less commonly with mucin-producing adenocarcinomas. The precise mechanism involved in the production of RBC-specific autoantibodies associated with these malignancies is not understood. It has been suggested that mucins secreted by some adenocarcinomas may alter the RBC antigens, making them more immunogenic to the host *(1)*.

Paraneoplastic cutaneous and muscular syndromes, such as pemphigus, polymyositis (PPM), or dermatomyositis (PDM), are associated with a variety of tumors (Table 1). Although autoantibodies are prominent in all three conditions, cell-mediated immunity, in particular by CD8[+] T lymphocytes, appears to be an important pathogenic mechanism in PPM *(47)*. The mechanism by which malignant tumors influence the development of these paraneoplastic syndromes is not defined. Researchers have suggested that these syndromes may be the result of cross-reacting antibodies to similar antigens in tumor cells, muscle and skin *(2,43)*.

Table 1
Autoimmune-Related Paraneoplastic Syndrome

Syndrome	Tumors	Clinical features	Antibody-defined antigens and potential roles	Ref.
Neurological:				
Paraneoplastic Encephalomyelitis/ Sensory Neuropathy	Small cell lung cancer	Sensory and memory loss; cerebellar, brainstem, motor, or autonomic dysfunction	Neuron-specific RNA-binding proteins (Hu antigens; 35–40 kDa) that may regulate cell proliferation; found in the cerebral cortex, limbic system, brainstem, cerebellum, spinal cord, and dorsal-root ganglion	7–11
Paraneoplastic Cerebral Degeneration	Small cell lung, ovarian and breast cancers	Ataxia of gait; appendicular ataxia; loss of Purkinje cells (pathology)	Purkinje cell-specific proteins (Yo antigens; 34–38 and 62–64 kDa) that may bind DNA and regulate gene expression	12–16
Paraneoplastic Opsoclonus-Myoclonus-Ataxia (POMA)	Neuroblastomas in children; small cell lung, fallopian or breast cancers in adults	Involuntary saccadic eye movements (dancing eyes); truncal and limbic myoclonus (dancing feet); and ataxia	Neuron-specific RNA-binding protein, referred to as Nova-1 (55 kDa) and defined by anti-Ri, that may be responsible for postmigratory maturation of neurons; associated with a mix of brainstem, cerebellar, and/or motor neurons	6,7,17
Cancer-Associated Retinopathy (CAR)	Primarily small lung cell cancers; also prostate, breast or gynecologic cancers	Blurred vision; flashing lights, loss of peripheral and color vision; night blindness	Recoverin, a photoreceptor-specific protein (23–26 kDa) that binds calcium and is involved in signal transduction via cGMP; disruption of signalling results in photoreceptor degeneration	18–24
Paraneoplastic Stiff-Man Syndrome	Breast cancers	Painful muscle cramps and stiffness	Amphiphysin, a protein found in the cytoplasm of all nerve terminals, that binds to dynamin and is involved in vesicle recycling	6,25–28
Lambert-Eaton Myasthenic Syndrome (LEMS)	Small cell lung cancers in 60% of cases	Muscle weakness, depressed tendon reflexes, dysfunction of autonomic nervous system (e.g., dry mouth sexual impotence, constipation)	Voltage-gated calcium channels of presynaptic motor end plates; specifically down-regulated by autoantibodies in SCLC cell lines, which may result in marked reduction of acetylcholine (Ach) release	6,29,30
Myasthenia Gravis (MG)	Thymic epithelial tumors	Progressive muscle weakness and excessive fatigue	Ach receptor (α-subunit) found at the motor end plate of the neuromuscular junction (NMJ); striated muscle proteins (e.g., titin); and neurofilaments; loss of receptors due to complement-mediated lysis; can be compensated to some extent by increased release of Ach at the NMJ	6,31–33

Hematological:

Disease	Associated conditions	Clinical features	Antigen/mechanism	References
Autoimmune Hemolytic Anemia (AIHA)	Chronic lymphocytic leukemia (CLL), non-Hodgkin's lymphoma (NHL), and Hodgkin's disease; less commonly with mucin-producing adenocarcinomas	Hemolysis; anemia due to sequestration of red blood cells in the spleen and destruction by macrophage	Erythrocyte membrane proteins; mucins produced by some tumors may alter red blood cell antigens, making them immunogenic to the host	1,34,35
Cold Agglutinin Disease (CAD)	Waldenström's macroglobulinemia or NHL	Anemia due to sequestration of antibody-tagged red blood cells in the liver	I red cell antigen	35

Cutaneous and Muscular:

Disease	Associated conditions	Clinical features	Antigen/mechanism	References
Paraneoplastic Pemphigus	NHL; less commonly with CLL, benign thymoma, sarcoma, Waldenstrom's macroglobulinemia and bronchogenic squamous cell carcinoma	Painful, extensive skin and mucosal ulcerations	Bullous pemphigoid antigen (230 kDa), desmoplakins-I and -II (250 and 210 kDa, respectively) and as yet an unidentified antigen (190 kDa); found in hemidesmosomes, cytoplasmic plaques or extracellular portions of desmosomes associated with the intercellular junction systems of the skin	2,36–40
Paraneoplastic Polymyositis/ Dermatomyositis (PPM/PDM)	Breast and ovarian cancers in women; lung and gastrointestinal cancers in men	Muscle weakness and elevated muscle enzymes; muscle pain and tenderness in more acute cases; in PDM, erythematous rash involving the face and appendicular joints	Receptors associated with the skin and muscles; in PDM, proteins associated with the microvasculature of muscles appear to be the most important immune targets	41–47

3. THERAPY-RELATED AUTOIMMUNITY IN HUMANS

3.1. Cytokine-Induced Autoimmunity

Cytokines, such as the interferons or interleukins, are normally produced by mononuclear leucocytes and usually exert their effects on cells in the local environment. They exhibit pleiotropic biologic effects, which often synergize, add to, or antagonize the effects of other cytokines. Over the past decade, cytokines have been used clinically in the treatment of a variety of malignant diseases, including hairy cell leukemia, renal cell carcinoma, malignant melanoma, Kaposi's sarcoma, and chronic myelogenous leukemia *(48)*. Results of some studies have indicated that patients undergoing therapy with interferons (IFNs) or interleukin-2 (IL-2) develop varied autoimmune syndromes, which often represent exacerbations of previously latent autoimmunity *(49)*. This is not surprising, considering that large pharmacologic doses have been systemically administered in these therapeutic modalities. Schattner suggests that the multiple activities of these cytokines, when used in nonphysiological doses, may cause an imbalance in immune responses and lead to autoimmune reactions. IFN-α and IL-2, which have been widely used in the treatment of malignant diseases, will be reviewed briefly.

3.1.1. IFN-α

IFN-α is a potent immune modulator that influences cellular proliferation and differentiation. A number of autoimmune diseases, including thyroiditis *(50)*, systemic lupus erythematosus *(51)*, psoriasis *(52)*, autoimmune hemolytic anemia *(53)*, and idiopathic thrombocytopenic purpura *(54)*, have been induced *de novo* or exacerbated by treatment with IFN-α. In the largest study reported to date, 19% of patients (25 of 135) with malignant carcinoid tumors treated with IFN-α-developed autoimmune diseases *(50)*. IFN-α may directly trigger production of pathogenic autoantibodies or up-regulate the expression of Class I and II MHC molecules, which may increase presentation of self-antigens to the immune system (51). The increased self-antigen presentation, coupled with IFN-α-enhanced B-lymphocyte function and production of autoantibodies, could account for the observed autoimmunity.

3.1.2. IL-2

IL-2, another potent immunomodulator, has been used in the clinic to increase tumoricidal activity by the induction of lymphokine-activated killer cells (LAKs). Treatment of malignancies with IL-2 has induced *de novo* autoimmune responses, reactivated quiescent autoimmunity and exacerbated a variety of autoimmune diseases *(48)*. These include hypothyroidism *(55)*, autoimmune hemolytic anemia *(56)*, diabetes mellitus *(57)*, chronic inflammatory arthritis resembling rheumatoid arthritis *(58)* and vasculitis *(59)*. Several mechanisms have been proposed to account for the effects of IL-2 on the development of autoimmune diseases. Autoreactive T- and B-lymphocytes, which are believed to be immunologically inactive (anergic), are present in healthy individuals

(57). IL-2 may abrogate anergy to self-antigens, which could induce organ-specific autoimmune diseases. The activation of anergic clones may result in the production of autoantibodies or of autoreactive cytotoxic T-lymphocytes, either of which may exert destructive effects on normal tissues.

3.2. Graft-vs-Tumor Effect: Induction of Tumor Autoimmunity

Autologous bone marrow transplantation (BMT), which involves intensive high-dose chemotherapy followed by infusion of cryopreserved autologous bone marrow, is a therapeutic option for the treatment of lymphohematopoietic malignancies and solid tumors, such as leukemias, lymphomas, and metastatic breast cancers *(60).* Tumor recurrence continues to be the primary cause of treatment failures, even though long-term disease-free survival can be attained in a relatively high percentage of cases. The rate of tumor recurrence in patients who receive allogeneic BMT is significantly lower than the rate of those who receive autologous BMT *(61,62).* This enhanced antitumor effect develops in approximately 50–70% of allogeneic BMT patients, and it may be due to the development of graft-versus-host disease (GVHD) that eliminates some of the tumor burden in these patients. It is thought that mature donor lymphocytes from the marrow graft, which respond to foreign major and/or minor histocompatibility (MHC/MiHC) antigens of the recipient, also recognize and destroy residual tumor cells *(60).* This antitumor response is referred to as the graft-versus-tumor (GVT) effect. If GVHD is prevented in these patients by removal of T-cells from the graft, there is a significant increase in the number of patients who relapse *(63).*

Although a GVT effect is normally absent in autologous BMT, an autoimmune GVHD-like syndrome can be observed after autologous BMT by treating patients with cyclosporin-A (CsA) alone or with CsA and IFN-γ *(64,65).* Treatment of patients with both CsA and IFN-γ increases the severity of the autologous GVHD. The in vitro studies on patients with non-Hodgkin's lymphoma or Hodgkin's disease undergoing autologous BMT and CsA treatment have detected autoreactive cytolytic T-cells in patients experiencing cutaneous GVHD *(65).* The cytolytic cells were capable of lysing pretransplant lymphocytes from the patients as well as lymphocytes from healthy third party donors. The lytic activity was blocked by treating target lymphocytes with antibodies directed against Class II MHC molecules. Lymphocytes obtained after resolution of the GVHD-like syndrome were no longer reactive against the patient's own pretransplant lymphocytes or lymphocytes from healthy donors. CsA is thought to inhibit clonal deletion of autocytotoxic thymic T-cells, which recognize self antigens in the context of MHC Class II antigens (including Class II antigens on tumor cells), while IFN-γ upregulates the expression of MHC Class II molecules on many cell types, including tumor cells *(64).* It is understandable, therefore, that CsA induces the GVHD-like syndrome and IFN-γ augments this effect. The approach of inducing an autoimmune syndrome to eliminate residual tumor cells appears promising *(60),* although it is too early to determine the overall efficacy of this type of treatment in lowering the relapse rate of lymphoid malignancies and solid tumors.

4. AUTOIMMUNE DISEASES ASSOCIATED WITH TUMOR VACCINE MODELS

A number of tumor vaccine strategies aimed at increasing the tumor immunogenicity and more specifically targeting immune effector cells to the tumor are currently under investigation. These strategies can be divided into two categories: nonspecific tumor vaccines and tumor antigen-based vaccines. Transgenic (TG) mouse models are frequently being utilized to evaluate the efficacy of some tumor vaccines.

4.1. Nonspecific Vaccines

These strategies are designed to overcome immunological tolerance to TAA without inducing severe autoimmune disease. Some investigators have attempted to increase the immunogenicity of tumors by transfecting tumor cells with cytokines or co-stimulatory molecules. Cytokines transfected into tumor cells include IL-2 *(66)*, IL-6 *(67)*, GM-CSF *(68)*, and IFN-γ *(69)*. The cDNA encoding a costimulatory gene, such as B7, is often cotransfected into tumors as part of these strategies *(70)*. Although the success rate varies depending on the nature of the tumor target and the immunization strategy, immunization with transfected tumor cells has usually been observed to increase the immunogenicity of the tumor, decrease the ability of the tumor to metastasize, and provide protection against parental tumors. A potential drawback of these vaccine strategies is that they may induce an immune response against self antigens expressed by both the tumor and normal tissue. Often, there has been no evaluation of autoimmune diseases in these studies.

4.2. Tumor Antigen Vaccines

Tumor vaccines directed against TSAs are less complex than those directed against TAAs because there is no attempt to disrupt the mechanisms of immunological tolerance. Vaccines directed against TSAs are unlikely to produce autoimmune disease because the antigens are expressed by tumor cells, but not by normal tissue. Human TAAs generally have substantially different sequences from the corresponding TAAs in other species. Moreover, differences in MHC antigens and in other genes that regulate the immune responses of humans and other species make it difficult to directly correlate the cause of autoimmune disease in different species. Therefore, preclinical studies in mice *(71)* using human TAAs may not adequately address the issue of immunological tolerance and autoimmunity to self-proteins. Table 2 lists some of the animal models currently used to study tumor vaccine efficacy.

Mdm2 (murine double minute) is a TAA overexpressed by a number of transformed murine cells. Dahl et al. demonstrated that unimmunized mice contain

Table 2
Animal Models Used to Evaluate Tumor Immunotherapy

	Animal model	Tumor type	Antigen	Ref.
Tumor-specific antigen	SCID mouse reconstituted with human lymphocytes	Human tumor		72
	Normal mouse	Syngenic tumor	p53	73,74
Tumor-associated antigen	SCID mouse (transgenic for TAA to evaluate autoimmunity reconstituted with human lymphocytes	Human tumor	CD 30	75
			TAG72	76
	Mouse trangenic for human TAA	Syngenic tumor expressing human TAA	MUC1	77
			FBL-*env*	78
	Normal mouse	Syngenic tumor expressing murine homolog of TAA	gp75	79,80
			P1A	81

cytolytic T-lymphocytes (CTLs) specific for mdm2, cyclin D1, and p53. CTLs specific for mdm2 recognized target cells infected with vaccinia virus expressing the cDNA for mdm2 *(82)*. This study did not evaluate the reactivity of the CTLs with nontransformed cells expressing mdm2, or the ability of the CTLs to provide tumor protection without serious autoimmune side effects in vivo. The induction of autoreactive CTLs underscores the potential utility of peptide-based tumor vaccine strategies.

A limited number of in vivo studies have evaluated autoimmunity and antitumor immunity resulting from TAA-specific antibodies and CTLs. HER2/neu is a TAA that is overexpressed by a number of malignancies, including breast and ovarian cancers. Disis et al. *(83)* demonstrated that rats immunized with peptides from HER2/neu produced T-cells specific for rat HER2/neu peptides. Antibodies produced by immunization with the rat HER2/neu protein were reactive with lysates from SKBR3, a human breast cancer cell line that over-expresses HER2/neu. The immunized rats showed no evidence of autoimmune disease, as evaluated by the absence of lymphocyte infiltration in tissues that normally express HER2/neu. These studies did not address whether immunization provides protection from tumor growth or metastasis.

Several evaluations of autoimmunity have been conducted with gp75, a TAA that has 90% amino acid identity in mice and humans, and is expressed by both melanoma cells and melanocytes. Hara et al. *(80)* found that injection of TA99, an antibody reactive with gp75, lead to tumor rejection and depigmentation of coat color following depilation. These results support the hypothesis that tumor rejection in this model is mediated by antibodies, and that these antibodies are reactive with gp75 expressed by normal cells. Natftzger et al. *(79)* demonstrated that immunization of mice with murine gp75 produced by insect cells or with human gp75, but not wildtype gp75, resulted in production of antibodies directed against murine gp75. The immunizations also protected mice from gp75-expressing B16F10 tumors. In contrast, no protection was seen with the gp75-negative melanoma SK-MEL-131. Mice immunized with gp75 purified from insect cells developed depigmentation of coat color without depilation, although histological analysis revealed no infiltrates of mononuclear cells. Changes in pigmentation were not observed in the eye, an organ known to express gp75.

The autoimmune consequences of producing tumor immunity with the murine tumor rejection antigen P1A has been examined in vivo *(81)*. P1A is expressed by P815 cells, a murine mastocytoma cell line, as well as by other tumor types and by normal testes and placenta. Male and pregnant female mice immunized with P1A-expressing P815 cells induced CTLs specific for P1A. Histological analyses of testes from mice immunized with L1210 cells, which also express P1A, revealed no inflammation or lymphocytic infiltrate. Similarly, placentae from immunized pregnant females showed normal gestation. In the testes and placenta, P1A expression is limited to spermatogonia and labyrinthine trophoblast cells, respectively. Human spermatogonia and trophoblast cells lack expression of MHC Class I molecules. The authors *(81)* concluded that the absence of Class I MHC expression enables these cells to escape attack by CTLs specific for P1A.

4.3. Transgenic Mouse Models of Tumor Vaccine Efficacy

Transgenic mice expressing TSA or TAA molecules are useful in vivo models to investigate tolerance and autoimmunity in vaccination against tumors. The most informative models are those in which the TAA is overexpressed in the appropriate tissues. One example of a TG model used to evaluate tolerance and autoimmunity has been described by Hu et al. *(78)*, using FBL tumor cells derived from a Friend virus-induced erythroleukemia of C57BL/6 mice. Two tumor antigens derived from this virus, the *env*- and *gag*-encoded viral proteins, have been characterized. Mice transgenic for the *env*-protein were developed using a lymphoid-specific promotor, resulting in expression of the *env*-protein in the spleen, thymus, and peripheral B- and T-cells. Both unimmunized TG and non-TG mice died within 20 days of challenge with FBL tumor cells. In contrast, the non-TG mice survived when immunized with *env*-prior to challenge, whereas the TG mice died by day 20. TG mice could be protected from progressive tumor growth if T-cells from immunized non-TG mice were injected with cyclophosphamide prior to challenge with FBL cells. Neither the immunization protocol nor the transfer of T-cells from immunized mice to the TG mice induced detectable autoimmune disease in the lymphoid tissues. These results indicate that *env*-TG mice are tolerant to *env*-protein. Although this model does not use a human TAA, the results suggest the usefulness of TG model systems for evaluating tolerance to TAA and the autoimmune consequences of anti-TAA immunity.

C57Bl/6 mice transgenic for the human TAA MUC1 (MUC1.Tg) have been developed, in which MUC1 is expressed in a temporal and spatial pattern similar to seen in humans. MUC1.Tg mice developed progressively growing tumors following challenge with a syngeneic melanoma cell line, the MUC1-expressing B16 cell line. In contrast, wildtype mice produced smaller and slow-growing tumors when challenged with the same dose of the MUC1-expressing B16 cells. Tumors obtained from wildtype mice were negative for MUC1 protein expression, while tumors from MUC1.Tg mice retained the MUC1 expression. MUC1-specific antibodies (IgM, IgG1, and IgG3) were also detected in wildtype mice, but not in MUC1.Tg mice. These results suggest that the MUC1.Tg mice are tolerant to MUC1. Studies are underway to evaluate the mechanisms that regulate this tolerance, and to explore the possibility of breaking tolerance with adoptive cellular therapy, using immune cells from wildtype mice.

5. TOLERANCE AND TUMOR IMMUNITY

The last decade has provided a greater understanding of the mechanisms that regulate immunological tolerance to self antigens. Much effort has been invested in elucidating the regulatory steps that fail in the course of autoimmune disease. The results of several experimental models of autoimmunity suggested the existence of autoreactive B- and T-lymphocytes. This led to the hypothesis that antiself-responses can be used for tumor immunotherapy. Popular topics for investigation included the extent of detection of autoreactive T- and B-lymphocyte within the thymus and bone marrow, reversal of anergy by peripheral lymphocytes, and the concept of autoimmune-mediated tumor regression. In this section, we will consider the immunological barriers that preclude tumor antigen recognition.

5.1. Overcoming Central T-Cell Tolerance

The dominant tolerogenic mechanisms affecting T-lymphocytes are intrathymic positive and negative selection *(84–86)*. Neither of these processes is entirely effective. For example, autoreactive T-cells can escape thymic deletion and exist in the peripheral T-cell pool. One explanation for this is that the thymus may not express all self-proteins, in effect being unable to tolerate potentially self-reactive T-cells. Another possibility is that the immune system does not achieve tolerance to all epitopes of self antigens and may react only with the most immunodominant epitopes. Thymic epithelial cells process and present self proteins to tolerate the developing T-cells compartments. Self-proteins that do not form stable complexes with thymic MHC molecules or those that are expressed with low frequency (subdominant or cryptic epitopes) may not induce T-cell tolerance, permitting autoreactive clones to exist in the mature T-cell repertoire *(87–89)*.

Effective immunization with TAA requires that the organism recognize and respond to a nonmutated self-protein expressed on both tumor and normal tissue.

Fulminant immune reactions toward self-proteins are difficult to produce, except in instances leading to autoimmune disease. For example, immunization with a single epitope of myelin basic protein (MBP) initially induces a restricted T-cell response in a murine model of multiple sclerosis, experimental autoimmune encephalomyelitis. Over the course of this disease, the pattern of T-cell reactivity broadens to include several cryptic epitopes contained within MBP *(90–92)*. Other models of B- and T-cell-mediated autoimmunity have a similar process: priming of autoreactive T-cells with cryptic self-epitopes can produce autoimmunity that expands to previously nonimmunogenic epitopes on self-proteins *(93)*. These findings have encouraged the exploration of preclinical models designed to induce antiself immunity that will eventually translate into an effective cancer therapy. Recently, five T-cell epitopes in the gp100 melanoma antigen with relatively low HLA-A2 binding affinity have been characterized. These contain nondominant amino acid residues for several of the anchor positions that contribute to HLA-A2 binding *(94)*. This finding is consistent with the hypothesis that nonmutated melanoma T-cell epitopes may serve as cryptic self-epitopes found within the TAA gp100.

Immunization with subdominant or cryptic epitopes has been tested as a means to create autoimmune reactivity against tumors overexpressing a TAA. For example, rats immunized with the cellular oncogene product HER2/neu did not develop immunity, however, rats immunized with selected HER2/neu peptides developed specific B- and T-cell responses to HER2/neu *(83)*. One interpretation is that the dominant epitopes within the HER2/neu protein effectively tolerized all HER-2/neu responsive T-cells. In contrast, the immune response produced by HER2/neu peptide immunogens may have resulted from subdominant epitopes within the HER2/neu protein that by themselves are unable to induce effective thymic and peripheral T-cell tolerance. These findings suggest that the T-cells reactive with the HER2/neu subdominant epitope escaped thymic deletion and remained responsive in the periphery. Stimulation of T-cell responses to TAA that are also expressed in normal tissues may cause a certain level of autoimmunity. Should this be the case, the destructive consequences of inducing antitumor T-cell responses that react with normal cells will need to be weighed against the benefit of providing tumor immunity.

5.2. Tumor Immunity and the Breakdown of Peripheral T-Cell Tolerance

The immune system has both intrathymic and extrathymic (peripheral) mechanisms to control autoreactive T-cells *(95,96)*. As dicussed above, it is possible to overcome at least some mechanisms that enforce peripheral T-cell tolerance. Several categories of peripheral T-cell tolerance exist, including: lack of costimulation, activation-induced cell death, and suppressor T-cells.

T-cell expansion and differentiation require TCR engagement (signal 1) and noncognate interactions between CD28 on the T-cell and B7-1 or B7-2 on the antigen-presenting cell (APC) (signal 2). Activation of TCR/CD28 is important to the development of normal humoral responses, transplant rejection, ini-

Table 3
Characteristics of Tumor Cells Expressing Costimulatory Molecules

Tumor line/model	Costimulatory molecule	Tumorgenicity	Effector cell	Wt protection	Ref.
Murine melanoma, K1735	B7.1	Weak	CD8	Yes	*111*
Murine melanoma BC16 and BC22 derived from K1735	E7 of HPV-16 B7.1	Weak	CD8	Yes	*112*
Murine T-lymphoma, EL-4	B7.1	Weak	ND	Yes	*113*
Murine sarcoma, SaI	B7.1 and MHC Class II	Weak	CD4	Yes	*114*
Murine plasmacytoma, J558	B7.1	Weak	CD8	No	*99*
Murine melanoma B16-BL6	B7.1	Weak	ND	Yes	*115*
Murine melanoma B16	B7.1	Strong	NA	No	*113*
Murine fibrosarcoma Ag104	B7.1	Strong	NA	No	*113*
Murine mastocytoma P815	B7.2	Weak	CD8	Yes	*116*
Murine fibrosarcoma MCA102	B7.2	Strong	NA	No	*116*
Murine mammary adenocarcinoma TS/A	B7.1 ICAM-1	Strong	CD4 CD8	Yes	*117*

tiation of autoimmune disease, and enhanced tumor immunogenicity *(97)*. A number of investigators have adopted strategies in which tumor cells are genetically manipulated to express costimulatory molecules, thus gaining the capacity to stimulate tumor-specific T-cells in vivo *(98)*. Tumor cells expressing costimulatory molecules are usually better immunogens than parental tumor cells (Table 3). Mice challenged with J558-B7 cells, an MHC class II-negative tumor cell line transfected with B7-1, induced CD8$^+$ T-cell-dependent, CD4$^+$ T-cell-independent tumor rejection *(99)*. Mice challenged with J558 cells transfected with the expression vector alone (J558-Neo) had a significantly higher incidence of tumors, indicating that the expression of B7-1 was responsible for tumor rejection. Results of in vitro cytotoxicity assays demonstrated that B7-1 was not the target antigen recognized by these antitumor CTLs. Unlike many of the experimental models described in Table 3, J558-B7 cells were unable to induce immunity to J558-Neo cells, indicating that there is little or no bystander effect in this tumor model.

The greater immunogenicity of the B7-1-transfected tumor cells compared to control-transfected tumor cell is reminiscent of the results obtained in several autoimmunity models in which nonlymphoid antigens (e.g., tissue-specific transgene products) did not elicit autoimmune reactions unless they were coexpressed with costimulatory molecules, such as B7-1 or B7-2 *(100,101)*. The results of these studies share a common feature: the induction of T-cell-mediated autoimmunity or tumor immunity relies on the expression of the antigen and costimulatory molecules in the appropriate context. A major theme emerging from confluence of results concerning pathogenesis of autoimmunity and the induction of tumor immunity is that autoreactive and tumor-specific clones do exist, and given the proper stimulation, can be activated.

5.3. Autoimmunity and the Breakdown of B-Cell Tolerance

The production of high affinity IgG antibodies is a T-cell-dependent process. For this reason, it has been postulated that T-cell tolerance is required to effectively tolerize the B-cell response *(102)*. However, B-lymphocytes are more than passive players in the immune response. They participate cooperatively with T-cells during various stages of immunological selection, activation, differentiation, and effector function. Studies in several experimental models have demonstrated that B-cell tolerance can be overcome, in some cases, with pathological consequences.

Table 1 lists several antibody-mediated autoimmune disorders associated with neoplasia. B-cell-mediated autoimmune diseases that have no apparent association with cancer may result from: the release of extrathymic or sequestered autoantigens; the failure to suppress self-reactive B-cell clones; polyclonal B-cell activation; or a bypass of T-cell tolerance *(96)*. Observations that certain types of tumor cells can cull and activate self-reactive B-cells raises several questions related to induction of self-reactive antibodies, including: 1) by what mechanisms can tumors cause self-reactive B-cell stimulation, 2) what is the degree of tumor immunity provided by the self-reactive antibodies, and 3) can TAA vaccines be administered to induce B-cell mediated tumor autoimmunity?

The postulate that immature self-reactive B-cells are physically eliminated within the bone marrow is supported by abundant evidence *(103–107)*. Deletion of B-cells reactive to cell surface antigens eliminates the possibility of their subsequent participation in an immune response; however, not every autoreactive B-cell clone is eliminated. The somatic mechanisms that contribute to the generation of diversity in B-cells make it possible to continuously develop autoreactive specificities. Thus, functional inactivation by processes such as anergy are important to the maintenance of peripheral B-cell tolerance *(103,104)*. Autoantibodies, such as DNA antibodies, are normally present in the serum of healthy individuals, presumably due to the incomplete deletion or incomplete inactivation of peripheral anti-DNA B-cells. A mouse transgenic (TG) for anti-DNA immunoglobulin was developed to address the question of B-cell tolerance towards disease-associated targets, such as DNA. Most TG B-cells bound DNA, yet they failed to secrete anti-DNA antibodies, suggesting that the DNA-reactive B-cells were not clonally eliminated, but instead, were developmentally arrested *(103)*.

Several studies report the expression of immunoglobulin transgene products to self- or pseudo-self-antigens without autoimmune consequences *(103–106)*. Mice transgenic for an autoantibody to erythrocytes were produced to create an experimental model for autoimmune hemolytic anemia *(107)*. The functional inactivations B-cells in these mice was incomplete. Both deletion and anergy of autoreactive B-cells were observed, although a significant fraction of mice developed hemolytic anemia. It was proposed that the autoimmune phenomenon was a result of the pathogenicity of the germline-encoded autoantibody. The results of this study suggesed that autoreactive B-cells are capable of inducing autoimmune disease under certain circumstances.

5.4. Tumor Immunity and the Breakdown of B-Cell Tolerance

Tumor immunotherapy protocols generally evaluate the induction of CTLs, rather than the production of antibodies directed towards TSA or TAA. Few experimental models exist to evaluate the efficacy of active, antibody-mediated tumor immunity. Recent analyses of human antibody-tumor antigen recognition patterns, however, have provided some insights into the regulation of B-cell tolerance to tumor antigens.

The tumor suppressor gene p53 has multiple mutational "hot spots." Patients with colorectal cancer, which express mutant p53 or Ras, have detectable antibodies to p53 or Ras. However, these antibodies are directed towards the nonmutated p53 or Ras domains, areas that represent the self-protein *(108,109)*. The presence of p53 antibodies in patients with colorectal cancer has been correlated with poor prognosis, although the causal aspects of this relationship are not well understood. This example illustrates that much of the detectable antibody response to a mutant oncoprotein can be directed against normal self proteins. Thus, the B-cell compartment retains a certain degree of self-reactivity towards tumor antigens.

The growth factor receptor HER2/neu is overexpressed in approximately 30% of breast and ovarian cancers. HER2/neu specific antibodies can be found in patients with HER2/neu positive tumors *(109)*. The function of these antibodies is unknown; however, study of a HER2/neu transgenic (TG) mouse model suggest that the antibodies may be therapeutic *(110)*. Injection of HER2/neu antibodies into HER2/neu TG mice prevented tumor growth in 50% of the mice that ordinarily would develop HER2/neu positive tumors. It appears that the antitumor efficacy of the HER2/neu antibody treatment involved a reduction in the HER2/neu signal transduction capacity *(110)*.

Passive antibody infusions may be used to evaluate the efficacy of antibody-mediated tumor immunity. For example, administration of a mouse MAb against the tyrosinase-related protein 1 (gp75) induced the rejection of both subcutaneous and lung metastases of the B16F10 tumor in a murine model *(79,80)*. Passive transfer of antibodies directed towards gp75, a melanocyte differentiation antigen, induced a degree of autoimmunity to melanocytes, resulting in alterations of coat color. In humans, administration of TAA-specific antibodies is often limited by nonspecific antibody interactions, host immune responses to the antibodies, and rapid antibody clearance.

6. CONCLUSIONS AND PERSPECTIVES

It is clear that inflammatory and autoimmune reactions can occur secondary to the development of cancer. In some cases, these conditions may aid in the destruction of tumor cells, even though they cause some degree of autoimmunity. Moreover, it is anticipated that future studies of tumor vaccine preparations, particularly effective vaccines, will have autoimmune consequences for the patient. Thus, tumor immunity and autoimmunity are in many ways similar processes to which there are both desirable and undesirable outcomes.

It is possible that some inflammatory conditions that are currently unexplained may be associated with antitumor responses. For example, a high percentage of patients with chronic ulcerative colitis ultimately develop colon tumors. It has been postulated that the colon tumors are secondary to the chronic inflammation that occurs at those sites, however, it is equally possible that the chronic inflammation at sites of ulcerative colitis are in part caused by autoimmune responses against premalignant or malignant cells that have arisen at that site and express an array of mutated gene products that serve as rejection antigens for the immune system. There are reports of the detection of mutated oncogenes (k-Ras) or of immune responses to mutated tumor suppressor genes (p53) in some cases of chronic pancreatitis *(118–120)*. Thus, an important subject that should be investigated in the future is to determine if unusual inflammatory reactions in otherwise unexplained cases represent autoimmune reactions against malignant or premalignant cells.

A conclusion that was controversial in the past but is now more widely accepted is that most individuals retain the ability to mount antiself immune responses, and that a combination of central and peripheral immune mechanisms are important in regulating these responses. Further research leading to a better understanding of the regulation of tolerance and immunity should provide us with tools and concepts that will help in treating both cancer and autoimmune disease.

REFERENCES

1. Cobo, F., Pereira, A., Nomdedeu, B., Gallart, T., Ordi, J., Torne, A., et al. (1996) Ovarian dermoid cyst-associated autoimmune hemolytic anemia: A case report with emphasis on pathogenic mechanisms. *J. Clin. Pathol.* **105**, 567–571.
2. Plotz, P. H. (1983) Autoantibodies are anti-idiotype antibodies to anti-viral antibodies. *Lancet* **2**, 824–829.
3. Van Roenn, J., Harris, J.E., and Braun, D. P. (1987) Suppressor cell function in solid tumor cancer patients. *J. Clin. Oncol.* **5**, 150–159.
4. Saikia, N. K. (1972) Extraction of pemphigus antibodies from a lymphoid neoplasm and its possible relationship to pemphigus vulgaris. *Br. J. Dermatol.* **86**, 411–414.
5. Bataille, R., Klein, B., Durie, B. G. M., and Sany, J. (1989) Interrelationship between autoimmunity and B-lymphoid cell oncogenesis in humans. *Clin. Exp. Rheumatol.* **7**, 319–328.

6. Lang, B. and Vincent, A. (1996) Autoimmunity to ion-channels and other proteins in paraneoplastic disorders. *Curr. Opin. Immunol.* **8,** 865–871.

7. Darnell, R. B. (1996) Onconeural antigens and the paraneoplastic neurologic disorders: At the intersection of cancer, immunity, and the brain. *Proc. Natl. Acad. Sci. USA* **93,** 4529–4536.

8. Anderson, N. E., Rosenblum, M. K., Graus, F., Wiley, R. G., and Posner, J. B. (1988) Auto-antibodies in paraneoplastic syndromes in small cell lung cancer. *Neurology* **38,** 1391–1398.

9. Furneaus, H. F., Reich, L., and Posner, J. B. (1990) Autoantibody synthesis in the central nervous system of patients with paraneoplastic syndromes. *Neurology* **40,** 1085–1091.

10. Liu, J., Dalmau, J., Szabo, A., Rosenfeld, M., Huber, J., and Furneaux, H. (1995) Paraneoplastic encephalomyelitis antigens bind to the AU-rich elements of mRNA. *Neurology* **45,** 544–550.

11. Richardson, G. E. and Johnson, B. E. (1992) Paraneoplastic syndromes in lung cancer. *Curr. Opin. Oncol.* **4,** 323–333.

12. Henson, R. A. and Urich, H. (1982) Cortical cerebellar degeneration, in *Cancer and the Nervous System* (Henson, R. A. and Urich, H., eds.), Blackwell Scientific, London, pp. 346–367.

13. Cunningham, J., Graus, F., Anderson, N., and Posner, J. B. (1986) Partial characterization of the Purkinje cell antigens in paraneoplastic cerebellar degeneration. *Neurology* **36,** 1163–1168.

14. Anderson, N. E., Rosenblum, M. K., and Posner, J. B. (1988) Paraneoplastic cerebellar degeneration: Clinical immunological correlations. *Ann. Neurol.* **24,** 559–567.

15. Furneaux, H. M., Rosenblum, M. K., Dalmau, J., Wong, E., Woodruff, P., Graus, F., et al. (1990) Selective expression of Purkinje-cell antigens in tumor tissue from patients with paraneoplastic cerebellar degeneration. *N. Engl. J. Med.* **322,** 844–1851.

16. Fathallah-Shaykh, H., Wolf, S., Wong, E., Posner, J. B., and Furneaux, H. M. (1991) Cloning of a leucine-zipper protein recognized by the sera of patients with antibody-associated paraneoplastic cerebellar degeneration. *Proc. Natl. Acad. Sci. USA* **88,** 3451–3454.

17. Fueyo, J., Ferrer, I., Valldeoriola, F., and Graus, F. (1993) The expression of a neuronal nuclear antigen (Ri) recognized by the human anti-Ri autoantibody in the developing rat nervous system. *Neurosci. Lett.* **162,** 141–144.

18. Thirkill, C. E. (1996) Lung cancer-induced blindness. *Lung Cancer* **14,** 253–264.

19. Lafeuillade, A., Quilichini, R., Chiozza, R., Pellegrino, P., and Thirkill, C. E. (1993) Paraneoplastic retinopathy (CAR syndrome) revealing prostatic cancer. *Presse Med.* **22,** 35.

20. Thirkill, C. E. (1994) Cancer associated retinopathy, the CAR syndrome. *Neuro-ophthalmol.* **14,** 297–323.

21. Dizhoor, A. M., Ray, S., Kumar, S., Niemi, G., Spencer, M., Brolley, D., et al. (1991) Recoverin: a calcium sensitive activator of retinal rod guanylate cyclase. *Science* **251,** 915–918.

22. Polans, A. S., Burton, M. D., Halet, T. L., Crabb, J. W., and Palczewski, K. (1993) Recoverin, but not visinin, is an autoantigen in the human retina identified with a cancer-associated retinopathy. *Invest. Ophthalmol. Vis. Sci.* **34,** 81–90.

23. Lem, J., Flannery, J. G., Li, T., Applebury, M. L., Farber, D. B., and Simon, M. I. (1992) Retinal degeneration is rescued in transgenic *rd* mice by expression of the cGMP phosphodiesterase beta subunit. *Proc. Natl. Acad. Sci. USA* **89**, 4422–4426.

24. Smith, D. P., Ranganathan, R., Hardey, R. W., Marx, J., Tsuchida, T., and Zuker, C. S. (1991) Photoreceptor deactivation and retinal degeneration mediated by a photoreceptor-specific protein kinase C. *Science* **254**, 1478–1484.

25. Moersch, F. P. and Woltman, H. W. (1956) Progressive fluctuating muscular rigidity and spasm ("stiff-man syndrome"): report of a case and some observations in 13 other cases. *Mayo Clin. Proc.* **31**, 421–427.

26. Folli, F., Solimena, M., Cofiell, R., Austoni, M., Tallini, G., Fassetta, G., et al. (1993) Autoantibodies to a 128-kd synaptic protein in three women with the stiff-man syndrome and breast cancer. *N. Engl. J. Med.* **328**, 546–551.

27. Grimaldi, L. M. E., Martino, G., Braghi, S., Quattrini, A., Furlan, R., Bosi, E., et al. (1993) Heterogeneity of autoantibodies in stiff-man syndrome. *Ann. Neurol.* **34**, 57–64.

28. David, C., McPherson, P. S., Mundigl, O., and De Camilla, P. (1996) A role of amphiphysin in synaptic vesical endocytosis suggested by its binding to dynamin in nerve terminals. *Proc. Natl. Acad. Sci. USA* **93**, 331–335.

29. O'Neill, J. H., Murray, N. M., and Nesom-Davis, J. (1988) The Lambert-Eaton myasthenic syndrome. A review of 50 cases. *Brain* **111**, 577–596.

30. Viglione, M. P., O'Shaughnessy, J., and Kim, Y. I. (1995) Inhibition of calcium currents and exocytosis by Lambert-Eaton syndrome antibodies in human lung cancer cells. *J. Physiol.* **488**, 303–317.

31. Vincent, A. (1994) Aetiological factors in development of myasthenia gravis. *Adv. Neuroimmunol.* **4**, 355–371.

32. Marx, A., Wilisch, A., Schultz, A., Greiner, A., Magi, B., Pallini, V., et al. (1996) Expression of neurofilaments and of a titin epitope in thymic epithelial tumors: implications for the pathogenesis of myasthenia gravis. *Am. J. Pathol.* **148**,1839–1850.

33. Kaminski, H. J., Fenstermaker, R. A., Abdul-Karim, F. W., Clayman, J., and Ruff, R. L. (1993) Acetylcholine receptor subunit gene expression in thymic tissue. *Muscle Nerve* **16**, 1332–1337.

34. Evers, J., Albert, F., Bazar, L., Sulica, V., and Sacher, R. A. (1992) Autoimmune hemolytic anemia presenting in Sezary syndrome: report of a case and review of the literature. *Acta Haematol.* **88**, 46–49.

35. Frenkel, E. P., Bick, R. L., and Rutherford, C. J. (1996) Anemia of malignancy. *Hematol./Oncol. Clin. North Am.* **10**, 861–873.

36. Joly, P., Thomine, E., Gilbert, D., Verdier, S., Delpech, A., Prost, C., et al. (1994) Overlapping distribution of autoantibody specificities in paraneoplastic pemphigus and pemphigus vulgaris. *J. Invest. Dermatol.* **103**, 65–72.

37. Masayuki, A., Klaus-Kovtun, V., and Stanley, J. R. (1991) Autoantibodies against a novel epithelial cadherin in pemphigus vulgaris, a disease of cell adhesion. *Cell* **67**, 869–877.

38. Anhalt, G. J., Kim, S. C., Stanley, J. R., Korman, N. J., Jabs, D. A., Kory, M., et al. (1990) Paraneoplastic pemphigus. An autoimmune mucocutaneous disease associated with neoplasia. *N. Engl. J. Med.* **323**, 1729–1735.

39. Helm, T. N., Camisa, C., Valenzuela, R., and Allen, C. M. (1993) Paraneoplastic pemphigus. A distinct autoimmune vesiculobullous disorder associated with neoplasia. *Oral Surg. Oral Med. Oral Pathol.* **75**, 209–213.

40. Camisa, C., Helm, T. N., Liu, Y. C., Valenzuela, R., Allen, C., Bona, S., et al. (1992) Paraneoplastic pemphigus: a report of three cases including one long-term survivor. *J. Am. Acad. Dermatol.* **27**, 547–553.
41. Mastaglia, F. L. and Ojeda, V. J. (1985) Inflammatory myopathies: Part 1. *Ann. Neurol.* **17**, 217– 227.
42. Barnes, B. E. (1976) Dermatomyositis and malignancy. A review of the literature. *Ann. Intern. Med.* **84**, 68–76.
43. Callen, J. P. (1982) The value of malignancy evaluation in patients with dermatomyositis. *J. Am. Acad. Dermatol.* **6**, 253–259.
44. Callen, J. P. (1984) Myositis and malignancy. *Clin. Rheum. Dis.* **10**, 117–130.
45. Emslie-Smith, A. M. and Engel, A. G. (1990) Microvascular changes in early and advanced dermatomyositis: a quantitative study. *Ann. Neurol.* **27**, 343–334.
46. Kissel, J. T., Mendell, J. R., and Rammohan, K. W. (1986) Microvascular deposition of complement membrane attack complex in dermatomyositis. *N. Engl. J. Med.* **314**, 331–334.
47. Targoff, I. N. (1993) Humoral immunity in polymyositis/dermatomyositis. *J. Invest. Dermatol.* **100**, 116S–123S.
48. Vial, T. and Descotes, J. (1995) Immune-mediated side-effects of cytokines in humans. *Toxicology* **105**, 31–57.
49. Schnatter, A. (1994) Lymphokines in autoimmunity-A critical review. *Clin. Immunol. Immunopathol.* **70**, 177–189.
50. Ronnblom, L. E., Alm, G. V., and Oberg, K. E. (1991) Autoimmunity after alpha-interferon therapy for malignant carcinoid tumor. *Ann. Intern. Med.* **1151**, 178–183.
51. Ronnblom, L. E., Alm, G. V., and Oberg, K. E. (1990) Possible induction of systemic lupus erythematosus by interferon-a treatment in a patient with a malignant carcinoid tumor. *J. Intern. Med.* **227**, 207–210.
52. Wolfe, J. T., Singh, A., Lessin, S. R., Jaworsky, C., and Rook, A. H. (1995) De novo development of psoriatic plaques in patients receiving interferon alfa for treatment of erythrodermic cutaneous T-cell lymphoma. *J. Am. Acad. Dermatol.* **32**, 887–893.
53. Pangalis, G. and Griva, E. (1988) Recombinant alfa-2b interferon therapy in untreated stages A and B chronic lymphocytic leukemia. *Cancer* **1**, 869–872.
54. Abdi, E. A., Brien, W., and Venner, P. M. (1986) Auto-immune thrombocytopenia related to interferon therapy. *Scan. J. Haematol.* **36**, 515–519.
55. Atkins, M. B., Mier, J. W., Parkinson, D. R., Gould, J. A., Berkman, E. M., and Kaplan, M. M. (1988) Hypothyroidism after treatment with interleukin-2 and lymphokine-activated killer cells. *N. Engl. J. Med.* **318**, 1557–1563.
56. Perez, R., Padavic, K., Krigel, R., and Weiner, L. (1991) Antierythrocyte auto-antibody formation after therapy with interleukin-2 and gamma-interferon. *Cancer* **67**, 2512–2517.
57. Soni, N., Meropol, N. J., Porter, M., and Caligiur, M. A. (1996) Diabetes mellitus induced by low-dose interleukin-2. *Cancer Immunol. Immunother.* **43**, 59–62.
58. Massorotti, E. M., Canaso, J., Mier, J. W., and Atkins, M. B. (1992) Chronic inflammatory arthritis following treatment with high dose interleukin-2 for malignancy. *Am. J. Med.* **92**, 693–697.
59. Engelhardt, M., Rump, J. A., Hellerich, U., Mertelsmann, R., and Lindemann, A. (1995) Leukocytoclastic vasculitis and long-term remission in a patient with

secondary AML and post-remission treatment with low dose interleukin-2. *Annu. Hematol.* **70,** 227–230.

60. Hess, A. D., Jones, R. J., Morris, L. E., Noga, S. J., Vogelsang, G. B., and Santos, G. W. (1992) Autologous graft-versus-host disease: a novel approach for antitumor immunotherapy. *Hum. Immunol.* **34,** 219–224.

61. Weiden, P. L., Flournoy, N., Thomas, E. D., Prentice, R., Fefer, A., Buckner, C. D., et al. (1979) Antileukemic effect of graft-versus-host disease in human recipients of allogeneic-marrow grafts. *N. Engl. J. Med.* **100,** 1068–1073.

62. Ringden, O., Rozman, C., Speck, B., Truitt, R. I., Zwaan, F. E., and Bortin, M. M. (1990) Graft-versus-leukemia reactions after bone marrow transplantation. *Blood* **75,** 555–562.

63. Martin, P. and Kernan, N. (1990) T cell depletion for the prevention of graft-versus-host disease, in *Graft-versus-Host Disease* (Burakoff, S. J., Deeg, N. J., Ferrara, J., and Atkinson, K., eds.), Marcel Dekker, New York, p. 371.

64. Kennedy, M. J., Vogelsang, G. B., Jones, R. J., Farmer, E. R., Hess, A. D., Altomonte, V., et al. (1994) Phase I trial of interferon gamma to potentiate cyclosporine-induced graft-versus-host disease in women undergoing autologous bone marrow transplantation for breast cancer. *J. Clin. Oncol.* **12,** 249–257.

65. Jones, R. J., Vogelsang, G. B., Hess, A. D., Farmer, E. R., Mann, R. B., Geller, R. B., et al. (1989) Induction of graft-versus-host disease after autologous bone marrow transplantation. *Lancet* **1,** 754–757.

66. Abdel-Wahab, Z., Dar, M. M., Hester, D., Vervaert, C., Gangavalli, R., Barber, J., et al. (1996) Effect of irradiation on cytokine production, MHC antigen expression, and vaccine potential of interleukin-2 and interferon-gamma gene-modified melanoma cells. *Cellular Immunol.* **171,** 246–254.

67. Mullen, C. A., Petropoulos, D., and Lowe, R. M. (1996) Treatment of microscopic pulmonary metastases with recombinant autologous tumor vaccine expressing interleukin 6 and *Escherichia coli* cytosine deaminase suicide genes. *Cancer Research* **56,** 1361–1366.

68. Levitsky, H. I., Montgomery, J., Ahmadzadeh, M., Staveley-O'Carroll, K., Guarnieri, F., Longo, D. L., et al. (1996) Immunization with granulocyte-macrophage colony stimulating factor-transduced, but not B7-1-transduced, lymphoma cells primes idiotype-specific T cells and generates potent systemic antitumor immunity. *J. Immunol.* **156,** 3858–3865.

69. Zatloukal, K., Schmidt, W., Cotten, M., Wagner, E., Stingl, G., and Birnstiel, M. L. (1993) Somatic gene therapy for cancer: the utility of transferrinfection in generating 'tumor vaccines'. *Gene* **135,** 199–207.

70. Fujii, H., Inobe, M., Kimura, F., Murata, J., Murakami, M., Onishi, Y., et al. (1996) Vaccination of tumor cells transfected with the B7-1 (CD80) gene induces the anti-metastatic effect and tumor immunity in mice. *Int. J. Cancer.* **66,** 219–224.

71. Herlyn, D., Somasundaram, R., Li, W., and Jacob, L. (1995) Animal models of human derived cancer vaccines. *Cell Biophys.* **27,** 15–30.

72. Williams, S. S., Alosco, T. R., Croy, B. A., and Bankert, R. B. (1993) The study of human neoplastic disease in severe combined immunodeficient mice. *Lab. Animal Science* **43,** 139–146.

73. Ciernik, I. F., Berzofsky, J. A., and Carbone, D. P. (1996) Induction of cytotoxic T lymphocytes and antitumor immunity with DNA vaccines expressing single T cell epitopes. *J. Immunol.* **156,** 2369–2375.

74. Mayordomo, J. I., Loftus, D. J., Sakamoto, H., De Cesare, C. M., Appasamy, P. M., Lotze, M. T., et al. (1996) Therapy of murine tumors with p53 wild-type and mutant sequence peptide-based vaccines. *J. Exp. Med.* **183,** 1357–1365.
75. Renner, C., Jung, W., Sahin, U., Denfeld, R., Pohl, C., Trümper, L., et al. (1994) Cure of xenografted human tumors by bispecific monoclonal antibodies and human T cells. *Science* **264,** 833–835.
76. Qi, Y., Moyana, T., Matte, G., Wilkinson, A., Bresalier, R., and Xiang, J. (1995) Immunolocalization of hepatic metastases of human colonic cancer by chimeric anti-TAG72 antibody in SCID mice. *J. Surg. Oncol.* **59,** 3–9.
77. Rowse, G., Tempero, R., VanLith, M., Hollingsworth, M. A., and Gendler, S. (1998) Immunological tolerance and tumor immunity in MUC1 transgenic mice. *Cancer Res.* **58,** 315–321.
78. Hu, J., Kindsvogel, W., Busby, S., Bailey, M. C., Shi, Y., and Greenberg, P. D. (1993) An evaluation of the potential to use tumor-associated antigens as targets for antitumor T cell therapy using transgenic mice expressing a retroviral tumor antigen in normal lymphoid tissues. *J. Exp. Med.* **177,** 1681–1690.
79. Naftzger, C., Takechi, Y., Kohda, H., Hara, I, Vijayasaradhi, S., and Houghton, A. N. (1996) Immune response to a differentiation antigen induced by altered antigen: a study of tumor rejection and autoimmunity. *Proc. Natl. Acad. Sci. USA* **93,** 14,809–14,814.
80. Hara, I., Takechi, Y., and Houghton, A. N. (1995) Implicating a role for immune recognition of self in tumor rejection: passive immunization against the brown locus protein. *J. Exp. Med.* **182,** 1609–1614.
81. Uyttenhove, C., Godfraind, C., Lethe', B., Amar-Costesec, A., Renauld, J-C., Gajewski, T. F., et al. (1997) The expression of mouse gene P1A in testis does not prevent safe induction of cytolytic T cells against a P1A-encoded tumor antigen. *Int. J. Cancer.* **70,** 349–356.
82. Dahl, A. M., Beverley, P. C. L., and Stauss, H. J. (1996) A synthetic peptide derived from the tumor-associated protein mdm2 can stimulate autoreactive, high avidity cytotoxic T lymphocytes that recognize naturally processed protein. *J. Immunol.* **157,** 239–246.
83. Disis, M. L., Gralow, J. R., Bernhard, H., Hand, S. L., Rubin, W. D., and Cheever, M. A. (1996) Peptide-based, but not whole protein, vaccines elicit immunity to HER-2/neu, an oncogenic self-protein. *J. Immunol.* **156,** 3151–3158.
84. Bevan, M. J., Hogquist, K. A., and Jameson, S. C. (1994) Selecting the T cell receptor repertoire. *Science* **264,** 796–797.
85. von Boehmer, H. (1994) Positive selection of lymphocytes. *Cell* **76,** 219–228.
86. Anderson, G., Moore, N. C., Owen, J. J. T., and Jenkinson, E. J. (1996) Cellular interactions in thymocyte development. *Annu. Rev. Immunol.* **14,** 73–100.
87. Mamula, M. J. and Craft, J. (1994) The expression of self antigenic determinants: implications for tolerance and autoimmunty. *Curr. Opion. Immunol.* **6,** 882–886.
88. Mamula, M. J. (1993) The inability to process a self-peptide allows autoreactive T cells to escape tolerance. *J. Exp. Med.* **177,** 567–571.
89. Moudgil, K. D. and Sercarz, E. E. (1994) The T cell reportiore against cryptic self determinants and its involvement in autoimmunity and cancer. *Clinical Immunol. Immunpathol.* **73,** 283–289.
90. Vanderlugt, C. J. and Miller, S. D. (1996) Epitope spreading. *Curr. Opin. Immunol.* **8,** 831–836.

91. McRae, B. L., Vanderlugt, C. L., Dal Canto, M. C., and Miller, S. D. (1995) Functional evidence for epitope spreading in the relapsing pathology of EAE in the SJL/J mouse. *J. Exp. Med.* **182,** 75–85.
92. James, J. A., Gross, T., Scofield, R. H., and Harley, J. B. (1995) Immunoglobulin epitopes spreading and autoimmune disease after peptide immunization: Sm B/B'-derived PPPGMRPP and PPPGIRGP induce spliceosome autoimmunity. *J. Exp. Med.* **181,** 453–461.
93. Lou, Y. and Tung, K. S. K. (1993) T cell peptide of a self-protein elicits autoantibody to the protein antigen. *J. Immunol.* **151,** 5790–5799.
94. Kawakami, Y., Eliyaha, S., Jennings, C., Sakaguchi, K., Kang, X., Southwood, S., et al. (1995) Recognition of multiple epitopes in a human melanoma antigen gp100 by tumor-infiltrating T lymphocytes associated with in vivo tumor regression. *J. Immunol.* **154,** 3961–3968.
95. Mondino, A., Khoruts, A., and Jenkins, M. K. (1996) The anatomy of T-cell activation and tolerance. *Proc. Natl. Acad. Sci. USA* **93,** 2245–2252.
96. Goodnow, C. C. (1996) Balancing immunity and tolerance: deleting and tuning lymphocyte repertoires. *Proc. Natl. Acad. Sci. USA* **93,** 2264–2271.
97. Lenschow, D. J., Walunas, T. L., and Bluestone, J. A. (1996) CD28/B7 system of T cell costimulation. *Annu. Rev. Immunol.* **14,** 233–258.
98. Pardoll, D. (1993) New strategies for enhancing the immunogenicity of tumors. *Curr. Opin. Immunol.* **5,** 719–725.
99. Ramarathinam, L., Castle, M., Wu, Y., and Liu, Y. (1994) T cell costimulation by B7/BB1 induces CD8 T cell-dependent tumor rejection: an important role of B7/BB1 in the induction, recruitment, and effector function of antitumor cells. *J. Exp. Med.* **179,** 1205–1214.
100. Miller, J. F. and Flavell, R. A. (1994) T-cell tolerance and autoimmunity in transgenic models of central and peripheral tolerance. *Curr. Opin. Immunol.* **6,** 892–899.
101. Guerder, S., Meyerhoff, J., and Flavell, R. (1994) The role of the T cell costimulator B7-1 in autoimmuntiy and the induction and maintenance of tolerance to peripheral antigen. *Immunity* **1,** 155–166.
102. Klinman, N. R. (1996) The 'clonal selection hypothesis' and current concepts of B cell tolerance. *Immunity* **5,** 189–195.
103. Erikson, J., Radic, M. Z., Camper, S. A. Hardy, R. R., Carmack, C., and Weigert, M. (1991) Expression of anti-DNA immunoglubulin transgenes in non-autoimmune mice. *Nature* **349,** 331–334.
104. Goodnow, C. C., Crosbie, J., Adelstein, S., Lavoie T. B., Smithgill, S. J., Brink, R. A., et al. (1988) Altered immunoglobulin expression and functional silencing of self-reactive B lymphocytes. *Nature* **334,** 676–679.
105. Russell, D. M., Dembic, Z., Morahan, G., Miller, J. F. A. P., Burki, K., and Nemazee, D. Peripheral deletion of self-reactive B cells. *Nature* **354,** 308–311.
106. Nemazee, D. A. and Burki, K. (1989) Clonal deletion of B lymphocytes in a transgenic mouse bearing anti-MHC class I antibody genes. *Nature* **337,** 562–566.
107. Okamoto, M. Murakami, M., Shimizu, A., Ozaki, S., Tsubata, T., Kumagai, S., et al. (1992) A transgenic model of autoimmune hemolytic anemia. *J. Exp. Med.* **175,** 71–79.
108. Schlichtholz, B., Legros, Y., Gillet, C., Marty, M., Lane, D., Calve, F., et al. (1992) The immune response to p53 in breast cancer patients is directed against immunodominant epitopes unrelated to the mutational hot spot. *Cancer Res.* **52,** 6380–6384.

109. Disis, M. and Cheever, M. A. (1996) Oncogenic proteins as tumor antigens. *Curr. Opin. Immunol.* **8,** 637–642.
110. Katsumata, M., Okudaira, T., Samanta, A., Clark, D. P., Drebin, J. A., Jolicoeur, P., et al. (1995) Prevention of breast tumor development in vivo by downregulation of the p815^{neu} receptor. *Nat. Med.* **1,** 644–648.
111. Townsend, S. E. and Allison, J. P. (1993) Tumor rejection after direct costimulation of CD8+ T cells by B7-transfected melanoma cells. *Science* **259,** 368–370.
112. Chen, L., Ashe, S., Brady, W. A., Hellstrom, I., Hellstrom, K. E., Ledbetter, J. A., et al. (1992) Costimulation of antitumor immunity by the B7 counterreceptor for the T lymphocyte molecules CD28 and CTLA-4. *Cell* **71,** 1093–1102.
113. Chen, L., McGowen, P., Ashe, S., Johnston, J., Li, Y., Hellstrom, I., and Hellstrom, K. E. (1994) Tumor immunogenicity determines the effect of B7 costimulation of T cell-mediated tumor immunity. *J. Exp. Med.* **179,** 523–532.
114. Basker, S., Ostrand-Rosenburg, S., Nabavi, N., Nadler, L. M., Freeman, G. J., and Glimcher L. H. (1993) Constitutive expression of B7 restores immunogencity of tumor cells expressing truncated major histocompatibility complex class II molecules. *Proc. Natl. Acad. Sci. USA* **90,** 5687–5690.
115. Fujii, H., Inobe, M., Kimura, F., Murata, J., Murakami, M., Onishi, Y., et al. (1996) Vaccination of tumor cells transfected with B7-1 (CD80) gene induces the antimetastatic effect and tumor immunity in mice. *Int. J. Cancer* **66,** 219–224.
116. Yang, G., Hellstrom, K. E., Hellstrom, I., and Chen L. (1995) Antitumor immunity elicited by tumor cells transfected with B7-2, a second ligand for CD28/CTLA-4 costimulatory molecules. *J. Immunol.* **154,** 2794–2800.
117. Cavallo, F., Martin-Fontecha, A., Bellone, M., Heltai, M., Gatti, E., Tornaghi, P., et al. (1995) Co-expression of B7-1 and ICAM-1 on tumors is required for rejection and the establishment of a memory response. *Eur. J. Immunol.* **25,** 1154–1162.
118. Rivera, J. A., Rall, C. J., Graeme-Cook, F., Fernandez-del-Castillo, C., Shu, P., Lakey, N., et al. (1997) Analysis of K-ras oncogene mutations in chronic pancreatitis with ductal hyperplasia. *Surgery* **121,** 42–49.
119. Uehara, H., Nakaizumi, A., Baba, M., Iishi, H., Tatsuta, M., Kitamura, T., et al. (1996) Diagnosis of pancreatic cancer by K-ras point mutation and cytology of pancreatic juice. *Am. J. Gastroenterol.* **91,** 1616–1621.
120. Raedle, J., Oremek, G., Welker, M., Roth, W. K., Caspary, W. F., and Zeuzem, S. (1996) p53 autoantibodies in patients with pancreatitis and pancreatic carcinoma. *Pancreas* **13,** 241–246.

23

The Dual Relationship Between Thymectomy and Autoimmunity

The Kaleidoscope of Autoimmune Disease

Yaniv Sherer, Yaron Bar-Dayan, and Yehuda Shoenfeld

1. INTRODUCTION

Autoimmune diseases are conditions in which the immune system damages the normal components of the individual. The etiology of autoimmune diseases is multifactorial and includes genetic, immune, hormonal and environmental factors (1), which are all combined to create the break in self-tolerance. Self-tolerance is normally maintained due to the balance between effector and suppressor T-cells (2). When this fragile equilibrium is distorted, either by activation of pathogenic effector T-cells, or by depletion of suppressor T-cells, the organism is prone to develop an autoimmune disease. The role of the thymus in these diseases is yet to be fully clarified, but this organ is widely accepted to be a major player in the maintenance of self-tolerance. Thus, on the one hand, the thymus helps prevent the development of autoimmunity, and on the other hand, it may participate in the initiation of autoimmune disease under certain conditions. Understanding the clinical and immunological response to thymectomy could shed light on the role of the thymus in autoimmune diseases. In this paper, we review the therapeutic as well as the pathogenic effects of thymectomy, which is intended to emphasize and clarify the pivotal role of the thymus in autoimmune diseases.

2. THYMECTOMY—REMOVAL OF THE "ATTACKER"

Thymectomy has a therapeutic effect in some autoimmune conditions. The rationale behind thymectomy as a treatment for these diseases is that the thymus may be one of the major contributor of the cells and molecules that attack self-antigens. Removal of the thymus, therefore, might cause clinical improvement or even disappearance of disease symptoms. In real life, however, the removal of the thymus results in either clinical improvement or in no significant change.

Contemporary Immunology: Autoimmune Reactions
Edited by: S. Paul © Humana Press Inc., Totowa, NJ

2.1. Removal of the "Attacker"—
Induction of Clinical Improvement

The combination of clinical improvement in the course of some autoimmune diseases following thymectomy, and of frequent changes in thymus histology and lymphocytes subpopulations in autoimmune diseases, suggest that the thymus is strongly involved in the disease pathogenesis. The way in which the thymus alters the immunological environment and makes it prone to develop an autoimmune disease differs from one disease to another. Intrathymic tolerance breakage due to environmental stimuli combined with various genetic predispositions is commonly accepted to play a pivotal role in disease pathogenics. It is reasonable to anticipate, therefore, that thymus removal may alter the pathogenic events. The beneficial effects of thymectomy on the course of autoimmune diseases are summarized as follows:

2.1.1. Myasthenia Gravis

Myasthenia gravis is an autoimmune disease, resulting from the production of antibodies against the acetylcholine receptor (3–5). Ten to 15% of myasthenic patients have a thymoma, and up to 60% of cases display thymic hyperplasia (4,6–7). Abnormal T-lymphocytes in circulation, bearing both helper and suppressor/cytotoxic T-cell markers (double-marker cells), are found at significantly higher levels in patients with thymomas and thymic hyperplasia than in patients with a normal thymus (8). Another interesting finding is the hyperproduction of IL-6 by thymic epithelial cells from myasthenic patients compared to controls (9). IL-6 is a possible autocrine growth factor for thymic epithelial cells, and the activity of this molecule may help explain the presence of lymphoid follicles characteristic of thymic hyperplasia in myasthenia gravis. The presence of mRNA coding for the α-subunit of the acetylcholine receptor in thymic epithelial cells may provide an explanation for the autosensitization against this protein in myasthenia gravis (7). In order to link this phenomenon to the pathogenesis of myasthenia gravis, Wakkach et al. (7) proposed two possibilities: either the acetylcholine receptor is tolerated in most disease-free individuals, and a breakdown of tolerance occurs in myasthenia gravis patients or the acetylcholine receptor is ignored in all individuals owing to its weak expression, thus allowing the acetylcholine receptor-reactive T-cells to persist. A triggering event in the thymus of myasthenic patients could activate these cells and initiate the autoimmune response as a consequence.

Thymectomy is a regular procedure in patients with myasthenia gravis, and its effectiveness in these patients is not questionable. Thymectomy should be offered to all myasthenia gravis patients unless they are older than 50 yr, have purely ocular disease, minimal symptoms or juvenile myasthenia (4,10). The results of thymectomy in myasthenia gravis patients include clinical improvement, along with a decline in antiacetylcholine receptor antibody titer (11). There is a better response to thymectomy among patients with thymic hyperplasia rather than with thymoma, as will be discussed further later.

2.1.2. Ulcerative Colitis

Ulcerative colitis is an inflammatory disease of the colon of unknown origin. It is often characterized by the formation of lymphoid follicles in the thymus *(12)*. Mucosal cytotoxic lymphocytes *(13)* can be detected as can the phenomenon of antibody-dependent cell mediated cytotoxicity *(14)*, both of which have been demonstrated to play an important role in mucosal destruction. Moreover, thymic growth factors in these patients can alter the micro-environment in the thymus, and in some cases retrovirus markers have been detected in the thymic epithelial cells *(14)*. These result support an impaired intrathymic maturation in ulcerative colitis, which may result in functional abnormalities of lymphocytes exiting from this organ into the periphery. In a series of ulcerative colitis patients, thymectomy induced a high percentage of remission, and decreased the anticolon antibody activity *(15)*. Although thymectomy seems to be effective in ulcerative colitis, it is not yet accepted as a regular treatment.

2.1.3. Multiple Sclerosis

The lymphocyte response to mitogens is depressed in multiple sclerosis *(16)* and exacerbations of this disease are associated with a decrease in T-suppressor lymphocytes. Thymectomy can result in beneficial effects in multiple sclerosis patients superior to steroids, and it may also increase the steroid-sensitivity in the postsurgery phase *(17)*. A good clinical response to thymectomy is more readily seen in patients with relapsing-remitting multiple sclerosis (MS) than in patients with chronic-progressive disease. The latter patients rarely show clinical improvement following thymectomy *(18)*.

2.1.4. Systemic Lupus Erythematosus

Far from being the treatment of choice in systemic lupus erythematosus, thymectomy is contraindicated in this disease *(19)*. However, there are a few reports of good clinical outcomes in thymectomized patients, especially in patients with concomitantly occurring thymoma and systemic lupus erythematosus *(20,21)*. The unpredictable response to thymectomy in lupus patients is best exemplified by the report of Zandman–Goddard et al. *(20)*. They have reported two patients, with the combination of thymoma and lupus, who have shown opposite clinical responses to thymectomy. The first patient is at remission six years after thymectomy, while the second patient, following the same procedure, became unresponsive, despite high dose steroid therapy.

2.2. Removal of the "Attacker"—No Significant Change

The fact that the thymus plays a role in the pathogenesis of autoimmune diseases does not necessarily imply that its removal will have a beneficial value. This is exemplified by the response of myasthenia gravis patients to thymectomy. As was mentioned previously, the clinical response to thymectomy is disappointing in the presence of thymoma, as opposed to the good clinical response in the presence of thymic hyperplasia *(10,22)*. The best response to thymectomy is seen in young patients with thymic hyperplasia, intermediate antibody titer, and expressing the HLA-A1, B8, and DRW3 markers *(10)*. Approximately 80% of such patients are expected to have significant clinical improvement or to be in complete remission following thymectomy *(4)*. However, subjects with the combination of thymic hyperplasia and myasthenia gravis are more likely to develop another autoimmune disease following thymus removal compared to subjects with thymoma and myasthenia gravis undergoing the procedure.

Spuler et al. *(22)* suggest that hyperplastic thymus tissue, but not thymomas, is a major source of B-cells producing antiacetylcholine receptor antibodies, which may be why removal of hyperplastic thymus tissue results in a reduction of the autoantibody titer and in clinical improvement. On the other hand, removal of thymomas rarely reduces the autoantibody titer. The major site of autoantibody production in thymoma-associated myasthenia gravis is still not known, although the regional lymph nodes or the spleen are potential candidates. As opposed to normal and hyperplastic thymus tissue, both of which express the acetylcholine receptor in epithelial cells, there is no acetylcholine receptor expression in thymomas *(22–23)*. Instead, a 153-kD protein (p153), distinct from the acetylcholine receptor but recognized by monoclonal antibodies against an epitope of the α-subunit of the receptor, was identified in epithelial cells in thymomas *(23–25)*. It is likely that T cells are sensitized intrathymically against epitopes of p153, and thus acquire the ability to recognize structurally related epitopes in the acetylcholine receptor *(22)*. These cross-reactive T-cells, functioning as T-helper lymphocytes, may activate B-cells peripherally to produce antiacetylcholine receptor autoantibodies. When fragments of either thymoma or lymphofollicular hyperplastic thymic tissues from thymectomized myasthenia gravis patient were transplanted into SCID mice, the hyperplastic thymic transplants provoked the formation of high titers of antibodies to the acetylcholine receptors, whereas the thymoma transplants did not (22).

It is evident, therefore, that the clinical response to thymectomy depends on the specific nature of the involvement of the thymus in disease pathogenesis. Thymectomy induces varying responses in different patients with the same disease. The fact that thymectomy has a beneficial effect in patients with relapsing-remitting MS, but not in patients with chronic-progressive disease, may be a consequence of the different pathogenic mechanisms in the two forms of this disease. In both patterns of MS, as in myasthenia gravis, the thymus may contribute to disease formation in different ways. The removal of the "attacker" effect, thus, may result in either a good clinical response or no significant change at all (Table 1). Alternatively, the thymus may be an innocent bystander with respect to disease pathogenesis, therefore, its removal will be without effect. With respect to the choice of therapies for individual patients, the response to thymectomy depends on the extent and way in which the thymus was involved in initiating the disease. Future studies should provide a better understanding of these processes, and help identify patients who have the best chance of achieving remission of their symptoms by thymectomy.

Table 1
The Varying Effects of Thymectomy
on the Course of Autoimmune Disease in Humans

Response to thymectomy	Mechanism	Diseases
Clinical improvement	Removal of the "attacker"	Myasthenia gravis Ulcerative colitis Multiple sclerosis Systemic lupus erythematosus[a]

No significant change	Removal of either the
	    "attacker" or an
	    innocent bystander
		Myasthenia gravis
		Multiple sclerosis

Clinical deterioration	Removal of the "protector"	Systemic lupus erythematosus

Disease switch	Removal of both the
	    "attacker" of one disease
	    and the "protector" of
	    another
		Pemphigus[b]
		Systemic lupus
		    erythematosus[b]

[a] Only a few reports. Thymectomy is not recommended in systemic lupus erythematosus.
[b] These diseases developed following thymectomy for another condition.

3. THYMECTOMY—REMOVAL OF THE "PROTECTOR"

When considering the role of the thymus in autoimmune diseases, one must keep in mind that the thymus is the most important organ responsible for self-tolerance. Under normal conditions the thymus functions as a "protector" against development of autoimmune diseases. As a result, thymectomy might sometimes result in clinical deterioration instead of improving the clinical status of the patient with autoimmune disease. In some cases, the thymectomy can even create a new autoimmune disease that replaces the old one. Even when thymectomy is indicated for another reason (i.e., thymoma), it can sometimes lead to additional autoimmunity reactions (Table 1).

3.1. Evidence for the Protective Role
of the Thymus Against Autoimmunity

The protective role of the intact thymus against development of autoimmune disease has been described by several authors. Bonomo et al. *(26)* claimed that in the adult intrathymic tolerization to components of self-peptides complexed to major histocompatibility Class II antigens on antigen-presenting cells prevents organ-specific autoimmune disease. Further, in the course of using prophylactic intrathymic islet allografts during the prehyperglycemic phase of diabetes, Brayman et al. *(27)* showed that exposure of thymic T-cells to islet antigens prevented hyperglycemia and beta-cell destruction in the diabetes-prone BioBreeding rats. Khoury et al. *(28–29)* reported the prevention of experimental

Table 2
The Effect of Neonatal Thymectomy
on Animal Models of Autoimmune Diseases

Induction or acceleration of the disease

Diabetes in female PVG/c rats *(31)*[a]
Autoimmune gastritis: murine *(32)*, BALB/c nu/+ mice *(33)*
SLE in NZB/W mice *(20)*
Autoallergic sialadenitis in C3H/He mice *(34)*[b]
Thyroiditis in Buffalo strain rat (35) and PVG/c strain mice *(36)*[a]
Autoimmune cholangitis in A/J mice *(37)*[a]
Autoimmune hepatitis in C3H/HeN mice *(38)*
Multiple organ autoimmune reactions in mice *(39,40)*

Prevention or improvement of the disease
Diabetes in genetically diabetic rats *(30)*
SLE in MRL/*lpr* mice *(41)*

[a] Thymectomy was combined with sublethal irradiation.
[b] Thymectomy was combined with immunization of the animal with antigen extracts.

autoimmune encephalomyelitis (an experimental model for the study of multiple sclerosis) by intrathymic injection of major basic protein (MBP) or its major encephalitogenic peptide (p71-90) (systemic immunization with MBP causes disease formation). Similarly, intravenous injection of the thymic dendritic cells incubated with p71-90 prevented the disease. In thymectomized animals, the intravenous injection of thymic dendritic cells did not prevent the disease. The authors concluded that autoreactive antigen-specific (MBP-specific) T-cells circulate through the thymus, interact via the T-cell receptor with MBP peptides presented by thymic dendritic cells, and thereby become tolerized to MBP.

3.2. Thymectomy-Lessons from Animal Models

Neonatal thymectomy is associated with the induction and acceleration of autoimmune disease, and, to a lesser extent, with prevention and amelioration of autoimmune disease, in several animal models of autoimmune disease summarized in Table 2 *(20,30–41)*. It is important to emphasize that neonatal thymectomy was not enough to influence the disease course in some of the animal models; an effect was achieved in these models only by combining thymectomy and sublethal irradiation *(31,36)*, or by combining thymectomy and immunization of the animals with the autoantigen *(34,37)*.

3.3. Possible Mechanisms for the Induction
of Autoimmune Diseases Following Neonatal Thymectomy

These are as follows.

1. Removal of the thymus reduces the level (or activity) of suppressor T-cells which produce cytokines responsible for suppressing the clonal expansion of the effector autoreactive T-cells *(32,33,39,40)*.

2. Thymectomy breaks self-tolerance by creating a disequilibrium between Th1 and Th2 CD4 cells. Autoimmune diseases mediated by autoreactive CD4 T-cells can potentially be prevented by diverting the cells to differentiate into regulatory Th2 effector cells *(42)*. There are many factors which contribute in vivo to the decision of stimulated CD4 T-cells to develop into Th1 versus Th2 cells. Self-tolerance can be induced by the expression of peripheral self-proteins on thymic epithelial cells. The intrathymic expression of proteins causes a reduction of the Th1 activity, with no decrease in Th2 activity *(43)*. There is no opportunity in thymectomized individuals for such self-tolerization mechanisms to occur on an ongoing basis, enhancing the possibility of autoimmune reactions.

3. Bonomo et al. *(44)* propose an alternative hypothesis for the development of post-thymectomy autoimmune reactions, which is based on the following observations and assumptions.

   a. The peripheral lymphoid tissues of neonatal animals contain a population of autoreactive T-cells that escape from the thymus during the first days of life. This may be owing to the low expression of major histocompatibility molecules on the surface of antigen presenting cells in the newborn thymus, a process that may favor positive rather than the negative selection of T-cells. Another contribution to aberrant selection processes may be provided by low levels of T-cell receptor expression.

   b. The autoreactive T-cells act in a nonspecific way to initiate an inflammatory reaction in the target organ, thus creating a microenvironment in which the organ-specific T-cells can be easily activated.

   c. The activated cells migrate to different peripheral organs, where they encounter their specific antigens expressed by antigen presenting cells. The resultant inflammation enhances aberrant expression of major histocompatibility antigens and costimulatory molecules, both on professional and nonprofessional antigen presenting cells. This process eventually leads to organ-specific disease.

   d. During the first week of life, the thymus is an "open organ" which allows peripheral cells to recirculate back into it. The recirculation of autoreactive T-cells is absent in the three-day-old thymectomized mice. Following thymectomy, prematurely exported cells cannot recirculate back into the thymus and cannot be deleted. Further, the "homeless" cells begin to express different cell-surface molecules aberrantly, which facilitates their homing to sites different from the normal homing pattern in the euthymic mice.

   e. Neonatal thymectomy decreases the number of peripheral T-cells by approximately 80%. This results in an increase in the ratio of the autoreactive T-cells and other T-cell subpopulations with regulatory functions. The change in the T-cell profile enhances the frequency of interactions between the T-cells and the antigen presenting cells and thus aggravates the autoimmune process.

The induction of autoimmune syndromes following neonatal thymectomy represent an autoimmune "physiological" model, in which disease occurs (in most cases) in the absence of immunization with foreign proteins. Thus, these models support the belief that an intact thymus is of great importance in maintaining self-tolerance. It is then understandable why thymectomy as treatment may sometimes achieve clinical deterioration instead of improvement.

3.4. The Thymus and the "Kaleidoscope of Autoimmunity" (Disease Switch)

The term "disease switch" implies the appearance of an autoimmune disease following thymectomy carried out for the treatment of a different autoimmune disease. Although this phenomenon is quite rare (45–49), its existence suggests that the thymus facilitates the development of one autoimmune disease and simultaneously prevents the appearance of another.

The most fascinating report about this phenomenon was probably that of Grinlinton et al. (49). They reported a pair of monozygotic twins who were concordant for myasthenia gravis, but became discordant for systemic lupus erythematosus following thymectomy. The first twin developed recurrent transverse myelitis and optic neuritis, while the other twin developed skin rash and persistent leukopenia. Both twins developed autoimmune thyroid disease but the former developed thyrotoxicosis, as opposed to the latter, who developed hypothyroidism. There are also several reports of patients who developed pemphigus or systemic lupus erythematosus following thymectomy (45–48).

These observations indicate that in systemic lupus erythematosus, as in myasthenia gravis and probably other autoimmune conditions, there are several pathogenic mechanisms underlying the disease. The role of the thymus is evidently variable depending on the specific presentation in different patients. Thymectomy may have opposite effects on patients with the same disease. Therefore, when considering the benefits and risks of thymectomy, one must keep in mind that thymectomy can cause adverse effects depending on where the patient is located in the "kaleidoscope of autoimmunity." Sometimes, the new disease induced by thymectomy may be worse than the disease for which the thymectomy is indicated.

In conclusion, thymectomy may have opposite effects on the course of autoimmune diseases. Several considerations suggest that the relationship between the thymus and autoimmune diseases is bipolar. These include changes in thymic histology and T-cell subpopulations over the course of disease, the effects of thymectomy in animal models and the clinical course of autoimmune diseases in humans after thymectomy. On the one hand, the thymus may be the initiator, alone or combined with other agents, that triggers the development of certain autoimmune diseases. On the other hand, with respect to other autoimmune diseases, the thymus may be no more than an innocent bystander, or it may even be actively involved in decreasing their severity. Therefore, thymectomy as a treatment for autoimmune diseases may result thymectomy in clinical improvement, deterioration, no significant change, or switch to another disease.

4. SUMMARY

The etiology of autoimmune diseases is multifactorial and includes genetic, immune, hormonal and environmental factors. The role of the thymus in autoimmune diseases is not fully elucidated. However, it has a major role in self tolerance maintenance. On the one hand, the thymus helps to prevent the development of autoimmunity, and on the other hand, under certain conditions, it may participate in the initiation of autoimmune diseases. Thymectomy has opposite effects on the course of different autoimmune diseases. Thymectomy has a therapeutic effect in myasthenia gravis, MS, and ulcerative colitis. In certain patients, however, it might have no effect on the clinical course of these diseases. In other autoimmune diseases (i.e., systemic lupus erythematosus), removal of the thymus can cause a clinical deterioration instead of an improvement. Moreover, removal of the thymus can cause a switch from one autoimmune disease to another. These observations suggest that the thymus can be visualized either as an "attacker" of self-antigens or as a "protector" against disease. The "attacker" and "protector" roles are not entirely mutually exclusive. Sometimes thymectomy can ameliorate one autoimmune condition and induce the appearance of another.

ACKNOWLEDGMENT

The work was supported by the Freda and Leon Schaller Grant for Research in Autoimmunity.

REFERENCES

1. Shoenfeld, Y. and Isenberg, D. (1989) Concluding remarks: the Mosaic of Autoimmunity, in *The Mosaic of Autoimmunity* (Shoenfeld, Y. and Isenberg, D., eds.), Elsevier, Amsterdam, pp. 509–511.
2. Tung, K. S. (1994) Mechanism of self-tolerance and events leading to autoimmune disease and autoantibody response. *Clin. Immunol. Immunopathol.* **73**, 275–282.
3. Baraka, A. (1993) Anesthesia and myasthenia gravis. *Middle East J. Anesthes.* **12**, 9–35.
4. Havard, C. W. H. and Fonseca, V. (1990) New treatment approaches to myasthenia gravis. *Drugs* **39**, 66–73.
5. Keys, P. A. and Blume, R. P. (1991) Therapeutic strategies for myasthenia gravis. *DICP* **25**, 1101–1108.
6. Tsuchiya, M., Asakura, H., and Yoshimatsu, H. (1989) Thymic abnormalities and autoimmune diseases. *Keio. J. Med.* **38**, 383–402.
7. Wakkach, A., Guyon, T., Bruand, C., Tzartos, S., Cohen-Kaminsky, S., and Berrih-Aknin, S. (1996) Expression of acetylcholine receptor genes in human thymic epithelial cell. *J. Immunol.* **157**, 3752–3760.
8. Matsui, M. and Kameyama, M. (1986) A double-label flow cytometric analysis of the simultaneous expression of OKT4 and Leu2a antigens on circulating T lymphocytes in myasthenia gravis. *J. Neuroimmunol.* **11**, 311–319.

9. Cohen-Kaminsky, S., Devergne, O., Delattre, R. M., Klingel-Schmitt. I., Emilie. D., Galanaud, P., et al. (1993) Interleukin-6 overproduction by cultured thymic epithelial cells from patients with myasthenia gravis is potentially involved in thymic hyperplasia. *Eur. Cytokine Netw.* **4**, 121–132.

10. Nyberg, H. R. and Gjerstad, L. (1988) Immunopharmacological treatment in myasthenia gravis. *Transplant Proc.* **20**, 201–210.

11. De Bates, M. H. (1994) Autoimmune diseases against cell surface receptors: myasthenia gravis, a prototype anti-receptor disease. *Nether. J. Med.* **45**, 294–301.

12. Mizuno, Y., Muraoka, M., Shimabukuro, K., Toda, K., Migagawa, K., Yoshimatsu, H., et al. (1990) Inflammatory bowel diseases and thymus disorder: reactivity of thymocytes with monoclonal antibodies. *Bull. Tokyo Dent. Coll.* **31**, 137–141.

13. Bendixen, G. (1969) Cellular hypersensitivity to components of intestinal mucosa in ulcerative colitis and Crohn's disease. *Gut* **10**, 631–636.

14. Tsuchiya, M., Asakura, H., and Yoshimatsu, H. (1989) Thymic abnormalities and autoimmune diseases. *Keio J. Med.* **38**, 383–402.

15. Tsuchiya, M., Hibi, T., Watanabe, M., Ohara, M., Ogata, H., Iwao, Y., et al. (1991) Thymectomy in ulcerative colitis: a report of cases over a 13 year period. *Thymus* **17**, 67–73.

16. D'Andrea, V., Meco, G., Corvese, F., Baselice, P. F., and Ambrogi, V. (1989) The role of the thymus in multiple sclerosis. *Ital. J. Neurol. Sci.* **10**, 43–48.

17. Vein, A. M., Khomak, W.Y., Belokrinkij, D. V., Skrab, O. S., Golubkov, V. A., Ippolitov, I. Ch., et al. (1981) Thymectomy in multiple sclerosis. *Sov. Med.* **12**, 42–45.

18. Trotter, J. L., Cliffort, B. D., Montgomery, E. B., and Ferguson, T. B. (1985) Thymectomy in multiple sclerosis: a three year follow-up. *Neurology* **35**, 1049–1051.

19. D'Andrea, V., Malinovsky, L., Ambrogi, V., Artico, M., Capuanolg, L. G., Buccolini, F. et al. (1993) Thymectomy as treatment of autoimmune diseases other than myasthenia gravis. *Thymus* **21**, 1–10.

20. Zandman, X., Goddard, G., Lorber, M., and Shoenfeld, Y. (1995) Systemic lupus erythematosus and thymoma- a double-edged sword. *Int. Arch. Allergy Immunol.* **108**, 99–102.

21. Steven, M. M., Westedt, M. L., Euldering, F., Hazevoet, H. M., Dijkman, J. H., and Cats, A. (1984) SLE and invasive thymoma: report of two cases. *Ann. Rheum. Dis.* **43**, 825–828.

22. Spuler, S., Sarropoulos, A., Mark, A., Hohlfeld, R., and Wekerle, H. (1996) Thymoma-associated myasthenia gravis. Transplantation of thymoma and extrathymomal thymic tissue into SCID mice. *Am. J. Pathol.* **148**, 1359–1365.

23. Geuder, K. I., Marx, A., Witzemann, V., Schalke, B., Kirchner, T., and Muller-Hermelink, H. K. (1992) Genomic organization and lack of the nicotinic acetylcholine receptor subunit genes in myasthenia gravis-associated thymoma. *Lab. Invest.* **66**, 452–458.

24. Marx, A., Osborn, M., Tzartos, S., Geuder, K. I., Schalke, B., Nix, W., et al. (1992) A striational muscle antigen and myasthenia gravis-associated thymomas share anacetylcholine-receptorepitope. *Dev. Immunol.* **2**, 77–84.

25. Marx, A., O'Connor, R., Geuder, K. I., Kirchner, T., and Muller-Hermelink, H. K. (1990) Characterization of a protein with an acetylcholine receptor-epitope from myasthenia gravis-associated thymomas. *Lab. Invest.* **62**, 279–286.

26. Bonomo, A., Kehn, P. J., Payer, E., Rizzo, L., Cheever, A. W., and Shevach, E. M. (1995) Pathogenesis of post-thymectomy autoimmunity. Role of syngeneic MLR-reactive T cells. *J. Immunol.* **154**, 6602–6611.

27. Brayman, K. L., Nakai, I., Field, M. J., Lloveras, J. J., Jessurun, J., Najarian, J. S., et al. (1992) Evaluation of intrathymic islet transplantation in the prediabetic period. *Surgery* **112**, 319–326.

28. Khoury, S. J., Gallon, L., Chen, W., Betres, K., Russell, M. E., Hancock, W. W., et al. (1995) Mechanisms of acquired thymic tolerance in experimental auto-immune encephalomyelitis: thymic dendritic-enriched cells induce specific periph-eral T cell unresponsiveness in vivo. *J. Exp. Med.* **182**, 357–366.

29. Khoury, S. J., Sayegh, M. H., Hancock, W. W., Gallon, L., Carpenter, C. B., and Weiner, H. L. (1993) Acquired tolerance to experimental autoimmune encephalo-myelitis by intrathymic injection of myelin basic protein or its major encephalito-genic peptide. *J. Exp. Med.* **178**, 559–566.

30. Zoneraich, S. (1994) Unraveling the conundrums of the diabetic heart diagnosed in 1876: prelude to genetics. *Can. J. Cardiol.* **10**, 945–950.

31. Penhale, W. J., Stumbles, P. A., Huxtable, C. R., Sutherland, R. J., and Pethick, D. W. (1990) Induction of diabetes in PVG/c strain rats by manipulation of the immune system. *Autoimmunity* **7**, 169–179.

32. Toh, B. H., van-Driel, I. R., and Gleeson, P. A. (1992) Autoimmune gastritis: toler-ance and autoimmunity to the gastric H+/K+ ATPase (proton pump). *Autoimmu-nity* **13**, 165–172.

33. Fukuma, K., Sakaguchi, S., Kuribayashi, K., Chen, W. L., Morishita, R., Sekita, K., et al. (1988) Immunologic and clinical studies on murine experimental auto-immune gastritis induced by neonatal thymectomy. *Gastroenterology* **94**, 274–283.

34. Hayashi, Y. and Hirokawa, K. (1989) Immunopathology of experimental auto-allergic sialadenitis in C3H/He mice. *Clin. Exp. Immunol.* **75**, 471–476.

35. Cohen, S. B. and Weetman, A. P. (1987) Characterization of different types of experi-mental autoimmune thyroiditis in the Buffalo strain rat. *Clin. Exp. Immunol.* **69**, 25–32.

36. Stott, D. I., Hassman, R., Neilson, L., and McGregor, A. M. (1988) Analysis of the spectrotypes of autoantibodies against thyroglobulin in two rat models of auto-immune thyroiditis. *Clin. Exp. Immunol.* **73**, 269–275.

37. Kobashi, H., Yamamoto, K., Yoshioka, T., Tomita, M., and Tsuji, T. (1994) Nonsuppurative cholangitis is induced in neonatally thymectomized mice: a pos-sible animal model for primary biliary cirrhosis. *Hepatology* **19**, 1424–1430.

38. Myozaki, M., Kamiyasu, M., Miura, T., Watanabe, Y., Nakanishi, T., and Yamashita, U. Induction of autoimmune hepatitis and autoantibodies to liver anti-gens by neonatal thymectomy in mice. *Clin. Exp. Immunol.* **104**, 133–143.

39. Moncayo, R. and Moncayo, H. E. (1992) Autoimmunity and the ovary. *Immunol. Today* **13**, 255–258.

40. Tung, K. S. and Lu, C. Y. (1991) Immunologic basis of reproductive failure. *Monogr. Pathol.* **33**, 308–333.

41. Shoenfeld, Y. and Isenberg, D. (1989) Hormonal components and autoimmune diseases, in *The Mosaic of Autoimmunity* (Shoenfeld, Y. and Isenberg, D., eds.), Elsevier, Amsterdam, pp. 271–278.

42. Lo, D., Reilly, C., Marconi, L. A., Ogata, L., Wei, Q., Prud-homme, G., et al. (1995) Regulation of CD4 T cell reactivity to self and non-self. *Int. Rev. Immunol.* **13**, 147–160.

43. Antonia, S. J., Geiger, T., Miller, J., and Flavell, R. A. (1995) Mechanisms of immune tolerance induction through the thymic expression of a peripheral tissue-specific protein. *Int. Immunol.* **7**, 715–725.

44. Bonomo, A., Kehn, P. J., and Shevach, E. M. (1995) Post-thymectomy autoimmunity: abnormal T-cell homeostasis. *Immunol. Today* **16,** 61–67.
45. Younus, J. and Ahmed, A. R. (1990) The relationship of pemphigus to neoplasia. *J. Am. Acad. Dermatol.* **23,** 498–502.
46. Mevorach, D., Perrot, S., Buchanan, N. M., Khamashta, M., Laoussadi, S., Hughes, G. R. et al. (1995) Appearance of systemic lupus erythematosus after thymectomy: four case reports and review of the literature. *Lupus* **4,** 33–37.
47. Petersen, P. and Lund, J. (1969) Systemic lupus erythematosus following thymectomy for myasthenia gravis. *Dan. Med. Bull.* **16,** 179–181.
48. Goldman, M., Herode, A., Borenstein, S., and Zanen, A. (1984) Optic neuritis, transverse myelitis, and anti-DNA antibodies nine years after thymectomy for myasthenia gravis. *Arthritis Rheum.* **27,** 701–703.
49. Grinlinton, F. M., Lynch, N. M., and Hart, H. H. (1991) A pair of monozygotic twins who are concordant for myasthenia gravis but became discordant for systemic lupus erythematosus post-thymectomy. *Arthritis Rheum.* **34,** 916–919.

24

Mechanisms of Action of Intravenous Immunoglobulin (IVIg) in Immune-Mediated Diseases

K. A. Nagendra Prasad, Michel D. Kazatchkine, and Srinivas V. Kaveri

1. INTRODUCTION

Intravenous immunoglobulin (IVIg) for therapeutic use is normal poly-specific immunoglobulin-G prepared from plasma pools of large numbers of healthy donors. The fundamental characteristics of immunoglobulin preparations relevant to their immunomodulatory and anti-inflammatory properties include 1) an intact Fc portion, which allows for appropriate interactions of IVIg with serum proteins (e.g., complement components) and with Fcγ receptors, 2) a relative distribution of IgG subclasses in the IVIg preparation that is similar to the distribution found in normal serum, 3) a normal half-life of the infused IgG in recipients, and 4) a large number of binding sites (variable regions) of antibodies, as a consequence of pooling IgG of several thousands of donors in IVIg. Thus, the broad spectrum of antibody reactivities present in IVIg comprises antibodies to pathogens and foreign antigens, and antibodies to self antigens ("natural autoantibodies") which are normally present in human serum, including antibodies to the idiotypes of immunoglobulins. As discussed later, anti-idiotypic antibodies in IVIg that are directed against autoantibodies are directly relevant to the immunoregulation of autoimmune disease.

2. MECHANISMS OF ACTION OF IVIg

The potential of IVIg therapy for the treatment of autoimmune and inflammatory disorders is increasing steadily (Table 1). The therapeutic utility of IVIg is supported by evidence on the immunomodulatory properties of normal immunoglobulin, originating from clinical trials and experimental models of disease. This chapter reviews the available information on the mechanisms by which IVIg exerts its immunoregulatory effects. A better understanding of these mechanisms is essential for improving the strategy of clinical trials and designing appropriate schedules of administration of IVIg. Further, a mechanistic understanding will enable the design of the "second generation" of IVIg preparations capable

Contemporary Immunology: Autoimmune Reactions
Edited by: S. Paul © Humana Press Inc., Totowa, NJ

Table 1
Autoimmune and Systemic Inflammatory Diseases
in Which IVIg is Reported to be Beneficial

Hematologic disorders
  Idiopathic Thrombocytopenic Purpura (ITP)
  Autoimmune Neutropenia.
  Autoimmune Hemolytic Anemia
  Autoimmune Erythroblastopenia
  Pure white cell aplasia
  Hemophilia Associated with Antihemophilic Factor Inhibitor
Autoimmune Rheumatic Disorders
  SLE
  Rheumatoid Arthritis (RA) (and Felty's Syndrome)
  Juvenile Chronic Arthritis (JCA)
  Polymyositis, Dermatomyositis
  ANCA-positive Systemic Vasculitis
  Kawasaki Disease
  Sjögren Syndrome
Neurologic diseases
  Guillain-Barr Syndrome (GBS)
  Chronic Inflammatory Demyelinating Polyneuropathy (CIDP)
  Myasthenia Gravis
  Monoclonal Gammapathy with anti-MAG activity
  Multiple Sclerosis
  Seizure Disorders
Endocrinologic Diseases
  Insulin-Dependent Diabetes Mellitus (IDDM)
  Thyroid Ophthalmopathy
Antiphospholipid Syndrome and recurrent spontaneous abortions
Dermatologic Diseases: Bullous Pemphygoid
Ophthalmology: Birdshot Retinopathy
Graft Versus Host Disease
Respiratory Diseases: Asthma

of selectively immunomodulating the autoimmune diseases, and it will help define the functions of normal immunoglobulins in immune homeostasis.

The proposed mechanisms of action of IVIg are listed in Table 2. One or several of these mechanisms may be simultaneously operative to yield the therapeutic benefits of IVIg. Some of these mechanisms are dependent on interactions between the Fc portion of IgG and the Fc receptors on phagocytes and lymphocytes. Other mechanisms of action of IVIg are primarily dependent on the variable (V) regions of infused antibodies. The distinction between Fc-dependent

Table 2
Mechanisms of Action of IVIg

Fc receptor-mediated effects
  Fc receptor blockade
  Fc receptor-mediated signaling
Anti-inflammatory effects
Attenuation of complement-mediated tissue damage
  Changes in the structure and solubility of immune complexes
  Induction of anti-inflammatory cytokines
  Neutralization of microbial toxins
  Neutralization of autoantibodies by anti-idiotypes
  Neutralization of superantigens
  Selection of immune repertoires
  Modulation of T-cell and monocytic cytokine production
  Control of expansion (or down-regulation) and of activation

and V region-dependent mechanisms is somewhat artificial, however, since many of the biological functions of IgG are amplified, or indeed made possible, by the cooperative interactions between Fc fragments and Fc receptors on cells targeted by the relevant V regions.

3. Fc RECEPTOR-MEDIATED EFFECTS

The functional blockade of Fc receptors on splenic macrophages by infused immunoglobulin probably accounts for a major component of the beneficial effect of IVIg in peripheral autoimmune cytopenias. Thus, the infusion of IVIg was shown to decrease the clearance of autologous erythrocytes coated with anti-D IgG in vivo *(1)*. Monocytes from patients with idiopathic thrombocyctic purpura receiving IVIg have been shown to exhibit a decreased ability to form Fc-dependent rosettes in vitro. Furthermore, the correction of acute auto-immune thrombocytopenia with kinetics and efficacy similar to those of intact IVIg has been achieved by intravenous infusion of Fc fragments prepared from IVIg and by infusion of monoclonal antibody (MAb) to FcγRIII *(2)*.

In addition to blocking the availability of Fcγ receptors to IgG, the binding of Fc of IgG to Fcγ receptors may trigger intracellular signaling and thereby affect the functions of B-cells, T-cells, and monocytes *(3)*. It has been shown, for example, that the interaction of IVIg with Fcγ receptors on normal peripheral blood mononuclear cells induces the release of the soluble FcγRIII (CD16) both in vitro and in vivo. The relevance of these observations to the therapeutic effects of IVIg in autoimmune disease, however, is unknown at present.

4. ANTI-INFLAMMATORY EFFECTS OF IVIG

Infusion of IVIg has been shown to result in a rapid and dramatic decrease in the systemic and local signs of inflammation in several conditions, including

Table 3
Evidence for the Presence in IVIg
of Antibodies Against V Regions of Autoantibodies

F(ab')$_2$ fragments of IVIg inhibit autoantibody activity
Autoantibody activity is selectively retained on affinity columns of F(ab')$_2$ fragments of IVIg coupled to Sepharose
IVIg shares anti-idiotypic reactivity against idiotypes of autoantibodies with heterologous anti-idiotypic antibodies
Infusion of IVIg results in the selective down- or up-regulation of B-cell clones that are complementary (i.e., idiotypically "connected") to V regions of IVIg

Kawasaki syndrome, dermatomyositis, and juvenile rheumatoid arthritis. Several mechanisms may potentially account for the anti-inflammatory effects of IVIg, including inhibition of complement-mediated damage, changes in the inflammatory potential of circulating immune complexes, and modulation of the relative production of pro-inflammatory and anti-inflammatory cytokines.

4.1. Attenuation of Complement-Mediated Tissue Damage

The ability of IVIg to interfere with complement activation was demonstrated in in vivo models of complement-dependent hepatic clearance of IgM-sensitized guinea pig erythrocytes *(4)* and anti-Forssman antibody-mediated shock in guinea pigs, a model in which rabbit IgG antibodies to endothelial cells induce acute complement-mediated tissue damage *(5)*. In the latter model, the median duration of survival was increased five fold and mortality was prevented in 38% of the animals. In both systems, IVIg was shown to prevent C3 and C4 uptake by IgG- and IgM-coated targets. The effect was not dependent on the interference by IVIg with the early steps of classical pathway activation (no inhibition of C1 uptake), but rather, on the ability of IVIg to bind the activated C3b and C4b fragments and to thereby prevent their binding to targets of complement activation. The *in situ* evidence that IVIg modulates complement attack in a human autoimmune disease has come from the demonstration of decreased deposition of C3b and C5b-9 complexes in small vessels of IVIg-treated patients with dermatomyositis *(6)*. Recent data indicate that the capacity of normal immunoglobulins to inhibit C3 and C4 uptake by immune complexes is not restricted to the IgG class. On a molar basis, monomeric serum IgA and IgM are even more active than IgG in inhibiting complement activation *(7)*.

4.2. Induction of Anti-Inflammatory Cytokines

The ability of IVIg to modulate the production and the functions of pro-inflammatory cytokines probably plays a key role in the early effects of IVIg observed in acute inflammatory conditions. In tissue culture, the addition of IVIg induces normal human peripheral blood monocytes to produce and release IL-1ra *(8,9)*. The effect is selective in that IVIg triggers gene transcription and secretion of IL-1ra (as well as of IL-8), without inducing the production

Table 4
Evidence for the Selection of Immune
Repertoires in Recipients of Normal Immunoglobulin

V regions of immunoglobulins select preimmune B-cell repertoires in the bone marrow and in peripheral tissues.

Infusion of IVIg results in transient or long-term suppression of disease-related B-cell clones in patients with autoimmune diseases. IVIg or homologous IgG prevents or delays autoimmune manifestations in experimental models of autoimmune diseases.

Infusion of IVIg in autoimmune patients is associated with selective down-regulation or stimulation of autoimmune clones that react with IVIg through V regions.

Infusion of IVIg in autoimmune patients restores the kinetics of spontaneous fluctuations of serum autoantibody levels to a pattern similar to those found in healthy individuals.

of IL-1α, IL-1β, TNF-α, or IL-6. The effect of IVIg requires both the Fc and F(ab')$_2$ portions of IgG. It has been suggested previously that IVIg suppresses lipopolysaccharide-induced production of TNF-a and IL-1 through an increase in intracellular levels of cAMP following the binding of IVIg with Fcγ receptors on monocytes *(10)*. Little information is available on the changes in patterns of cytokine production in patients upon administration of IVIg, mainly owing to the present limitations of methods to assess cytokine production in vivo. A marked increase in plasma levels of IL-1ra resulting in a 1000-fold molar excess of IL-1ra over IL-1β has been reported in some patients in a recent study *(11)*.

Normal IgG has been shown to contain natural antibodies against IL-1α, TNF-α, and IL-6 *(12–14)*. Such natural anticytokine antibodies may be involved in the inhibition of cytokine-mediated effects if they are produced in excess in systemic inflammatory disorders. We have recently shown that IVIg contain antibodies to IL-4 receptors, as assessed by ELISA and BIAcore technology using recombinant IL-4 receptor.

5. NEUTRALIZATION OF AUTOANTIBODIES BY ANTI-IDIOTYPES

Interactions between IVIg and the variable regions of autoantibodies provide the basis for the ability of IVIg to neutralize circulating autoantibodies, resulting in short term decrease in serum autoantibody titers. In the long term, such interactions may potentially regulate both the activity and proliferation of autoreactive B-cell clones. The evidence demonstrating that IVIg contains antibodies capable of recognizing the idiotypes of disease-associated and of natural autoantibodies is summarized in Table 3.

We have shown that intact IVIg and the F(ab')$_2$ fragments of IVIg neutralize the functional activity of various autoantibodies and inhibit the binding of the autoantibodies to their respective autoantigens in vitro. Inhibition of autoantibody activity by IVIg has been reported in the case of autoantibodies to factor VIII *(15)*, thyroglobulin, DNA, intrinsic factor *(16)*, peripheral nerves *(17)*, neutrophil cytoplasmic antigens *(18)*, platelet gpIIb and IIIa *(19)*, the acetylcholine receptor *(20)*, endothelial cells *(21)*, phospholipids *(22)*, nephritic factor *(23)*, and retinal autoantigens *(24)*. More recently, it was shown that IVIg contains antibodies directed to the cross-reactive 4B4 idiotype that is strongly associated with Sjögren's syndrome *(25)*. In patients with antifactor VIII autoimmune disease and with antinuclear cytoplasmic antigen-positive vasculitis, a positive correlation is observed between the ability of IVIg to neutralize autoantibody activity in vitro and that of IVIg to decrease autoantibody titers in treated patients in vivo *(26,27)*.

Direct evidence that the IVIg contain anti-idiotypes to autoantibodies came from affinity chromatography experiments using columns of $F(ab')_2$ fragments of IVIg coupled to Sepharose, in which a 1.5-fold to a 50-fold increase in specific autoantibody activity was observed in the acid eluates of the columns, demonstrating that $F(ab')_2$ fragments of IVIg specifically bind idiotypic determinants located in or close to the antigen-binding site of the autoantibodies *(16,28)*. Immunoblotting analysis of the interactions between antiendothelial cell autoantibodies, endothelial cell extracts and IVIg further demonstrated that the IVIg reacts selectively with certain antibody species within the polyclonal population of anti-endothelial cell autoantibodies *(29)*. We have also shown that IVIg binds anti-factor VIII autoantibodies and anti-thyroglobulin autoantibodies with characteristics similar to those of defined mouse and rabbit antiidiotypic reagents, providing further evidence that IVIg contains anti-idiotypes to autoantibodies *(28,30)*. Finally, IVIg was shown to bind to a synthetic peptide derived from the CDR2/FR3 region of the V1 S107 heavy chain *(31)*. This peptide [T15H(50-73)] originates from the V region of the T15 idiotype of mouse and human anti-phosphorylcholine antibodies, and represents an evolutionarily conserved structure *(32,33)*. T15(50-73) serves as the binding site in the "self-binding" phenomenon observed in certain antibodies (*see* Kohler and Müller, Chapter 13). The IVIg possesses the potential, therefore, to perturb the self-binding events, perhaps with regulatory implications.

The presence of antibodies in IVIg that are idiotypically "connected" with IgG and IgM autoantibodies reflects the normal, physiological situation, in which anti-idiotypic antibodies to antibodies are conceived to regulate the expression of the immune repertoire *(34,35)*. Complementary interactions between the V regions of the different antibodies present in IVIg may result in additive or synergistic enhancement of similar interactions occurring in autologous antibodies. Alternatively, the IVIg anti-idiotypic activities might inhibit certain specific autologous interactions *(36)*.

6. NEUTRALIZATION OF SUPERANTIGENS

IVIg inhibits superantigen-elicited T-cell activation, e.g., by staphylococcal toxin superantigens, which are the targets for specific anti-superantigen antibodies present in IVIg *(37)*. Further, we recently observed that the presence of IVIg in cultures of normal peripheral blood mononuclear cells stimulated with SEB superantigen rescued the CD3 blast cells from apoptosis, which express the Vβ T-cell marker and expand in the presence of SEB *(38)*. These observations are potentially relevant in interpreting the effect of IVIg in certain diseases which may be triggered by bacterial superantigens (e.g., Kawasaki disease).

7. SELECTION OF IMMUNE REPERTOIRES

Natural autoantibodies serve to regulate the self-reactivity in healthy individuals. Several lines of evidence derived from studies in normal mice and from clinical observations in recipients of therapeutic IgG indicate that IVIg, which, by mass, is primarily composed of natural IgG antibodies, selects expressed B-cell and T-cell repertoires in vivo. The evidence is summarized in Table 4. If pathological autoimmunity emerges because of a failure of the immunological control mechanisms, the beneficial effects of treatment with IVIg can be hypothesized to be owing to restoration of the physiological regulation mechanisms. In this hypothesis, IVIg can be seen as a substitutional therapy aimed at compensating for a deficiency in regulatory molecules and/or cells.

7.1. Antibodies in IVIg Against Functional Membrane Molecules of Lymphocytes

In addition to binding to idiotypes of soluble immunoglobulins, IVIg reacts with a number of membrane molecules of T-cells, B-cells, and monocytes. The recognition of membrane antigens relevant for control of autoreactivity and induction of self tolerance provides, thus, provides yet another mechanistic basis for understanding the complex regulatory functions of IVIg, e.g., on lymphocyte proliferation, differentiation and cytokine production. Thus, IVIg has been shown to contain antibodies to the variable and constant regions of the human αβ T-cell receptor, cytokine receptors, CD5, CD4, HLA Class I antigens, and adhesion molecules. The binding of IVIg to the TCR variable and constant regions has been documented in studies using synthetic peptides derived from the TCR. Overlapping synthetic hexadecapeptides of human TCR β YT35 were used to assess the binding of IVIg by ELISA in one study *(39)*. By using affinity purification methods, an anti-Vβ8-enriched antibody fraction was purified from IVIg that displayed high levels of binding to specific Vβ8 TCR peptides. The presence of autoantibodies to defined human TCR peptides imparts to IVIg the potential for modulating specific T-cell immune responses.

Antibodies to CD5 were identified based on the ability of F(ab')$_2$ fragments of IVIg to inhibit the binding of CD5 MAb to a CD5-expressing human T-cell line and to mouse cells that expressed human CD5 following stable transfection with CD5 cDNA *(40)*. Antibodies to CD4 have been characterized in IVIg using both immunochemical and functional approaches *(41)*. F(ab)$_2$ fragments of IVIg were found to bind to recombinant human CD4, as assessed by ELISA, immunoblotting and real time analysis of complex formation using the BIAcore technology. Anti-CD4 antibodies were isolated from IVIg by affinity chromatography on a recombinant CD4-Sepharose column and shown to bind human CD4$^+$ T-cells. The affinity-purified anti-CD4 antibodies from IVIg inhibited the proliferative responses of lymphocytes in mixed lymphocyte culture and the in vitro infection of CD4$^+$ T-cells with HIV. We have recently shown that IVIg contains antibodies to the B07.75-84 peptide, which corresponds to a nonpolymorphic determinant of HLA Class I molecules *(42)*. IVIg and F(ab')$_2$ fragments of IVIg bound to the peptide, as well as to purified soluble HLA antigens and to HLA antigens expressed on human T-cells. Antibodies to a CD8 peptide isolated from IVIg by affinity chromatography were shown to inhibit CD8-mediated, HLA Class I-restricted cytolysis of an influenza peptide-primed target cell by an influenza virus-specific human T-cell line. The presence in IVIg of antibodies to critical regions of HLA Class I molecules suggests the capability of IVIg to modulate Class I-restricted cellular interactions in the immune response. Of interest in this regard, are recent observations that administration of IVIg decreases the plasma titer of cytotoxic anti-Class I antibodies, allowing, in certain cases, superior survival of allotransplants in hyperimmunized dialyzed patients with a positive cross match.

8. PERSPECTIVES

The IgG immunoglobulin molecule bears the potential for V region-mediated and Fc-mediated interactions with a large number of soluble molecules and membrane components that are involved in the control of inflammation and in maintaining homeostasis of autoreactivity. IVIg carries an even broader functional potential, since it represents a pool of natural antibodies from the plasma of large numbers of healthy donors. Other postulated biological roles of natural antibodies include participation in natural defenses against infectious agents and tumors, removal of senescent/altered self molecules *(43,44)*, transport of other biologically active molecules such as cytokines *(45)*, and transport and presentation of antigens for T-cell stimulation (46). An additional role for natural antibodies can be conceived from observations that the antibodies display catalytic activity *(47–50)*. The existence of a polyreactive enzymatic activity in individuals who are not deliberately immunized, and a lowered catalytic activity in patients with autoimmune disease such as rheumatoid arthritis imply that antibody-dependent catalysis may play a functional role in autoimmune manifestations *(50)*. Thus, the potential catalytic activity of natural antibodies in IVIg may explain at least in part its ameliorative effect in autoimmune diseases.

Delineating which of the mechanisms described above is predominantly involved in an individual disease may provide in the future the means for targeted intervention using engineered human immunoglobulins; that is, unless the intrinsic complexity of polyclonal IgG is required for achieving immunomodulation of a system that is otherwise regulated in such a fine and subtle fashion under physiological conditions.

REFERENCES

1. Fehr, J., Hofmann, V., and Kappeler, U. (1982) Transient reversal of thrombocytopenia in idiopathic thrombocytopenic purpura by high-dose intravenous gammaglobulin. *N. Engl. J. Med.* **306**, 1254–1258.
2. Clarkson, S. B., Bussel, J. B., Kimberly, R. P., Valinsky, J. E., Nachman, R. L., and Unkeless, J. C. (1986) Treatment of refractory immune thrombocytopenic purpura with an anti-Fc gamma-receptor antibody. *N. Engl. J. Med.* **314**, 1236–1239.
3. Fridman, W. (1993) Regulation of B-cell activation and antigen presentation by Fc receptors. *Curr. Opin. Immunol.* **5**, 355–360.
4. Basta, M., Langlois, P. F., Marques, M., Frank, M. M., and Fries, L. F. (1989) High-dose intravenous immunoglobulin modifies complement-mediated in vivo clearance. *Blood* **74**, 326–333.
5. Basta, M., Kirshbom, P., Frank, M. M., and Fries, L. F. (1989) Mechanism of therapeutic effect of high-dose intravenous immunoglobulin. Attenuation of acute, complement-dependent immune damage in a guinea pig model. *J. Clin. Invest.* **84**, 1974–1981.
6. Basta, M. and Dalakas, M. C. (1994) High-dose intravenous immunoglobulin exerts its beneficial effect in patients with dermatomyositis by blocking endomysial deposition of activated complements fragments. *J. Clin. Inv.* **94**, 1729–1735.
7. Miletic, V. D., Hester, C. G., and Frank, M. M. (1996) Regulation of complement activity by Immunoglobulin. *J. Immunol.* **156**, 749–757.
8. Poutsiaka, D. D., Clark, B. D., Vannier, E., and Dinarello, C. A. (1991) Production of IL-receptor antagonist and IL-1β by peripheral blood mononuclear cells is differentially regulated. *Blood* **78**, 1275–1279.
9. Ruiz de Souza, V., Carreno, M. P., Kaveri, S. V., Ledur, A., Sadeghi, H., Cavaillon, J. M., et al. (1995) Selective induction of interleukin-1 receptor antagonist and interleukin-8 in human monocytes by normal polyspecific IgG (intravenous immunoglobulin). *Eur. J. Immunol.* **25**, 1267–1273.
10. Shimozato, T., Iwata, M., Kawada, H., and Tamura, N. (1991) Human immunoglobulin preparation for intravenous use induces elevation of cellular cyclic adenosine 3': 5'-monophosphate levels, resulting in suppression of tumor necrosis factor alpha and interleukin-1 production. *Immunology* **72**, 497–501.
11. Aukrust, P., Froland, S. S., Liabakk, N. B., Muller, F., Nordoy, I., Haug, C., et al. (1994) Release of cytokines, soluble cytokine receptors, and interleukin-1 receptor antagonist after intravenous immunoglobulin administration in vivo. *Blood* **84**, 2136–2143.
12. Bendtzen, K., Svenson, M., Jonsson, V., and Hippe, E. (1990) Autoantibodies to cytokines - friends or foes? *Immunol. Today* **11**, 167–169.
13. Svenson, M., Hansen, M. B., and Bendtzen, K. (1990) Distribution and characterization of autoantibodies to interleukin 1α in normal human sera. *Scand. J. Immunol.* **32**, 695–701.
14. Abe, Y., Horiuchi, A., Miyake, M., and Kimura, S. (1994) Anti-cytokine nature of human immunoglobulin: one possible mechanism of the clinical effect of intravenous therapy. *Immunol. Rev.* **139**, 5–19.
15. Sultan, Y., Kazatchkine, M. D., Maisonneuve, P., and Nydegger, U. E. (1984) Anti-idiotypic suppression of autoantibodies to Factor VIII (antihaemophilic factor) by high-dose intravenous gammaglobulin. *Lancet* **ii**, 765–768.

16. Rossi, F. and Kazatchkine, M. D. (1989) Antiidiotypes against autoantibodies in pooled normal human polyspecific Ig. *J. Immunol.* **143,** 4104–4109.
17. van Doorn, P. A., Rossi, F., Brand, A., van Lint, M., Vermeulen, M., and Kazatchkine, M. D. (1990) On the mechanism of high dose intravenous immunoglobulin treatment of patients with chronic inflammatory demyelinating polyneuropathy. *J. Neuroimmunol.* **29,** 57–64.
18. Rossi, F., Jayne, D. R. W., Lockwood, C. M., and Kazatchkine, M. D. (1991) Antiidiotypes against anti-neutrophil cytoplasmic antigen autoantibodies in normal human polyspecific IgG for therapeutic use and in the remission sera of patients with systemic vasculitis. *Clin. Exp. Immunol.* **83,** 298–303.
19. Berchtold, P., Dale, G. L., Tani, P., and McMillan, R. (1989) Inhibition of autoantibody binding to platelet glycoprotein IIb/IIIa by anti-idiotypic antibodies in intravenous immunoglobulins. *Blood* **74,** 2414–2417.
20. Liblau, R., Gajdos, P., Bustarret, F. A., Habib, R. E., Bach, J. F., and Morel, E. (1991) Intravenous gammaglobulin in myasthenia gravis: Interaction with anti-acetylcholine receptor autoantibodies. *J. Clin. Immunol.* **11,** 128–131.
21. Ronda, N., Haury, M., Nobrega, A., Kaveri., S. V., Coutinho, A., and Kazatchkine, M. D. (1994) Analysis of natural and disease-associated autoantibody repertoires: anti-endothelial cell IgG autoantibody activity in the serum of healthy individuals and patients with systemic lupus erythematosus. *Int. Immunol.* **6,** 1651–1660.
22. Caccavo, D., Vaccaro, F., Ferri, G. M., Amoroso, A., and Bonomo, L. (1994) Antiidiotypes against antiphospholipid antibodies are present in normal polyspecific immunoglobulins for therapeutic use. *J. Autoimmunity* **7,** 537–548.
23. Fremeaux-Bacchi, V., Maillet, F., Berlan, L., and Kazatchkine, M. D. (1992) Neutralizing antibodies against C3Nef in intravenous immunoglobulin. *Lancet* **340,** 63–64.
24. Kazatchkine, M. D., Dietrich, G., Hurez, V., Ronda, N., Bellon, B., Rossi, F., and Kaveri, S. V. (1994) V Region-mediated selection of autoreactive repertoires by intravenous immunoglobulin (IVIg). *Immunol. Rev.* **139,** 79–107.
25. Dekeyser, F., Kazatchkine, M. D., Rossi, F., Dang, H., and Talal, N. (1996) Pooled human immunoglobulins contain anti-idiotypes with reactivity against the 4B4/P36 cross-reactive idiotype. *Clin. Exp. Rheumatol.* **14,** 587–591.
26. Rossi, F., Sultan, Y., and Kazatchkine, M. D. (1988) Anti-idiotypes against autoantibodies and alloantibodies to Factor VIII:C (anti-haemophilic factor) are present in therapeutic polyspecific normal immunoglobulins. *Clin. Exp. Immunol.* **74,** 311–316.
27. Jayne, D. R. W., Davies, M., Fox, C., and Lockwood, C. M. (1991) Treatment of systemic vasculitis with pooled intravenous immunoglobulin. *Lancet* **ii,** 1137–1139.
28. Dietrich, G. and Kazatchkine, M. D. (1990) Normal immunoglobulin G (IgG) for therapeutic use (intravenous Ig) contain antiidiotypic specificities against an immunodominant, disease-associated, cross-reactive idiotype of human anti-thyroglobulin autoantibodies. *J. Clin. Invest.* **85,** 620–625.
29. Ronda, N., Haury, M., Nobrega, A., Coutinho, A., and Kazatchkine, M. D. (1994) Selectivity of recognition of variable (V) regions of autoantibodies by intravenous immunoglobulin (IVIg). *Clin. Immunol. Immunopathol.* **70,** 124–128.
30. Kaveri, S. V., Wang, H. T., Rowen, D., Kazatchkine, M. D., and Kohler, H. (1993) Monoclonal anti-idiotypic antibodies against human anti-thyroglobulin autoantibodies recognize idiotopes shared by disease-associated and natural anti-thyroglobulin autoantibodies. *Clin. Immunol. Immunopathol.* **69,** 333–340.

31. Kaveri, S. V., Kang, C. Y., and Kohler, H. (1990) Natural mouse and human antibodies bind to a peptide derived from a germline variable heavy chain: evidence for evolutionary conserved self-binding locus. *J. Immunol.* **145,** 4207–4213.
32. Kang, C.-Y., Brunck, T. K., Kieber-Emmons, T., Blalock., J. E., and Kohler, H. (1988) Inhibition of self-binding antibodies (autobodies) by a Vh-derived peptide. *Science* **240,** 1034–1036.
33. Halpern, R., Kaveri, S. V., and Kohler, H. (1991) Human anti-phosphorylcholine antibodies share idiotopes and are self-binding. *J. Clin. Invest.* **88,** 476–482.
34. Adib, M., Ragimbeau, J., Avrameas, S., and Ternynck, T. (1990) IgG autoantibody activity in normal mouse serum is controlled by IgM. *J. Immunol.* **145,** 3807–3813.
35. Hurez, V., Kaveri, S. V., and Kazatchkine, M. D. (1993) Expression and control of the natural autoreactive IgG repertoire in normal human serum. *Eur. J. Immunol.* **23,** 783–789.
36. Dietrich, G., Algiman, M., Sultan, Y., Nydegger, U. E., and Kazatchkine, M. D. (1992) Origin of anti-idiotypic activity against anti-factor VIII autoantibodies in pools of normal human immunoglobulin G (IVIg). *Blood* **79,** 2946–2951.
37. Takei, S., Arora, Y., and Walker, S. M. (1993) Intravenous immunoglobulin contains specific antibodies inhibitory to activation of T cells by staphylococcal toxin superantigens. *J. Clin. Invest.* **91,** 602–607.
38. Baudet, V., Hurez, V., Lapeyre, C., Kaveri, S. V., and Kazatchkine, M. D. (1996) Intravenous immunoglobulin (IVIg) enhances the selective expansion of Vβ3+ and Vβ17+ αβ T cells induced by superantigen. *Scand. J. Immunol.* **43,** 277–282.
39. Marchalonis, J. J., Kaymaz, H., Dedeoglu, F., Schlutter, S. F., Yocum, D. E., and Edmundson, A. B. (1992) Human autoantibodies reactive with synthetic auto-antigens from T cell receptor β chain. Proc. Natl. Acad. Sci. USA **89,** 3325-3329.
40. Vassilev, T., Gelin, C., Kaveri, S. V., Zilber, L., Boumsell, L., and Kazatchkine, M. D. (1993) Antibodies to the CD5 molecule in normal human immunoglobulins for therapeutic use (intravenous immunoglobulins, IVIg). *Clin. Exp. Immunol.* **92,** 369–372.
41. Hurez, V., Kaveri, S. V., Mouhoub, A., Dietrich, G., Mani, J. C., Klatzmann, D., and Kazatchkine, D. (1994) Anti-CD4 activity of normal human immunoglobulins G for therapeutic use (Intravenous immunoglobulin, IVIg). *Therap. Immunol.* **1,** 269–278.
42. Kaveri, S., Vassilev, T., Hurez, V., Lengagne, R., Lefranc, C., Cot, S., et al. (1996) Antibodies to a conserved region of HLA class I molecules, capable of modulating CD8 T cell-mediated function, are present in pooled normal immunoglobulin for therapeutic use (IVIg). *J. Clin. Invest.* **97,** 865–869.
43. Schlesinger, J. S. and Horwitz, M. A. (1994) A role for natural antibody in the pathogenesis of leprosy: antibody in non-immune serum mediates C3 fixation to the mycobacterium leprae surface and hence phagocytosis by human mononuclear phagocytes. *Infect. Immunol.* **62,** 280–289.
44. Giger, U., Sticher, B., Naef, R., Burger, R., and Lutz, H. U. (1995) Naturally occuring human anti-band 3 antoantibodies accelerate clearance of erythrocytes in guinea pigs. *Blood* **85,** 1920–1926.
45. Hansen, M. B., Svenson, M., Abbell, K., Yasukawa, K., Diamant, M., and Bendtzen, K. (1995) Influence of interleukin-6 autoantibodies on IL-6 binding to cellular receptors. *Eur. J. Immunol.* **25,** 348–354.

46. Thornton, B., Vetvicka, P. V., and Ross, G. D. (1994) Natural antibody and complement-mediated antigen processing and presentation by B lymphocytes. *J. Immunol.* **152,** 1727–1737.

47. Paul, S., Volle, D. J., Beach, C. M., Johnson, D. R., Powell, M. J., and Massey, R. J. (1989) Catalytic hydrolysis of vasoactive intestinal peptide by human autoantibody. *Science* **244,** 1158–1162.

48. Shuster, A. M., Gololobov, G. V., Kvashuk, O. A., Bogomolova, A. E., Smirnov, I., and Gabibov, A. G. (1992) DNA hydrolyzing autoantibodies. *Science* **256,** 665–669.

49. Paul, S. (1994) Catalytic activity of anti-ground state antibodies, antibody subunits, and human autoantibodies. *Appl. Biochem. Biotechnol.* **47,** 41–43.

50. Kalaga, R., Li, L., O'Dell, J. R., and Paul, S. (1995) Unexpected presence of polyreactive catalytic antibodies in IgG from unimmunized donors and decreased levels in rheumatoid arthritis. *J. Immunol.* **155,** 2695–2702

25

Mucosal Immunization
for Induction of Tolerance to Autoantigens

Bao-Guo Xiao and Hans Link

1. BACKGROUND

Mucosal immunology is one of the most rapidly developing and exciting fields of immunology. Mucosal immunization offers several important advantages over parenteral immunization, including higher efficacy to achieve both mucosal and systemic immunity, minimization of adverse effects, easy delivery, and inexpensiveness. Mucosal immunology has a history that dates back more than 2000 yr, and many of the important phenomena have been dealt with in two recent reviews (1,2). The modern concept was developed by the Russian scientist Alexandre Besredka in 1919. He showed the existence of a protective immune system functioning in the gut fairly independently of systemic immunity, which utilizes secretory IgA (sIgA) as the major effector substance. In addition to inducing local sIgA antibody secretion and cell-mediated immune responses, mucosal administration of antigens also results in a state of peripheral immunological tolerance in several experimental animal models. Figure 1 shows schematically the two major defense mechanisms in the mucosal membrane. This phenomenon is often referred to as "mucosal tolerance" and has been observed in the human fed (immunized) with several antigens including classical immunogens such as keyhole-limpet hemocyanin (KLH). In order to join forces in terms of basic and practical research, an International Society for Mucosal Immunology (SMI) has been organized to promote this important field (3).

2. ONTOGENY OF ORALLY INDUCED TOLERANCE

Oral administration of myelin basic protein (MBP) to adult but not neonatal animals protects against the development of experimental autoimmune encephalomyelitis (EAE) induced by immunization with neuronal extracts. As opposed to the adult animals, oral MBP did not induce the deletion or unresponsiveness of autoreactive lymphocytes. To the contrary, the neonatal animals treated with oral MBP displayed enhanced disease expression during adulthood (4), suggesting that immaturity of the immunoregulatory network in the gut permits sensitization to autoantigens, a phenomenon that might contribute to the pathogenesis of autoimmune diseases in later life.

Contemporary Immunology: Autoimmune Reactions
Edited by: S. Paul © Humana Press Inc., Totowa, NJ

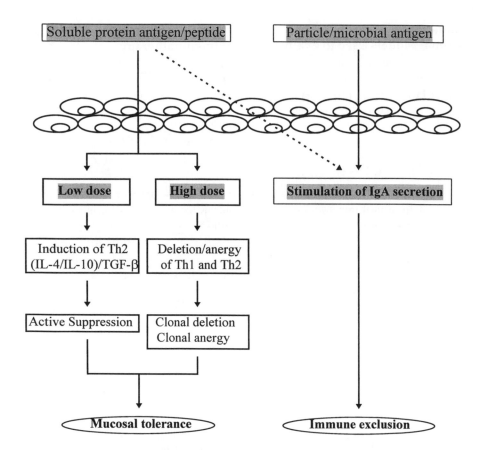

Fig. 1. Schematic depiction of two major defense mechanisms in the mucosal membrance. First-line defense is principally mediated by stimulating IgA secretion in cooperation with various nonspecific protective factors. Secretory immunity is stimulated mainly by particulate or live microbial antigens. Solublc antigen induces mucosal tolerance, depending on the antigen dose used. A low dose of antigen preferentially activates TGF-β and Th2 cells, which suppress Th1-cell function. By contrast, a high dose of antigen directly anergizes or deletes antigen-specific T-cells, including Th1 and Th2.

It is conceivable that when certain environmental antigens are exposed to the immature (neonatal) intestinal barrier, they prime the immune system rather than induce oral tolerance, as occurs in the adult. The immunological priming effects of orally introduced MBP in newborn mice gradually decrease until approximately the fourth week of life, at which time tolerance is induced. The kinetics of oral priming vs. tolerance induction by MBP during ontogeny correlate with the delayed-type hypersensitivity (DTH) responses to MBP, and are similar to the tolerogenic effects of feeding another protein, ovalbumin (OVA), in the neo-natal period *(5)*. Events occurring in the mucosa-associated lymphoid tissue (MALT) may contribute intimately in the failure to induce oral tolerance in the neonatal period. MHC Class II molecules appear in the MALT of the rat at around four weeks of age. The absence of these T-cell regulatory molecules may restrict the elicitation of regulatory cells associated with oral tolerance in adults. Recent studies provide evidence for the presence of MHC molecules on gut epithelial cells that selectively stimulate regulatory T-cells in peripheral blood *(6)*. MHC expression in MALT might thus contribute to the induction of oral tolerance. Alternatively, induction of the regulatory cells involved in oral tolerization may be controlled by other markers or cells with a distinctive ontogenic kinetics of expression in the MALT. This would explain the age-related and route of entry-dependent mechanisms of the antigen-driven tolerization phenomenon.

3. THE PHYSIOLOGICAL FUNCTION OF MUCOSAL ORGAN-SPECIFIC AUTOIMMUNITY

Orally administered antigen encounters the MALT, a very well-developed immune network that evolved not only to protect the host from ingested pathogens, but also to develop the inherent property of preventing the host from reacting in harmful ways to ingested proteins. The mucous membranes are endowed with powerful mechanical and physicochemical cleansing mechanisms that degrade and repel most foreign matter. In a healthy human adult, various MALTs together form the largest mammalian lymphoid organ system. The MALT has three main functions: 1) to protect mucous membranes against colonization and invasion by potentially dangerous microbes, 2) to prevent the systemic uptake of undegraded antigens, including foreign proteins derived from ingested food, and 3) to prevent the development of potentially harmful immune responses to these antigens if they do reach the body interior. It follows that upon encounter with this plethora of antigenic stimuli present in food, the MALT must economically utilize the appropriate immunological effector mechanisms and regulate their intensity to avoid bystander tissue damage and immunological exhaustion.

The issue of how antigens are taken up, processed and presented by antigen-presenting cells (APCs) at mucosal surfaces is fundamental for understanding the induction of mucosal immune response and oral tolerance. One route of antigen entry to mucosal surfaces involves the M-cells, which are located in follicle-associated epithelium. The M-cells are derived from the stem cell compartment of the epithelial layer and their development depends on the presence of lymphoid cells *(7)*. In contrast to the intestinal epithelial cells, which take up soluble antigens efficiently, the M-cells appear to be specialized for binding and transporting particulate antigens. Consistent with this role, the surface of the M-cells appears to be specialized for endocytosis.

Dendritic cells (DCs) are also important for antigen sampling at mucosal surfaces. In the normal respiratory tract, a submucosal network of DCs functions as a surveillance system to monitor inhaled antigens, and intricate cross-regulation takes place between DCs, alveolar macrophages and T-cells within the respiratory mucosa. DCs are inert locally, but they are responsible for transporting autoantigens to regional lymph nodes, where leakage of processed peptides from the MHC Class II to the Class I pathway may provide stimulation of CD8$^+$ regulatory T-cells *(8)*.

4. MUCOSAL TOLERANCE IN AGGRESSIVE ORGAN-SPECIFIC AUTOIMMUNITY

One of the most interesting questions in immunology is how we can survive encounter with so many potential antigens at the mucosal surfaces without raising aberrant immune responses. The answer is that the antigens are often capable of inducing systemic unresponsiveness as a result of mucosal tolerance mechanisms. Mucosal tolerance can potentially affect all types of immune responses, including systemic antibody responses. The observed effects are generally variable, however, depending on the animal species, the age, the nature of the antigens, and the route of administration (gastric, buccal, nasal, or rectal).

4.1. Oral Route

The phenomenon of oral tolerance was first reported in 1911 by Wells *(9)*, who showed that orally administered hen egg protein imparted resistance to anaphylaxis in guinea pigs induced by the previously ingested protein. Merrill Chase *(10)* reported that oral administration of certain haptens resulted in the suppression of systemic responses to the fed antigen. In the 1970s, there was much research activity in this area, focused on the effects of feeding a variety of protein antigens and on the mechanism of suppression of the immune response. Multiple feedings were observed to be superior to a single oral dose for tolerance induction. In the case of EAE, a minimum of 10 mg MBP administered orally was necessary for tolerance induction. Larger oral doses (20 or 100 mg) of MBP provided the best protection from EAE, while lower doses (0.4 mg) exacerbated the clinical course of disease *(11)*.

4.2. Nasal Route

An alternative route towards induction of mucosal tolerance is via the nose. This route presents certain advantages over the oral route. It avoids the encounter of the antigens with the acidic and proteolytic environment of the stomach. Therefore, nasal administration appears to be more effective than oral administration in inducing tolerance at low antigen doses *(12)*. We demonstrated that Torpedo acetylcholine receptor (AChR) given orally in mg doses or nasally in µg doses to Lewis rats prior to immunization with AChR prevented clinical signs of experimental autoimmune myasthenia gravis (EAMG) and suppressed AChR-specific B- and T-cell-mediated immune responses *(13)*. Nasal deposition of MBP peptides (Acl-9 or Acl-11) was effective for induction ofthe unresponsiveness, whereas oral administration is relatively ineffective, as assessed in an H-2u mouse model *(14)*. Although dose-related differences between the oral and nasal routes are evident, the final immunological effects and the implications for disease development are similar using the two routes.

4.3. The Protein, Peptide, and Altered Peptide

Over the past two decades, several variables important for the induction of oral tolerance have been identified. The antigens used to induce mucosal tolerance include various protein antigens, heterologous red blood cells and certain killed viruses. The fact that lymphocytes respond differently to different forms of the antigen was first revealed by Dresser and colleagues more than 30 yr ago *(15)*. Concerning induction of antigen-specific peripheral tolerance by oral antigen, MBP from different species has been observed to achieve cross-species tolerance, and the tolerance displays a species-related hierarchy *(16,17)*. This has suggested the existence of tolerogenic epitopes in the MBP molecule distinct from the encephalitogenic epitopes *(17)*. The evident cross-epitope suppressor effect mediated in the local microenvironment is an additional advantage of the oral tolerance induction strategy. In our own experiments, AChR from Torpedo, MBP from bovine spinal cord, guinea pig MBP (GP MBP), and peptides of the P2 protein of peripheral nervous system (PNS) myelin successfully induced oral and nasal tolerance to subsequent immunization with AChR, MBP and bovine PNS myelin (BPM), respectively, in Lewis rats. The existence of MBP determinants capable of preferentially eliciting systemic immunological suppression has also been suggested from the results of feeding both the disease-inducing fragment (residues 44–89) and the nonencephalitogenic MBP fragments (residues 1–37 and 90–170) generated by pepsin digestion *(18)*.

In certain systems, the specificity of orally induced tolerance in EAE may involve species-specific determinants on the MBP molecule *(19)*. Rats fed GP MBP were protected from EAE induced by GP MBP, but not by feeding with rat or human MBP. Rats fed rat MBP were not protected from EAE induced with MBP from any of three species *(16)*. The specificity of orally induced tolerance is suggested to be determined by residues 68–88 as indicated by studies on synthetic peptides derived from GP MBP and rat MBP, which differ by a single amino acid (serine/threonine substitution at position 80). Only Lewis rats fed GP MBP peptide 68–88 were protected from EAE induced with GP 68–88 or rat 68–88. In contrast, feeding rat MBP peptide 68–88 did not protect against EAE induced by challenge with either peptide *(16)*. These findings suggest that small structural differences in MBP can produce dramatically different clinical outcome, a consideration with important implications for the design of clinical trials in multiple sclerosis (MS). It is clear that the affinity of self-antigens for the MHC plays an important role in dictating the fate of peripheral autoreactive T-cells *(20)*. High affinity peptides are more likely to induce tolerance, whereas low affinity peptides will allow autoreactive cells to persist in healthy individuals *(21)*. While the details of the individual systems need to be worked out, these studies underline the therapeutic potential of peptides with different MHC affinity in the treatment of autoimmune disease.

Table 1
Peptides Used in Experimental Autoimmune Diseases for Induction of Mucosal Tolerance

Peptides		Animal models						Ref.
		EAE	EAMG	EAN	EAU	IDDM	CIA	
MBP	68–88	(R)(O)[a]						*16*
	21–40	(R)(O)[a]						*87*
	71–90	(R)(O)[a]						*87*
	Ac1–9	(M)(N)[a]						*14*
	68–86	(R)(N)[a]						Not published
	87–99	(R)(N)[a]						
AChR	α61–76		(R)(N)[b]					Not published
	α100–116		(R)(N)[b]					
	α146–162		(R)(N)[b]					
	δ354–367		(R)(N)[b]					
P2	57–81			(R)(N)				Not published
S-Ag	342–355				(R)(O)			*34*
Insulin	B-(9–23)					(M)(N)		*71*
Collagen	184–198						(R)(N)	*71*
	250–270						(M)(O)	*88*

[a] Inhibition of disease.
[b] No effect.
(R), rat; (M), mouse; (O), oral; (N), nasal.

Recently, the development of structurally modified peptides, i.e., peptides containing amino acid replacements and truncated peptides, has pointed to an additional means to modulate the immune response. While previous concepts held that in a single T-cell clone, the activation of the TCR is an all-or-none event, recent data indicate that TCR engagement with altered peptides can lead to varying biological consequences. Thus, altered peptides can cause secretion of cytokines without stimulating cellular proliferation *(22)*. This phenomenon has also been demonstrated in the case of human MBP-specific T-cell clones *(23)*. Moreover, structurally altered peptides derived from the autoantigen and from an unrelated protein have been shown to influence the development of EAE, possibly through changes in cytokine secretion *(24)*. Several groups have found that the induction of disease can be prevented by coimmunization with autoantigens and a synthetic MHC binding peptide *(25)*, possibly as a result of competition for autoantigen binding and presentation by MHC class II molecules *(26)*. The use of altered peptides has revealed an additional effect, termed TCR antagonism. The altered peptides can bind the MHC and deliver a negative signal through the TCR. Thus, the peptides do not function as mere competitive blockers, but actually transmit a signal to the T-cell that is nonproliferative while retaining the activity to modulate certain T-cell functions such as cytokine secretion *(27,28)*. The TCR antagonist peptides can thus be seen as actively inducing a nonproliferative immune response capable of reversing ongoing EAE induced by adoptive transfer of MBP-reactive $CD4^+$ cells *(24)*. Table 1 lists the peptides that have been used for mucosal tolerance induction to achieve protection against autoimmune diseases.

4.4. Double and Triple Tolerance

One characteristic of the autoimmune diseases is that the affected humans and animals tend to develop more than one disease covering a common spectrum of clinical symptoms *(29)*. Myasthenia gravis (MG) patients occasionally show the presence of concurrent autoimmune disorders such as systemic lupus erythematosus, rheumatoid arthritis, or MS. The associated development of organ-specific and systemic autoimmune diseases suggests a general inherited predisposition to aggressive autoimmunity, which might arise from breakdown of a common mechanism of immunological self-tolerance. This hypothesis makes it interesting to attempt the induction of simultaneous tolerance against several autoimmune diseases by targeting the key cells responsible for immunological damage, and perhaps approach the ideal of preventing autoimmune diseases by achieving long lasting, nontoxic and specific effects on autoaggressive cells alone. In our previous experiments, tolerance against EAMG + EAE was achieved by oral administration of an AChR + MBP combination *(30)*. In recent experiments, we administered a combination of AChR + MBP + peripheral nerve myelin via the nasal route prior to systemic immunization with these antigens. This maneuver effectively suppressed the incidence and severity of the combined clinical picture consisting of EAMG + EAE + experimental allergic neuritis (EAN) observed in the control anamals. The macrophage infiltration in sections of muscle, spinal cord and sciatic nerve was reduced, and the T- and B-cell autoreactivities to the three antigens were down-regulated *(31)*.

4.5. The Mechanism of Mucosal Tolerance Induction

The "effector" mechanisms of orally induced tolerance have been studied extensively in autoimmune models, particularly EAE. These mechanisms appear to be determined primarily by the dose of the fed antigen. Low antigen doses favor the generation of regulatory cells that suppress the specific immune response in the target organ, whereas high antigen doses induce an antigen-specific anergic/deletional state in the peripheral immune system. Low doses of orally administered antigen are taken up by mucosa-associated antigen-presenting cells. These cells, through complex cellular interactions, preferentially induce regulatory T-cells to secrete suppressive cytokines, such as TGF-β, IL-4, and IL-10 (Fig. 2). High doses of orally administered antigen, on the other hand, appear to pass through the gut and enter the systemic circulation, either as intact or processed protein, and induce unresponsiveness of T-cells primarily through clonal energy/deletion. Both low and high dose of orally administered antigen elicit effects specific for the given antigen.

CD8$^+$ suppressor T-cells play a central role in recognizing nonautoantigenic epitopes in the context of class I MHC molecules. These cells appear to be activated in an antigen-specific manner by oral immunization, and their activation

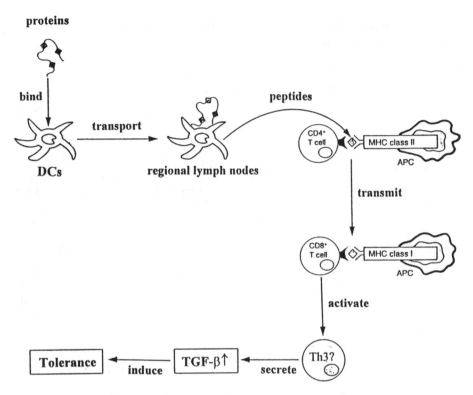

Fig. 2. A possible mechanism of TGF-β-mediated mucosal tolerance to auto-antigens. Dendritic cells (DCs) transport autoantigens to regional lyrnph nodes where leakage of processed peptides from MHC Class II to the Class I pathway may provide stimulation of CD8⁺ regulatory T-cells (Th3?). These cells secrete TGF-β and induce mucosal tolerance.

is suggested to result in nonspecific bystander suppression effects via secretion of the anti-inflammatory cytokine TGF-β *(32)*. The bystander suppression effect can be achieved by adoptive transfer of CD8⁺ T-cells from orally tolerized rats (33). The tolerogenic cells may include γ/δ T-cells *(34)*, the vast majority of which express CD8 in the rat. A remarkable observation was that the CD8⁺ cells isolated from orally tolerized animals can alter their phenotype to CD4⁺ T-cells during activation, while retaining their ability to suppress experimental autoimmune uveitis (EAU) *(35)*.

The ability to impart protection against disease is not a unique feature of the CD8⁺ cells. Oral tolerance was successfully induced in CD8-depleted animals, as demonstrated by less severe clinical disease and reduced T-cell proliferation, although there was lower TGF-β production by the cells in vitro *(36)*. It appears that CD4⁺ T-cells can mediate active suppression in orally tolerized mice in the absence of CD8⁺ T cells.

Further evidence for the role of CD4⁺ T-cells has been derived from studies on T-cell clones isolated from the mesenteric lymph nodes of SJL mice that had been orally tolerized to MBP *(37)*. These clones were CD4$^+$ and were structurally identical with Th1 encephalitogenic CD4$^+$ clones as assessed from T-cell receptor usage, MHC restriction pattern and epitope recognition properties. However, these cells secreted TGF-β together with varying amounts of IL-4 and IL-10, and they were capable of suppressing EAE induced with either MBP or myelin proteolipid protein (PLP) *(37)*.

The effect of orally administered MBP on the humoral immune response to MBP has been studied. A significant decrease of MBP-specific serum IgG and IgA, but not IgM, was observed in MBP-fed rats, suggesting a lack of maturation of the primary antibody response *(38)*. It is likely that an absence of specifically derived T-cell factors, e.g., IL-4 and IL-5, may be responsible, at least in part, for the interruption in class switching from IgM to IgG/IgA antibodies. In contrast to the decreased levels of MBP-specific serum IgA, increased levels of salivary IgA specific for the fed antigen was observed *(38)*. This observation argues for the occurrence of a compartmentalized B-cell response such that MBP specific B-cells remain selectively localized in the mucosal sites.

Bystander suppression has been described from the study of regulatory cells after oral administration of low MBP doses (Fig. 2) *(8,39)*. Bystander suppression solves a major conceptual problem related to designing antigen-specific and T-cell-specific therapy for inflammatory autoimmune diseases, such as MS, type I diabetes and rheumatoid arthritis, in which the autoantigen is unknown, and which involve reactivities to multiple autoantigens in various target tissues. In animal models of autoimmune diseases, there is intraantigenic and interantigenic spreading of autoreactivity at the target organ during the course of chronic inflammation *(40,41)*. In human autoimmune disease, reactivities to multiple autoantigens in the target tissue have been found. For example, in MS, immune responses to at least four myelin antigens, MBP, PLP, myelin-associated glycoprotein (MAG), and myelin oligodendrocyte glycoprotein (MOG), are known to occur *(42)*. Because regulatory cells induced by oral antigen secrete antigen-nonspecific cytokines as a consequence of the induction, it is not necessary to know the primary antigen responsible for initiating organ-specific inflammatory disease. Bystander suppression is evident from observations that PLP peptide-induced EAE can be inhibited by feeding MBP *(43)*. Also, MBP-specific T-cell clones from orally tolerized animals which secrete TGF-β suppress PLP-induced disease. Suppression of PLP peptide-induced disease was achieved by feeding MBP peptides 1–11 and 89–101, thereby clearly demonstrating antigen-driven bystander suppression in the target organ in the SJL mouse *(43)*. Other examples include the suppression of adjuvant-induced and antigen-induced arthritis by feeding type II collagen, and the suppression of insulitis in the NOD mouse by feeding glucagon *(44)*.

5. CLINICAL APPLICATIONS

The immune system is often defined by its ability to distinguish between pathogenic and self-antigens, to which it is functionally tolerant. A variety of

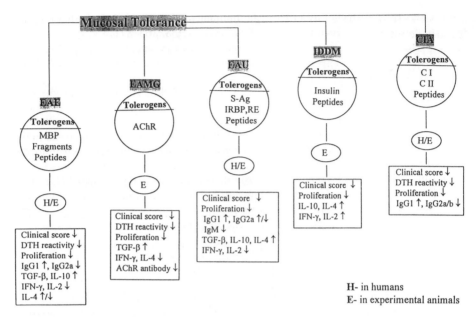

Fig. 3. Mucosal tolerance induced by orally or nasally administered autoantigens or peptides in different autoimmune diseases and their experimental animal counterparts.

mechanisms are involved in tolerance, including central and peripheral deletion, anergy, and suppression. The fact that autoimmune diseases occur so frequently, coupled with observations that autoreactive T-cells can be readily recruited from peripheral lymphoid organs, indicates that self-tolerance is often incomplete *(45)*.

Therapeutic approaches to autoimmune disease still rely heavily on the application of various nonspecific immunosuppressive drugs. These drugs are often severely toxic and they may compromise the normal effector functions of lymphocytes involved in immune surveillance and protective immunity. Thus, the management of autoimmune conditions can be greatly improved if there are ways to target the autoreactive T-cells more specifically.

Many studies have demonstrated that mucosally administered autoantigens and peptides can suppress autoimmune disease in different experimental animal models (Fig. 3). What are the foundations for further consideration of mucosal tolerance induction as an immunotherapy for autoimmune disease? It is well known that subsets of CD4+ T-cells regulate various immune responses through the production of distinct cytokines *(46)*. Th1 cells produce IL-2 and IFN-γ, resulting in macrophage activation and IgG2a isotype antibody production. Th2 cells produce IL-4, IL-6, and IL-10, which activate certain humoral immune responses like IgG1 and IgE antibody production. Th1 cells appear to play a pivotal role in destructive inflammatory reaction and in autoimmune disease, whereas Th2 cells appear to counteract the Th1 cell functions. Mucosal tolerance via administration of autoantigens and their peptide derivatives can convert the Th1-dominated tissue-damaging response to a Th2-dominated anti-inflammatory response, and induce regulatory cells to secrete antigen-nonspecific cytokines following antigen-specific triggering.

6. MUCOSALLY INDUCED TOLERANCE TO AUTOIMMUNE DISEASES IN EXPERIMENTAL MODELS

6.1. EAE

The largest amount of work on oral tolerance has been undertaken in EAE. Oral administration of MBP suppresses EAE in the Lewis rat and the SJL mouse. When MBP is administered orally at low doses, suppression of EAE in Lewis rat is mediated by $CD8^+$ T-cells that adoptively transfer protection and suppress in vitro proliferative responses by releasing TGF-β when stimulated with the tolerizing antigen *(11)*. Furthermore, oral administration of MBP is associated with increased expression of TGF- β in the brain *(47)*, and administration of anti-TGF-β in vivo abrogates the protective effects of orally administered MBP *(11)*. Oral administration of MBP also results in a reduction in IL-2 and IFN-γ without a concomitant increase in Th2 cytokines or TGF-β *(48)*.

We observed that nasal administration of MBP dose-dependently suppressed EAE in DA rats. In rats receiving 60 µL of 1000 µg MBP/mL nasally per day for 10 d prior to immunization, EAE was completely prevented (Fig. 4A). This was accompanied by strongly reduced levels of MBP-reactive, IFN-γ secreting Th1-like cells, indicating suppression of Th1 responses in tolerized rats *(49)*.

Nasal administration of MBP also reduced the serum levels of anti-MBP IgG2b antibodies, further suggesting a downregulated MBP-specific Th1 response in tolerized rats. Tolerized rats also showed significantly increased levels of anti-MBP IgGI antibodies. This indicates a IgG2b to IgG1 switch. Further evaluation of the cellular cytokine expression upon restimulation with MBP in vitro suggested that the levels of cells expressing mRNA for TGF-β and IL-4 (but not Il-10) were increased in tolerized rats. This observation is consistent with an IL-4-mediated Th1 to Th2 switch in the tolerized rats *(49)*.

6.2. EAMG

Oral induction of tolerance with AChR to EAMG has been established *(50)*. EAMG, an experimental model of MG in humans, is considered as an antibody-mediated autoimmune disease. Since the antibody response to AChR is T-cell dependent, treatment directed at AChR-specific T-cells should be effective in EAMG. Oral administration of AChR produces striking and clinically significant inhibition of both humoral and cellular immune responses characteristic of EAMG *(51,52)*.

AChR administered orally to Lewis rats in mg doses or nasally in µg doses prior to immunization with AChR prevented clinical signs of EAMG, and suppressed the AChR-specific B- and T-cell responses *(52,53)*. The development of tolerance was related to suppression of IFN-γ mRNA and IL-4 mRNA

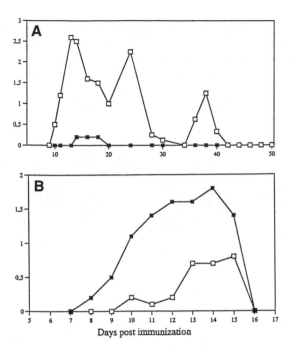

Fig. 4. Effect of nasal administration of MBP, or/and peptides prior to immunization and post immunization in Lewis and DA rats. (A) Nasal administration of bovine MBP suppressed EAE in DA rats. DA rats received 60 μL of a solution containing 1000 μg/mL of bovine MBP for 10 consecutive days prior to immunization with syngenic spinal cord homogenate (SCM) (100 mg/rat) + incomplete Freund's adjuvant (IFA) (■). Protracted-relapsing EAE with typical course was observed in control rats (□). (B) Nasal administration of bovine MBP exacerbated ongoing EAE in DA rats. DA rats were immunized with reduced amount of immunogen (syngenic SCH + IFA; 50 mg/rat). Control DA rats receiving PBS by the nasal route (■) developed slight EAE, while rats receiving MBP administered nasally at day 7 postimmunization (□) showed enhanced severity of EAE.

expression, but strong augmentation of TGF-β mRNA expression, implying that active suppression mechanisms could be important factors involved in orally and nasally induced tolerance to EAMG *(53,54)*. The Th2-related IL-4 expression is necessary for antibody synthesis and class switches. We observed that the levels of AChR-reactive, IL-4 mRNA-expressing cells were lower in certain lymphoid organs of rats that had been orally or nasally tolerized to EAMG. These observations imply that induction of tolerance to EAMG by oral or nasal administration of AChR might partly be a result of suppression of AChR-reactive IL-4 producing Th2 cells and up-modulation of AChR-reactive TGF-β producing cells.

Selected peptides of AChR have also been employed in an effort to induce mucosal tolerance in EAMG that is mediated by antibodies against AChR. The effects of nasal administration of different doses of four peptides (α61-76;

α100-116; αl46-162, and δ354-367) of Torpedo AChR subunits were evaluated. None of these peptides, neither alone nor in combination, induced tolerance to EAMG. There were no differences in levels or affinities of anti-AChR antibodies between the groups (not published).

6.3. EAN

Nasal administration of the soluble neuritogenic bovine P2-peptide 57-81 (60 μg/rat/d, for 10 consecutive d) before immunization of Lewis rats with BPM resulted in suppression of EAN, and in prevention of EAN relapse upon challenge with BPM. Proliferative responses and IFN-γ mRNA expression of lymph node cells were suppressed in P2 peptide 57-81 tolerized rats compared to control rats, while levels of IL-4 and TGF-β mRNA expressing cells were markedly upregulated. P2 peptide 58-81 administered from d 11 post-immunization, i.e., after clinical EAN had been established, and for 10 consecutive d, was also effective in treating EAN that had been induced with BPM. Nasal administration of P2-peptide 57-81 (300 μg/rat/d for 10 consecutive d), also effectively suppressed the severity and shortened clinical EAN in a dose dependent manner *(55)*.

6.4. EAU

EAU is an established model for human posterior uveitis. Bovine retinal extract (RE) is a heterologous mixture of highly uveitogenic proteins including S-antigen (S-Ag), interphotoreceptor retinal binding protein (IRBP) and rhodopsin. RE is a potent inducer of EAU. Tolerance to S-Ag induced EAU has been achieved in susceptible animals by oral administration of mg quantities of S-Ag *(56)*. As has been shown for EAE, the mechanisms responsible for the reduction of the ocular inflammation in EAU are different, depending on the dose of S-Ag administered orally, with low doses favoring suppression and high doses favoring energy *(57)*. Tolerance to EAU involving the putative suppressor cells appears to require production of both IL-4 and IL-10, whereas the tolerance involving anergy may not require the presence of these cytokines *(58)*. Adoptively transfered γ/δ T-cells from orally tolerized rats have been observed to mediate suppression of uveitis in an antigen-specific fashion. The effect of orally administered Escherichia coli expressing S-Ag on the development of EAU induced with S-Ag in Lewis rats has recently been evaluated. Feeding rats with 1 mg bacteria on d 7, 5, 3, 2, and 1 prior to immunization with S-Ag caused a significant suppression of the disease, accompanied by decreased proliferative response of lymphocytes to S-Ag in vitro *(59)*. Nasal inoculation of Lewis rats with RE or S-Ag prior to immunization with RE was observed to suppress both the severity and the incidence of clinical EAU *(60,61)*. Inhalation of S-Ag protected only against subsequent challenge with S-Ag and not against other autoantigens present in RE, whereas inhalation of whole RE protected against S-Ag-induced EAU *(60)*. The antibody response in tolerized rats consisted predominantly of anti-S-Ag IgG2a, accompanied by suppression of anti-S-Ag IgM antibodies.

6.5. IDDM

It is now well established that insulin-dependent diabetes mellitus (IDDM) is an autoimmune disorder in which the insulin-producing beta cells are specifically destroyed. Although the available data indicate that T-cells are the predominant mediators of beta cell destruction, overt diabetes is often preceded by the appearance of circulating antibodies to a number of beta cell products. The nonobese diabetic (NOD) mouse, which develops IDDM with many similarities to human IDDM, is considered to be a good model of type I diabetes. This model has been studied to identify immune mechanisms capable of suppressing the disease process and to develop new approaches for immunotherapy of IDDM *(62)*. An orally administered pancreatic autoantigen would theoretically represent an ideal therapeutic intervention in IDDM. In NOD mice, the pathogenesis of diabetes is suggested to involve Th1 cells, which secrete IL-2, IFN-γ and TNF-α and are thought to promote cell-mediated immunity *(63)*. Oral administration of insulin or insulin β-chains can delay and suppress the development of insulitis and diabetes in NOD mice. Following oral administration of insulin, a selective expansion of Th2 cells occurs in the pancreas. T-cell lines generated from NOD mice fed and immunized with insulin β-chain secrete IL-4 and IL-10 *(64)*. Nasal administration of β-(9-23) epitopes (residues 9-23 of the β-chain), resulted in a marked delay in the onset of diabetes in NOD mice. This protective effect is associated with a reduced T-cell proliferative response to β-(9-23) *(65)*.

The BB rat is also used as model for human IDDM. Diabetes-resistant (DR) BB rats are nonlymphopenic descendants of DP-BB forebears. The cumulative incidence of spontaneous diabetes in these rats is <1%, but the susceptibility to IDDM induction is retained *(66)*. Oral insulin does not prevent or delay autoimmune IDDM in BB rats *(67)*. The reason for the discrepancy between the observations in the BB rat and NOD mouse is not known. It is possible that the immunological mechanisms underlying oral tolerance are dependent on species-specific or strain-specific characteristics of IDDM that are presently not well understood.

6.6. AA

Adjuvant arthritis (AA) is an extensively studied form of experimental arthritis resembling rheumatoid arthritis in a number of aspects. AA can be induced in susceptible (Lewis) rats by immunization with mycobacterial antigens together with Freund's complete adjuvant. It can be concluded from several studies that T-cell responses play an important immunomodulatory role in the induction of AA. Oral administration of type I collagen can suppress AA *(68)*. M36, a mycobacterial peptide, is the immunodominant T-cell epitope for induction of arthritis. Nasal administration of M36 resulted in a delayed onset of arthritis, a lower maximum arthritis score, and a lower lymphocyte proliferative response to M36 *(69)*.

As in the AA model, it has been shown that collagen-induced arthritis (CIA) can be prevented by oral administration of soluble-type II collagen (CII) in the rat *(70)*. Nasal delivery of CII, like oral delivery, can prevent the progression of arthritis *(70)*. The synthetic peptide 184–198 of bovine type II collagen is capable of inducing tolerance to CIA after nasal administration *(71)*. The nasal delivery of the immunodominant bCB11.61-75 peptide in a total dose of 250 µg gave comparable protection against CIA *(70)*.

In summary, experimental model systems have been applied in the last few years to elucidate the mechanisms by which mucosal induction of tolerance induces protection from subsequent as well as ongoing autoimmune disease. Successful treatment of disease via mucosal autoantigen delivery has been reported in diverse experimental models. In order to achieve effective suppression of the clinical course of established and relapsing EAE, multiple oral doses of MBP were required *(11)*. In another report, multiple oral administration of MBP or myelin to rats and guinea pigs starting at recovery from the acute phase of EAE resulted in reduced clinical and histopathological changes *(72)*. Oral AChR administration to treat ongoing EAMG resulted in inhibition of the clinical manifestation of EAMG, concomitant with an enhancement of the AChR-antibody response *(73)*, underlining that the antibody response is not always pathogenic. In our experiments, similar results were observed in treating ongoing EAMG. Rats receiving high dose of AChR (600 µg/rat) developed relatively mild muscular weakness and reduced loss of muscle AChR, whereas anti-AChR antibody IgG levels were elevated compared to the control EAMG rats receiving PBS *(74)*.

Although mucosal tolerance induction is generally effective in protecting against subsequent experimental autoimmune diseases, the success in suppressing ongoing disease is somewhat variable. The possibility of the simultaneous use of synergistic agents or immune enhancers to broaden the effectiveness of mucosal autoantigen delivery is attractive. IFN-β works synergistically with orally administered autoantigen to reduce clinical EAE in both mice and rats *(75)*. Orally, but not systemically administered, lipopolysaccharide (LPS) enhances the protection to EAE achieved by orally administered MBP *(76)*. In the EAE model, IL-4 secreting Th2-type cells may play an important role in oral tolerization. Immunohistochemical studies in the Lewis rat EAE showed that oral MBP feeding is associated with increased expression of TGF-β in the brain without an increase of IL-4 expression, whereas MBP plus LPS feeding produces increased expression of both cytokines *(75)*. When the protein tolerogen is coupled to recombinant cholera toxin-B subunit and orally administered, a marked enhancement of tolerance to the protein has been observed *(76)*.

7. MUCOSAL ANTIGEN ADMINISTRATION FOR TREATMENT OF AUTOIMMUNE DISEASES IN HUMANS

Based on the long history of oral tolerance and the apparent safety of mucosal tolerance in experimental animal models, clinical trials have been initiated in MS, rheumatoid arthritis (RA) and uveitis *(77)*. In RA, a phase II trial involved 60 patients in a double-blind placebo-controlled design in which patients received

100 μg of oral type II collagen (CII) daily for the first month, followed by 500 μg daily for three months. The treated patients showed a significant decrease in joint swelling and disease index, and reduced anti-CII antibody titres *(78)*. One double-blind phase III trial of oral CII treatment on 280 RA patients has been completed, with negative results (Weiner, personal communication). Details of this study including subgrouping anti-CII antibody titres are awaited.

Based on the currently popular hypothesis that MS is related to autoaggressive immunity to myelin components, bovine myelin administration has been used to treat the disease. In phase I/II studies, daily administration of bovine myelin was reported to be well tolerated *(77,79)*. T-cell lines were generated from 34 patients with relapsing-remitting MS, 17 of whom received bovine myelin by the oral route daily. The frequency of MBP and PLP stimulated T-cell lines secreting TGF-β was augmented in myelin-fed compared to nontreated patients *(79)*. These data could implicate that oral autoantigen administration results in altered cytokine secretion including the secretion of anti-inflammatory TGF-β in a human disease with putative autoimmune background. Despite these promising observations, a double-blind phase III trial, in which 504 patients with MS were randomized by sex and DR type, failed to show any clear clinical benefit of bovine myelin administration beyond the placebo effect (Weiner, personal communication). Results fiom MRI, being a surrogate marker for MS and performed during the treatment course, are awaited.

The problem in MS is that an "MS antigen" has not yet been identified. In addition to MBP and PLP, myelin antigens of possible immunogen in an autoaggressive attack also include MAG, MOG and 2',3'-cyclic nucleotide 3'-phosphohydrolase (CNPase) *(80)*. Other non-myelin components have been identified as putative autoantigens in the induction of the abnormal immune responses demonstrable in MS. They include αB-crystallin that is a heat shock protein, the neuronal protein S-100β and glial fibrillary acidic protein (GFAP). Furthermore, dramatically enhanced T- and B-cell immunity to several viruses is found in MS patients' cerebrospinal fluid, i.e. in the immediate vicinity of the diseased CNS *(81)*. Taken together, MS could be a less suitable candidate for mucosal tolerance than diseases where the antigen is well known and the hypothesis of an autoimmune background is better founded.

In uveitis, a double-blind trial of bovine S-Ag and a S-Ag mixture is currently in progress. Trials are planned both in juvenile and new-onset diabetes in which oral insulin, insulin derivates, or other islet-cell antigens will be administered. Ongoing trials in patients who undergo organ transplantation should be even more promising on a theoretical basis.

Whether clinical trials with antigens in treating MS or RA, or other autoimmune diseases will be successful will depend on a number of variables, including 1) optimal dose, 2) route of administration, since it may be more effective to chose the nasal route and, thereby, avoiding acidic and proteolytic gastric environment, 3) time of administration during the disease course, 4) type of antigen administered, such as peptide or altered peptide, and 5) combined administration of antigen and certain cytokines such as IL-4, IL-10 or TGF-β1. The ultimate outcome of successful immunotherapy by mucosal tolerance induction will be determined, in part, by an interplay of these variables.

Mechanisms involved in autoimmune disease are more complicated than a simple change of the Th1-Th2 balance *(82)*. Recently, the results of two additional studies revealed: 1) oral administration of large amounts of OVA may increase—rather than prevent—the disease in a murine models of IDDM *(82)* and 2) intraperitoneal administration of soluble MOG resulted in subsequent development of a hyperacute form of EAE in a marmoset model of MS induced by MOG *(84)*. We also observed that nasal administration of bovine MBP enhances clinical signs of ongoing EAE induced in DA rats by immunization with GP spinal cord homogenate (Fig. 4B). The complexities in the treatment of autoimmune diseases by antigen administration indicate that clinicians must carefully evaluate and monitor the effects of the oral or nasal treatments, as we move from experimental diseases into the clinic.

8. FUTURE DIRECTIONS

The molecular and cellular events involved in the induction of oral tolerance in humans are not understood. Because of the enormous potential medical importance in the prevention and treatment of autoimmune diseases, further studies of mucosal tolerance induction are warranted. Specifically, 1) the relative efficacy of the oral, nasal, and rectal immunization routes should be compared, 2) the types and forms of relevant antigens necessary to achieve optimal tolerization should be examined further, 3) optimal antigen-delivery systems, such as covalent linkage of antigens to the cholera toxin-B (CTB) subunit, should be evaluated to maximize tolerance while minimizing the doses that are sufficient to make the mucosal induction of tolerance an economically feasible approach, and 4) immunization protocols that can selectively enhance or suppress the desired type of immune response should be explored. As expected, mucosally delivered viral and bacterial vaccines induce mucosal, and often systemic synthesis of antibodies. Less is known about the T-cell-mediated protective responses and induction of cytotoxic T-cells as a consequence of mucosal immunization in humans.

Prevention and treatment are two different stories. In ongoing autoimmune diseases, most T-cells are activated and can be easily expanded when exposed to the autoantigen. Administration of oral antigen to treat ongoing EAMG has yielded encouraging results, but the treatment methods will require modifications so as to bias the immune system effectively towards AChR unresponsiveness, while avoiding a stimulation of the destructive autoimmune response. Treatment of ongoing disease may require the development of a modified molecule with lower immunogenic potential than the native protein. An ongoing study is designed to determine whether modified natural or recombinant AChR are effective agents in the oral treatment of MG *(73)*.

The possibility of using synergists in conjunction with oral tolerance induction is an attractive means to broaden the efficacy of the treatment. Using CTB subunit-coupled MBP, one can dramatically decrease the amount of antigen needed for preventing EAE, thereby reducing the possibility that the tolerizing antigens acts as immunogen for induction of destructive responses. Certain beneficial regulatory cytokines have been considered as potential synergists. Oral administration of IFN-β enhances the suppressive effects of oral MBP *(75)*. In addition to the autoantigen and its derivative peptides, several groups have used peptides derived from the T-cell receptor to prevent and treat EAE *(85,86)*. It appears that multiple weapons, alone or in combination, can be developed to combat unwanted autoimmune responses accurately and effectively.

9. SUMMARY

Mucosal administration of autoantigens can result in the development of peripheral immunological tolerance. Depending on the dose of administered antigen, energy/deletion of antigen-specific T-cells (higher doses) and/or selective expansion of cells producing immunosuppressive cytokines (TGF-β, IL-4, and IL-10) (lower doses) serve as the two major mechanisms. At comparable antigen dose, induction of tolerance is more effectively obtained by nasal as opposed to the oral route. The ability of mucosal tolerance induction in preventing subsequent diseases is clearly superior to symptomatic treatment of the disease. To broaden and enhance its efficacy, studies are warranted to evaluate if and how mucosal tolerance induction can be combined with administration of anti-inflammatory cytokines. A series of studies has demonstrated that mucosal tolerance can be induced in several experimental models of autoimmune diseases (EAE, EAMG, EAU, IDDM, and AA) by oral and/or nasal antigen administration. Based on the experimental experience with mucosal tolerance induction and its apparent safety, further trials in human autoimmune diseases are necessary, despite the negative results recently obtained in MS and RA by oral feeding with bovine myelin and CII, respectively.

REFERENCES

1. Mestecky, J. and McGhee, J. R. (1989) Oral immunization: past and present, in *New strategies for oral immunization. Current Topics in Microbiology and Immunology* (Mestecky, J., and McGhee, J. R., eds.), vol. 146, Berlin: Springer-Verlag, pp. 3–11.
2. Bienenstock, J. (1991) A non-historical overview of mucosal immunology, in *Frontiers of mucosal immunology. Proceedings of the Sixth International Congress of Mucosal Immunology* (Tsuchita, M., Nagura, H., Hibi, T., and Moro, I., eds.), vol. 1. Amsterdam, Excerpta Medica/Elsevier, pp. XV–XVIII.
3. Brandtzaeg, P. (1995) The SMI—An international society for mucosal immunology. *Immunologist* **3**, 67–69.
4. Miller, A., Lider, O., Abramsky, O., and Weiner, H. L. (1994) Oral administration of myelin basic protein in neonates primes for immune responses and enhances experimental autoimmune encephalomyelitis in adult animals. *Eur. J. Immunol.* **24**, 1026–1032.

5. Hanson, D. G. (1981) Ontogeny of orally induced tolerance to soluble proteins in mice. I. Priming and tolerance in newborns. *J. Immunol.* **127,** 1518-1524.

6. Mayer, L. and Shlien, R. (1987) Evidence for function of Ia molecules on gut epithelial cells in man. *J. Exp. Med.* **166,** 1471–1483.

7. Kagnoff, M. F. (1996) Mucosal immunology: new frontiers. *Immunol. Today* **17,** 57–60.

8. Holt, P. G. (1994) Immunoprophylaxis of atopy: light at the end of the tunnel? *Immunol. Today* **15,** 484–489.

9. Wells, H. G. (1991) Studies on the chemistry of anaphylaxis (III). Experiments with isolated proteins, especially those of the hen's egg. *J. Infect. Dis.* **9,** 147–171.

10. Chase, M. W. (1946) Inhibition of experimental drug allergy by prior feeding of the sensitized agent. *Proc. Soc. Exp. Biol. Med.* **61,** 257–259.

11. Meyer, A. L., Benson, J. M., Gienapp, I. E., Cox, K. L., and Whitacre, C. C. (1996) Suppression of murine chronic relapsing experimental autoimmune encephalomyelitis by the oral administration of myelin basic protein. *J. Immunol.* **157,** 4230–4238.

12. Hirabayashi, Y., Kurata, H., Funato, H., Nagamine, T., Aizawa, C., Tamura, S., et al. (1990) Comparison of intranasal inoculation of influenza HA vaccine combined with cholera toxin B subunit with oral or parenteral vaccination. *Vaccine* **8,** 243–248.

13. Ma, C. G., Zhang, G. X., Xiao, B. G., Wang, Z. Y., Link, J., Olsson, T. et al. (1996) Mucosal tolerance to experimental autoimmune myasthenia gravis is associated with down-regulation of AChR-specific IFN-γ-expressing Th1-like cells and up-regulation of TGF-β mRNA in mononuclear cells. *Ann. NY Acad. Sci.* **778,** 273–287.

14. Metzler, B. and Wraith, D. C. (1992) Inhibition of experimental autoimmune encephalomyelitis by inhalation but not oral administration of the encephalitogenic peptide: influence of MHC binding affinity. *Int. Immunol.* **5,** 1159–1165.

15. Dresser, D. W. (1962) Specific inhibition of antibody production. I. Protein overloading paralysis. *Immunology* **5,** 161–168.

16. Javed, N. H., Gienapp, I. E., Cox, K. L., Whitacre, C. C. (1995) Exquisite peptide specificity of oral tolerance in experimental autoimmune encephalomyelitis. *J. Immunol.* **155,** 1599–1605.

17. Miller, A., Lider, O., Al-Sabbagh, A., and Weiner, H. L. (1992) Suppression of experimental autoimmune encephalomyelitis by oral administration of myelin basic protein. V. Hierarchy of suppression by myelin basic protein from different species. *J. Neuroimmunol.* **39,** 243–250.

18. Higgins, P. J. and Weiner, H. L. (1988) Suppression of experimental autoimmune encephalomyelitis by oral administration of myelin basic protein and its fragments. *J. Immunol.* **140,** 440–445.

19. Bitar, D. M. and Whitacre, C. C. (1988) Suppression of experimental autoimmune encephalomyelitis by the oral administration of myelin basic protein. *Cell Immunol.* **11,** 364–370.

20. Liu, G. Y. and Wraith, D. C. (1995) Affinity for class II MHC determines the extent to which soluble peptides tolerize autoreactive T cells in naive and primed adult mice - implications for autoimmunity. *Int. Immunol.* **7,** 1255–1263.

21. Joosten, I., Wauben, M. H. M., Holewijn, M. C., Reske, K., Pedersen, F. L., Roosenboommn, C. F. P., et al. (1994) Direct binding of autoimmune disease related T cell epitopes to purified Lewis rat MHC class II molecules. *Int. Immunol.* **6,** 751–759.

22. Evavold, B. D., Sloan, L. J., and Allen, P. M. (1993) Tickling the TCR: selective T-cell functions stimulated by altered peptide ligands. *Immunol. Today* **14,** 602–609.
23. Windhagen, A., Scholz, C., Hollsberg, P., Fukaura, H., Sette, A., and Hafler, D. A. (1995) Modulation of cytokine patterns of human autoreactive T cell clones by a single amino acid substitution of their peptide ligand. *Immunity* **2,** 373–380.
24. Karin, N., Mitchell, D. J., Brocke, S., Ling, N., and Steinman, L. (1994) Reversal of experimental autoimmune encephalomyelitis by a soluble peptide variant of a myelin basic protein epitope: T cell receptor antagonism and reduction of interferon gamma and tumor necrosis factor alpha production. *J. Exp. Med.* **180,** 2227–2237.
25. Adorini, L. and Nagy, Z. A. (1990) Peptide competition for antigen presentation. *Immunol. Today* **11,** 21–24.
26. Guery, J. C., Sette, A., Leighton, J., Dragomir, A., and Adorini, L. (1992) Selective immunosuppression by administration of major histocompatibility complex (MHC) class 11-binding peptides. I. Evidence for in vivo MHC blockade preventing T cell activation. *J. Exp. Med.* **175,** 1345–1352.
27. Alexander, J., Ruppert, J., Snoke, K., and Sette, A. (1994) TCR antagonism and T cell tolerance can be independently induced in a DR-restricted, hemagglutinin-specific T cell clone. *Int. Immunol.* **6,** 363–367.
28. Franco, A., Southwood, S., Arrhenius, T., Kuchroo, V. K., Grey, H. M., Sette, A., et al. (1994) T-cell receptor antagonist peptides are highly effective inhibitors of experimental allergic encephalomyelitis. *Eur. J. Immunol.* **24,** 940–946.
29. Sakaguchi, S., Toda, M., Asano, M., Itoh, M., Moores, S. S., and Sakaguchi, N. (1996) T cell-mediated maintenance of nature self-tolerance: its breakdown as a possible cause of various autoimmune diseases. *J. Autoimmun.* **9,** 211–220.
30. Wang, Z. Y., He, B., Qiao, J., and Link, H. (1995) Suppression of experimental autoimmune myasthenia gravis and experimental allergic encephalomyelitis by oral administration of acetylcholine receptor and myelin basic protein: double tolerance. *J. Neuroimmunol.* **63,** 79–86.
31. Shi, F. D., Bai, X. F., Xiao, B. G., van der Meide, P. H., and Link, H. (1998) Nasal administration of multiple antigens suppresses experimental autoimmune myasthenia gravis. encephalomyelitis and neuritis. *J. Neurol. Sci.* **155,** 1–12.
32. Miller, A., Lider, O., Roberts, A. B., Sporn, M. B., and Weiner, H. L. (1992) Suppressor T cells generated by oral tolerization to myelin basic protein suppress both in vitro and in vivo immune responses by the release of transforming growth factor-β after antigen-specific triggering. *Proc. Natl. Acad. Sci. USA* **89,** 421–425.
33. Lider, O., Santos, L. M. B., Lee, C. S. Y., Higgins, P. J., and Weiner, H. L. (1989) Suppression of experimental autoimmune encephalomyelitis by oral administration of myelin basic protein II. Suppression of disease and in vitro immune responses is mediated by antigen-specific CD8 T lymphocytes. *J. Immunol.* **142,** 748–752.
34. Wildner, G., Hunig, T., and Thurau, S. R. (1996) Orally induced. Peptide-specific γ/δ TCR+ cell suppress experimental autoimmune uveitis. *Eur. J. Immunol.* **26,** 2140–2148.
35. Caspi, R. R., Kuwabara, T., and Nussenblatt, R. B. (1988) Characterization of a suppressor cell line which downgrades experimental autoimmune uveoretinitis in the rat. *J. Immunol.* **140,** 2579–2584.

36. Chen, Y., Inobe, J., and Weiner, H. L. (1995) Induction of oral tolerance to myelin basic protein in CD8-depleted mice: both CD4$^+$ and CD8$^+$ cells mediated active suppression. *J. Immunol.* **155,** 910–916.
37. Chen, Y., Kuchroo, V. K., Inobe, J., Hafler, D. A., and Weiner, H. L. (1994) Regulatory T cell clones induced by oral tolerance: suppression of autoimmune encephalomyelitis. *Science* **265,** 1237–1240.
38. Fuller, K. A., Pearl, D., and Whitacre, C. C. (1990) Oral tolerance in experimental autoimmune encephalomyelitis: serum and salivary antibody responses. *J. Neuroimmunol.* **28,** 15–26.
39. Miller, A., Lider, O., and Weiner, H. L. (1991) Antigen-driven bystander suppression after oral administration of antigens. *J. Exp. Med.* **174,** 791–798.
40. Lehmann, P., Forsthuber, T., Miller, A., and Sercarz, E. E. (1992) Spreading of T-cell autoimmunity to cryptic determinants of an autoantigen. *Nature* **358,** 155–157.
41. Tisch, R., Yang, X. D., Singer, S. M., Liblau, R. S., Fuggei, L., and McDevitt, H. O. (1993) Immune response to glutamic acid decarboxylase correlates with insulitis in non-obese diabetic mice. *Nature* **366,** 72–75.
42. Lu, C. Z., Fredrikson, S., Xiao, B. G., and Link, H. (1993) Interleukin-2 secreting cells in multiple sclerosis and controls. *J. Neurol. Sci.* **120.** 99–106.
43. Al-Sabbagh, A., Miller, A., Santos, L. M. B., and Weiner, H. L. (1994) Antigen-driven tissue-specific suppression following oral tolerance: orally administered myelin basic protein suppresses proteolipid protein-induced experimental autoimmune encephalomyelitis in the SJL mouse. *Eur. J. Immunol.* **24,** 2104–2109.
44. Weiner, H. L., Friedman, A., Miller, A., Khoury, S. J., Al-Sabbagh, A., Santos, L. M. B., et al. (1994) Oral tolerance: immunologic mechanisms and treatment of animal and human organ-specific autoimmune diseases by oral administration of autoantigens. *Annu. Rev. Immunol.* **12,** 809–837.
45. Schluesener, H. J. and Wekerle, H. (1985) Autoaggressive T lymphocyte lines recognizing the encephalitogenic region of myelin basic protein: in vitro selection from unprimed rat T lymphocyte populations. *J. Immunol.* **135,** 3128–3133.
46. Paul, W. E. and Seder, R. A. (1994) Lymphocyte responses and cytokines. *Cell* **76,** 241–251.
47. Khoury, S. J., Hancock, W. W., and Weiner, H. L. (1992) Oral tolerance to myelin basic protein and natural recovery from experimental autoimmune encephalomyelitis is associated with downregulation of inflammatory cytokines and differential upregulation of tranforming growth factor-β, interleukin-4 and prostaglandin E expression in the brain. *J. Exp. Med.* **176,** 1355–1364.
48. Chen, Y., Inobe, J. I., Marks, R., Gonnella, P., Kuchroo, V. K., and Weiner, H. L. (1995) Peripheral deletion of antigen-reactive T cells in oral tolerance. *Nature* **376,** 177–180.
49. Bai, X. F., Shi, F. D., Xiao, B. G., Li, H. L., van der Meide, P. H., and Link, H. (1997) Nasal administration of myelin basic protein prevents relapsing experimental autoimmune encephalomyelitis in DA rats by activating regulatory cells expressing IL-4 and TGF-β mRNA. *J. Neuroimmunol.* **80,** 65–75.
50. Wang, Z. Y., Qiao, J., and Link, H. (1993) Suppression of experimental autoimmune myasthenia gravis by oral administration of acetylcholine receptor. *J. Neuroimmunol.* **44,** 209–214.

51. Okumura, S., McIntosh, K., and Drachman, D. B. (1994) Oral administration of acetylcholine receptor: effects on experimental myasthenia gravis. *Ann. Neurol.* **36,** 704–713.
52. Wang, Z. Y., Huang, J., Olsson, T., He, B., and Link, H. (1995) B cell responses to acetylcholine receptor in rats orally tolerized against experimental autoimmune myasthenia gravis. *J. Neurol. Sci.* **128,** 167–174.
53. Ma, C. G., Zhang, G. X., Xiao, B. G., Link, J., Olsson, T., and Link, H. (1995) Suppression of experimental autoimmune myasthenia gravis by nasal administration of acetylcholine receptor. *J. Neuroimmunol.* **58,** 51–60.
54. Wang, Z. Y., Link, H., Ljungdahl, A., Hojeberg, B., Link, J., He, B., et al. (1994) Induction of interferon-γ, interleukin-4 and transforming growth factor-β in rats orally tolerized against experimental autoimmune myasthenia gravis. *Cell Immunol.* **157,** 353–368.
55. Zhou, L. P., Zhu, Jie., Deng, G. M., Levi, M., Wahren, B., Diab, A., et al. Treatment with bovine P2 protein peptide 57-81 by nasal route is effective in EAN. *J. Neuroimmunol.,* in press.
56. Nussenblatt, R. B., Caspi, R. R., Mahdi, R. Chan, C. C., Roberge, F., Lider, O., et al. (1990) Inhibition of S-Ag induced experimental autoimmune uveoretinitis by oral induction of tolerance with S-Ag. *J. Immunol.* **144,** 1689–1695.
57. Gregerson, D. S., Obritsch, W. F., and Donoso, L. A. (1993) Oral tolerance in experimental autoimmune uveoretinitis: distinct mechanisms of resistance are induced by low versus high-dose feeding protocols. *J. Immunol.* **151,** 5751–5761.
58. Caspi, R. R., Stiff, L. R., Morawetz, R., Miller-Rivero, N. E., Chan, C. C., Wiggert, B., et al., (1996) Cytokine-dependent modulation of oral tolerance in a murine model of autoimmune uveitis. *Ann. NY Acad. Sci.* **778,** 315–324.
59. Singh, V. K., Anand, R., Sharma, K., and Agarwal, S. S. (1996) Suppression of experimental autoimmune uveitis in Lewis rats by oral administration of recombinant Escherichia coli expressing retinal S-antigen. *Cell Immunol.* **172,** 158–162.
60. Dick, A. D., Cheng, Y. F., McKinnon, A., Liversidge, J., and Forrester, J. V. (1993) Nasal administration of retinal antigens suppresses the inflammatory response in experimental allergic uveoretinitis. *Brit. J. Ophthalmol.* **77,** 171–175.
61. Dick, A. D., Cheng, Y. F., Liversidge, J., and Forrester, J. V. (1994) Intranasal administration of retinal antigens suppresses retinal antigen-induced experimental autoimmune uveoretinitis. *Immunology* **82,** 625–631.
62. Shizuru, A., Edwards-Taylor, C., Banks, B. A., Gregory, A. K., and Fathman, C. G. (1988) Immunotherapy of the NOD mouse: treatment with an antibody to T-helper lymphocytes. *Science* **240,** 659–662.
63. Liblau, R. S., Singer, S. M., and McDevitt, H. O. (1995) Th1 and Th2 CD4+ T cells in the pathogenesis of organ-specific autoimmune diseases. *Immunol. Today* **16,** 34–38.
64. Maron, R., Blogg, N. S., Polanski, M., Hancock, W., and Weiner, H. L. (1996) Oral tolerance to insulin and the insulin B-chain. *Ann. NY Acad. Sci.* **778,** 347–357.
65. Daniel, D. and Wegmann, D. R. (1996) Protection of nonobese diabetic mice from diabetes by intranasal or subcutaneous administration of insulin peptide B-(9-23). *Proc. Natl. Acad. Sci. USA* **93,** 956–960.
66. Crisa, L., Mordes, P., and Rossini, A. A. (1992) Autoimmune diabetes mellitus in the BB rat. *Diabetes Metab. Rev.* **8,** 4–37.

67. Mordes, J. P., Schirf, B., Roipko, D., Greiner, D. L., Weiner, H. L., Nelson, P., et al. (1996) Oral insulin does not prevent insulin-dependent diabetes mellitus in BB rats. *Ann. NY Acad. Sci.* **778,** 418–421.
68. Zhang, Z. J., Lee, C. S. Y., Lider, O., and Weiner, H. L. (1990) Suppression of adjuvant arthritis in Lewis rats by oral administration of type II collagen. *J. Immunol.* **145,** 2489–2493.
69. Prakken, B. J., van der Zee, R., Anderton, S. M., van Kooten, P., Kuis, W., and van Eden, W. (1996) Tolerance to an arthritogenic T-cell epitope of hsp65 and the regulation of experimental arthritis. *Ann. NY Acad. Sci.* **778,** 425–426.
70. Staines, N. A., Harper, N., Ward, F. J., Thompson, H. S. G., and Bansal, S. (1996) Arthritis: animal models of oral tolerance. *Ann. NY Acad. Sci.* **778,** 297–305.
71. Staines, N. A., Harper, N., Ward, F. J., Malmstrorn, V., Holmdahl, R., and Bansal, S. (1996) Mucosal tolerance and suppression of collagen-induced arthritis (CIA) induced by nasal inhalation of synthetic peptide 184–198 of bovine type II collagen (CII) expressing a dominant T cell epitope. *Clin. Exp. Immunol.* **103,** 368–375.
72. Brod, S. A., Al-Sabbagh, A., Sobel, R. A., Hafler, D. A., and Weiner, H. L. (1991) Suppression of experimental autoimmune encephalomyelitis by oral administration of myelin antigens. IV. Suppression of chronic relapsing disease in the Lewis rat and strain 13 guinea pig. *Ann. Neurol.* **29,** 615–622.
73. Drachman, D. B., Okumura, S., Adams, R. N., and McIntosh, K. R.. (1996) Oral tolerance in myasthenia gravis. *Ann. NY Acad. Sci.* **778,** 258–272.
74. Shi, F. D., Bai, X. F., Li, H. L., Huang, Y. M., van der Meide, P. H., and Link, H. (1998) Nasal tolerance in experimental autoimmune myasthenia gravis (EAMG): induction of protective tolerance in primed animals. *Clin. Exp. Immunol.* **111,** 506–512.
75. Nelson, P. A., Akselband, Y., Dearborn, S. M., Al-Sabbagh, A., Tian, Z. J., Gonnella, P. A., et al. (1996) Effect of oral beta interferon on subsequent immune responsiveness. *Ann. NY Acad. Sci.* **778,** 145–155.
76. Sun, J. B., Holmgren, C., and Czerkinsky, C. (1994) Cholera toxin B subunit: an efficient transmucosal carrier-delivery system for induction of peripheral immunological tolerance. *Proc. Natl. Acad. Sci. USA* **91,** 10,795–10,799.
77. Weiner, H. L. (1994) Oral tolerance. *Proc. Natl. Acad. Sci. USA* **91,** 10,762-10,765.
78. Gimsa, U., Sieper, J., Braun, J., and Mitchison, N. A. (1997) Type 11 collagen serology: a guide to clinical responsiveness to oral tolerance? *Rheumatol. Int.* **16,** 237–240.
79. Fukaura, H., Kent, S. C., Pietrusewicz, M. J., Khoury, S. J., Weiner, H. L., and Hafler, D. A. (1996) Antigen-specific TGF-βI secretion with bovine myelin oral tolerization in multiple sclerosis. *Ann.. NY. Acad Sci.* **778,** 251–257.
80. Sun, J. B. (1993) Autoreactive T and B cells in nervous system diseases. *Acta Neurol. Scand.* **87(Suppl. 142),** 1–56.
81. Link, H., Sun, J. B., Wang, Z. Y., Xu, Z., Love, A., Fredrikson, S., et al. (1992) Virus-reactive and autoreactive T cells are accumulated in cerebrospinal fluid in multiple sclerosis. *J. Neuroimmunol.* **38,** 63–73.
82. McFarland, H. F. (1996) Complexities in the treatment of autoimmune disease. *Science* **274,** 2037–2038.
83. Blanas, E., Carbone, F. R., Allison, J., Miller, J. F. A. P., and Heath, W. R. (1996) Induction of autoimmune diabetes by oral administration of autoantigen. *Science* **274,** 1707–1709.

84. Genain, C. P., Abel, K. Belmar, N., Villinger, F., Rosenberg, D. P., Linington, C., et al. (1996) Late complications of immune deviation therapy in a nonhuman primate. *Science* **274,** 2054–2057.

85. Vandenbark, A. A., Hashim, G., and Offner, H. (1989) Immunization with a synthetic T-cell receptor V-region peptide protects against experimental autoimmune encephalomyelitis. *Nature* **341,** 541–544.

86. Howell, M. D., Winters, S. T., Olee, T., Powell, H. C., Carlo, D. J., and Brostoff, S. W. (1989) Vaccination against experimental allergic encephalomyelitis with T cell receptor peptides. *Science* **246,** 668–670.

87. Miller, A., Al-Sabbagh, A., Santos, L. M. B., Das, M. P., and Weiner, H. L. (1993) Epitopes of myelin basic protein that trigger TGF-β release after oral tolerization are distinct from encephalitogenic epitopes and mediate epitope-driven bystander suppression. *J. Immunol.* **151,** 7307–7315.

88. Khare, S. D., Krco, C. J., Pawelski, J. R., Griffiths, M. M., Luthra, H. S., and David, C. S. (1994) Oral administration of human collagen peptide 250-270 suppresses collagen-induced arthritis in DBA/I mice by inhibiting a Th1 response. *Arth. Rheum.* **37(Suppl.),** S398.

Index